Rapid Review
Pathology

Rapid Review Series

Series Editor
Edward F. Goljan, MD

Behavioral Science, Second Edition
Vivian M. Stevens, PhD; Susan K. Redwood, PhD; Jackie L. Neel, DO;
Richard H. Bost, PhD; Nancy W. Van Winkle, PhD; Michael H. Pollak, PhD

Biochemistry, Second Edition
John W. Pelley, PhD; Edward F. Goljan, MD

Gross and Developmental Anatomy, Second Edition
N. Anthony Moore, PhD; William A. Roy, PhD, PT

Histology and Cell Biology, Second Edition
E. Robert Burns, PhD; M. Donald Cave, PhD

Microbiology and Immunology, Second Edition
Ken S. Rosenthal, PhD; James S. Tan, MD

Neuroscience
James A. Weyhenmeyer, PhD; Eve A. Gallman, PhD

Pathology, Second Edition
Edward F. Goljan, MD

Pharmacology, Second Edition
Thomas L. Pazdernik, PhD; Laszlo Kerecsen, MD

Physiology
Thomas A. Brown, MD

USMLE Step 2
Michael W. Lawlor, MD, PhD

USMLE Step 3
David Rolston, MD; Craig Nielsen, MD

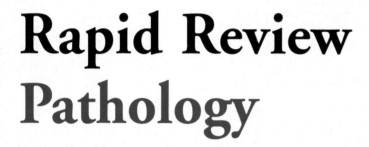

Rapid Review
Pathology

SECOND EDITION

Edward F. Goljan, MD
Professor and Chair
Department of Pathology
Oklahoma State University Center for Health Sciences
College of Osteopathic Medicine
Tulsa, Oklahoma

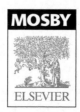

MOSBY

ELSEVIER

MOSBY
ELSEVIER

1600 John F. Kennedy Blvd.
Suite 1800
Philadelphia, PA 19103-2899

RAPID REVIEW PATHOLOGY, Second Edition   ISBN-13: 978–0–323–04414–1
Copyright © 2007, 2004 by Mosby, Inc., an affiliate of Elsevier Inc.   ISBN-10: 0–323–04414–X

Library of Congress Cataloging-in-Publication Data
Goljan, Edward F.
  Pathology / Edward F. Goljan—2nd ed.
    p. ; cm.—(Rapid review series)
  ISBN-13: 978–0–323–04414–1   ISBN-10: 0–323–04414–X
    1. Pathology—Outlines, syllabi, etc. 2. Pathology—Examinations, questions, etc. I. Title. II. Series.
    [DNLM: 1. Pathology—Examination Questions. 2. Pathology—Outlines. QZ 18.2 G626p 2007]
  RB120.G654 2007
  616.07076—dc22

                                                                            2006046689

ISBN-13: 978–0–323–04414–1
ISBN-10: 0–323–04414–X

Publishing Director: Linda Belfus
Acquisitions Editor: James Merritt
Developmental Editor: Katie DeFrancesco
Design Direction: Steven Stave

Printed in Canada
Last digit is the print number: 9   8   7   6   5   4

To my wife, Joyce. Without you my life would truly be incomplete. Also to the memory of my son Keith, who I miss very much, but will see again.

EFG

Series Preface

The First Editions of the *Rapid Review Series* have received high critical acclaim from students studying for the United States Medical Licensing Examination (USMLE) Step 1 and high ratings in *First Aid for the USMLE Step 1*. The Second Editions continue to be invaluable resources for time-pressed students. As a result of reader feedback, we have improved upon an already successful formula. We have created a learning system, including a print and electronic package, that is easier to use and more concise than other review products on the market.

SPECIAL FEATURES

Book

- **Outline format:** Concise, high-yield subject matter is presented in a study-friendly format.
- **High-yield margin notes:** Key content that is most likely to appear on the exam is reinforced in the margin notes.
- **Visual elements:** NEW to this edition, full-color images have been added to enhance your study and recognition of key pathology images. Abundant two-color schematics and summary tables enhance your study experience.
- **Two-color design:** Colored text and headings make studying more efficient and pleasing.
- **Two practice examinations:** Two sets of 50 USMLE Step 1–type clinically oriented, multiple-choice questions (including images where necessary) and complete discussions (rationales) for all options are included.

New! Online Study and Testing Tool

- **350 USMLE Step 1–type MCQs:** Clinically oriented, multiple-choice questions that mimic the current board format are presented. These include images where necessary, and complete rationales for all answer options. All the questions from the book are included so you can study them in the most effective mode for you!
- **Test mode:** Select from randomized 50-question sets or by subject topics for an exam-like review session. This mode features a 60-minute timer to simulate the actual exam, a detailed assessment report that can be printed or saved to your hard drive, and direct links to all or only incorrect questions. The links include your answer, the correct answer, and full rationales for all answer options, so you can fully analyze your test session and learn from your mistakes.
- **Study mode:** Like the test mode, in the study mode you can select from randomized 50-question sets or by subject topics to create a dynamic study session. This mode features unlimited attempts at each question, instant feedback (either on selection of the correct answer or when using the "Show Answer" feature), complete rationales for all answer options, and a detailed progress report that can be printed or saved to your hard drive.
- **Online access:** Online access allows you to study from an internet-enabled computer wherever and whenever it is convenient. This access is activated through registration on www.studentconsult.com with the pincode printed inside the front cover.

Student Consult

- **Full online access:** You can access the complete text and illustrations of this book on www.studentconsult.com.
- **Save content to your PDA:** Through our unique Pocket Consult platform, you can clip selected text and illustrations and save them to your PDA for study on the fly!
- **Free content:** An interactive community center with a wealth of additional valuable resources is available.

Acknowledgment of Reviewers

The publisher expresses sincere thanks to the medical students and faculty who provided many useful comments and suggestions for improving both the text and the questions. Our publishing program will continue to benefit from the combined insight and experience provided by your reviews. For always encouraging us to focus on our target, the USMLE Step 1, we thank the following:

Richard M. Awdeh, Yale University School of Medicine

Joy A. Baldwin, University of Vermont College of Medicine

John Cowden, Yale University School of Medicine

Andrew Deak, Northeastern Ohio Universities College of Medicine

Tracey DeLucia, Loyola University Chicago Stritch School of Medicine

Steven Engman, Loyola University Chicago Stritch School of Medicine

Michael Hoffman, University of Medicine and Dentistry New Jersey, Robert Wood Johnson School of Medicine

James Massullo, Northeastern Ohio Universities College of Medicine

Sarah Schlegel, University of Connecticut School of Medicine

Tina Tran, Virginia Commonwealth University School of Medicine

Acknowledgments

The second edition of this book is the culmination of more than 23 years of teaching medical students and 11 years of teaching USMLE Step 1 board review courses in pathology and USMLE Step 2 board reviews in medicine. This edition has been extensively revised. There are more tables, more schematics, more pictures (all in high-quality color), more margin notes, and there is more high-yield information. All of the original 350 questions have been extensively revised and some replaced. The outline format has been adhered to and is "less dense" than in the previous edition. The material in the book is not only useful for performing well on USMLE Step 1, but is also very useful for subjects (e.g., cardiovascular, etc.) covered in the USMLE step 2 exam.

I especially want to thank Ivan Damjanov, MD, PhD. Many of his photographs are included in the book. The quality of the photographs exemplifies his incredible breadth and depth of knowledge and experience in the field of pathology. He is also one of very few academic and practicing pathologists who understand the importance of integrating pathology with the basic and clinical sciences. Ivan, I truly value your friendship and support.

Special thanks to Katie DeFrancesco from Elsevier, who kept track of all the major changes in the second edition and did not restrict me in the amount of new material added to the book. I also thank Matt Chansky, illustrator, who translated my thoughts into figures that will clearly help medical students understand difficult subjects.

Edward F. Goljan, MD

Contents

CHAPTER 1

Cell Injury

I. Tissue Hypoxia

A. Hypoxia

1. Hypoxia refers to inadequate oxygenation of tissue.
   a. Oxygen (O_2) is an electron acceptor in the mitochondrial oxidative pathway.
   b. Inadequate oxygen decreases synthesis of adenosine triphosphate (ATP).
2. Several types of hypoxia produce O_2-related changes reported with arterial blood gas measurements (Table 1-1).
   - O_2 diffuses from the alveoli, to plasma ($\uparrow$ Pao_2), and to red blood cells (RBCs), where it attaches to heme groups ($\uparrow$ Sao_2).

Hypoxia: inadequate oxygenation

B. Causes of tissue hypoxia

1. Ischemia
   a. Decreased arterial blood flow or venous blood flow
   b. Examples—coronary artery atherosclerosis, thrombosis of splenic vein
2. Hypoxemia
   a. Decrease in Pao_2
   b. Causes
      (1) Respiratory acidosis
         (a) Carbon dioxide (CO_2) retention in the lungs produces a corresponding decrease in Pao_2.
         (b) Examples include depression of the medullary respiratory center (e.g., barbiturates), paralysis of diaphragm, chronic bronchitis.
      (2) Ventilation defects
         (a) Impaired O_2 delivery to alveoli
            - Example—respiratory distress syndrome (RDS) with collapse of the distal airways
         (b) No O_2 exchange in lungs that are perfused but *not* ventilated
         (c) Diffuse disease (RDS) produces intrapulmonary shunting of blood
            - Administration of 100% O_2 does *not* increase the Pao_2.
      (3) Perfusion defects
         (a) Absence of blood flow to alveoli
            - Example—pulmonary embolus
         (b) No O_2 exchange in lungs that are ventilated but *not* perfused
         (c) Produces an increase in pathologic dead space
            - Administration of 100% O_2 increases the Pao_2.
      (4) Diffusion defects
         (a) Decreased O_2 diffusion through the alveolar-capillary interface
         (b) Examples—interstitial fibrosis, pulmonary edema

Most common cause of hypoxia: coronary artery atherosclerosis

$\uparrow$ Alveolar Pco_2 = $\downarrow$ Pao_2

Ventilation defect: perfused but not ventilated

Perfusion defect: ventilated but not perfused

TABLE 1-1:
Terminology
Associated with
Oxygen Transport
and Hypoxia

Term	Definition	Contributing Factors	Significance
PaO_2	Pressure keeping O_2 dissolved in plasma of arterial blood	Percentage of O_2 in inspired air, atmospheric pressure, normal O_2 exchange	Reduced in hypoxemia
SaO_2	Average percentage of O_2 bound to Hb	PaO_2 and valence of heme iron in each of the four heme groups Fe^{2+} binds to O_2; Fe^{3+} does not	$SaO_2 < 80\%$ produces cyanosis of skin and mucous membranes
O_2 content	Total amount of O_2 carried in blood	Hb concentration in red blood cells (most important factor), PaO_2, SaO_2	Hb is the most important carrier of O_2

Fe^{2+}, ferrous iron; Fe^{3+}, ferric iron; Hb, hemoglobin; O_2, oxygen; PaO_2, partial pressure of arterial oxygen; SaO_2, arterial oxygen saturation.

3. Hemoglobin (Hb)-related abnormalities
    a. Anemia
        (1) Decreased Hb concentration
        (2) Causes
            (a) Decreased production of Hb (e.g., iron deficiency)
            (b) Increased destruction of RBCs (e.g., hereditary spherocytosis)
            (c) Decreased production of RBCs (e.g., aplastic anemia)
            (d) Increased sequestration of RBCs (e.g., splenomegaly)
        (3) Normal PaO_2 and SaO_2

Anemia: normal PaO_2 and SaO_2

MetHb: heme Fe^{3+}

    b. Methemoglobinemia
        (1) Methemoglobin (metHb) is Hb with oxidized heme groups (Fe^{3+}).
        (2) Causes
            (a) Oxidizing agents
                • Examples—nitrite- or sulfur-containing drugs, such as nitroglycerin and trimethoprim-sulfamethoxazole
            (b) Deficiency of metHb reductase
                • Reductase normally converts ferric iron, Fe^{3+}, to ferrous iron, Fe^{2+}
        (3) Pathogenesis of hypoxia
            (a) Fe^{3+} cannot bind O_2
            (b) Normal PaO_2, decreased SaO_2

> Patients with methemoglobinemia have chocolate-colored blood and cyanosis. Skin color does *not* return to normal after administration of O_2. Treatment is methylene blue (activates metHb reductase) and ascorbic acid (reduces Fe^{3+} to Fe^{2+}).

    c. Carbon monoxide (CO) poisoning
        (1) Produced by incomplete combustion of carbon-containing compounds

    (2) Caused by automobile exhaust, smoke inhalation, wood stoves

    (3) Pathogenesis of hypoxia

        (a) CO competes with O_2 for binding sites on Hb, which decreases Sao_2 *without* affecting Pao_2.

        (b) It inhibits cytochrome oxidase in the electron transport chain (ETC).

        (c) It causes a left shift in the O_2-binding curve (OBC).

    (4) Clinical findings

        (a) Cherry-red discoloration of skin and blood

        (b) Headache (first symptom), coma, necrosis of the globus pallidus

> CO poisoning: normal Pao_2, ↓ Sao_2

> Treat CO poisoning with 100% O_2.

d. Factors causing a left shift in the OBC

    (1) Decreased 2,3-bisphosphoglycerate (BPG)

        • Intermediate of glycolysis via conversion of 1,3-BPG to 2,3-BPG

    (2) CO, alkalosis, metHb, fetal Hb, hypothermia

> At high altitudes, the atmospheric pressure is decreased; however, the percentage of O_2 in the atmosphere remains the same. Hypoxemia stimulates peripheral chemoreceptors (e.g., carotid body) causing respiratory alkalosis, which shifts the OBC to the left. However, alkalosis activates phosphofructokinase in glycolysis causing increased production of 1,3-BPG, which is converted to 2,3-BPG. This right shifts the OBC, leading to increased release of O_2 to tissue.

e. Enzyme inhibition of oxidative phosphorylation

    (1) Synthesis of ATP is decreased.

    (2) CO and cyanide (CN) inhibit cytochrome oxidase in the ETC.

        (a) CN poisoning may result from drugs (e.g., nitroprusside) and combustion of polyurethane products in house fires.

        (b) CN poisoning is treated with amyl nitrite (produces metHb which combines with CN) followed by thiosulfate (CN converted to thiocyanate).

> CO and CN inhibit cytochrome oxidase.

f. Uncoupling of oxidative phosphorylation

    (1) Uncoupling proteins carry protons pumped from the ETC into the mitochondrial matrix.

        (a) Bypass of ATP synthase causes decreased synthesis of ATP.

        (b) Examples include thermogenin in brown fat in newborns, dinitrophenol used in synthesizing TNT.

    (2) Oxidative energy is released as heat rather than as ATP.

        • Danger of developing hyperthermia with dinitrophenol

> Agents such as alcohol and salicylates act as mitochondrial toxins. They damage the inner mitochondrial membrane, causing protons to move into the mitochondrial matrix. Like dinitrophenol, hyperthermia is also a common complication in alcohol and salicylate poisoning.

> Mitochondrial toxins: alcohol, salicylates

C. **Tissues susceptible to hypoxia**

1. Watershed areas between two blood supplies
   a. The blood supply from the two vessels does *not* overlap.
   b. Examples
      (1) Area between the distribution of the anterior and middle cerebral arteries
      (2) Area between the distribution of the superior and inferior mesenteric arteries (i.e., splenic flexure)

2. Subendocardial tissue
   a. Coronary vessels penetrate the epicardial surface.
   b. Subendocardial tissue receives the *least* amount of O_2.

Neurons: most adversely affected cell in tissue hypoxia

ST-segment depression on ECG: sign of subendocardial ischemia

> Factors decreasing coronary artery blood flow (e.g., coronary artery atherosclerosis) produce subendocardial ischemia, which is manifested by chest pain (i.e., angina) and ST-segment depression in an electrocardiogram (ECG). Increased thickness of the left ventricle (i.e., hypertrophy) in the presence of increased myocardial demand for O_2 (e.g., exercise) can also produce subendocardial ischemia.

3. Renal cortex and medulla
   a. The straight portion of the proximal tubule in the cortex is most susceptible to hypoxia.
   b. The $Na^+/K^+/2Cl^-$ cotransport channel in the thick ascending limb of the renal medulla is most susceptible to hypoxia.

D. **Consequences of hypoxic cell injury**

1. Decreased synthesis of ATP
2. Anaerobic glycolysis is used for ATP synthesis and is accompanied by several changes:
   a. Activation of phosphofructokinase caused by low citrate levels and increased adenosine monophosphate
   b. Net gain of 2ATP
   c. Decrease in intracellular pH caused by an excess of lactate
   d. Impaired Na^+,K^+-ATPase pump
      • Diffusion of Na^+ and H_2O into cells causes cellular swelling (potentially reversible with restoration of O_2).
3. Decreased protein synthesis due to detachment of ribosomes (potentially reversible)
4. Irreversible cell changes
   a. Impaired calcium (Ca^{2+})-ATPase pump
   b. Increased cytosolic Ca^{2+}, having two causes:
      (1) Enzyme activation
         (a) Phospholipase increases cell and organelle membrane permeability.
         (b) Proteases damage the cytoskeleton.
         (c) Endonucleases cause fading of nuclear chromatin (karyolysis).
      (2) Reentry of Ca^{2+} into mitochondria
         • Increases mitochondrial membrane permeability, with release of cytochrome *c* (activates apoptosis)

Lactate decreases intracellular pH and denatures structural and enzymic proteins.

Cytochrome *c*: activates apoptosis

II. Free Radical Cell Injury

A. Definition of free radicals

1. Compounds with a single unpaired electron in an outer orbital
2. Degrade nucleic acids and membrane molecules
   a. DNA fragmentation and dissolution
   b. Lipid peroxidation of polyunsaturated lipids in cell membranes

Free radicals: damage membranes and DNA

B. Types of free radicals

1. O_2-derived free radicals
   a. Superoxides ($O_2^{\bullet}$)
   b. Hydroxyl ions ($OH^{\bullet}$)
   c. Peroxides (H_2O_2)
2. Drug and chemical free radicals
   a. Free radicals are produced in the liver cytochrome P-450 system.
   b. Examples include acetaminophen and carbon tetrachloride.

C. Neutralization of free radicals

1. Superoxide dismutase neutralizes superoxide free radicals.
2. Glutathione peroxidase (enhances glutathione) neutralizes peroxide, hydroxyl, and acetaminophen free radicals.
3. Catalase neutralizes peroxide free radicals.
4. Vitamin antioxidants (ascorbic acid, vitamin E, β-carotenes) block the formation of free radicals and degrade free radicals.

Glutathione peroxidase: present in pentose phosphate pathway

D. Examples of free radical injury

1. Acetaminophen free radicals
   a. May cause diffuse chemical hepatitis
      (1) Liver cell necrosis occurs around the central veins.
      (2) Treatment with *N*-acetylcysteine increases synthesis of glutathione for neutralization of drug free radicals.
   b. May cause renal papillary necrosis
      • Necrosis occurs in association with the use of nonsteroidal anti-inflammatory agents.

Acetaminophen: most common cause of drug-induced fulminant hepatitis

2. Carbon tetrachloride free radicals
   • Produce liver cell necrosis with fatty change
3. Ischemia/reperfusion injury
   a. Occurs with restoration of blood flow to ischemic myocardium and cerebral tissue
   b. $O_2^{\bullet}$ and cytosolic Ca^{2+} irreversibly damage previously injured cells after restoration of blood flow.

Reperfusion injury: $O_2^{\bullet}$ and ↑ in cytosolic Ca^{2+}

4. Retinopathy of prematurity
   • Blindness may occur in the treatment of respiratory distress syndrome with an O_2 concentration > 50%.
5. Iron overload disorders
   a. Examples include hemochromatosis and hemosiderosis.
   b. Intracellular iron produces $OH^{\bullet}$, which damage parenchymal cells.
      • Examples of injury include cirrhosis, exocrine/endocrine pancreatic dysfunction, diffuse skin pigmentation.

III. Injury to Cellular Organelles

A. Mitochondria

1. Release of cytochrome *c* from injured mitochondria initiates apoptosis.
2. Injurious agents include alcohol, salicylates, and increased cytosolic Ca^{2+}.

B. Smooth endoplasmic reticulum (SER)

1. Induction of enzymes of the liver cytochrome P-450 system
   a. Caused by alcohol, barbiturates, and phenytoin
   b. Causes SER hyperplasia and increased drug detoxification, with lower-than-expected therapeutic drug levels
2. Inhibition of enzymes of the cytochrome P-450 system
   a. Caused by proton receptor blockers (e.g., omeprazole) and macrolides (e.g., erythromycin)
   b. Results in decreased drug detoxification, with higher-than-expected therapeutic drug levels

C. Lysosomes

1. Primary lysosomes
   a. Hydrolytic enzymes destined for primary lysosomes are marked with mannose 6-phosphate in the Golgi apparatus.
   b. Marked enzymes are transferred to primary lysosomes.

> Inclusion (I)-cell disease is a rare inherited condition in which lysosomal enzymes lack the mannose 6-phosphate marker. Therefore, primary lysosomes do *not* contain the hydrolytic enzymes necessary to degrade complex substrates. Undigested substrates accumulate as large inclusions in the cytosol. Symptoms include psychomotor retardation and early death.

   c. Deficiency of lysosomal enzymes occurs in lysosomal storage diseases.
      (1) Complex substrates accumulate in lysosomes.
      (2) Example—Gaucher's disease with deficiency of glucocerebrosidase causes accumulation of glucocerebrosides in the lysosome.
2. Secondary lysosomes (phagolysosomes)
   a. Arise from fusion of primary lysosomes with phagocytic vacuoles
   b. Defective in Chédiak-Higashi syndrome (CHS)

> CHS is an autosomal recessive disease with a defect in membrane fusion. This results in fusion of azurophilic granules in the primary lysosomes of leukocytes (giant granules) and inability of primary lysosomes to fuse with phagosomes to produce secondary phagolysosomes. There is increased susceptibility to infection (particularly *Staphylococcus aureus*) due to defects in chemotaxis (directed migration), degranulation, and bactericidal activity.

D. Cytoskeleton

1. Mitotic spindle defects
   • Examples—vinca alkaloids and colchicine bind to tubulin in microtubules, which interferes with the assembly of the mitotic spindle.
2. Intermediate filament defects

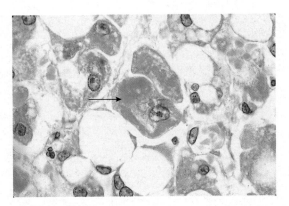

1-1: *Mallory bodies. Hyaline (eosinophilic) inclusions (arrow) are present in the cytosol of hepatocytes. (From Kumar V, Fausto N, Abbas A: Robbins and Cotran's Pathologic Basis of Disease, 7th ed. Philadelphia, WB Saunders, 2004, p 34, Fig. 1-34A.)*

      a. Ubiquitin binds to damaged intermediate filaments and marks them for degradation in proteasomes in the cytosol.

> Ubiquitin: marker for intermediate filament degradation

      b. Mallory bodies
         • Damaged ("ubiquinated") cytokeratin intermediate filaments in hepatocytes in alcoholic liver disease (Fig. 1-1)
      c. Lewy bodies
        (1) Damaged neurofilaments in idiopathic Parkinson's disease
        (2) Eosinophilic cytoplasmic inclusions in degenerating substantia nigra neurons
   3. Rigor mortis
     • Myosin heads become locked to actin filaments as a result of a lack of ATP.

IV. Intracellular Accumulations
  A. Types of accumulations (Table 1-2)
    1. Excess of exogenous or endogenous pigments
    2. Excess of normal cell constituents
    3. Excess of exogenous or endogenous abnormal substances
  B. Fatty change in the liver
    1. Cytosolic accumulation of triglyceride
    2. Mechanisms of fatty change

> Most common cause of fatty change: alcohol

      a. Increased glycerol 3-phosphate (G3-P)
        (1) Intermediate of glycolysis
        (2) Substrate for triglyceride synthesis
        (3) Metabolic intermediates of alcohol metabolism
          • Increased reduced nicotinamide adenine dinucleotide (NADH), a product of alcohol metabolism, accelerates conversion of dihydroxyacetone phosphate to G3-P.

> Glycerol 3-phosphate: substrate for triglyceride synthesis

      b. Increased fatty acid synthesis
        • Example—acetyl coenzyme A, the end product of alcohol metabolism, is used to synthesize fatty acids.

TABLE 1-2: Intracellular Accumulations

Substance	Clinical Significance
Endogenous Accumulations	
Bilirubin	Kernicterus: fat-soluble unconjugated bilirubin derived from Rh hemolytic disease of newborn; bilirubin enters basal ganglia nuclei of brain, causing permanent damage
Cholesterol	Xanthelasma: yellow plaque on eyelid; cholesterol in macrophages Atherosclerosis: cholesterol-laden smooth muscle cells and macrophages (i.e., foam cells); components of fibrofatty plaques
Glycogen	Diabetes mellitus: increased glycogen in proximal renal tubule cells (cells are insensitive to insulin and become overloaded with glycogen) Von Gierke's glycogenosis: deficiency of glucose-6-phosphatase; glycogen excess in hepatocytes and renal tubular cells
Hemosiderin and ferritin	Iron overload disorders (e.g., hemochromatosis): excess hemosiderin deposition in parenchymal cells, leading to free radical damage and organ dysfunction (e.g., cirrhosis); increase in serum ferritin Iron deficiency: decrease in ferritin and hemosiderin
Melanin	Addison's disease: destruction of the adrenal cortex; hypocortisolism leads to an increase in ACTH causing excess synthesis of melanin and diffuse pigmentation of the skin and mucosal membranes
Triglyceride	Fatty liver: triglyceride in hepatocytes pushes the nucleus to the periphery
Exogenous Accumulations	
Anthracotic pigment	Coal worker's pneumoconiosis: phagocytosis of black anthracotic pigment (coal dust) by alveolar macrophages ("dust cells")
Lead	Lead poisoning: lead deposits in nuclei of proximal renal tubular cells (acid-fast inclusion) contribute to nephrotoxic changes in the proximal tubule

ACTH, adrenocorticotropic hormone; GI, gastrointestinal.

    c. Decreased β-oxidation of fatty acids
- Causes include alcohol, hypoxia, and diphtheria toxin.

    d. Increased mobilization of fatty acids from adipose tissue
- Causes include alcohol and starvation.

    e. Decreased synthesis of apolipoprotein B-100
- Causes include carbon tetrachloride and decreased protein intake (e.g., kwashiorkor).

    f. Decreased hepatic release of very low density lipoprotein
- Causes include carbon tetrachloride and decreased protein intake.

3. Morphology

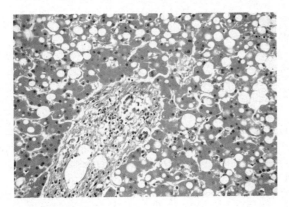

1-2: *Fatty change of the liver. Vacuoles containing triglyceride are noted in most of the hepatocytes. The nucleus is displaced to the periphery. (From Kumar V, Fausto N, Abbas A: Robbins and Cotran's Pathologic Basis of Disease, 7th ed. Philadelphia, WB Saunders, 2004, p 36, Fig. 1-36B.)*

      b. Clear space pushing the nucleus to the periphery (Fig. 1-2)

C. Iron (see Table 1-2)
   1. Ferritin
      a. Major soluble iron storage protein
      b. Stored in bone marrow macrophages (most abundant site) and hepatocytes
      c. Small amounts circulate in serum
         • Directly correlates with ferritin stores in the bone marrow
   2. Hemosiderin
      a. Insoluble product of ferritin degradation in lysosomes
      b. Does *not* circulate in serum
      c. Appears as golden brown granules in tissue
      d. Appears as blue granules when stained with Prussian blue

D. Pathologic calcification
   1. Dystrophic calcification
      a. Deposition of calcium phosphate in necrotic tissue
      b. Normal serum calcium and phosphate
      c. Examples—calcified atherosclerotic plaque, calcification in pancreatitis (Fig. 1-14)
   2. Metastatic calcification
      a. Deposition of calcium phosphate in normal tissue
      b. Due to increased serum calcium and/or phosphate
         (1) Causes of hypercalcemia—primary hyperparathyroidism, malignancy-induced hypercalcemia
         (2) Causes of hyperphosphatemia—renal failure, primary hypoparathyroidism
           • Excess phosphate drives calcium into normal tissue.
      c. Examples of metastatic calcification
         (1) Calcification of renal tubular basement membranes in the collecting ducts (nephrocalcinosis)
         (2) Basal ganglia calcification in hypoparathyroidism

Serum ferritin: ↓ in iron deficiency anemia

Hemosiderin: ferritin degradation product

Dystrophic calcification: calcification of necrotic tissue

Metastatic calcification: calcification of normal tissue

Atrophy: ↓ size of tissue or organ

V. Adaptation to Cell Injury: Growth Alterations

A. Atrophy

1. Decrease in size of a tissue or organ
2. Causes of atrophy
   a. Decreased hormone stimulation
      - Example—hypopituitarism causing atrophy of target organs, such as the thyroid and adrenal cortex
   b. Decreased innervation
      - Example—skeletal muscle atrophy following loss of lower motor neurons in amyotrophic lateral sclerosis
   c. Decreased blood flow
      - Example—cerebral atrophy due to atherosclerosis of the carotid artery
   d. Decreased nutrients
      - Example—total calorie deprivation in marasmus
   e. Increased pressure
      - Example—atrophy of the renal cortex and medulla in hydronephrosis (Fig. 1-3)
   f. Occlusion of secretory ducts
      - Example—thick ductal secretions in cystic fibrosis cause atrophy of exocrine glands

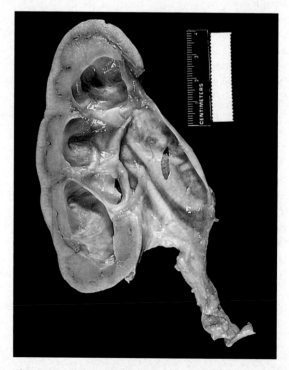

1-3: *Hydronephrosis of the kidney. There is marked dilation of the renal pelvis and calyces with thinning of the overlying cortex and medulla due to compression atrophy. (From Kumar V, Fausto N, Abbas A: Robbins and Cotran's Pathologic Basis of Disease, 7th ed. Philadelphia, WB Saunders, 2004, p 1013, Fig. 20-56.)*

3. Mechanisms of atrophy
   a. Shrinkage of cells due to increased catabolism of cell organelles (e.g., mitochondria) and reduction in cytosol
      (1) Organelles and cytosol form autophagic vacuoles.
      (2) Autophagic vacuoles fuse with primary lysosomes for enzymatic degradation.
      (3) Undigested lipids are stored as residual bodies.

> Brown atrophy is a tissue discoloration that results from lysosomal accumulation of lipofuscin ("wear and tear" pigment). Lipofuscin is an indigestible lipid derived from lipid peroxidation of cell membranes, which may occur in atrophy and free radical damage of tissue.

   b. Loss of cells by apoptosis
B. **Hypertrophy**
   1. Increase in cell size
   2. Causes of hypertrophy
      a. Increased workload
         (1) Left ventricular hypertrophy in response to an increase in afterload (resistance) or preload (volume) (Fig. 1-4)
         (2) Skeletal muscle hypertrophy in weight training

Hypertrophy: ↑ cell size

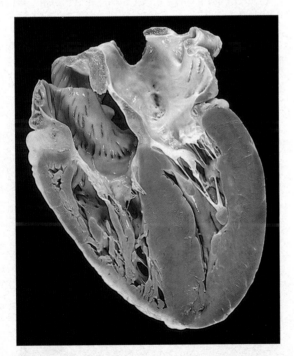

1-4: *Left ventricular hypertrophy, showing the thickened free left ventricular wall (right side) and the thickened interventricular septum. The right ventricle wall (left side) is of normal thickness. (From Kumar V, Fausto N, Abbas A: Robbins and Cotran's Pathologic Basis of Disease, 7th ed. Philadelphia, WB Saunders, 2004, p 561, Fig. 12-3A.)*

(3) Smooth muscle hypertrophy in the urinary bladder in response to urethral obstruction (e.g., prostate hyperplasia)

(4) Surgical removal of one kidney with compensatory hypertrophy (and hyperplasia) of the other kidney

b. Increased hormonal stimulation
  • Example—enlargement of the gravid uterus due to smooth muscle hypertrophy (and hyperplasia) from estrogen stimulation

3. Mechanisms of cardiac muscle hypertrophy
  a. Induction of genes for synthesis of growth factors, nuclear transcription, and contractile proteins
  b. Increase in cytosol, number of cytoplasmic organelles, and DNA content

C. Hyperplasia

Hyperplasia: ↑ number of cells

1. Increase in the number of normal cells
2. Causes of hyperplasia
  a. Hypersecretion of trophic hormones
    (1) Acromegaly due to an increase in growth hormone and insulin growth factor-1 (Fig. 22-1)
    (2) Endometrial gland hyperplasia due to hyperestrinism (Fig. 21-8)
    (3) Benign prostatic hyperplasia due to an increase in dihydrotestosterone (Fig. 1-5)
    (4) Gynecomastia (male breast tissue) due to increased estrogen
    (5) Polycythemia due to an increase in erythropoietin
  b. Chronic irritation
    • Example—thickened epidermis from constant scratching
  c. Chemical imbalance
    • Example—hypocalcemia stimulates parathyroid gland hyperplasia

3. Mechanisms of hyperplasia

Cell types: labile, stable, permanent

  a. Dependent on the regenerative capacity of different types of cells
  b. Labile cells (stem cells)
    (1) Divide continuously

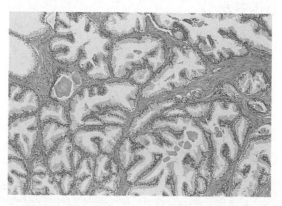

1-5: *Benign prostatic hyperplasia. The prostatic glands show infolding into the glandular spaces. (From Damjanov I, Linder J: Pathology: A Color Atlas. St. Louis, Mosby, 2000, p 249, Fig. 12-32.)*

(2) Examples—stem cells in the bone marrow, crypts of Lieberkühn, and basal cells in the epidermis

(3) May undergo hyperplasia as an adaptation to cell injury

c. Stable cells (resting cells)

(1) Divide infrequently, because they are normally in the Go (resting) phase

(2) Must be stimulated (e.g., growth factors, hormones) to enter the cell cycle

(3) Examples—hepatocytes, astrocytes, smooth muscle cells

(4) May undergo hyperplasia or hypertrophy as an adaptation to cell injury

d. Permanent cells (nonreplicating cells)

(1) Highly specialized cells that cannot replicate

(2) Examples—neurons and skeletal and cardiac muscle cells

(3) May undergo hypertrophy (only muscle)

D. Metaplasia

1. Replacement of one fully differentiated cell type by another

- Substituted cells are less sensitive to a particular stress.

2. Types of metaplasia

a. Metaplasia from squamous to glandular epithelium

(1) Example—distal esophagus epithelium shows an increase in goblet cells and mucus-secreting cells in response to acid reflux

(2) This is called Barrett's esophagus (Fig. 17-5)

b. Metaplasia from glandular to other types of glandular epithelium

(1) Example—pylorus and antrum epithelium shows an increase in goblet cells and Paneth cells in response to *Helicobacter pylori*–induced chronic atrophic gastritis

(2) This is called intestinal metaplasia (Fig. 1-6).

c. Metaplasia from glandular to squamous epithelium

(1) Mainstem bronchus epithelium develops squamous metaplasia in response to irritants in cigarette smoke.

Metaplasia: one cell type replaces another

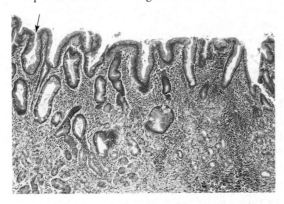

1-6: *Intestinal metaplasia of the gastric mucosal epithelium in chronic gastritis. The arrow shows clear spaces in the mucosal epithelium representing goblet cells, which are normally present in the intestine. (From Kumar V, Fausto N, Abbas A: Robbins and Cotran's Pathologic Basis of Disease, 7th ed. Philadelphia, WB Saunders, 2004, p 815, Fig. 17-14.)*

(2) Endocervical epithelium develops squamous metaplasia in response to the acid pH in the vagina.

    d. Metaplasia from transitional to squamous epithelium
- Example—*Schistosoma hematobium* infection in the urinary bladder causes transitional epithelium to undergo squamous metaplasia.

3. Mechanism of metaplasia
    a. Reprogramming stem cells in response to signals:
      (1) Hormones (e.g., estrogen)
      (2) Vitamins (e.g., retinoic acid)
      (3) Chemical irritants (e.g., cigarette smoke)
    b. Sometimes reversible if the irritant is removed

E. Dysplasia

1. Disordered cell growth
2. Risk factors for dysplasia
    a. Hyperplasia (see section V)
    b. Metaplasia (see section V)
    c. Infection
    - Example—human papillomavirus type 16, causing squamous dysplasia of the cervix
    d. Chemicals
    - Example—irritants in cigarette smoke, causing squamous metaplasia to progress to squamous dysplasia in the mainstem bronchus
    e. Ultraviolet light
    - Example—solar damage of the skin, causing squamous dysplasia

3. Microscopic features of dysplasia (Fig. 1-7)
    a. Nuclear features
      (1) Increased mitotic activity, with normal mitotic spindles
      (2) Increased nuclear size and chromatin
    b. Disorderly proliferation of cells with loss of cell maturation as cells progress to the surface

4. Dysplasia may or may not progress to cancer if the irritant is removed.

VI. Cell Death
- Cell death occurs when cells or tissues are unable to adapt to injury.

A. Necrosis

1. Death of groups of cells, often accompanied by an inflammatory infiltrate
2. Coagulation necrosis
    a. Preservation of the structural outline of dead cells
    b. Mechanism of coagulation necrosis
      (1) Denaturation of enzymes and structural proteins
        (a) Intracellular accumulation of lactate or heavy metals (e.g., lead, mercury)

Dysplasia: disordered cell growth

Dysplasia may progress to cancer.

Coagulation necrosis: preservation of structural outlines

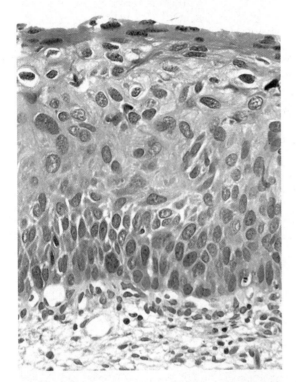

1-7: *Squamous dysplasia of the cervix, a precursor of squamous cell carcinoma. There is a lack of orientation of the squamous cells throughout the upper two thirds of the epithelium. Many of the nuclei are enlarged, are hyperchromatic, and have irregular nuclear margins. (From Kumar V, Fausto N, Abbas A: Robbins and Cotran's Pathologic Basis of Disease, 7th ed. Philadelphia, WB Saunders, 2004, p 1075, Fig. 22-19C.)*

       (b) Exposure of cells to ionizing radiation
     (2) Inactivation of intracellular enzymes prevents dissolution (autolysis) of the cell.
  c. Microscopic features (Fig. 1-8)
     (1) Indistinct outlines of cells within dead tissue
     (2) Absent nuclei or karyolysis (fading of nuclear chromatin)
  d. Infarction
     (1) Gross manifestation of coagulation necrosis secondary to the sudden occlusion of a vessel
     (2) Usually wedge-shaped if dichotomously branching vessels (e.g., pulmonary artery) are occluded
     (3) Pale (ischemic) type
       • Increased density of tissue (e.g., heart, kidney, spleen) prevents RBCs from diffusing through necrotic tissue (Fig. 1-9).
     (4) Hemorrhagic (red) type
       • Loose-textured tissue (e.g., lungs, small bowel) allows RBCs to diffuse through necrotic tissue (Fig. 1-10).

Infarctions: pale and hemorrhagic types

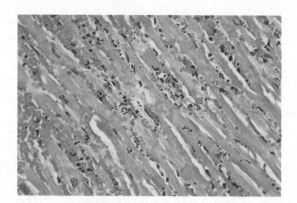

1-8: *Acute myocardial infarction (MI) showing coagulation necrosis. This section of myocardial tissue is from a 3-day-old acute MI. The outlines of the myocardial fibers are intact; however, they lack nuclei and cross-striations. A neutrophilic infiltrate is present between some of the dead fibers. (From Damjanov I, Linder J: Pathology: A Color Atlas. St. Louis, Mosby, 2000, p 375, Fig. 17-15.)*

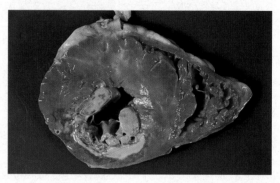

1-9: *Acute myocardial infarction (MI) showing a pale infarction of the posterior wall of the left ventricle (bottom left). (From Damjanov I, Linder J: Anderson's Pathology, 10th ed. St. Louis, Mosby, 1996, p 374, Fig. 17-13.)*

> Dry gangrene of the toes in individuals with diabetes mellitus is a form of infarction that results from ischemia. Coagulation necrosis is the primary type of necrosis present in the dead tissue (Fig. 1-11).

3. Liquefactive necrosis
   a. Necrotic degradation of tissue that softens and becomes liquified
   b. Mechanisms
      • Lysosomal enzymes released by necrotic cells or neutrophils cause liquefaction of tissue.
   c. Examples
      (1) Central nervous system infarction
         • Autocatalytic effect of hydrolytic enzymes generated by neuroglial cells produces a cystic space (Fig. 1-12).

Cerebral infarction: liquefactive *not* coagulative necrosis

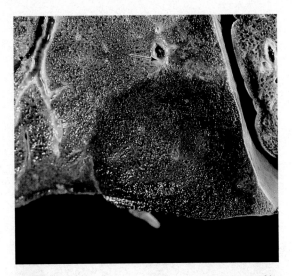

1-10: *Hemorrhagic infarction of the lung. There is a roughly wedge-shaped area of hemorrhage extending to the pleural surface. The arrow shows an embolus in one of the pulmonary artery tributaries. (From Kumar V, Fausto N, Abbas A: Robbins and Cotran's Pathologic Basis of Disease, 7th ed. Philadelphia, WB Saunders, 2004, p 138, Fig. 4-19A.)*

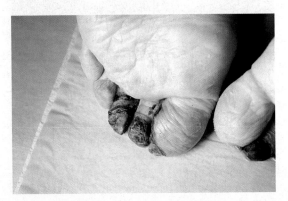

1-11: *Dry gangrene of the toes. Dry gangrene involves the first four toes. The dark black areas of gangrene are bordered by light-colored, parchment-like skin. (From Damjanov I: Pathology for the Health-Related Professions, 2nd ed. Philadelphia, WB Saunders, 2000, p 18, Fig. 1-24.)*

    (2) Abscess in a bacterial infection
- Hydrolytic enzymes generated by neutrophils liquefy dead tissue.

> Wet gangrene of the toes of individuals with diabetes mellitus is a superimposed anaerobic infection (e.g., *Clostridium perfringens*) of dead tissue. Liquefactive necrosis is the primary type of necrosis.

  4. Caseous necrosis
    a. Variant of coagulation necrosis associated with acellular, cheese-like (caseous) material

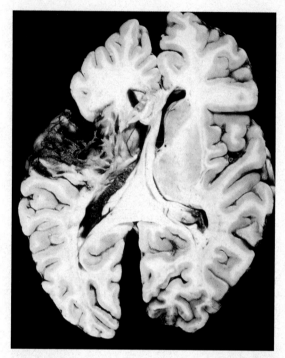

1-12: *Cerebral infarction showing liquefactive necrosis of the cerebral cortex leaving a large cystic cavity. (From Kumar V, Fausto N, Abbas A: Robbins and Cotran's Pathologic Basis of Disease, 7th ed. Philadelphia, WB Saunders, 2004, p 1365, Fig. 28-16.)*

Tuberculosis: most common cause of caseous necrosis

Enzymatic fat necrosis: acute pancreatitis

    b. Mechanism
- Caseous material is formed by the release of lipid from the cell walls of *Mycobacterium tuberculosis* and systemic fungi (e.g., *Histoplasma*) after destruction by macrophages.

    c. Microscopic features
      (1) The acellular material in the center of a granuloma contains activated macrophages, CD4 helper T cells, and multinucleated giant cells (Fig. 1-13).
      (2) Some granulomas do *not* exhibit caseation (e.g., sarcoidosis).

5. Enzymatic fat necrosis
    a. Peculiar to adipose tissue located around an acutely inflamed pancreas
    b. Mechanisms
      (1) Activation of pancreatic lipase (e.g., alcohol excess) causing hydrolysis of triglyceride in fat cells
      (2) Conversion of fatty acids into soap (saponification)
- Combination of fatty acids and calcium

    c. Gross appearance
- Chalky yellow-white deposits are primarily located in peripancreatic and omental adipose tissue (Fig. 1-14).

    d. Microscopic appearance
- Pale outlines of fat cells filled with basophilic-staining calcified areas

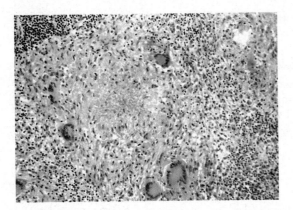

1-13: *Caseous granuloma showing a central area of acellular, necrotic material surrounded by activated macrophages (epithelioid cells), lymphocytes, and multiple multinucleated Langhans-type giant cells. (From Kumar V, Fausto N, Abbas A: Robbins and Cotran's Pathologic Basis of Disease, 7th ed. Philadelphia, WB Saunders, 2004, p 83, Fig. 2-33.)*

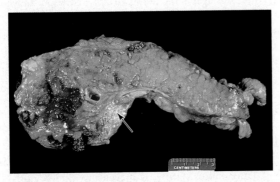

1-14: *Enzymatic fat necrosis in acute pancreatitis. Dark areas of hemorrhage are present in the head of the pancreas (left side), and focal areas of pale fat necrosis (arrow) are present in the peripancreatic fat. (From Kumar V, Fausto N, Abbas A: Robbins and Cotran's Pathologic Basis of Disease, 7th ed. Philadelphia, WB Saunders, 2004, p 943, Fig. 19-5.)*

    e. Traumatic fat necrosis
       (1) Occurs in fatty tissue (e.g., female breast tissue) as a result of trauma
       (2) *Not* enzyme-mediated
  6. Fibrinoid necrosis
    a. Limited to small muscular arteries, arterioles, venules, and glomerular capillaries
    b. Mechanism
      • Deposition of pink-staining proteinaceous material in damaged vessel walls due to damaged basement membranes

c. Associated conditions
- Immune vasculitis (e.g., Henoch-Schönlein purpura), malignant hypertension

B. Apoptosis

Apoptosis: programmed cell death

1. Programmed, enzyme-mediated cell death
2. Examples
   a. Destruction of cells during embryogenesis
      - Example—loss of müllerian structures in a male fetus due to Sertoli cell synthesis of müllerian inhibitory factor
   b. Hormone-dependent atrophy of tissue
      - Example—endometrial cell breakdown after withdrawal of estrogen and progesterone in the menstrual cycle
   c. Death of tumor cells by cytotoxic CD8 T cells, corticosteroid destruction of lymphocytes
3. Mechanisms of apoptosis

Caspases: group of cysteine proteases

   a. Signals initiate apoptosis by activating caspases:
      (1) Binding of tumor necrosis factor to its receptor
      (2) Withdrawal of growth factors or hormones
      (3) Injurious agents including viruses, radiation, free radicals that damage DNA
      (4) *BAX* gene, cytochrome *c*
   b. Genes regulating apoptosis

TP53 suppressor gene: "guardian" of the cell

      (1) *TP53* suppressor gene
         (a) Temporarily arrests the cell cycle in the G_1 phase to repair DNA damage (aborts apoptosis)
         (b) Promotes apoptosis if DNA damage is too great by activating the *BAX* apoptosis gene

BAX gene: apoptosis gene

      (2) *BCL2* gene family

BCL2 gene: anti-apoptosis gene

         - Manufactures gene products that inhibit apoptosis (i.e., antiapoptosis gene) by preventing mitochondrial leakage of cytochrome *c* into the cytosol
   c. Changes in the cell
      (1) Activation of endonuclease leads to nuclear pyknosis ("ink dot" appearance) and fragmentation.
      (2) Activation of protease leads to the breakdown of the cytoskeleton.
      (3) Formation of cytoplasmic buds on the cell membrane
         - Buds contain nuclear fragments, mitochondria, and condensed protein fragments.
      (4) Formation of apoptotic bodies by the breaking off of cytoplasmic buds
      (5) Phagocytosis of apoptotic bodies by neighboring cells or macrophages
4. Microscopic appearance of apoptosis
   a. Cell detachment from neighboring cells
   b. Deeply eosinophilic-staining cytoplasm (Fig. 1-15)
   c. Pyknotic, fragmented, or absent nucleus
   d. Minimal or no inflammatory infiltrate surrounding the cell

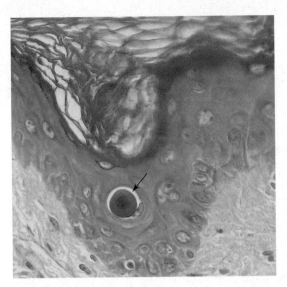

1-15: *Apoptosis in the epidermis. The arrow shows a clear space in the epidermis containing an intensely eosinophilic staining cell with a small, dense nucleus. (From Kumar V, Fausto N, Abbas A: Robbins and Cotran's Pathologic Basis of Disease, 7th ed. Philadelphia, WB Saunders, 2004, p 28, Fig. 1-26A.)*

TABLE 1-3:
Enzyme Markers of Cell Death

Enzyme	Diagnostic Use
Aspartate aminotransferase (AST)	Marker of diffuse liver cell necrosis (e.g., viral hepatitis) Mitochondrial enzyme preferentially increased in alcohol-induced liver disease
Alanine aminotransferase (ALT)	Marker of diffuse liver cell necrosis (e.g., viral hepatitis) More specific for liver cell necrosis than AST
Creatine kinase MB (CK-MB)	Isoenzyme increased in acute myocardial infarction or myocarditis
Amylase and lipase	Marker enzymes for acute pancreatitis Lipase more specific than amylase for pancreatitis Amylase also increased in salivary gland inflammation (e.g., mumps)

C. **Enzyme markers of cell death**
1. Tissues release certain enzymes that indicate the type of tissue involved and extent of injury.
2. Table 1-3 lists clinically significant enzyme markers.

Inflammation and Repair

I. Acute Inflammation

- Transient and early response to injury that involves release of chemical mediators, causing stereotypic vessel and leukocyte responses

A. Cardinal signs of inflammation (Fig. 2-1)

1. Rubor (redness) and calor (heat)
   - Histamine-mediated vasodilation of arterioles
2. Tumor (swelling)
   - Histamine-mediated increase in permeability of venules
3. Dolor (pain)
   - Prostaglandin (PG) E_2 sensitizes specialized nerve endings to the effects of bradykinin and other pain mediators.

B. Stimuli for acute inflammation

1. Infections (e.g., bacterial or viral infection)
2. Immune reactions (e.g., reaction to a bee sting)
3. Other stimuli
   - Tissue necrosis (e.g., acute myocardial infarction), trauma, radiation, burns

C. Sequential vascular events

1. Vasoconstriction of arterioles
   - Neurogenic reflex that lasts only seconds
2. Vasodilation of arterioles
   a. Histamine and other vasodilators (e.g., nitric oxide) relax vascular smooth muscle, causing increased blood flow.
   b. Increased blood flow increases hydrostatic pressure.

3. Increased permeability of venules
   a. Histamine and other mediators contract endothelial cells producing endothelial gaps.
   b. A transudate (protein and cell-poor fluid) moves into the interstitial tissue.
4. Swelling of tissue (edema)
   - Net outflow of fluid surpasses lymphatic ability to remove fluid.
5. Reduced blood flow
   - A decrease in hydrostatic pressure is caused by outflow of fluid into the interstitial tissue.

D. Sequential cellular events

- The events described will emphasize neutrophil events in acute inflammation due to a bacterial infection (e.g., *Staphylococcus aureus*).

1. Neutrophils are the primary leukocytes in acute inflammation (Fig. 2-2).
2. Margination

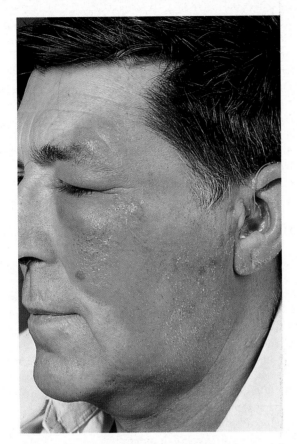

2-1: *Signs of acute inflammation. The patient has erysipelas of the face due to group A streptococcus. Signs of acute inflammation that are present in the photograph include redness (rubor) and swelling (tumor). The infection is associated with warm skin (calor) and pain (dolor). (From Forbes C, Jackson W: Color Atlas and Text of Clinical Medicine, 2nd ed. St. Louis, Mosby, 2003, p 37, Fig. 1-106.)*

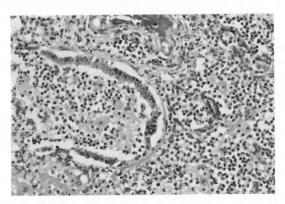

2-2: *Acute inflammation. Histologic section of lung in bronchopneumonia showing sheets of neutrophils with multilobed nuclei. (From Damjanov I: Pathology for the Health-Related Professions, 2nd ed. Philadelphia, WB Saunders, 2000, p 182, Fig. 8-8.)*

a. RBCs aggregate into rouleaux ("stacks of coins") in venules.

b. Neutrophils are pushed from the central axial column to the periphery (margination).

3. Rolling

a. Due to activation of selectin adhesion molecules on the surface of neutrophils and endothelial cells

b. Neutrophils loosely bind to selectins and "roll" along the endothelium.

4. Adhesion

a. Adhesion molecules firmly bind neutrophils to endothelial cells.

b. Neutrophil adhesion molecules

(1) β_2-Integrins (CD11a:CD18)

(2) Adhesion molecule activation is mediated by C5a and leukotriene B_4 (LTB$_4$).

(3) Catecholamines, corticosteroids, and lithium inhibit activation of adhesion molecules.

• This causes an increase in the peripheral blood neutrophil count (neutrophilic leukocytosis).

(4) Endotoxins enhance activation of adhesion molecules.

• This causes a decrease in the peripheral blood neutrophil count (neutropenia).

c. Endothelial cell adhesion molecules

(1) Intercellular adhesion molecule (ICAM) and vascular cell adhesion molecule (VCAM) bind to integrins on the surface of neutrophils.

(2) ICAM and VCAM activation is mediated by interleukin 1 (IL-1) and tumor necrosis factor (TNF).

d. Leukocyte adhesion deficiency (LAD)

(1) Autosomal recessive disorders

(2) LAD type 1 is a deficiency of CD11a:CD18.

(3) LAD type 2 is a deficiency of a selectin that binds neutrophils.

(4) Clinical findings

(a) Delayed separation of the umbilical cord (>1 month)

• Neutrophil enzymes are important in cord separation.

(b) Severe gingivitis, poor wound healing, peripheral blood neutrophilic leukocytosis

5. Transmigration (diapedesis)

a. Neutrophils dissolve the basement membrane and enter interstitial tissue.

b. Fluid rich in proteins and cells (i.e., exudate) accumulates in interstitial tissue.

c. Functions of exudate

(1) Dilute bacterial toxins

(2) Provide opsonins (assist in phagocytosis), antibodies, and complement

6. Chemotaxis

a. Neutrophils follow chemical gradients that lead to the infection site.

b. Chemotactic mediators bind to neutrophil receptors.

• Mediators include C5a, LTB$_4$, bacterial products, and IL-8.

Selectins: responsible for "rolling" of neutrophils

β_2-Integrins: neutrophil adhesion molecules

Delayed separation umbilical cord: selectin or CD11a:CD18 deficiency

Chemotaxis: directed migration of neutrophils

c. Binding causes the release of calcium, which increases neutrophil motility.

7. Phagocytosis
  a. Multistep process:
    (1) Opsonization
    (2) Ingestion
    (3) Killing
  b. Opsonization
    (1) Opsonins attach to bacteria.
      (a) Opsonins include IgG, C3b fragment of complement, and other proteins (e.g., C-reactive protein).
      (b) Neutrophils have membrane receptors for IgG and C3b.
    (2) Opsonization enhances neutrophil recognition and attachment to bacteria.
    (3) Bruton's agammaglobulinemia is an opsonization defect.
  c. Ingestion
    (1) Neutrophils engulf (phagocytose) and then trap bacteria in phagocytic vacuoles.
    (2) Primary lysosomes empty hydrolytic enzymes into phagocytic vacuoles producing phagolysosomes.
      • In Chédiak-Higashi syndrome (see Chapter 1), a defect in membrane fusion prevents phagolysosome formation.
  d. Bacterial killing
    (1) O_2-dependent myeloperoxidase (MPO) system (Fig. 2-3)
      (a) Only present in neutrophils and monocytes (*not* macrophages)
      (b) Production of superoxide free radicals ($O_2^{\bullet}$)
        • NADPH oxidase converts molecular O_2 to $O_2^{\bullet}$, which releases energy called the respiratory, or oxidative, burst.
      (c) Production of peroxide (H_2O_2)
        • Superoxide dismutase converts $O_2^{\bullet}$ to H_2O_2, which is neutralized by glutathione peroxidase.
      (d) Production of bleach ($HOCl^{\bullet}$)
        • MPO combines H_2O_2 with chloride (Cl^-) to form hypochlorous free radicals ($HOCl^{\bullet}$), which kill bacteria.
      (e) Chronic granulomatous disease and MPO deficiency are examples of diseases that have a defect in the O_2-dependent MPO system.

Chronic granulomatous disease (CGD), an X-linked recessive disorder, is characterized by deficient NADPH oxidase in the cell membranes of neutrophils and monocytes. The reduced production of $O_2^{\bullet}$ results in an absent respiratory burst. Catalase-positive organisms that produce H_2O_2 (e.g., *Staphylococcus aureus*) are ingested but *not* killed, because the catalase degrades H_2O_2. Myeloperoxidase is present, but $HOCl^{\bullet}$ is *not* synthesized because of the absence of H_2O_2. Catalase-negative

---

Opsonins: IgG and C3b

Bruton's agammaglobulinemia: opsonization defect

Chédiak-Higashi syndrome: cannot form phagolysosomes

O_2-dependent MPO system: most potent microbicidal system

End-product O_2-dependent MPO system: bleach

Chronic granulomatous disease: absent NADPH oxidase and respiratory burst

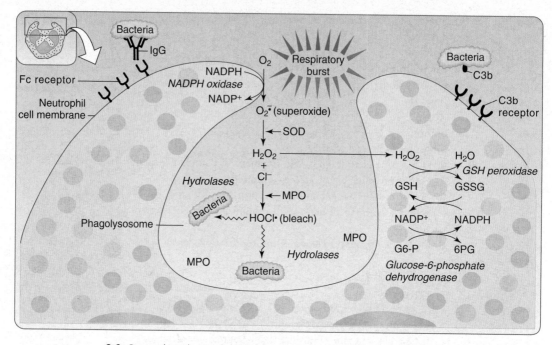

2-3: *Oxygen-dependent myeloperoxidase system. A series of biochemical reactions occurs in the phagolysosome, resulting in the production of hypochlorous free radicals (bleach; HOCl•) that destroy bacteria. GSH, reduced glutathione; G6-P, glucose 6-phosphate; GSSG, oxidized glutathione; H_2O_2, peroxide; MPO, myeloperoxidase; $NADP^+$, oxidized form of nicotinamide adenine dinucleotide phosphate; NADPH, reduced nicotinamide adenine dinucleotide phosphate; 6PG, 6-phosphogluconate; SOD, superoxide dismutase.*

organisms (e.g., *Streptococcus* species) are ingested and killed when myeloperoxidase combines H_2O_2 with Cl⁻ to form HOCl•. The classic screening test for CGD is the nitroblue tetrazolium test (NBT). In this test, leukocytes are incubated with a colorless NBT dye, which is converted to a blue color if the respiratory burst is intact. This test has been replaced by other more sensitive tests.

Myeloperoxidase (MPO) deficiency, an autosomal recessive disorder, differs from CGD in that both $O_2^{•-}$ and H_2O_2 are produced (normal respiratory burst). The absence of MPO prevents synthesis of HOCl•.

MPO deficiency: normal respiratory burst

(f) Deficiency of NADPH (e.g., glucose-6-phosphate dehydrogenase deficiency) produces a microbicidal defect.
(2) O_2-independent system
(a) Refers to bacterial killing from substances located in leukocyte granules
(b) Examples—lactoferrin (binds iron necessary for bacterial reproduction) and major basic protein (eosinophil product that is cytotoxic to helminths)

TABLE 2-1:
Sources and Functions of Chemical Mediators

Mediator	Source(s)	Function(s)
Arachidonic Acid Metabolites		
Prostaglandins	Macrophages, endothelial cells, platelets PGH_2: major precursor of PGs and thromboxanes	PGE_2: vasodilation, pain, fever PGI_2: vasodilation; inhibition of platelet aggregation
Thromboxane A_2	Platelets Converted from PGH_2 by thromboxane synthase	Vasoconstriction, platelet aggregation, bronchoconstriction
Leukotrienes (LTs)	Converted from arachidonic acid by lipoxygenase-mediated hydroxylation	LTB_4: chemotaxis and activation of neutrophil adhesion molecules LTC_4, LTD_4, LTE_4: vasoconstriction, increased vessel permeability, bronchoconstriction
Bradykinin	Product of kinin system activation by activated factor XII	Vasodilation, increased vessel permeability, pain, bronchoconstriction
Chemokines	Leukocytes, endothelial cells	Activate neutrophil chemotaxis
Complement	Synthesized in liver	C3a, C5a (anaphylatoxins): stimulate mast cell release of histamine C3b: opsonization C5a: activation of neutrophil adhesion molecules, chemotaxis C5–C9 (membrane attack complex): cell lysis
Cytokines IL-1, TNF	Lymphocytes, macrophages, endothelial cells	Initiate PGE_2 synthesis in anterior hypothalamus, leading to production of fever Activate endothelial cell adhesion molecules Increase liver synthesis of acute-phase reactants, such as ferritin, coagulation factors (e.g., fibrinogen), and C-reactive protein Increase release of neutrophils from bone marrow
IL-6		Increase liver synthesis of acute phase reactants
IL-8		Chemotaxis
Histamine	Mast cells (primary cell), platelets, enterochromaffin cells	Vasodilation, increased vessel permeability
Nitric Oxide (NO)	Macrophages, endothelial cells Free radical gas released during conversion of arginine to citrulline by NO synthase	Vasodilation, bactericidal
Serotonin	Mast cells, platelets	Vasodilation, increased vessel permeability

IL, interleukin; PG, prostaglandin; TNF, tumor necrosis factor.

E. **Chemical mediators (Table 2-1)**
1. They derive from plasma, leukocytes, local tissue, bacterial products.
   - Example—arachidonic acid mediators are released from membrane phospholipids in macrophages, endothelial cells, and platelets (Fig. 2-4).
2. They have short lives (e.g., seconds to minutes).

Histamine: most important chemical mediator of acute inflammation

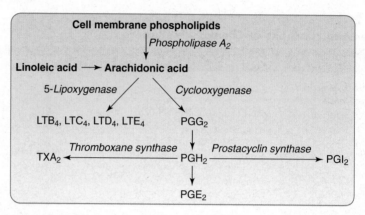

Cell membrane phospholipids

$\downarrow$ *Phospholipase A_2*

Linoleic acid $\longrightarrow$ **Arachidonic acid**

5-Lipoxygenase   *Cyclooxygenase*

LTB_4, LTC_4, LTD_4, LTE_4 PGG_2

Thromboxane synthase $\downarrow$ *Prostacyclin synthase*

$TXA_2 \longleftarrow$ ————— PGH_2 ————— $\longrightarrow PGI_2$

$\downarrow$

PGE_2

2-4: *Arachidonic acid metabolism. Arachidonic acid is released from membrane phospholipids. It is converted into prostaglandins (PGs), thromboxane A_2 (TXA$_2$), and leukotrienes (LTs).*

3. They may have local and systemic effects.
   - Example—histamine may produce local signs of itching or systemic signs of anaphylaxis.
4. They have diverse functions.
   a. Vasodilation
      - Examples—histamine, nitric oxide, PGI_2
   b. Vasoconstriction
      - Example—thromboxane A_2 (TXA_2)
   c. Increase vessel permeability
      - Examples—histamine, bradykinin, LTC_4-D_4-E_4, C3a and C5a (anaphylatoxins)
   d. Produce pain
      - Examples—PGE_2, bradykinin
   e. Produce fever
      - Examples—PGE_2, IL-1, TNF
   f. Chemotactic
      - Examples—C5a, LTB_4, IL-8

F. **Consequences of acute inflammation**
   1. Complete resolution
      a. Occurs with mild injury to cells that have the capacity to enter the cell cycle (e.g., labile and stable cells)
      b. Examples—first-degree burn, bee sting
   2. Tissue destruction and scar formation
      a. Occurs with extensive injury or damage to permanent cells
      b. Example—third-degree burns
   3. Progression to chronic inflammation

G. **Types of acute inflammation**
   - Location, cause, and duration of inflammation determine the morphology of an inflammatory reaction.
   1. Purulent (suppurative) inflammation

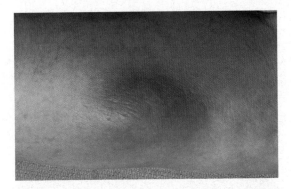

2-5: *Purulent (suppurative) inflammation. The photograph shows a skin abscess (furuncle) due to* Staphylococcus aureus. *Abscesses are pus-filled nodules located in the dermis. (From Lookingbill D, Marks J: Principles of Dermatology, 3rd ed. Philadelphia, WB Saunders, 2000, p 257, Fig. 16-2A.)*

  a. Localized proliferation of pus-forming organisms, such as *Staphylococcus aureus* (e.g., skin abscess; Fig. 2-5)

  b. *S. aureus* contains coagulase, which cleaves fibrinogen into fibrin and traps bacteria and neutrophils.

 2. Fibrinous inflammation

  a. Due to increased vessel permeability, with deposition of a fibrin-rich exudate

  b. Example—fibrinous pericarditis (Fig. 2-6)

 3. Pseudomembranous inflammation

  a. Bacterial toxin-induced damage of the mucosal lining, producing a shaggy membrane composed of necrotic tissue

  b. Example—pseudomembranes associated with *Clostridium difficile* in pseudomembranous colitis (Fig. 2-7)

   • *Corynebacterium diphtheriae* produces a toxin causing pseudomembrane formation in the pharynx and trachea.

H. Role of fever in inflammation

 1. Right-shifts oxygen-binding curve

  • More O_2 is available for the O_2-dependent MPO system.

 2. Provides a hostile environment for bacterial and viral reproduction

II. Chronic Inflammation

 • Inflammation of prolonged duration (weeks to years) that most often results from persistence of an injury-causing agent

A. Causes of chronic inflammation

 1. Infection

  • Examples—tuberculosis, leprosy, hepatitis C

 2. Autoimmune disease

  • Examples—rheumatoid arthritis, systemic lupus erythematosus

 3. Sterile agents

  • Examples—silica, uric acid, silicone in breast implants

B. Morphology

 1. Cell types

S. aureus: most common cause of a skin abscess

Infection: most common cause of chronic inflammation

Monocytes and macrophages: primary leukocytes in chronic inflammation

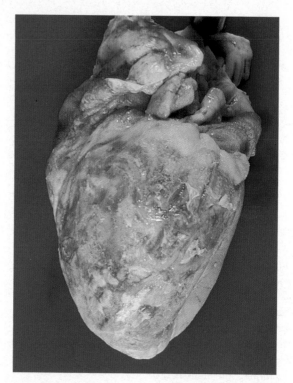

2-6: *Fibrinous inflammation. The epicardial surface of the heart is covered by a shaggy layer of fibrin material. (From Damjanov I: Pathology for the Health-Related Professions, 2nd ed. Philadelphia, WB Saunders, 2000, p 31, Fig. 2-12.)*

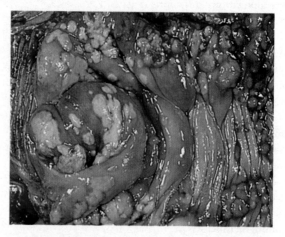

2-7: *Pseudomembranous inflammation. There is necrosis and a yellow-colored exudate covering the mucosal surface of the colon due to a toxin produced by Clostridium difficile. (From Grieg: Color Atlas of Surgical Diagnosis. London, Mosby-Wolfe, 1996, p 202, Fig. 26-10.)*

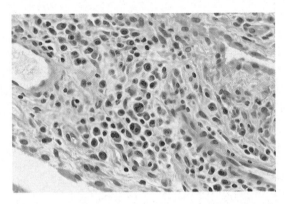

2-8: *Chronic inflammation. This tissue shows an infiltrate of predominantly plasma cells (cells with eccentric nucleus and perinuclear clearing) and lymphocytes. (From Damjanov I, Linder J: Anderson's Pathology, 10th ed. St. Louis, Mosby, 1996, p 390, Fig. 18-7B.)*

- Monocytes and macrophages, lymphocytes and plasma cells, eosinophils (Fig. 2-8)
2. Necrosis
   - *Not* as prominent a feature as in acute inflammation
3. Destruction of parenchyma
   - Loss of functional tissue, with repair by fibrosis
4. Formation of granulation tissue
   a. Highly vascular tissue composed of newly formed blood vessels (i.e., angiogenesis) and activated fibroblasts
      (1) Essential for normal wound healing
      (2) Converted into scar tissue
   b. Fibronectin is required for granulation tissue formation.
      (1) Cell adhesion glycoprotein located in the extracellular matrix (ECM)
         - Binds to collagen, fibrin, and cell surface receptors (e.g., integrins)
      (2) Chemotactic factor that attracts fibroblasts (synthesize collagen) and endothelial cells (form new blood vessels, angiogenesis)
         - Vascular endothelial growth factor (VEGF) and basic fibroblast growth factor (FGF) are important in angiogenesis.
5. Granulomatous inflammation
   - Specialized type of chronic inflammation
   a. Causes
      (1) Infections
         (a) Examples—tuberculosis and systemic fungal infection (e.g., histoplasmosis)
         (b) Usually associated with caseous necrosis (i.e., soft granulomas)
            - Caseation is due to lipid released from the cell wall of dead pathogens.
      (2) Noninfectious causes
         (a) Examples—sarcoidosis and Crohn's disease
         (b) Noncaseating (i.e., hard granulomas)

Granulation tissue: converted to scar tissue

Fibronectin: key adhesion glycoprotein in ECM

Cell types in a granuloma: macrophages and CD4 helper T cells

Epithelioid cells: macrophages activated by γ-interferon from CD4 T_H cells

b. Morphology
  (1) Pale, white nodule with or without central caseation
  (2) Usually well-circumscribed (see Fig. 1-13)
  (3) Cell types
    (a) Epithelioid cells (activated macrophages), mononuclear (round cell) infiltrate (CD4 helper T cells, or T_H cells of the T_H1 type)
    (b) Multinucleated giant cells formed by fusion of epithelioid cells
      • Nuclei usually located at the periphery
  (4) Pathogenesis of a tuberculous granuloma (Box 2-1)

III. Tissue Repair
  #### A. Factors involved in tissue repair
    1. Parenchymal cell regeneration
    2. Repair by connective tissue (fibrosis)
  #### B. Parenchymal cell regeneration
    1. Depends on the ability of cells to replicate
      a. Labile cells (e.g., stem cells in epidermis) and stable cells (e.g., fibroblasts) can replicate (see Chapter 1).
      b. Permanent cells *cannot* replicate.
        • Cardiac and striated muscle are replaced by scar tissue (fibrosis).
    2. Depends on factors that stimulate parenchymal cell division and migration
      • Stimulatory factors include loss of tissue and production of growth factors (Table 2-2).
    3. Cell cycle (Fig. 2-9)
      a. Phases of the cell cycle
        (1) G_0 phase
          • Resting phase of stable parenchymal cells
        (2) G_1 phase
          • Synthesis of RNA, protein, organelles, and cyclin D

G_1 phase: most variable phase in cell cycle

BOX 2-1

SEQUENCE OF FORMATION OF A TUBERCULOUS GRANULOMA

- The tubercle bacillus *Mycobacterium tuberculosis* undergoes phagocytosis by alveolar macrophages (processing of bacterial antigen).
- Macrophages present antigen to CD4 T cells in association with class II antigen sites.
- Macrophages release interleukin (IL) 12 (stimulates formation of T_H1 class cells) and IL-1 (causes fever; activates T_H1 cells).
- T_H1 cells release IL-2 (stimulates T_H1 proliferation), γ-interferon (activates macrophages to kill tubercle bacillus; epithelioid cells), and migration inhibitory factor (causes macrophages to accumulate).
- Lipids from killed tubercle bacillus lead to caseous necrosis.
- Activated macrophages fuse and become multinucleated giant cells.

TABLE 2-2:
Factors Involved in Tissue Repair

Factor	Function(s)
Growth Factors	
Vascular endothelial cell growth factor (VEGF)	Stimulates angiogenesis
Basic fibroblast growth factor (BFGF)	Stimulates angiogenesis
Epidermal growth factor (EGF)	Stimulates keratinocyte migration
	Stimulates granulation tissue formation
Platelet-derived growth factor (PDGF)	Stimulates proliferation of smooth muscle, fibroblasts, endothelial cells
Hormones	
Insulin growth factor-1 (IGF-1)	Stimulates synthesis of collagen
	Promotes keratinocyte migration
Interleukins (IL)	
IL-1	Chemotactic for neutrophils
	Stimulates synthesis of metalloproteinases (i.e., trace metal containing enzymes)
	Stimulates synthesis and release of acute phase reactants from the liver

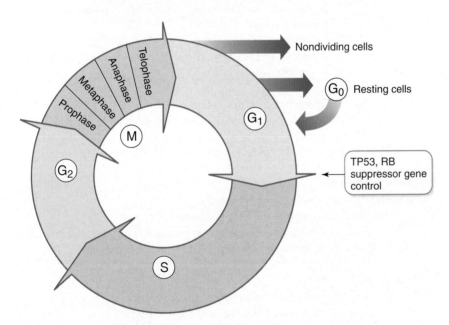

2-9: *Cell cycle. Refer to the description in the text. (From Burns ER, Cave MD: Rapid Review: Histology and Cell Biology. St. Louis, Mosby, 2004, p 36, Fig. 3-5.)*

(3) S (synthesis) phase
  • Synthesis of DNA, RNA, protein
(4) G_2 phase
  • Synthesis of tubulin, which is necessary for formation of the mitotic spindle

(5) M (mitotic) phase
   • Two daughter cells are produced.
b. Regulation of the G_1 checkpoint (G_1 to S phase)

   (1) Most critical phase of the cell cycle
   (2) Control proteins include cyclin-dependent kinase 4 (Cdk4) and cyclin D
      (a) Growth factors activate nuclear transcribing proto-oncogenes to produce cyclin D and Cdk4.
      (b) Cyclin D binds to Cdk4, forming a complex causing the cell to enter the S phase.
   (3) *RB* (retinoblastoma) suppressor gene
      (a) RB protein product arrests the cell in the G_1 phase.
      (b) Cdk4 phosphorylates the RB protein causing the cell to enter the S phase.

   (4) *TP53* suppressor gene
      (a) TP53 protein product arrests the cell in the G_1 phase by inhibiting Cdk4.
         • Prevents RB protein phosphorylation and, if necessary, provides time for repair of DNA in the cell

      (b) In the event that there is excessive DNA damage, the *BAX* gene is activated.
         • *BAX* gene inhibits the *BCL2* antiapoptosis gene (Chapter 1) causing release of cytochrome *c* from the mitochondria and apoptosis of the cell.
4. Restoration to normal
   a. Requires preservation of the basement membrane
   b. Requires a relatively intact extracellular matrix (ECM; i.e., collagen, adhesive proteins)

      • Laminin, the key adhesion protein in the basement membrane, interacts with type IV collagen, cell surface receptors, and components in the ECM.
C. **Repair by connective tissue (fibrosis)**
1. Occurs when injury is severe or persistent
   • Tissue in a third-degree burn *cannot* be restored to normal owing to loss of skin, basement membrane, and connective tissue infrastructure.
2. Steps in repair
   a. Requires neutrophil transmigration to liquefy injured tissue and then macrophage transmigration to remove the debris
   b. Requires formation of granulation tissue

      • Accumulates in the ECM and eventually produces dense fibrotic tissue (scar)
   c. Requires the initial production of type III collagen
      (1) Collagen is the major fibrous component of connective tissue.
      (2) It is a triple helix of cross-linked α-chains.

         • Lysyl oxidase cross-links points of hydroxylation (vitamin C–mediated) on adjacent α-chains.

(3) Cross-linking increases the tensile strength of collagen.
  • Type I collagen in skin, bone, and tendons has the greatest tensile strength.

> Ehlers-Danlos syndrome (EDS) consists of a group of mendelian disorders characterized by defects of type I and type III collagen synthesis and structure. Clinical findings include hypermobile joints, aortic dissection (most common cause of death), bleeding into the skin (ecchymoses), and poor wound healing (Fig. 2-10).

EDS: defects in type I and III collagen

d. Dense scar tissue produced from granulation tissue must be remodeled.
  (1) Remodeling increases the tensile strength of scar tissue.
  (2) Metalloproteinases (collagenases) replace type III collagen with type I collagen, increasing tensile strength to approximately 80% of the original.

Zinc: cofactor in collagenase

3. Primary and secondary intention wound healing (Box 2-2)
  a. Healing by primary intention
    (1) Approximation of wound edges by sutures
    (2) Used for clean surgical wounds
  b. Healing by secondary intention
    (1) Wound remains open
    (2) Used for gaping or infected wounds

D. Factors that impair healing
  1. Persistent infection
    a. Most common cause of impaired wound healing
    b. *Staphylococcus aureus* is the most common pathogen.
  2. Metabolic disorders
    • Example—diabetes mellitus increases susceptibility to infection by decreasing blood flow to tissue and increasing tissue levels of glucose.

Infections: most common cause of impaired wound healing

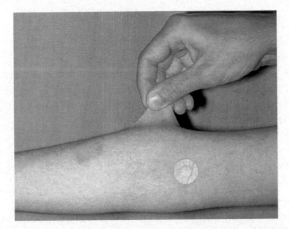

2-10: *Ehlers-Danlos syndrome. The patient shows extreme hyperelasticity of the skin. (From Forbes C, Jackson W: Color Atlas and Text of Clinical Medicine, 2nd ed. St. Louis, Mosby, 2003, p 150, Fig. 3-112.)*

BOX 2-2

WOUND HEALING BY PRIMARY AND SECONDARY INTENTION

Primary Intention

Day 1: fibrin clot (hematoma) develops. Neutrophils infiltrate the wound margins. There is increased mitotic activity of basal cells of squamous epithelium in the apposing wound margins.

Day 2: squamous cells from apposing basal cell layers migrate under the fibrin clot and seal off the wound after 48 hours. Macrophages emigrate into the wound.

Day 3: granulation tissue begins to form. Initial deposition of type III collagen begins but does *not* bridge the incision site. Macrophages replace neutrophils.

Days 4–6: granulation tissue formation peaks, and collagen bridges the incision site.

Week 2: collagen compresses blood vessels in fibrous tissue, resulting in reduced blood flow. Tensile strength is ~10%.

Month 1: collagenase remodeling of the wound occurs, with replacement of type III collagen by type I collagen. Tensile strength increases, reaching ~80% within 3 months. Scar tissue is devoid of adnexal structures (e.g., hair, sweat glands) and inflammatory cells.

Secondary Intention

Typically, these wounds heal differently from primary intention:

More intense inflammatory reaction than primary healing
Increased amount of granulation tissue formation than in primary healing
Wound contraction caused by increased numbers of myofibroblasts

---

3. Nutritional deficiencies
   a. Decreased protein (e.g., malnutrition)
   b. Vitamin C deficiency
      - Decreased hydroxylation of proline and lysine causes decreased tensile strength in collagen owing to loss of linkage sites between tropocollagen molecules (triple helix of α chains)
   c. Trace metal deficiency
      (1) Copper deficiency leads to decreased cross-linking of α-chains in collagen.
      (2) Zinc deficiency leads to defects in removal of type III collagen in wound remodeling.
4. Glucocorticoids
   a. Interfere with collagen formation and decrease tensile strength
   b. Occasionally used along with antibiotics to prevent scar formation (e.g., bacterial meningitis)

Vitamin C deficiency: decreased cross-linking of collagen

Glucocorticoids: prevent scar formation

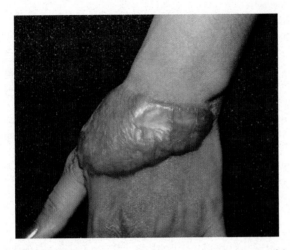

2-11: *Keloid formation. The patient shows a raised, thickened scar over the dorsum of the hand. (From Lookingbill D, Marks J: Principles of Dermatology, 3rd ed. Philadelphia, WB Saunders, 2000, p 115, Fig. 8-5A.)*

Keloids, the raised scars caused by excessive synthesis of type III collagen, are common in African Americans and may occur as the result of third-degree burns. Microscopically, keloids appear as irregular, thick collagen bundles that extend beyond the confines of the original injury (Fig. 2-11).

Keloids: excess type III collagen

E. Repair in other tissues
1. Liver
   a. Mild injury (e.g., hepatitis A)
      (1) Regeneration of hepatocytes
      (2) Restoration to normal is possible if cytoarchitecture is intact.
   b. Severe or persistent injury (e.g., hepatitis C)
      (1) Regenerative nodules develop that lack sinusoids and portal triads.
      (2) Increased fibrosis occurs around regenerative nodules.
         • Potential for cirrhosis

Severe injury liver: regenerative nodules and fibrosis

2. Lung
   a. Type II pneumocytes are the key repair cells of the lung.
   b. They replace damaged type I and type II pneumocytes.

Lung injury: type II pneumocyte is repair cell

3. Brain
   a. Astrocytes proliferate in response to an injury (e.g., brain infarction).
      • This is called gliosis.
   b. Microglial cells (macrophages) are scavenger cells that remove debris (e.g., myelin).

Brain injury: proliferation of astrocytes and microglial cells

4. Peripheral nerve transection
   a. Distal degeneration of the axon (called wallerian degeneration) and myelin sheath
   b. Proximal axonal degeneration up to the next node of Ranvier
   c. Macrophages and Schwann cells phagocytose axonal/myelin debris.

d. Muscle undergoes atrophy in ~15 days.

e. Nerve cell body undergoes central chromatolysis.
   (1) Nerve cell body swells.
   (2) Nissl bodies (composed of rough endoplasmic reticulum and free ribosomes) disappear centrally.
   (3) Nucleus is peripheralized.

Peripheral nerve transection: Schwann cell key cell in reinnervation

f. Schwann cells proliferate in the distal stump.

g. Axonal sprouts develop in the proximal stump and extend distally using Schwann cells for guidance.

h. Regenerated axon grows 2 to 3 mm/day.

i. Axon becomes remyelinated.

j. Muscle is eventually reinnervated.

5. Heart
   a. Cardiac muscle is permanent tissue.
   b. Damaged muscle is replaced by noncontractile scar tissue.

IV. Laboratory Findings Associated with Inflammation
A. Leukocytes
1. Acute inflammation (e.g., bacterial infection) (Fig. 2-12)
   a. Absolute neutrophilic leukocytosis

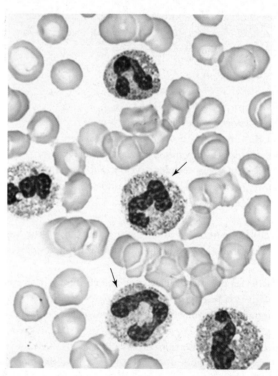

2-12: Absolute leukocytosis with left shift. Arrows point to band (stab) neutrophils, which exhibit prominence of the azurophilic granules (toxic granulation). Vacuoles in the cytoplasm represent phagolysosomes. (From Hoffbrand AV: Color Atlas: Clinical Hematology, 3rd ed. St. Louis, Mosby, 2000, p 115, Fig. 7-11A.)

       (1) Accelerated release of neutrophils from the bone marrow

       (2) Mediated by IL-1 and TNF

    b. Left shift

       • Defined as greater than 10% band (stab) neutrophils or the presence of earlier precursors (e.g., metamyelocytes)

    c. Toxic granulation

       • Prominence of azurophilic granules (primary lysosomes) in neutrophils

    d. Increase in serum IgM

       (1) Peaks in 7 to 10 days

       (2) Isotype switching (μ heavy chain replaced by γ heavy chain) in plasma cells to produce IgG peaks in 12 to 14 days.

> IgM: predominant immunoglobulin in acute inflammation

  2. Chronic inflammation (e.g., tuberculosis)

    a. Absolute monocytosis

    b. Increase in serum IgG

  3. Table 2-3 summarizes cells involved in inflammation.

  4. Peripheral blood effects of corticosteroid therapy

    a. Absolute neutrophilic leukocytosis

> IgG: predominant immunoglobulin in chronic inflammation

       • Inhibits activation of neutrophil adhesion molecules

    b. Lymphopenia

       (1) Sequesters B and T lymphocytes in lymph nodes

       (2) Signal for apoptosis of lymphocytes

    c. Eosinopenia

       • Sequesters eosinophils in lymph nodes

> Corticosteroid effect in blood: ↑ neutrophils; ↓ lymphocytes and eosinophils

B. Erythrocyte sedimentation rate (ESR)

  • ESR is the rate (mm/hour) of settling of RBCs in a vertical tube.

  1. ESR is increased in acute and chronic inflammation (e.g., rheumatoid arthritis).

  2. Plasma factor or RBC factors that promote rouleaux formation increase the ESR.

    a. Increase in fibrinogen (acute-phase reactant) in plasma decreases negative charge in RBCs, promoting rouleaux formation.

    b. Anemia promotes rouleaux formation.

       • Abnormally shaped RBCs (e.g., sickle cells) do *not* produce rouleaux.

> ↑ ESR: ↑ fibrinogen, anemia

C. C-reactive protein (CRP)

  1. Acute-phase reactant

  2. Clinical usefulness

    a. Sensitive indicator of necrosis associated with acute inflammation

       • CRP is increased in inflammatory (disrupted) atherosclerotic plaques and bacterial infections.

    b. Excellent monitor of disease activity (e.g., rheumatoid arthritis)

> CRP: marker of necrosis and disease activity

D. Serum protein electrophoresis in inflammation (Fig. 2-13)

TABLE 2-3:
Cells in Inflammation

Cell	Characteristics
Neutrophil	Key cell in acute inflammation Receptors for IgG and C3b: important in phagocytosis of opsonized bacteria Bone marrow neutrophil pools 　Mitotic pool: myeloblasts, promyelocytes, myelocytes 　Postmitotic pool: metamyelocytes, band neutrophils (stabs), segmented neutrophils Peripheral blood neutrophil pools 　Marginating pool: adherent to the endothelium (account for ~50% of peripheral blood pool) 　Circulating pool: measured in complete blood cell count (CBC) Causes neutrophilic leukocytosis 　Infections (e.g., acute appendicitis) 　Sterile inflammation with necrosis (e.g., acute myocardial infarction) 　Drugs inhibiting neutrophil adhesion molecules: corticosteroids, catecholamines, lithium
Monocytes and macrophages	Key cells in chronic inflammation Receptors for IgG and C3b Monocytes become macrophages: fixed (e.g., macrophages in red pulp), wandering (e.g., alveolar macrophages) Functions: phagocytosis, process antigen, enhance host immunologic response (secrete cytokines like IL-1, TNF) Causes of monocytosis: chronic inflammation, autoimmune disease, malignancy
B cells and T cells	Peripheral blood lymphocyte count: T cells 60–70%, B cells 10–20% of the total B cell function: become plasma cells when antigenically stimulated T cell functions: cellular immunity (type IV HSR), cytokines regulate B cells, defense against intracellular pathogens (e.g., tuberculosis) Causes of B/T lymphocytosis: viral infections
Plasma cells	Antibody-producing cells derived from B cells Morphology: well-developed rough endoplasmic reticulum (site of protein synthesis); bright blue cytoplasm under Wright-Giemsa stain; nucleus eccentrically located and has perinuclear clearing
Mast cells and basophils	Release mediators in acute inflammation and allergic reactions (type I HSR) Receptors for IgE Early release reaction: release of preformed mediators (i.e., histamine, chemotactic factors, proteases) Late phase reaction: new synthesis and release of PGs and LTs, which enhance and prolong the acute inflammatory process
Eosinophils	Receptors for IgE Red granules contain crystalline material; become Charcot-Leyden crystals in the sputum of asthmatics Preformed chemical mediators in granules 　Major basic protein (MBP) kills invasive helminths 　Histaminase neutralizes histamine 　Arylsulfatase neutralizes leukotrienes Functions 　Modulate type I HSR by neutralizing histamine and leukotrienes 　Destruction of invasive helminths: IgE receptors interact with IgE coating the surface of invasive helminths→ antibody-dependent cytotoxicity reaction (type II HSR) causes the release of MBP→ kills helminth Causes of eosinophilia 　Type I HSR reactions: allergic rhinitis, bronchial asthma 　Invasive helminthic infections *excluding* pinworms and adult worms in ascariasis, which are *not* invasive

HSR, hypersensitivity reaction; IL, interleukin; PG, prostaglandin; LT, leukotriene; TNF, tumor necrosis factor.

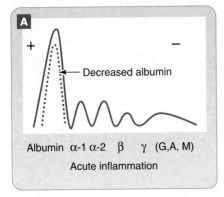 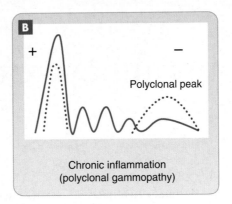

2-13: *Serum protein electrophoresis in acute inflammation (**A**) and chronic inflammation (**B**). Refer to the text for discussion.*

Clinical correlation: Proteins in serum are separated into individual fractions by serum protein electrophoresis (SPE). Charged proteins placed in a buffered electrolyte solution will migrate toward one or the other electrode when a current is run through the solution. Proteins with the most negative charges (e.g., albumin) migrate to the positive pole, or anode, and those with the most positive charges (e.g., γ-globulins) remain at the negatively charged pole, or cathode. Beginning at the anode, proteins separate into five major peaks on cellulose acetate—albumin, followed by α_1-, α_2-, β-, and γ-globulins. The γ-globulins in decreasing order of concentration are IgG, IgA, and IgM (IgD and IgE are in very low concentration).

1. Acute inflammation (see Fig. 2-13A)
   a. Slight decrease in serum albumin
      (1) Catabolic effect of inflammation
      (2) Amino acids are used by the liver to synthesize acute phase reactants.
   b. Normal γ-globulin peak
      • Serum IgM is increased in acute inflammation; however, it does *not* alter the configuration of the γ-globulin peak.
2. Chronic inflammation (see Fig. 2-13B)
   a. Greater decrease in serum albumin than in acute inflammation
   b. Increase in γ-globulins due to increase in IgG
      • Diffuse increase in the γ-globulin peak is due to many clones of benign plasma cells producing IgG (i.e., polyclonal gammopathy).

IgM: marker of acute inflammation

Polyclonal gammopathy: sign of chronic inflammation; ↑ IgG

Immunopathology

I. **Cells of the Immune System (Table 3-1)**
   A. **Innate (natural, nonspecific) immunity**
      1. Antigen-independent cells providing first defense against pathogens
      2. Types of cells
         a. Phagocytic cells (e.g., neutrophils, macrophages)
         b. Natural killer cells
   B. **Acquired (specific) immunity**
      1. Antigen-dependent activation and expansion of lymphocytes
      2. B lymphocytes produce antibodies (i.e., humoral immune response).
         a. IgM synthesis begins at birth.
            • Presence of IgM at birth may indicate congenital infection (e.g., cytomegalovirus).
         b. IgG synthesis begins at 2 months.
            • Presence of IgG at birth is maternally derived IgG.
      3. T cells are involved in cell-mediated immune responses.

II. **Major Histocompatibility Complex (MHC)**
   A. **Location**
      • Short arm of chromosome 6
   B. **Human leukocyte antigen (HLA) genes**
      • Code for HLA proteins that are unique to each individual
   C. **Class I MHC molecules**
      1. Coded by HLA-A, -B, and -C genes
      2. Present on the membranes of all nucleated cells
         • *Not* present on mature RBCs; present on platelets
      3. Recognized by CD8 T cells and natural killer cells
   D. **Class II MHC molecules**
      1. Coded by HLA-DP, -DQ, and -DR genes
      2. Present on antigen-presenting cells (APCs)
         • B cells, macrophages, dendritic cells
      3. Recognized by CD4 T cells
   E. **HLA association with disease**
      1. HLA-B27 with ankylosing spondylitis
      2. HLA-DR2 with multiple sclerosis
      3. HLA-DR3 and -DR4 with type 1 diabetes mellitus

Natural killer cells: large granular lymphocytes in peripheral blood

IgM and IgG synthesis: begin after birth

Class I MHC: present on nucleated cells

APCs: B cells, macrophages, dendritic cells

HLA-B27: ankylosing spondylitis

TABLE 3-1:
Types of Immune
Cells

Cell Type	Derivation	Location	Function

T cells
  CD4 (helper)
  CD8 (cytotoxic/
  suppressor)
	Bone marrow lymphocyte stem cells mature in thymus	Peripheral blood and bone marrow, thymus, paracortex of lymph nodes, Peyer's patches	CD4 cells: secrete cytokines (IL-2 → proliferation of CD4/CD8 T cells; γ-interferon → activation of macrophages); help B cells become antibody-producing plasma cells
			CD8 cells: kill virus-infected, neoplastic, and donor graft cells

B cells	Bone marrow stem cells	Peripheral blood and bone marrow, germinal follicles in lymph nodes, Peyer's patches	Differentiate into plasma cells that produce immunoglobulins to kill encapsulated bacteria (e.g., *Streptococcus pneumoniae*) Act as APCs that interact with CD4 cells
Natural killer cells	Bone marrow stem cells	Peripheral blood (large granular lymphocytes)	Kill virus-infected and neoplastic cells
Macrophages	Conversion of monocytes into macrophages in connective tissue	Connective tissue; organs (e.g., alveolar macrophages, lymph node sinuses)	Involved in phagocytosis and cytokine production Act as APCs
Dendritic cells	Bone marrow stem cells	Skin (Langerhans' cells), germinal follicles	Act as APCs

APC, antigen-presenting cell; IL, interleukin.

F. **HLA testing**
  1. Transplantation workup
     - Close matches of HLA-A, -B, and -D loci in both the donor and graft recipient increase the chance of graft survival.
  2. Determining disease risk
     - Example—HLA-B27–positive individuals have an increased risk of ankylosing spondylitis.

TABLE 3-2:
Hypersensitivity
Reactions

Reaction	Pathogenesis	Examples
Type I	IgE-dependent activation of mast cells	Atopic disorders: hay fever, eczema, hives, asthma, reaction to bee sting Drug hypersensitivity: penicillin rash or anaphylaxis

Type II	Antibody-dependent reaction	Complement-dependent reactions
		  Lysis: ABO mismatch, Goodpasture's syndrome, hyperacute transplantation rejection
		  Phagocytosis: warm (IgG) autoimmune hemolytic anemia, ABO and Rh hemolytic disease of newborn
		Complement-independent reactions
		  Antibody (IgG, IgE)-dependent cell-mediated cytotoxicity: natural killer cell destruction of neoplastic and virus-infected cells; helminth destruction by eosinophils
		  Antibodies directed against cell surface receptors: myasthenia gravis, Graves' disease

Type III	Deposition of antigen-antibody complexes	Systemic lupus erythematosus (DNA-anti-DNA) Rheumatoid arthritis (IgM-Fc receptor IgG) Serum sickness (horse antithymocyte globulin-antibody)
Type IV	Antibody-independent T cell–mediated reactions	Delayed type: contact dermatitis (e.g., poison ivy), tuberculous granuloma Cell-mediated cytotoxicity: killing of tumor cells and virus-infected cells

III. **Hypersensitivity Reactions (Table 3-2)**

A. **Type I (immediate) hypersensitivity**

- IgE antibody–mediated activation of mast cells (effector cells) produces an inflammatory reaction.

1. IgE antibody production (sensitization)

  a. Allergens (e.g., pollen, drugs) are first processed by APCs (macrophages or dendritic cells).

  b. APCs interact with CD4 T_H2 cells, causing interleukins (ILs) to stimulate B-cell maturation.

  c. IL-4 causes plasma cells to switch from IgM to IgE synthesis.

  d. IL-5 stimulates the production and activation of eosinophils.

2. Mast cell activation (reexposure)

  a. Allergen-specific IgE antibodies are bound to mast cells.

  b. Allergens cross-link IgE antibodies specific for the allergen on mast cell membranes.

  c. IgE triggering causes mast cell release of preformed mediators.

    (1) Early phase reaction with release of histamine, chemotactic factors for eosinophils, proteases

    (2) Produces tissue swelling and bronchoconstriction

  d. Late-phase reaction

    (1) Mast cells synthesize and release prostaglandins and leukotrienes.

    (2) Enhances and prolongs acute inflammatory reaction

Type I hypersensitivity: IgE activation of mast cells

Mast cells: early and late phase reactions

Desensitization therapy involves repeated injections of increasingly greater amounts of allergen, resulting in production of IgG antibodies that attach to allergens and prevent them from binding to mast cells.

3. Tests used to evaluate type I hypersensitivity
   a. Scratch test (best overall sensitivity)
      • Positive response is a histamine-mediated wheal-and-flare reaction after introduction of an allergen into the skin.
   b. Radioimmunosorbent test
      • Detects specific IgE antibodies in serum that are against specific allergens

Anaphylactic shock: potentially fatal type I hypersensitivity reaction

4. Clinical examples of type I hypersensitivity (see Table 3-2)

B. Type II (cytotoxic) hypersensitivity
   • Antibody-dependent cytotoxic reactions
   1. Complement-dependent reactions
      a. Lysis
         • Antibody (IgG or IgM) directed against antigen on the cell membrane activates the complement system, leading to lysis by the membrane attack complex.
      b. Phagocytosis
         • Fixed macrophages (e.g., in spleen) phagocytose hematopoietic cells (e.g., RBCs) coated by IgG antibodies and/or complement (C3b).
   2. Complement-independent reactions
      a. Antibody (IgG, IgE)-dependent cell-mediated cytotoxicity
         • Leukocytes with receptors for IgG or IgE lyse but do *not* phagocytose cells coated by antibodies.
      b. IgG autoantibodies directed against cell surface receptors
   3. Tests used to evaluate type II hypersensitivity
      a. Direct Coombs' test detects IgG and/or C3b attached to RBCs.
      b. Indirect Coombs' test detects antibodies in serum (e.g., anti-D).
   4. Clinical examples of type II hypersensitivity (see Table 3-2)

Type II hypersensitivity: antibody-dependent cytotoxic reactions

C. Type III (immunocomplex) hypersensitivity
   • Activation of the complement system by circulating antigen-antibody complexes (e.g., DNA-anti-DNA complexes)
   1. First exposure to antigen
      • Synthesis of antibodies
   2. Second exposure to antigen
      a. Deposition of antigen-antibody complexes
      b. Complement activation, producing C5a, which attracts neutrophils that damage tissue
   3. Arthus reaction
      a. Localized immunocomplex reaction
      b. Example—farmer's lung from exposure to thermophilic actinomycetes, or antigens, in air
   4. Test used to evaluate type III hypersensitivity
      a. Immunofluorescent staining of tissue biopsies
      b. Example—glomeruli in glomerulonephritis

Type III hypersensitivity: activation of complement by circulating antigen-antibody complexes

Antibody-mediated hypersensitivity reactions: type I, II, and III

5. Clinical examples of type III hypersensitivity (see Table 3-2)

D. Type IV hypersensitivity

- Antibody-independent T cell–mediated reactions (cellular immunity)
  1. Delayed reaction hypersensitivity
     - CD4 cells interact with macrophages (APCs with MHC class II antigens), resulting in cytokine injury to tissue.
  2. Cell-mediated cytotoxicity
     - CD8 T cells interact with altered MHC class I antigens on neoplastic, virus-infected, or donor graft cells, causing cell lysis.
  3. Test used to evaluate type IV hypersensitivity
     a. Patch test to confirm contact dermatitis
        - Example—suspected allergen (e.g., nickel) placed on an adhesive patch is applied to the skin to see if a skin reaction occurs.
     b. Skin reaction to *Candida*
  4. Clinical examples of type IV hypersensitivity (see Table 3-2)

IV. Transplantation Immunology

A. Factors enhancing graft viability

  1. ABO blood group compatibility between recipients and donors
  2. Absence of preformed anti-HLA cytotoxic antibodies in recipients
     - People must have previous exposure to blood products to develop anti-HLA cytotoxic antibodies.
  3. Close matches of HLA-A, -B, and -D loci between recipients and donors

B. Types of grafts

  1. Autograft (i.e., self to self)
     - Associated with the best survival rate
  2. Syngeneic graft (isograft)
     - Between identical twins
  3. Allograft
     - Between genetically different individuals of the same species

> The fetus is an allograft that is *not* rejected by the mother. Trophoblastic tissue may prevent maternal T cells from entering fetus.

  4. Xenograft
     a. Between two species
     b. Example—transplant of heart valve from pig to human

C. Types of rejection

- Transplantation rejection involves a humoral or cell-mediated host response against MHC antigens in the donor graft.
  1. Hyperacute rejection
     a. Irreversible reaction occurs within minutes.
     b. Pathogenesis
        (1) ABO incompatibility or action of preformed anti-HLA antibodies in the recipient directed against donor antigens in vascular endothelium
        (2) Type II hypersensitivity reaction

c. Pathologic finding
   - Vessel thrombosis
d. Example—blood group A person receives a blood group B heart.
2. Acute rejection
   a. Most common transplant rejection
   b. Reversible reaction that occurs within days to weeks
      (1) Type IV cell-mediated hypersensitivity
          (a) CD4 T cells release cytokines, resulting in activation of host macrophages, proliferation of CD8 T cells, and destruction of donor graft cells.
          (b) Extensive interstitial round cell lymphocytic infiltrate in the graft, edema, and endothelial cell injury
      (2) Antibody-mediated type II hypersensitivity reaction
          (a) Cytokines from CD4 T cells promote B-cell differentiation into plasma cells, producing anti-HLA antibodies that attack vessels in the donor graft.
          (b) Vasculitis with intravascular thrombosis in recent grafts
          (c) Intimal thickening with obliteration of vessel lumens in older grafts

> Acute rejection is potentially reversible with immunosuppressive agents, such as cyclosporine (blocks CD4 T-cell release of IL-2), OKT3 (monoclonal antibody against T-cell antigen recognition site), and corticosteroids (lymphotoxic). Immunosuppressive therapy is associated with an increased risk of cervical squamous cell cancer, malignant lymphoma, and squamous cell carcinoma of the skin (most common).

Acute rejection: most common type; type IV and type II hypersensitivity

3. Chronic rejection
   a. Irreversible reaction that occurs over months to years
   b. Pathogenesis
      (1) Not well characterized
      (2) Involves continued vascular injury with ischemia to tissue
   c. Blood vessel damage with intimal thickening and fibrosis

Chronic rejection: irreversible

D. Graft-versus-host (GVH) reaction
1. Causes
   a. Potential complication in bone marrow and liver transplants
   b. Potential complication in blood transfusions given to patients with a T-cell immunodeficiency and newborns.
2. Pathogenesis
   - Donor T cells recognize host tissue as foreign and activate host CD4 and CD8 T cells.
3. Clinical findings
   a. Bile duct necrosis (jaundice)
   b. Gastrointestinal mucosa ulceration (bloody diarrhea)
   c. Dermatitis

GVH reaction: jaundice, diarrhea, dermatitis

E. Types of transplants (Table 3-3)

TABLE 3-3:
Some Types of
Transplants

Type of Transplant	Comments
Cornea	Best allograft survival rate Danger of transmission of Creutzfeldt-Jakob disease
Kidney	Better survival with kidney from living donor than from cadaver
Bone marrow	Graft contains pluripotential cells that repopulate host stem cells Host assumes donor ABO group Danger of graft-versus-host reaction and cytomegalovirus infection

TABLE 3-4:
Autoantibodies in
Autoimmune
Disease

Autoantibodies	Disease	Test Sensitivity (%)
Antiacetylcholine receptor	Myasthenia gravis	90
Anti–basement membrane	Goodpasture syndrome	>90
Anticentromere	CREST syndrome	90
Antiendomysial and antigliadin	Celiac disease	95
Anti-insulin	Type 1 diabetes	50
Anti–islet cell		75
Anti–intrinsic factor	Pernicious anemia	60
Anti–parietal cell		90
Antimicrosomal	Hashimoto's thyroiditis	97
Antithyroglobulin		85
Antimitochondrial	Primary biliary cirrhosis	90–100
Antimyeloperoxidase	Microscopic polyangiitis	80 (p-ANCA)
Antiproteinase 3	Wegener's granulomatosis	>90 (c-ANCA)
Antiribonucleoprotein	Mixed connective tissue disease	100
Anti–thyroid-stimulating hormone receptor	Graves' disease	85

c-ANCA, cytoplasmic antineutrophil cytoplasmic antibody; p-ANCA, perinuclear antineutrophilic cytoplasmic antibody.

V. Autoimmune Diseases
- Autoimmune dysfunction is associated with a loss of self-tolerance, resulting in immune reactions directed against host tissue.
  A. Mechanisms of autoimmunity
  1. Release of normally sequestered antigens (e.g., sperm)
  2. Sharing of antigens between host and pathogen
  3. Defects in functions of helper or suppressor T cells
  4. Persistence of autoreactive T and B cells
  5. Presence of specific autoantibodies (Table 3-4)
  B. Systemic lupus erythematosus (SLE)
  - Connective tissue disease that mainly affects the blood, joints, skin, and kidneys
  1. Occurs predominantly in women of childbearing age
  2. Pathogenesis
     - Polyclonal B-cell activation, sustained estrogen activity, environmental triggers (e.g., sun, procainamide)

3. Clinical findings
   a. Hematologic
      • Autoimmune hemolytic anemia, thrombocytopenia, leukopenia
   b. Lymphatic
      (1) Generalized painful lymphadenopathy
      (2) Splenomegaly
   c. Musculoskeletal
      • Small-joint inflammation (e.g., hands) with absence of joint deformity
   d. Skin
      (1) Immunocomplex deposition along basement membrane
         • Produces liquefactive degeneration
      (2) Malar butterfly rash (Fig. 3-1)
   e. Renal
      • Diffuse proliferative glomerulonephritis (most common glomerulonephritis)

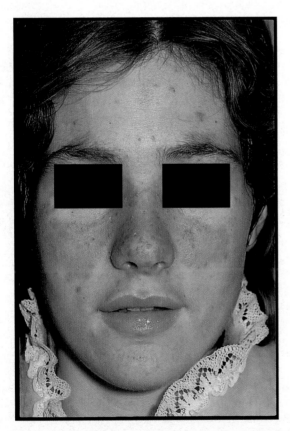

3-1: Malar rash in systemic lupus erythematosus showing the butterfly-wing distribution. (From Forbes C, Jackson W: Color Atlas and Text of Clinical Medicine, 2nd ed. St. Louis, Mosby, 2003, Fig. 3-77.)

Most common cardiac finding in SLE: fibrinous pericarditis with effusion

Procainamide: most common drug associated with drug-induced lupus

Drug-induced lupus: antihistone antibodies

Confirm SLE: anti-double-stranded DNA and anti-Sm antibodies

    f. Cardiovascular
      (1) Fibrinous pericarditis with or without effusion
      (2) Libman-Sacks endocarditis (sterile vegetations on mitral valve)
    g. Respiratory
      (1) Interstitial fibrosis of lungs
      (2) Pleural effusion with friction rub
    h. Pregnancy-related
      (1) Complete heart block in newborns
        • Caused by IgG anti-SS-A (Ro) antibodies crossing the placenta
      (2) Recurrent spontaneous abortions
        • Caused by antiphospholipid antibodies

4. Drug-induced lupus erythematosus
    a. Associated drugs
      • Procainamide, hydralazine
    b. Features that distinguish drug-induced lupus from SLE
      (1) Antihistone antibodies
      (2) Low incidence of renal and central nervous system (CNS) involvement
      (3) Disappearance of symptoms when the drug is discontinued

5. Laboratory findings in SLE
    a. Positive serum antinuclear antibody (ANA) (almost all cases)
      (1) Anti-double-stranded DNA antibodies and anti-Sm antibodies
        • Used to confirm the diagnosis of SLE, because they are highly specific for the disease (i.e., few false-positive results)
      (2) Anti-Ro antibodies are positive in 25% to 50% of cases.
    b. Antiphospholipid antibodies
      (1) Lupus anticoagulant and anticardiolipin antibodies
      (2) Damage vessel endothelium, producing vessel thrombosis
      (3) Increased incidence of strokes and recurrent spontaneous abortions

> Anticardiolipin antibodies may produce a false-positive syphilis serologic test by cross-reacting with cardiolipin in the rapid plasma reagin (RPR) and Venereal Disease Research Laboratory (VDRL) tests.

    c. Lupus erythematosus cell
      (1) Neutrophil containing phagocytosed altered DNA
      (2) *Not* specific for SLE
    d. Decreased serum complement
      • Used up with activation of complement system
    e. Immunocomplexes at the dermal-epidermal junction in skin biopsies
      • Immunofluorescent studies identify complexes in a band-like distribution along the dermal-epidermal junction.

C. Systemic sclerosis (scleroderma)
    • Excessive production of collagen that primarily targets the skin (scleroderma), gastrointestinal tract, lungs, and kidneys
1. Occurs predominantly in women of childbearing age
2. Pathogenesis

a. Small-vessel endothelial cell damage produces blood vessel fibrosis and ischemic injury.

b. T-cell release of cytokines results in excessive collagen synthesis.

3. Clinical findings

a. Raynaud's phenomenon

(1) Sequential color changes (normal to blue to red) caused by digital vessel vasculitis and fibrosis

(2) Digital infarcts

b. Skin

(1) Skin atrophy and tissue swelling beginning in the fingers and extending proximally

(2) Parchment-like appearance

(3) Extensive dystrophic calcification in subcutaneous tissue

(4) Tightened facial features (e.g., radial furrowing around the lips) (Fig. 3-2)

c. Gastrointestinal

(1) Dysphagia for solids and liquids

(a) No peristalsis in the lower two thirds of the esophagus (smooth muscle replaced by collagen)

(b) Lower esophageal sphincter relaxation with reflux

(2) Small bowel

(a) Loss of villi (malabsorption)

(b) Wide-mouthed diverticula (bacterial overgrowth)

Systemic sclerosis: excess collagen deposition

Raynaud's phenomenon: most common initial sign of systemic sclerosis

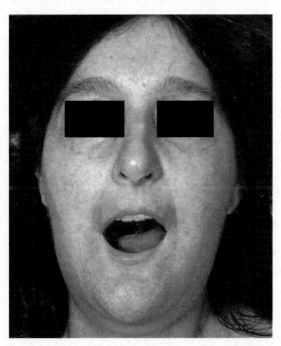

3-2: *Systemic sclerosis. The tightening of the skin around the mouth is caused by excess collagen. (From Forbes C, Jackson W: Color Atlas and Text of Clinical Medicine, 2nd ed. St. Louis, Mosby, 2003, Fig. 3-81.)*

Systemic sclerosis: anti-topoisomerase antibodies

CREST syndrome = calcinosis, *Raynaud's* phenomenon, esophageal dysfunction, sclerodactyly, telangiectasia

    d. Respiratory
       (1) Interstitial fibrosis of lungs
       (2) Respiratory failure (most common cause of death)
    e. Renal
       (1) Vasculitis involving arterioles (i.e., hyperplastic arteriolosclerosis) and glomeruli
       (2) Infarctions, malignant hypertension
  4. Laboratory findings in systemic sclerosis
    a. Serum ANA is positive in 70% to 90% of cases.
    b. Antitopoisomerase antibody is positive in 15% to 40% of cases.
  5. CREST syndrome
     • Limited sclerosis
    a. Clinical findings
       (1) C—calcification, centromere antibody
       (2) R—Raynaud's phenomenon
       (3) E—Esophageal dysmotility
       (4) S—sclerodactyly (i.e., tapered, claw-like fingers)
       (5) T—telangiectasis (i.e., multiple punctate blood vessel dilations)
    b. Laboratory findings
       • Anticentromere antibodies in ~90% of cases

D. Dermatomyositis (DM; with skin involvement) and polymyositis (PM; no skin involvement)
  1. Occurs predominantly in women 40 to 60 years of age
  2. Associated with risk of malignant neoplasms (15–20% of cases), particularly lung cancer
  3. Pathogenesis
    a. DM is associated with antibody-mediated damage.
    b. PM is associated with T cell–mediated damage.
  4. Clinical findings
    a. Muscle pain and atrophy
       • Shoulders are commonly involved.
    b. Heliotrope eyelids or "raccoon eyes" (purple-red eyelid discoloration)
  5. Laboratory findings
    a. Serum ANA is positive in fewer than 30% of cases.
    b. Increased serum creatine kinase
    c. Muscle biopsy shows a lymphocytic infiltrate.

DM/PM: ↑ serum creatine kinase

MCTD: antiribonucleoprotein antibodies

E. Mixed connective tissue disease (MCTD)
  1. Signs and symptoms similar to SLE, systemic sclerosis, and PM
  2. Renal disease is uncommon.
  3. Antiribonucleoprotein antibodies are positive in almost 100% of cases.

VI. Immunodeficiency Disorders
  • Defects in B cells, T cells, complement, or phagocytic cells
  A. Risk factors for immune disorders
    1. Prematurity
    2. Autoimmune diseases (e.g., systemic lupus erythematosus)

3. Lymphoproliferative disorders (e.g., malignant lymphoma)
4. Infections (e.g., human immunodeficiency virus [HIV])
5. Immunosuppressive drugs (e.g., corticosteroids)

B. **Congenital immunodeficiency disorders (Table 3-5)**
   1. B-cell disorders
      • Recurrent encapsulated bacterial infections (e.g., *Streptococcus pneumoniae*)
   2. T-cell disorders
      • Recurrent infections caused by intracellular pathogens (fungi, viruses, protozoa)
   3. Combined B- and T-cell disorders

C. **Acquired immunodeficiency syndrome (AIDS)**
   1. Modes of transmission
      a. Sexual transmission (>75% of cases)
         (1) Homosexual transmission (anal intercourse between men) is the most common cause in the United States.
         (2) Heterosexual transmission is the most common cause in developing countries.
         (3) Virus enters blood vessels or dendritic cells in areas of mucosal injury.
      b. Intravenous drug abuse
         • Rate of HIV infection is markedly increasing in female sex partners of male intravenous drug abusers.
      c. Other modes of transmission
         (1) Vertical transmission
            (a) Transplacental route, blood contamination during delivery, breast-feeding
            (b) Most pediatric cases of AIDS is due to transmission of virus from mother to child.
         (2) Accidental needlestick
            (a) Risk per accident is 0.3%.
            (b) Most common mode of infection in health care workers
         (3) Blood products
            • Risk per unit of blood is 1 per 2 million units of blood transfused.
      d. Body fluids containing HIV
         (1) Blood, semen, breast milk
         (2) Virus *cannot* enter intact skin or mucosa.
   2. Etiology
      a. RNA retrovirus
      b. HIV-1 is the most common cause in the United States.
      c. HIV-2 is the most common cause in developing countries.
   3. Pathogenesis
      a. HIV envelope protein (gp120) attaches to the CD4 molecule of T cells.
      b. HIV infects CD4 T cells, causing direct cytotoxicity.
      c. Infection of non–T cells

IgA deficiency: most common congenital immunodeficiency

AIDS: most common acquired immunodeficiency disease worldwide

AIDS: most common cause of death due to infection worldwide

Pediatric AIDS: most due to vertical transmission

TABLE 3-5:
Congenital
Immunodeficiency
Disorders

Disease	Defect(s)	Clinical Features
B-Cell Disorders		
Bruton's agammaglobulinemia	Failure of pre-B cells to become mature B cells Mutated tyrosine kinase X-linked recessive disorder	Sinopulmonary infections Maternal antibodies protective from birth to age 6 months ↓ Immunoglobulins
IgA deficiency	Failure of IgA B cells to mature into plasma cells	Sinopulmonary infections, giardiasis Anaphylaxis if exposed to blood products that contain IgA ↓ IgA and secretory IgA
Common variable immunodeficiency	Defect in B-cell maturation to plasma cells Adult immunodeficiency disorder	Sinopulmonary infections, GI infections (e.g., *Giardia*), pneumonia, autoimmune disease ↓ Immunoglobulins
T-Cell Disorder		
DiGeorge syndrome	Failure of third and fourth pharyngeal pouches to develop Thymus and parathyroids fail to develop	Hypoparathyroidism (tetany); absent thymic shadow on radiograph; PCP Danger of GVH reaction
Combined B- and T-Cell Disorders		
Severe combined immunodeficiency (SCID)	Adenosine deaminase deficiency; adenine toxic to B and T cells, ↓ deoxynucleoside triphosphate precursors for DNA synthesis Autosomal recessive disorder	Defective CMI ↓ Immunoglobulins Treatment: gene therapy, bone marrow transplant (patients with SCID do *not* reject allografts)
Wiskott-Aldrich syndrome	Progressive deletion of B and T cells X-linked recessive disorder	Symptom triad: eczema, thrombocytopenia, sinopulmonary infections Associated risk of malignant lymphoma Defective CMI ↓ IgM, normal IgG, ↑ IgA and IgE
Ataxia-telangiectasia	Mutation in DNA repair enzymes Thymic hypoplasia Autosomal recessive disorder	Cerebellar ataxia, telangiectasias of eyes and skin Risk of lymphoma and/or leukemia ↑ Serum α-fetoprotein

CMI, cell-mediated immunity; GVH, graft-versus-host; PCP, *Pneumocystis jiroveci* pneumonia.

(1) Can infect monocytes and macrophages in tissue (e.g., lung, brain)

(2) Can infect dendritic cells in mucosal tissue
- Dendritic cells transfer virus to B-cell germinal follicles.

(3) Macrophages and dendritic cells are reservoirs for virus.
- Loss of cell-mediated immunity

d. Reverse transcriptase

(1) Converts viral RNA into proviral double-stranded DNA

(2) DNA is integrated into the host DNA.

4. HIV and AIDS testing (Table 3-6)

5. Clinical findings

a. Acute phase
- Mononucleosis-like syndrome 3 to 6 weeks after infection

b. Latent (chronic) phase

(1) Asymptomatic period 2 to 10 years after infection

(2) CD4 T-cell count greater than 500 cells/μL

(3) Viral replication occurs in dendritic cells (reservoir cells) in germinal follicles of lymph nodes.

c. Early symptomatic phase

(1) CD4 T-cell count 200 to 500 cells/μL

(2) Generalized lymphadenopathy

(3) Non–AIDS-defining infections, including hairy leukoplakia, or Epstein-Barr virus (EBV)–caused glossitis, oral candidiasis

(4) Fever, weight loss, diarrhea

> HIV: cytotoxic to CD4 T cells; loss of cell-mediated immunity

> Anti-gp120: detected in ELISA test screen
>
> Western blot: confirms HIV

> Reservoir cell for HIV: follicular dendritic cells in lymph nodes

TABLE 3-6: Laboratory Tests Used in HIV and AIDS

Test	Use	Comments
ELISA	Screening test	Detects anti-gp120 antibodies Sensitivity ~100% Positive within 6–10 weeks
Western blot	Confirmatory test	Used if ELISA is positive or indeterminate Positive test: presence of p24 antigen and gp41 antibodies and either gp120 or gp160 antibodies ~100% specificity
p24 Antigen	Indicator of active viral replication Present before anti-gp120 antibodies	Positive prior to seroconversion and when AIDS is diagnosed (two distinct peaks)
CD4 T-cell count	Monitoring immune status	Useful in determining when to initiate HIV treatment and when to administer prophylaxis against opportunistic infections
HIV viral load	Detection of actively dividing virus Marker of disease progression	Most sensitive test for diagnosis of acute HIV before seroconversion

AIDS, acquired immunodeficiency syndrome; ELISA, enzyme-linked immunoabsorbent assay; HIV, human immunodeficiency virus.

TABLE 3-7:
Organ Systems Affected by AIDS

Organ System	Condition	Comments
Central nervous system (CNS)	AIDS-dementia complex	Caused by HIV Multinucleated microglial cells reservoir of virus
	Primary CNS lymphoma	Caused by EBV Most common extranodal site for lymphoma
	Cryptococcosis	Cause of CNS fungal infection
	Toxoplasmosis	Cause of space-occupying lesions
	CMV retinitis	Cause of blindness
Gastrointestinal	Esophagitis	Caused by *Candida,* herpesvirus, CMV
	Colitis	Caused by *Cryptosporidium,* CMV
Hepatobiliary	Biliary tract infection	Caused by CMV
Renal	Focal segmental glomerulosclerosis	Causes hypertension and nephrotic syndrome
Respiratory	Pneumonia	Caused by *Pneumocystis jiroveci* and *Streptococcus pneumoniae*
Skin	Kaposi sarcoma	Caused by HHV-8
	Bacillary angiomatosis	Caused by *Bartonella henselae*

AIDS, acquired immunodeficiency syndrome; CMV, cytomegalovirus; EBV, Epstein-Barr virus; HHV-8, human herpes virus type 8; HIV, human immunodeficiency virus.

Most common CNS fungal infection in AIDS: cryptococcosis

Most common malignancy in AIDS: Kaposi's sarcoma

CMV: most common cause of blindness in AIDS

d. AIDS (Table 3-7)
  (1) Criteria
    • HIV-positive with CD4 T-cell count of 200 cells/μL or less or an AIDS-defining condition
  (2) Most common AIDS-defining infections
    • *Pneumocystis jiroveci* pneumonia, systemic candidiasis
  (3) AIDS-defining malignancies
    • Kaposi's sarcoma (Fig. 3-3), Burkitt's lymphoma (EBV), primary CNS lymphoma (EBV)
  (4) Causes of death
    • Disseminated infections (cytomegalovirus, *Mycobacterium avium* complex)
e. Immunologic abnormalities
  (1) Lymphopenia (low CD4 T-cell count)
  (2) Cutaneous anergy (defect in cell-mediated immunity)
  (3) Hypergammaglobulinemia (due to polyclonal B-cell stimulation by EBV)
  (4) CD4:CD8 ratio <1
f. CD4 count and risk for certain diseases
  (1) 700 to 1500: normal
  (2) 200 to 500: oral thrush, herpes zoster (shingles), hairy leukoplakia
  (3) 100 to 200: *Pneumocystis jiroveci* pneumonia, dementia
  (4) Below 100: toxoplasmosis, cryptococcosis, cryptosporidiosis

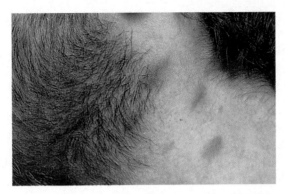

3-3: *Kaposi's sarcoma in HIV. Skin lesions are raised, red, and nonpruritic. (From Forbes C, Jackson W: Color Atlas and Text of Clinical Medicine, 2nd ed. St. Louis, Mosby, 2003, Fig. 1-48.)*

**TABLE 3-8:
Complement
Disorders**

Disorder	Comments
Hereditary angioedema	Autosomal dominant disorder with deficiency of C1 esterase inhibitor Continued C1 activation decreases C2 and C4 and increases their cleavage products, which have anaphylatoxic activity Normal C3 Swelling of face and oropharynx
C2 deficiency	Most common complement deficiency Association with septicemia (usually *Streptococcus pneumoniae*) and lupus-like syndrome in children
C6–C9 deficiency	Increased susceptibility to disseminated *Neisseria gonorrhoeae* or *N. meningitidis* infections
Paroxysmal nocturnal hemoglobinuria	Acquired stem cell disease Defect in molecule anchoring decay accelerating factor (DAF), which normally degrades C3 and C5 convertase on hematopoietic cell membranes Complement-mediated intravascular lysis of red blood cells (hemoglobinuria), platelets, and neutrophils

    (5) Below 50: CMV retinitis, *Mycobacterium avium* complex, progressive multifocal leukoencephalopathy, primary central nervous system lymphoma

  6. Pregnant women with AIDS
- Treatment with a reverse transcriptase inhibitor reduces transmission to newborns to less than 8%.

D. Complement system disorders (Table 3-8)
  1. Complement pathways
    a. Classic and alternative pathways
    b. C1 esterase inhibitor inactivates the protease activity of C1 in the classic pathway.

Hereditary angioedema: deficiency C1 esterase inhibitor

c. Membrane attack complex (C5–C9) is the final common pathway for both the classic and alternative pathways.

2. Testing of the complement system
   a. A decrease in C4 or C2 indicates activation of the classic pathway.
   b. A decrease in factor B indicates activation of the alternative pathway.
   c. A decrease in C3 indicates activation of either system.

VII. Amyloidosis

  A. Amyloid

    1. Fibrillar protein that forms deposits in interstitial tissue, resulting in organ dysfunction

    2. Characteristics
   a. Linear, nonbranching filaments in a β-pleated sheet
   b. Apple green–colored birefringence in polarized light with Congo red stain of tissue
   c. Eosinophilic staining with H&E (hematoxylin and eosin) stain
   d. Derived from various proteins

    3. Major types of amyloid proteins
   a. Amyloid light chain (AL)
      • Derived from light chains (e.g., Bence Jones protein)
   b. Amyloid-associated (AA)
      • Derived from serum associated amyloid (SAA), an acute phase reactant (see Chapter 2)
   c. β-Amyloid (Aβ)
      • Derived from amyloid precursor protein (protein product of chromosome 21)

  B. Types of amyloidosis (Table 3-9)

    1. Systemic
   a. Similar tissue involvement in both primary and secondary types
   b. Primary amyloidosis
      (1) AL amyloid disposition
      (2) Associated with multiple myeloma (30% of cases)
   c. Secondary (reactive)
      (1) AA amyloid

Amyloid: apple green birefringence in polarized light

β-Amyloid is associated with Alzheimer's disease in Down syndrome.

TABLE 3-9: Common Types of Amyloidosis and Associated Clinical Findings

Type of Amyloidosis	Clinical Findings
Primary and secondary	Nephrotic syndrome, renal failure (common cause of death) Arrhythmia, heart failure Macroglossia, malabsorption Hepatosplenomegaly Carpal tunnel syndrome
Senile cerebral	Dementia (Alzheimer's type) caused by toxic Aβ deposits in neurons Amyloid precursor protein coded by chromosome 21 Associated with Down syndrome

        (2) Associated with chronic inflammation (e.g., rheumatoid arthritis, tuberculosis)

  2. Localized

    a. Confined to a single organ (e.g., brain)

    b. Alzheimer's disease

      (1) Aβ

      (2) Most common cause of dementia

  3. Hereditary

    • Autosomal recessive disorder involving AA amyloid (e.g., familial Mediterranean fever)

C. Pathogenesis

  • Abnormal folding of normal or mutant proteins

D. Techniques used to diagnose amyloidosis

  1. Immunoelectrophoresis (to detect light chains) in primary amyloidosis

  2. Tissue biopsy (e.g., adipose, rectum)

Amyloid: abnormal folding of protein

Water, Electrolyte, Acid-Base, and Hemodynamic Disorders

I. **Water and Electrolyte Disorders**
A. **Body fluid compartments**
1. Total body water (TBW) is ~60% of the body weight in kg (Fig. 4-1).
a. Sodium (Na$^+$) is the major extracellular fluid (ECF) cation.
b. Potassium (K$^+$) is the major intracellular fluid (ICF) cation.
c. ECF is subdivided into the interstitial and vascular compartments.
2. Plasma osmolality (POsm)
a. Osmolality is the number of solutes in plasma (i.e., tonicity of ECF).
b. POsm = 2 (serum Na$^+$) + serum glucose/18 + serum blood urea nitrogen (BUN)/2.8 = 275–295 mOsm/kg
• POsm roughly correlates with the serum Na$^+$ concentration.
c. Urea diffuses freely between ECF and ICF.
3. Na$^+$ and glucose are limited to the ECF.
a. Changes in their concentration produce an osmotic gradient.
(1) Water shifts between the ECF and ICF compartments by osmosis.
(2) Water moves from a low to high solute concentration.
(3) Water shifts do *not* occur with alterations in urea concentration.
b. Hyponatremia (decreased POsm) causes water to shift from ECF to ICF (Fig. 4-2A).
c. Hypernatremia or hyperglycemia (increased POsm) cause water to shift from ICF to ECF (Fig. 4-2B).
B. **Isotonic, hypotonic, and hypertonic disorders**
1. Serum Na$^+$ concentration (mEq/L) reflects the ratio of total body Na$^+$ (TBNa$^+$) to total body water (TBW).
a. Serum Na$^+$ ~ TBNa$^+$/TBW
• TBNa$^+$ is the sum total of all the ECF Na$^+$ and is expressed in mg/kg of body weight.
b. Evaluation of TBNa$^+$ status
(1) Decreased TBNa$^+$ produces signs of volume depletion.
(a) Dry mucous membranes (Fig. 4-3)
(b) Decreased skin turgor (i.e., skin tenting when the skin is pinched)
(c) Drop in blood pressure and increase in pulse when sitting up from a supine position (i.e., positive tilt test)

Na$^+$, K$^+$: major ECF and ICF cations, respectively

Osmosis: water movement between ECF and ICF; controlled by serum Na$^+$

Serum Na$^+$ ~ TBNa$^+$/TBW

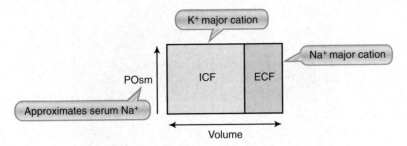

4-1: *Body fluid compartments. See text for discussion.*

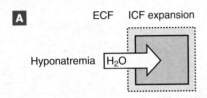

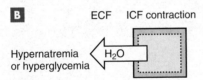

4-2: *Osmotic shifts in hyponatremia (**A**) and hypernatremia or hyperglycemia (**B**). See text for discussion.*

(2) Increased TBNa$^+$ may produce body cavity effusions (e.g., ascites) and dependent pitting edema (Fig. 4-4).

    (a) Dependent pitting edema is due to an excess of Na$^+$-containing fluid in the interstitial space.

        • Due to the low protein content in edema fluid, fluid obeys the law of gravity and moves to the most dependent portion of the body (e.g., ankles, if the person is standing).

    (b) An alteration in Starling pressures must be present to produce pitting edema and body effusions.

> Fluid movement across a capillary/venule wall into the interstitial space is driven by Starling pressures (*not* osmosis). The net direction of fluid movement depends on which Starling pressure is dominant. An increase in plasma hydrostatic pressure or a decrease in plasma oncotic pressure (i.e., serum albumin) causes fluid to diffuse out of capillaries and venules and into the interstitial space, resulting in dependent pitting edema and/or body cavity effusions.

    (c) In patients who have no Starling pressure alterations, pitting edema and body effusions are *not* likely to occur.

↓ TBNa$^+$: signs of volume depletion

↑ TBNa$^+$: pitting edema, body cavity effusions

Starling pressure alterations: control water movement in ECF compartment

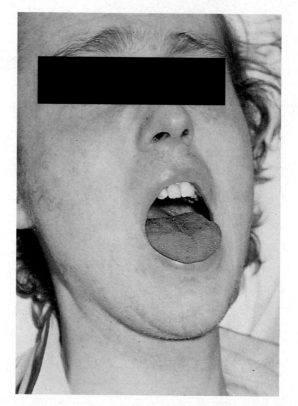

4-3: *Patient with signs of volume depletion. The mucosal surface of the tongue is dry. Additional findings on examination were hypotension, tachycardia, and decreased skin turgor. (From Forbes C, Jackson W: Color Atlas and Text of Clinical Medicine, 2nd ed. St. Louis, Mosby, 2003, Fig. 7-90.)*

(3) Normal TBNa$^+$ is associated with normal skin turgor and hydration.

2. Isotonic fluid disorders (Table 4-1)

   a. Isotonic loss of fluid

      (1) POsm and serum Na$^+$ are normal ($\downarrow$TBNa$^+$/$\downarrow$TBW).

         • The arrows represent the magnitude of change in TBNa$^+$ and TBW.

      (2) There is *no* osmotic gradient or fluid shift between ECF and ICF.

         • ECF volume contracts; however, the ICF volume remains normal.

      (3) Signs of volume depletion are present.

      (4) Examples include adult diarrhea, loss of whole blood.

> Normal (isotonic) saline (0.9%) approximates plasma tonicity (POsm). It is infused in patients to maintain the blood pressure when there is a significant loss of sodium-containing fluid (e.g., blood loss, diarrhea, sweat).

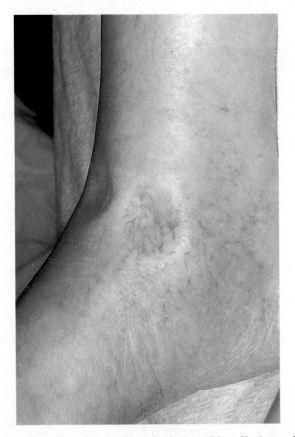

4-4: *Dependent pitting edema showing depressions in the skin around the ankle. Pitting edema is due to an increase in vascular hydrostatic pressure or a decrease in vascular oncotic pressure (hypoalbuminemia). (From Forbes C, Jackson W: Color Atlas and Text of Clinical Medicine, 2nd ed. St. Louis, Mosby, 2003, Fig. 5-8.)*

      b. Isotonic gain of fluid
         (1) POsm and serum Na^+ are normal ($\uparrow$TBNa$^+$/$\uparrow$TBW).
         (2) There is *no* osmotic gradient or fluid shift between ECF and ICF.
            • ECF volume expands; however, the ICF volume remains normal.
         (3) Pitting edema and body cavity effusions may be present.
         (4) Example is excessive infusion of isotonic saline.
    3. Hypotonic fluid disorders (see Table 4-1)
      a. Hyponatremia (decreased POsm) is always present.
         (1) Osmotic gradient is present.
         (2) Water shifts to the ICF compartment (expands).
      b. Hypertonic loss of Na^+ ($\downarrow\downarrow$TBNa$^+$/$\downarrow$TBW)
         (1) ECF volume contracts and ICF volume expands.
         (2) Signs of volume depletion appear.
         (3) Examples include increased renal loss of Na^+ (e.g., loop diuretic, Addison's disease, 21-hydroxylase deficiency).

Isotonic loss or gain: serum Na^+ normal

Hypotonic disorders: hyponatremia always present; ICF expansion

TABLE 4-1:
Isotonic and Hypotonic Disorders

Compartment Alteration	POsm/Na⁺	ECF Volume	ICF Volume	Conditions
Normal ECF and ICF	Normal	Normal	Normal	Normal hydration
Isotonic loss	Normal $\downarrow$TBNa⁺/$\downarrow$TBW	Contracted	Normal	Adult diarrhea Loss of whole blood
Isotonic gain	Normal $\uparrow$TBNa⁺/$\uparrow$TBW	Expanded Starling pressure alteration	Normal	Excessive isotonic (normal) saline
Hypertonic loss of Na⁺	Decreased $\downarrow\downarrow$TBNa⁺/$\downarrow$TBW	Contracted	Expanded	Loop diuretics Addison's disease 21-Hydroxylase deficiency
Gain of water	Decreased TBNa⁺/$\uparrow\uparrow$TBW	Expanded	Expanded	SIADH
Hypotonic gain of Na⁺	Decreased $\uparrow$TBNa⁺/$\uparrow\uparrow$TBW	Expanded Starling pressure alteration	Expanded	Right-sided heart failure Cirrhosis Nephrotic syndrome

ECF, extracellular fluid; ICF, intracellular fluid; POsm, plasma osmolality; SIADH, syndrome of inappropriate antidiuretic hormone; TB, total body; W, water.

Rapid intravenous fluid correction of hyponatremia with saline in an alcoholic may result in central pontine myelinolysis, an irreversible demyelinating disorder. As a general rule, all intravenous replacement of Na^+-containing fluid should be given slowly over the first 24 hours.

c. Gain of water ($TBNa^+/\uparrow\uparrow TBW$)
   (1) Expansion of ECF and ICF volumes
   (2) Normal skin turgor
   (3) Example—syndrome of inappropriate secretion of antidiuretic hormone (SIADH, e.g., small cell carcinoma of the lung)
d. Hypotonic gain of Na^+ ($\uparrow TBNa^+/\uparrow\uparrow TBW$)
   (1) Expansion of the ECF and ICF volumes
   (2) Caused by pitting edema states with Starling pressure alterations
      (a) Right-sided heart failure with increase in venous hydrostatic pressure
      (b) Cirrhosis and nephrotic syndrome with decrease in plasma oncotic pressure

Pitting edema states: right-sided heart failure, cirrhosis, nephrotic syndrome

In these pitting edema states, the cardiac output is decreased, which causes the release of catecholamines, activation of the renin-angiotensin-aldosterone system, stimulation of ADH release, and increased renal retention of Na^+. The kidney reabsorbs a slightly hypotonic, Na^+-containing fluid ($\uparrow\uparrow TBNa^+/\uparrow\uparrow TBW$). Because these pitting edema states have alterations in Starling pressures, the Na^+-containing fluid is redirected into the interstitial space, causing pitting edema and body cavity effusions.

4. Hypertonic fluid disorders (Table 4-2)
   a. Increased POsm is most often due to hypernatremia or hyperglycemia.
      (1) Osmotic gradient is present.
      (2) Water shifts out of the ICF (contracts) to the ECF.
   b. Hypotonic loss of Na^+ ($\downarrow TBNa^+/\downarrow\downarrow TBW$)
      (1) Contraction of the ECF and ICF volumes
      (2) Signs of volume depletion
      (3) Examples—sweating, osmotic diuresis (e.g., glucosuria), infant diarrhea
   c. Loss of water ($TBNa^+/\downarrow\downarrow TBW$)
      (1) Contraction of the ECF (mild) and ICF volumes
      (2) Normal skin turgor
      (3) Examples
         (a) Diabetes insipidus due to loss of ADH or refractoriness to ADH
         (b) Insensible water loss (e.g., fever)
   d. Hypertonic gain of Na^+ ($\uparrow\uparrow\uparrow TBNa^+/\uparrow TBW$)
      (1) ECF volume expands and ICF volume contracts.
      (2) Pitting edema and body cavity effusions may be present.
      (3) Examples include infusion of $NaHCO_3$ or Na^+-containing antibiotics.

Hypertonic disorder: hypernatremia or hyperglycemia; ICF contraction

TABLE 4-2:
Hypertonic Disorders

Compartment Alteration	POsm/Na$^+$	ECF Volume	ICF Volume	Conditions
Hypotonic loss of Na$^+$	Increased ↓TBNa$^+$/↓↓TBW	Contracted	Contracted	Osmotic diuresis: glucose Sweating Infant diarrhea
Loss of water	Increased TBNa$^+$/↓↓TBW	Contracted (mild)	Contracted	Insensible water loss: fever Diabetes insipidus
Hypertonic gain of Na$^+$	Increased ↑↑TBNa$^+$/↑TBW	Expanded	Contracted	Infusion of a Na$^+$-containing antibiotic Infusion of NaHCO$_3$
Hyperglycemia	Increased ↑Glucose ↓Na$^+$ (dilutional effect)	Contracted	Contracted	Diabetic ketoacidosis Hyperosmolar nonketotic coma

ECF, extracellular fluid; ICF, intracellular fluid; POsm, plasma osmolality; TB, total body; W, water.

   e. Hypertonic state due to hyperglycemia
      • Examples—diabetic ketoacidosis (DKA), hyperosmolar nonketotic coma
      (1) Water shifts from the ICF to the ECF compartment.
         (a) Dilutional effect on serum Na$^+$ causes hyponatremia.
         (b) Increased POsm (due to hyperglycemia) and hyponatremia (dilutional).
      (2) Signs of volume depletion
         • Glucosuria produces a hypotonic loss of water and Na$^+$ (osmotic diuresis), causing signs of volume depletion.
C. Potassium (K$^+$) disorders
   1. Functions of potassium
      a. Regulation of neuromuscular excitability and muscle contraction
      b. Regulation of insulin secretion

Hyperglycemia: ↑ POsm, ↓ serum Na$^+$

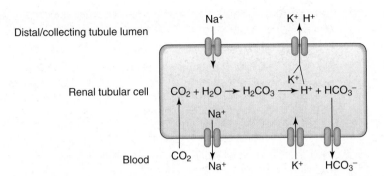

4-5: *Aldosterone-mediated Na⁺-K⁺ and H⁺ channels. These channels are located in the late distal and collecting ducts. Na⁺ is exchanged for K⁺, which is excreted in the urine. If K⁺ is depleted, Na⁺ is exchanged for H⁺ (protons), which is excreted in the urine. Loss of H⁺ causes a corresponding increase in reabsorption of HCO_3^- into the blood.*

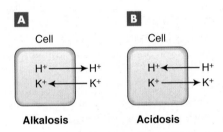

4-6: *Potassium (K^+) shifts related to alkalosis (**A**) and acidosis (**B**). See text for discussion.*

- Hypokalemia inhibits insulin secretion, while hyperkalemia stimulates insulin secretion.

2. Control of potassium
  a. Aldosterone
    (1) Increases the secretion of K^+ and H^+ in the late distal and collecting tubules (Fig. 4-5)
    (2) Increases reabsorption of K^+ by the H^+/K^+-ATPase pump in the collecting tubules
  b. Arterial pH
    (1) Alkalosis causes H^+ to move out of cells and K^+ into cells (Fig. 4-6A).
      - Potential for hypokalemia
    (2) Acidosis causes H^+ to move into cells (for buffering) and K^+ out of cells (Fig. 4-6B).
      - Potential for hyperkalemia

3. Hypokalemia (serum K^+ < 3.5 mEq/L)
  a. Causes of hypokalemia (Table 4-3)
  b. Clinical findings
    (1) Muscle weakness
      - Due to changes in the intracellular/extracellular K^+ membrane potential
    (2) U waves on an electrocardiogram (ECG, Fig. 4-7)

Alkalosis: K^+ shifts into cell

Acidosis: K^+ shifts out of cell

Loop and thiazide diuretics: most common cause of hypokalemia

Hypokalemia: ECG shows U wave

**TABLE 4-3:
Causes of
Hypokalemia**

Pathogenesis	Causes
Decreased intake	Elderly patients, eating disorders
Transcellular shift	Alkalosis Drugs enhancing Na^+/K^+-ATPase pump: insulin, β_2-agonists (e.g., albuterol)
Gastrointestinal loss	Diarrhea (~30 mEq/L in stool) Laxatives Vomiting (~5 mEq/L in gastric juice)
Renal loss	Loop and thiazide diuretics (most common cause) Osmotic diuresis: glucosuria Mineralocorticoid excess: primary aldosteronism, 11-hydroxylase deficiency, Cushing syndrome

(3) Polyuria
  (a) Collecting tubules are refractory to ADH (i.e., nephrogenic diabetes inspidus).
  (b) Tubule cells are distended with fluid (called vacuolar nephropathy).
(4) Rhabdomyolysis
  • Hypokalemia inhibits insulin, which decreases muscle glycogenesis, leading to rhabdomyolysis.
4. Hyperkalemia (serum $K^+ > 5.0$ mEq/L)
  a. Causes (Table 4-4)
  b. Clinical findings
    (1) Ventricular arrhythmias
      • Severe hyperkalemia (e.g., 7–8 mEq/L) causes the heart to stop in diastole.
    (2) Peaked T waves on an ECG (Fig. 4-8)
      • Due to accelerated repolarization of cardiac muscle
    (3) Muscle weakness
      • Hyperkalemia partially depolarizes the cell membrane which interferes with membrane excitability.

II. Acid-Base Disorders
  A. Primary alterations in arterial P_{CO_2} (Pa_{CO_2}, 33–45 mm Hg)
    1. Respiratory acidosis
      a. Causes of respiratory acidosis (Table 4-5)
      b. Pathogenesis
        (1) Alveolar hypoventilation with retention of CO_2
        (2) $Pa_{CO_2} > 45$ mm Hg
          • $\downarrow$ pH ~ $\uparrow HCO_3/\uparrow\uparrow P_{CO_2}$
      c. Metabolic alkalosis is compensation
        (1) Serum $HCO_3 \leq 30$ mEq/L in acute respiratory acidosis
        (2) Serum $HCO_3^- > 30$ mEq/L (indicates renal compensation) in chronic respiratory acidosis

Renal failure: most common cause of hyperkalemia

Hyperkalemia: ECG shows peaked T waves

Respiratory acidosis: $Pa_{CO_2} > 45$ mm Hg

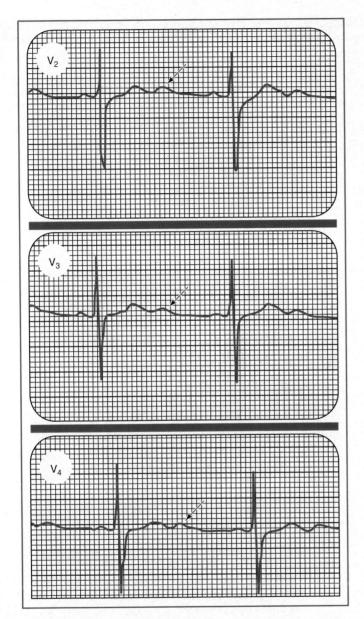

4-7: *Electrocardiogram showing hypokalemia. A positive wave after the T wave is called a U wave (arrows). U waves are a sign of hypokalemia. (From Goldman L, Bennet JC: Cecil Textbook of Medicine, 21st ed. Philadelphia, WB Saunders, 1999, Fig 102-7.)*

TABLE 4-4:
Causes of
Hyperkalemia

Pathogenesis	Causes
Tissue breakdown	Iatrogenic (e.g., venipuncture) Rhabdomyolysis (rupture of muscle)
Transcellular shift	Acidosis Drugs inhibiting Na^+/K^+-ATPase pump: β-blocker (e.g., propanolol), digitalis toxicity, succinylcholine
Decreased renal excretion	Renal failure (most common cause) Mineralocorticoid deficiency: Addison's disease, 21-hydroxylase deficiency, hyporeninemic hypoaldosteronism (destruction of juxtaglomerular apparatus) Drugs: spironolactone (inhibits aldosterone); triamterene, amiloride (inhibit Na^+ channels)

LEAD V$_3$

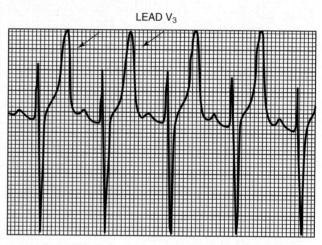

4-8: *Electrocardiogram showing hyperkalemia. Arrows show peaked T waves, which are a sign of hyperkalemia. (From Goldman L, Bennet JC: Cecil Textbook of Medicine, 21st ed. Philadelphia, WB Saunders, 1999, Fig 102-8A.)*

Compensation refers to respiratory and renal mechanisms that bring the arterial pH close to but *not* into the normal pH range (7.35–7.45). In primary respiratory acidosis and alkalosis, compensation is metabolic alkalosis and metabolic acidosis, respectively. In primary metabolic acidosis and alkalosis, compensation is respiratory alkalosis and respiratory acidosis, respectively. When the expected compensation remains in the normal range, an uncompensated disorder is present. If compensation moves outside the normal range but does *not* bring pH into the normal range, a partially compensated disorder is present. When compensation brings the pH into the normal range, full compensation is present, which rarely occurs.

TABLE 4-5:
Causes of
Respiratory
Acidosis and
Alkalosis

Anatomic Site	Respiratory Acidosis	Respiratory Alkalosis
CNS respiratory center	Depression of center: trauma, barbiturates	Overstimulation: anxiety, high altitude, normal pregnancy (estrogen/progesterone effect), salicylate poisoning, endotoxic (septic) shock, cirrhosis
Upper airway	Obstruction: acute epiglottitis (*Hemophilus influenzae*), croup (parainfluenza virus)	
Muscles respiration	Paralysis: ALS, phrenic nerve injury, Guillain-Barré syndrome, hypokalemia, hypophosphatemia ($\downarrow$ ATP)	Rib fracture: hyperventilation from pain
Lungs	Obstructive disease: chronic bronchitis, cystic fibrosis Other: pulmonary edema, ARDS, RDS, severe bronchial asthma	Restrictive disease: sarcoidosis, asbestosis Others: pulmonary embolus, mild bronchial asthma

ALS, amyotrophic lateral sclerosis; ARDS, acute respiratory distress syndrome; ATP, adenosine triphosphate; RDS, respiratory distress syndrome.

    d. Clinical findings
      (1) Somnolence
      (2) Cerebral edema (vasodilation of cerebral vessels)
  2. Respiratory alkalosis
    a. Causes of respiratory alkalosis (see Table 4-5)
    b. Pathogenesis
      (1) Alveolar hyperventilation with elimination of CO_2
      (2) $Paco_2 < 33\,mm\,Hg$
        • $\uparrow$ pH ~ $\downarrow$ HCO_3^-/$\downarrow\downarrow$ PCO_2
    c. Metabolic acidosis is compensation.
      (1) Serum $HCO_3 \geq 18\,mEq/L$ in acute respiratory alkalosis
      (2) Serum $HCO_3^- < 18\,mEq/L$ but $> 12\,mEq/L$ (indicates renal compensation) in chronic respiratory alkalosis
    d. Clinical findings
      (1) Light-headedness and confusion
      (2) Signs of tetany
        (a) Thumb adduction into the palm (carpopedal spasm)
        (b) Perioral twitching when the facial nerve is tapped (Chvostek sign)
        (c) Perioral numbness and tingling

Respiratory alkalosis: $Paco_2 < 33\,mm\,Hg$

Alkalosis increases the number of negative charges on albumin (more COO^- groups on acidic amino acids). Therefore, calcium is displaced from the ionized calcium fraction and is bound to albumin, causing a decrease in ionized calcium levels and signs of tetany.

TABLE 4-6:
Causes of Increased Anion Gap Metabolic Acidosis

Causes	Pathogenesis
Lactic acidosis	Most common type Any cause of tissue hypoxia with concomitant anaerobic glycolysis: e.g., shock, CN poisoning, CO poisoning, severe hypoxemia ($PO_2 < 35\,mmHg$), CHF, severe anemia (Hb < 6 g/dL) Alcoholism: increased synthesis of lactic acid as pyruvate is converted to lactate due to the excess of NADH in alcohol metabolism Liver disease: liver normally converts lactate to pyruvate; liver disease (e.g., hepatitis, cirrhosis) causes lactate to accumulate in blood
Ketoacidosis	Diabetic ketoacidosis (type 1 diabetes mellitus): leads to an accumulation of AcAc and β-OHB Alcoholism: acetyl CoA in alcohol metabolism is converted to ketoacids; increase in NADH causes AcAc to convert to β-OHB, which is *not* detected with standard tests for ketone bodies Starvation: acetyl CoA from β-oxidation of fatty acids is converted to ketoacids
Renal failure	Retention of organic acids: e.g., sulfuric and phosphoric acids
Salicylate poisoning	Salicylic acid is an acid; it is also a mitochondrial toxin that uncouples oxidative phosphorylation leading to tissue hypoxia and lactic acidosis; in some cases (usually adults), excess salicylate overstimulates the CNS respiratory center producing a primary respiratory alkalosis
Ethylene glycol poisoning	Ethylene glycol is in antifreeze; it is converted to glycolic and oxalic acid by alcohol dehydrogenase; oxalate anions combine with calcium to produce calcium oxalate crystals that obstruct renal tubules causing renal failure
Methyl alcohol poisoning	Methyl alcohol is present in window-washing fluid, Sterno, and solvents for paints; it is converted into formic acid by alcohol dehydrogenase; formic acid damages the optic nerve causing optic neuritis and the potential for permanent blindness

AcAc, acetoacetate; β-OHB, β-hydroxybutyrate; CHF, congestive heart failure; CN, cyanide; CO, carbon monoxide; Hb, hemoglobin; IV, intravenous.

B. **Primary alterations in HCO_3^- (22–28 mEq/L)**
- Applies to venous and arterial bicarbonate
1. Metabolic acidosis
   a. Increased anion gap (AG) type
      - Anion gap (AG) = serum Na^+ − (serum Cl^- + serum HCO_3^-) = 12 mEq +/− 2.
      (1) Excess H^+ ions of an acid are buffered by HCO_3^-, which decreases the serum HCO_3^-.
      (2) HCO_3^- loss is counterbalanced by the anions of the acid (e.g., lactate).
      (3) Example—serum Na^+ 130 mEq/L (135–147), serum Cl^- 88 mEq/L (95–105), serum HCO_3^- 10 mEq/L (22–28)
         - AG = 130 − (88 + 10) = 32 mEq/L (12 mEq/L +/− 2).
      (4) Causes of increased AG metabolic acidosis (Table 4-6)

↑ AG metabolic acidosis: anions of acid replace HCO_3^-

TABLE 4-7:
Causes of Normal Anion Gap Metabolic Acidosis

Causes	Pathogenesis
Diarrhea	Most common cause in children Loss of HCO_3^- in stool
Type I distal renal tubular acidosis	Inability to synthesize HCO_3^- in the H^+/K^+-ATPase pump in the collecting tubules Inability to secrete H^+ ions decreases titratable acidity (H_2PO_4) and NH_4Cl causing the urine pH to be >5.5 Causes: amphotericin, light chains in multiple myeloma Rx: oral administration of HCO_3^-
Type II proximal renal tubular acidosis	Renal threshold for reclaiming HCO_3^- is lowered from a normal of ~24 mEq/L to ~15 mEq/L Urine pH is initially >5.5 due to loss of filtered HCO_3^- in the urine; when the serum HCO_3^- is equal to the renal threshold, the proximal tubules reclaim HCO_3^-, causing the urine pH to drop to <5.5 Causes: carbonic anhydrase inhibitors (most common cause), primary hyperparathyroidism ($\uparrow$ PTH, $\downarrow$ proximal tubule HCO_3^- reclamation), proximal tubule nephrotoxic drugs/chemicals (e.g., aminoglycosides, heavy metals) Rx: thiazides to produce volume depletion, which increases the renal threshold for reclaiming HCO_3^-
Type IV renal tubular acidosis	Due to destruction of the JG apparatus: e.g., hyaline arteriolosclerosis of afferent arterioles in diabetes mellitus, acute or chronic tubulointerstitial inflammation (e.g., Legionnaire's disease) Produces hyporeninemic hypoaldosteronism Only RTA with hyperkalemia: due to hypoaldosteronism

JG, juxtaglomerular; PTH, parathyroid hormone; RTA, renal tubular acidosis; Rx, treatment.

b. Normal AG metabolic acidosis
   (1) Due to a loss of HCO_3^- or an inability to synthesize HCO_3^- in the kidneys
   (2) Cl^- anions increase to counterbalance the loss of HCO_3^- anions.
      • Produces a hyperchloremic normal AG metabolic acidosis
   (3) Example—serum Na^+ 136 mEq/L, serum Cl^- 110 mEq/L, serum HCO_3^- 14 mEq/L
      (a) AG = 136 − (110 + 14) = 12 mEq/L.
      (b) Drop of 10 mEq/L of HCO_3^- from normal (24 − 14 = 10) is counterbalanced by a gain of 10 mEq/L of Cl^- ions (100 + 10 = 110).
   (4) Causes of normal AG metabolic acidosis (Table 4-7)
c. Pathogenesis
   (1) Serum HCO_3^- < 22 mEq/L
      • $\downarrow$ pH ~ $\downarrow\downarrow$ HCO_3^-/$\downarrow$ Pco_2
   (2) Addition of an acid (increased AG type)
   (3) Loss of HCO_3^- or inability to synthesize HCO_3^- (normal AG type)
d. Respiratory alkalosis is compensation.

Normal AG metabolic acidosis: Cl^- anions replace HCO_3^-

Metabolic acidosis: HCO_3^- < 22 mEq/L

TABLE 4-8:
Causes of
Metabolic Alkalosis

Causes	Pathogenesis
Vomiting	Loss of hydrochloric acid Volume depletion increases proximal tubule reabsorption of Na^+, which increases reclamation of HCO_3^-; correction of volume depletion with 0.9% normal saline corrects the alkalosis (chloride-responsive)
Mineralocorticoid excess	Gain in bicarbonate Enhanced function of aldosterone-mediated Na^+-H^+ channels in the late distal and collecting ducts increases the synthesis of HCO_3^- leading to metabolic alkalosis (see Fig. 4-5); infusion of 0.9% normal saline does *not* correct the metabolic alkalosis (chloride-resistant) Causes: primary aldosteronism, 11-hydroxylase deficiency, Cushing syndrome
Thiazide and loop diuretics	Gain in bicarbonate Block in Na^+ reabsorption leads to augmented late distal and collecting tubule reabsorption of Na^+ and secretion of H^+, the latter increasing synthesis of HCO_3^-, leading to metabolic alkalosis (see Fig. 4-5); volume depletion also increases the proximal tubule reclamation of HCO_3^-, which maintains the metabolic alkalosis

e. Clinical findings
(1) Hyperventilation (Kussmaul breathing)
(2) Warm shock
• Acidosis vasodilates peripheral resistance arterioles.
(3) Osteoporosis
• Bone buffers excess H^+ ions.
2. Metabolic alkalosis
a. Causes of metabolic alkalosis (Table 4-8)
b. Pathogenesis
(1) Due to a loss of hydrogen ions (H^+) or a gain in HCO_3^-
(2) Serum $HCO_3^- > 28\,mEq/L$
• $\uparrow$ pH ~ $\uparrow\uparrow$ HCO_3^-/$\uparrow Pco_2$
c. Respiratory acidosis is compensation.
d. Clinical findings
(1) Increased risk for ventricular arrhythmias
• Metabolic alkalosis left-shifts the oxygen-binding curve and its compensation, respiratory acidosis, decreases arterial Po_2 causing hypoxia in cardiac muscle, which precipitates ventricular arrhythmias.
(2) Tetany (see respiratory alkalosis discussion)
C. Mixed acid-base disorders
1. Blend of two or more primary acid-base disorders occurring at the same time
2. Clues that suggest a mixed disorder
a. Presence of a normal pH due to a combination of a primary acidosis and a primary alkalosis:

Loop and thiazide diuretics: most common cause of metabolic alkalosis

Metabolic alkalosis: $HCO_3^- > 28\,mEq/L$

(1) Salicylate intoxication, particularly in adults
    (a) Salicylic acid produces a primary metabolic acidosis.
    (b) Salicylates overstimulate the respiratory center causing primary respiratory alkalosis.
(2) Patient with chronic bronchitis who is taking a loop diuretic
    (a) Chronic bronchitis produces a primary respiratory acidosis.
    (b) Loop diuretics produce a primary metabolic alkalosis.
  b. Extreme acidemia due to a primary metabolic acidosis plus a primary respiratory acidosis
    • Example—cardiorespiratory arrest with primary respiratory acidosis (no ventilation) and primary metabolic acidosis (lactic acidosis from hypoxia)

D. Selected electrolyte profiles (Table 4-9)
E. Selected arterial blood gas profiles (Table 4-10)

III. Edema
• Presence of increased fluid in the interstitial space of the ECF compartment
A. Types of edema fluid
1. Transudate
  a. Protein-poor (<3 g/dL) and cell-poor fluid
  b. Produces dependent pitting edema and body cavity effusions
2. Exudate
  a. Protein-rich (>3 g/dL) and cell-rich (e.g., neutrophils) fluid
  b. Produces swelling of tissue but *no* pitting edema
3. Lymphedema
  a. Protein-rich fluid
  b. Nonpitting edema
4. Glycosaminoglycans
  a. Increase in hyaluronic acid and chondroitin sulfate
  b. Nonpitting edema called myxedema
B. Pathophysiology of edema
1. Alteration in Starling pressure
  a. Produces a transudate
  b. Increased vascular hydrostatic pressure:
    (1) Pulmonary edema in left-sided heart failure
    (2) Peripheral pitting edema in right-sided heart failure
    (3) Portal hypertension in cirrhosis producing ascites
  c. Decreased vascular plasma oncotic pressure (hypoalbuminemia):
    (1) Malnutrition with decreased protein intake
    (2) Cirrhosis with decreased synthesis of albumin
    (3) Nephrotic syndrome with increased loss of protein in urine (>3.5 g/24 hours)
    (4) Malabsorption with decreased reabsorption of protein
  d. Renal retention of sodium and water
    (1) Increases hydrostatic pressure (increased plasma volume)
    (2) Decreases oncotic pressure (dilutional effect on albumin)
    (3) Examples—acute renal failure, glomerulonephritis

Salicylate intoxication: often mixture of primary metabolic acidosis and primary respiratory alkalosis

Edema: excess fluid in interstitial space

Transudate: protein-poor and cell-poor fluid
Exudate: protein-rich and cell-rich fluid

Pitting edema: transudate; ↑ hydrostatic pressure and/or ↓ oncotic pressure

**TABLE 4-9:
Selected Electrolyte
Profiles**

Serum Na$^+$ (mEq/L)	Serum K$^+$ (mEq/L)	Serum Cl$^-$ (mEq/L)	Serum HCO$_3^-$ (mEq/L)	Discussion
136–145	3.5–5.0	95–105	22–28	Normal ranges
118	3.0	84	22	SIADH: dilutional effect of excess water on all electrolytes
128	5.9	96	20	Addison's disease: lack of aldosterone causes loss of Na$^+$ (hyponatremia), retention of K$^+$ (hyperkalemia), and decreased synthesis of HCO$_3^-$ (metabolic acidosis; see Fig. 4-5)
130	2.9	80	36	Vomiting: loss of Na$^+$ and K$^+$ in vomitus (hyponatremia, hypokalemia); volume depletion causes increased reclamation of HCO$_3^-$ in proximal tubule (metabolic alkalosis)
				Loop and thiazide diuretics: hypertonic loss Na$^+$ in urine (hypernatremia); augmented exchange of Na$^+$ for K$^+$ (hypokalemia) and increased regeneration of HCO$_3^-$ in late distal Na$^+$/K$^+$ + H$^+$ channels (metabolic alkalosis, see Fig. 4-5)
152	2.8	110	33	Mineralocorticoid excess: primary aldosteronism; augmented exchange of Na$^+$ for K$^+$ (hypernatremia, hypokalemia), and increased synthesis of HCO$_3^-$ in late distal Na$^+$/K$^+$ + H$^+$ channels (metabolic alkalosis, see Fig. 4-5)

SIADH, syndrome of inappropriate antidiuretic hormone.

TABLE 4-10:
Selected Arterial
Blood Gas Profiles

pH	PaCO₂ (mm Hg)	HCO₃⁻ (mEq/L)	Discussion
7.35–7.45	33–45	22–28	Normal ranges
7.00	52	13	Mixed disorder (extreme acidemia): primary metabolic acidosis (HCO₃⁻ < 22 mEq/L) + primary respiratory acidosis (PaCO₂ > 45 mm Hg) Example: cardiorespiratory arrest
7.20	74	28	Acute respiratory acidosis, uncompensated (PaCO₂ > 45 mm Hg, HCO₃⁻ < 30 mEq/L) Examples: CNS respiratory center depression (e.g., barbiturate poisoning)
7.33	60	31	Chronic respiratory acidosis with partially compensated metabolic alkalosis (PaCO₂ > 45 mm Hg, HCO₃⁻ > 30 mEq/L) Examples: chronic bronchitis, cystic fibrosis
7.28	28	12	Metabolic acidosis with partially compensated respiratory alkalosis (HCO₃⁻ < 22 mEq/L, PaCO₂ < 33 mm Hg) Examples: disorders associated with increased and normal anion gap metabolic acidosis
7.42	22	14	Mixed disorder (normal pH): primary metabolic acidosis (HCO₃⁻ < 22 mEq/L) + primary respiratory alkalosis (PaCO₂ < 33 mm Hg) Example: salicylate poisoning, septic shock
7.50	47	35	Metabolic alkalosis with partially compensated respiratory acidosis (HCO₃⁻ > 28 mEq/L, PaCO₂ > 45 mm Hg) Causes: loop/thiazide diuretics, vomiting, mineralocorticoid excess
7.56	24	21	Acute respiratory alkalosis with partially compensated metabolic acidosis (PaCO₂ < 33 mm Hg, HCO₃⁻ < 22 mEq/L) Causes: anxiety, pulmonary embolus, normal pregnancy

CNS, central nervous system.

    2. Increased vascular permeability
      a. Produces an exudate
      b. Example—acute inflammation (e.g., tissue swelling following a bee sting)
    3. Lymphatic obstruction
      a. Produces lymphedema
      b. Examples
        (1) Lymphedema following modified radical mastectomy and radiation
        (2) Filariasis due to *Wuchereria bancrofti*
        (3) Scrotal and vulvar lymphedema due to lymphogranuloma venereum

(4) Breast lymphedema due to blockage of subcutaneous lymphatics by malignant cells
4. Increased synthesis of extracellular matrix components (e.g., glycosaminoglycans)
   a. T-cell cytokines stimulate fibroblasts to synthesize glycosaminoglycans.
   b. Example—pretibial myxedema and exophthalmos in Graves' disease

IV. Thrombosis

- A thrombus is an intravascular mass attached to the vessel wall and is composed of varying proportions of coagulation factors, RBCs, and platelets.

A. Pathogenesis of thrombi

1. Endothelial cell injury
   - Due to turbulent blood flow at arterial bifurcations or overlying atherosclerotic plaques; cigarette smoke
2. Stasis of blood flow
   - Sluggish blood flow due to prolonged bed rest or sitting
3. Hypercoagulability
   a. Activation of coagulation system
   b. Causes of hypercoagulability
      (1) Hereditary or acquired factor deficiencies
         - Example—hereditary antithrombin III deficiency or acquired deficiency due to oral contraceptives
      (2) Antiphospholipid syndrome
         - Due to lupus anticoagulant or anticardiolipin antibodies

B. Types of thrombi

1. Venous thrombi
   a. Pathogenesis
      (1) Stasis
         - Procoagulants (e.g., tissue thromboplastin) released from damaged endothelium cause localized activation of the coagulation system.
      (2) Hypercoagulable state
   b. Sites
      (1) Deep vein in the lower extremity below the knee
      (2) Other sites
         - Superficial saphenous, hepatic, and renal veins; dural sinuses
   c. Composition
      (1) Adherent, occlusive, dark red fibrin clot
         - Contains entrapped RBCs, white blood cells, and platelets
      (2) In the lower extremities, they propagate (extend) toward the heart.
         - Danger of pulmonary artery embolization
   d. Anticoagulants heparin and warfarin prevent formation of venous thrombi.
2. Arterial thrombi
   a. Pathogenesis
      (1) Endothelial cell injury due to turbulent blood flow
         - Platelets adhere to areas of injury.

Stasis of blood flow: venous thrombi

Most common site for venous thrombosis: deep vein in lower extremity below the knee

Heparin and warfarin: anticoagulants that prevent venous thrombosis

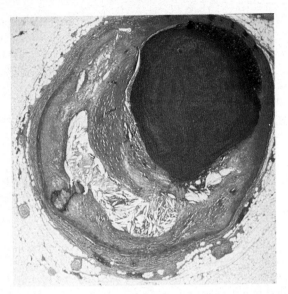

4-9: *Coronary artery thrombosis. In this specially stained cross-section of a coronary artery, collagen is blue and the thrombus is red. The red thrombus in the vessel lumen is composed of platelets held together by fibrin. Directly beneath the thrombus is a fibrous plaque, which stains blue. Beneath the plaque is necrotic atheromatous debris. (From Damjanov I, Linder J: Pathology: A Color Atlas. St. Louis, Mosby, 2000, p 21, Fig. 1-44.)*

       (2) Hypercoagulable state
  b. Sites
       (1) Elastic and muscular arteries
       (2) Majority of thrombi overlie atherosclerotic plaques
         • Example—coronary artery thrombosis (Fig. 4-9)
  c. Composition of thrombi in muscular arteries and aortic branches
       (1) Adherent, usually occlusive, gray-white fibrin clot composed of platelets
       (2) Aspirin and other inhibitors of platelet aggregation prevent formation of these thrombi.
  d. Composition of thrombi in the heart and aorta
       (1) Laminated thrombi with alternating pale and red areas (lines of Zahn)
        (a) Pale areas are composed of platelets held together by fibrin.
        (b) Red areas are composed predominantly of RBCs.
        (c) Mixed type of thrombus
       (2) Examples of thrombi in the heart
        (a) Thrombus in left ventricle due to a transmural myocardial infarction (mural thrombus)
        (b) Thrombus in left atrium in patients with mitral stenosis complicated by atrial fibrillation
       (3) Thrombi in the aorta usually develop in aneurysms.
        • Example—abdominal aortic aneurysm

Aspirin: prevents formation of arterial thrombi

Mixed thrombus: prevented by aspirin along with anticoagulant therapy

(4) Aspirin along with anticoagulant therapy helps to prevent these types of thrombi.
   e. Clinical findings in arterial thrombosis
     (1) Infarction (e.g., acute myocardial infarction, stroke)
     (2) Embolization
  3. Postmortem clot
   a. Fibrin clot of plasma (resembles chicken fat) *without* entrapped cells
   b. It is *not* attached to the vessel wall.

V. Embolism

- Detached mass (e.g., clot, fat, gas) that is carried through the blood to a distant site

A. Pulmonary thromboembolism (see Chapter 16)

Pulmonary thromboembolism: majority originate in femoral veins

  1. Site of origin
   a. Majority originate from the femoral vein (extension of deep vein thrombus).
   b. Others originate from the pelvic veins or vena cava.
  2. Clinical findings
   a. Sudden death
    - Due to a saddle embolus occluding the major pulmonary artery branches (Fig. 4-10)
   b. Pulmonary infarction
    (1) Small thromboemboli occlude medium-sized or small pulmonary arteries.
    (2) Less than 10% of thromboemboli produce infarction.
   c. Paradoxic embolism
    - Venous thromboembolus passes through an atrial septal defect into the systemic circulation.

B. Systemic embolism

  - Emboli traveling in the arterial system
  1. Causes of systemic embolism

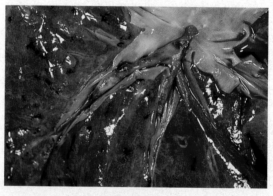

4-10: *Pulmonary embolus. The main branches of the pulmonary artery are occluded with large-caliber thromboemboli (saddle emboli). Most pulmonary thromboemboli come from the femoral vein. (From Damjanov I, Linder J: Pathology: A Color Atlas. St. Louis, Mosby, 2000, p 57, Fig. 4-26.)*

a. Thrombi from the left side of the heart (80% of cases)
   (1) Mural thrombus in left ventricle following acute myocardial infarction
   (2) Thrombus in the left atrium in mitral stenosis
      • Atrial fibrillation predisposes to atrial clot formation and embolization.
b. Atrial myxoma, vegetations from aortic or mitral valve

2. Sites of embolism
   a. Lower extremities (most common)
   b. Brain (via the middle cerebral artery)
   c. Small bowel (via the superior mesenteric artery)
   d. Spleen and kidneys

3. Clinical findings
   a. Pale infarctions in the digits, spleen, and kidneys
   b. Hemorrhagic infarctions in the brain and small bowel (see Chapter 1)

C. Fat embolism
1. Causes
   a. Most often due to traumatic fracture of the long bones (e.g., femur)
   b. Other causes include trauma to fat-laden tissues, fatty liver.

2. Pathogenesis
   a. Microglobules of fat from the bone marrow obstruct microvasculature
      • Produces ischemia and hemorrhage
   b. Fatty acids damage vessel endothelium.
      • Formation of platelet thrombi in areas of injury

3. Clinical findings
   a. Symptoms begin 24 to 72 hours after trauma.
   b. Restlessness, delirium, coma
   c. Dyspnea, tachypnea
      • Fat microglobules in pulmonary capillaries cause hypoxemia.
   d. Petechiae develop over the chest and upper extremities.
      • Due to thrombocytopenia from platelet adhesion to microglobules of fat
   e. Death results in less than 10% of cases.

D. Amniotic fluid embolism
1. Occurs during labor or immediately postpartum.
2. Pathogenesis
   a. Tears in placental membranes or uterine veins
   b. Infusion of amniotic fluid with procoagulants into the maternal circulation
3. Clinical findings
   a. Abrupt onset of dyspnea, cyanosis, hypotension, and bleeding
      (1) Dyspnea is due to pulmonary edema or acute respiratory distress syndrome.
      (2) Bleeding is due to disseminated intravascular coagulation (DIC).
      (3) Diagnosis is most often confirmed at autopsy.
         • Fetal squamous cells are present in the pulmonary vessels.
   b. Maternal mortality rate varies from 60% to 80%.

Systemic embolism: majority originate in left side of heart

Fat embolism: fracture of long bones

Amniotic fluid embolism: abrupt onset dyspnea, hypotension, bleeding (DIC)

E. Decompression sickness

- Form of gas embolism
1. Scuba and deep sea diving is the most common cause.
2. Pathogenesis
   a. Atmospheric pressure increases by 1 for every 33 ft of descent into water.
   b. Nitrogen gas is forced out of the alveoli and dissolves in blood and tissues.
   c. Rapid ascent causes nitrogen to expand and form gas bubbles in tissue and vessel lumens.
3. Clinical findings
   a. Pain develops in joints, muscles, and bones.
      - Called "the bends"
   b. Pneumothorax
      (1) Complication of a sudden rise to the surface
      (2) Due to rupture of a preexisting subpleural bleb
      (3) Causes dyspnea and pleuritic chest pain
   c. Pulmonary embolus
      (1) Pressure on the veins in the lower extremities produces stasis and thrombus formation.
      (2) Pulmonary thromboembolism occurs
      (3) Causes dyspnea and pleuritic chest pain
   d. Chronic changes
      - Aseptic necrosis in bones (femur, tibia, humerus) from bone infarctions
4. Treatment
   - Recompression (nitrogen forced into solution) followed by slow decompression

VI. Shock

- Shock is reduced perfusion of tissue, which results in impaired oxygenation of tissue.

A. Types of shock

1. Hypovolemic shock
   a. Due to excessive fluid loss (e.g., blood, sweat)
   b. Hemorrhage
      (1) Loss of greater than 20% of blood volume (~1000 mL) results in shock.
      (2) *No* initial effect on hemoglobin and hematocrit concentration
         (a) Absolute neutrophilic leukocytosis is the first hematologic sign.
         (b) Infusion of 0.9% saline immediately uncovers the RBC deficit.
      (3) Plasma is replaced first with fluid from the interstitial space.
         - Uncovers the RBC deficit within hours to days
      (4) RBC response in the bone marrow begins in 5 to 7 days.
   c. Pathophysiology of hypovolemic shock
      (1) Decreased cardiac output (CO)
         - Due to decreased volume of blood

Decompression sickness: nitrogen gas bubbles occlude vessel lumens

Pneumothorax and pulmonary embolism: complications of scuba diving

Hypovolemic shock: most often caused by blood loss

(2) Decreased left ventricular end-diastolic pressure (LVEDP)

(3) Increased peripheral vascular resistance (PVR)
  - Due to vasoconstriction of arterioles from catecholamines and angiotensin II, which are released in response to the decreased CO

d. Clinical findings in hypovolemic shock

(1) Cold, clammy skin due to vasoconstriction of skin vessels

(2) Hypotension; rapid, weak pulse (compensatory response to decreased CO)

2. Cardiogenic shock

a. Most commonly caused by an acute myocardial infarction

b. Pathophysiology of cardiogenic shock

(1) Decreased CO
  - Due to decreased force of contraction in the left ventricle

(2) Increased LVEDP
  - Blood accumulates in the left ventricle.

(3) Increased PVR
  - Same mechanism as in hypovolemic shock

c. Clinical findings in cardiogenic shock
  - Chest pain followed by signs similar to hypovolemic shock

3. Septic shock

a. Septicemia is most commonly due to gram-negative pathogens (e.g., *Escherichia coli*).

b. Pathogenesis

(1) Endotoxins damage endothelial cells.
  - Causes the release of vasodilators such as nitric oxide and prostaglandin I_2

(2) Endotoxins activate the alternative complement pathway.
  - Anaphylatoxins (C3a and C5a) are produced, which stimulate mast cell release of histamine (vasodilator)

(3) Interleukin 1 and tumor necrosis factor are released from macrophages.
  - Activate neutrophil adhesion molecules, causing neutrophil adherence to pulmonary capillaries

c. Pathophysiology of septic shock

(1) Initial increase in CO
  (a) Due to rapid blood flow through dilated arterioles, causing increased return of blood to the heart
  (b) Tissues are unable to extract oxygen, because of the increased blood flow.

(2) Decreased LVEDP
  - Due to neutrophil transmigration through the pulmonary capillaries into alveoli producing noncardiogenic pulmonary edema

(3) Decreased PVR
  - Due to vasodilation of peripheral resistance arterioles

d. Clinical findings in septic shock

(1) Warm skin, due to vasodilation of skin vessels

Hypovolemic shock: ↓ CO, ↓ LVEDP, ↑ PVR

Cardiogenic shock: most often caused by acute myocardial infarction

Cardiogenic shock: ↓ CO, ↑ LVEDP, ↑ PVR

Septic shock: most often caused by sepsis due to E. coli

Septic shock (initial phase): ↑ CO, ↓ LVEDP, ↓ PVR

TABLE 4-11: Summary of Pathophysiologic Findings in Hypovolemic, Cardiogenic, and Septic Shock

Type	CO	PVR	LVEDP
Hypovolemic	↓	↑	↓
Cardiogenic	↓	↑	↑
Endotoxic (septic)	↑	↓	↓

CO, cardiac output; LVEDP, left ventricular end-diastolic pressure; PVR, peripheral vascular resistance.

      (2) Bounding pulse, due to increased CO
      (3) Acute respiratory distress syndrome
         • Due to neutrophil transmigration into alveoli
      (4) Disseminated intravascular coagulation
         • Due to activation of the intrinsic and extrinsic coagulation system
    4. Summary of pathophysiologic findings in shock (Table 4-11)
B. Complications associated with shock
    1. Ischemic acute tubular necrosis
      • Coagulation necrosis of proximal tubule cells and cells in the thick ascending limb
    2. Multiorgan dysfunction
      • Most common cause of death
    3. Lactic acidosis due to tissue hypoxia

Multiorgan dysfunction: most common cause of death in shock

5 CHAPTER

Genetic and Developmental Disorders

I. Mutations
- Mutations are a permanent change in DNA.

A. Point mutations
- Mutation involving a change in a single nucleotide base within a gene
1. Silent mutation
   - Altered DNA codes for the *same* amino acid without changing the phenotypic effect
2. Missense mutation
   - Altered DNA codes for a *different* amino acid, which changes the phenotypic effect

> In both sickle cell trait and sickle cell disease, a missense mutation occurs when adenine replaces thymidine, causing valine to replace glutamic acid in the sixth position of the β-globin chain. As a result, RBCs spontaneously sickle in the peripheral blood if the amount of sickle hemoglobin is greater than 60%.

Missense mutation: sickle cell disease/trait

3. Nonsense mutation
   - Altered DNA codes for a stop codon that causes premature termination of protein synthesis

> In β-thalassemia major, a nonsense mutation produces a stop codon that causes premature termination of DNA transcription of the β-globin chain. Consequently, there is a marked decrease in the synthesis of hemoglobin A ($\alpha_2\beta_2$), resulting in a microcytic anemia.

β-Thalassemia major: nonsense mutation with stop codon

B. Frameshift mutation
1. Insertion or deletion of one or more nucleotides shifts the reading frame of the DNA strand
2. Example—in Tay-Sachs disease, a four-base insertion results in the synthesis of a defective lysosomal enzyme (hexosaminidase).

Frameshift mutation: Tay-Sachs disease

C. Trinucleotide repeat disorders
1. Errors in DNA replication
   - Cause amplification of a sequence of three nucleotides (e.g., CAG), which disrupts gene function
2. Associated with anticipation
   a. Increasing severity of clinical disease in each successive generation

Anticipation: additional trinucleotide repeats increases disease severity in future generations

b. Caused by the addition of more trinucleotide sequences during gametogenesis

c. Female carriers may be symptomatic
- Occurs if they have more paternally (than maternally) derived X chromosomes with trinucleotide repeats

d. Examples—fragile X syndrome, Huntington's disease, Friedreich's ataxia, myotonic dystrophy

II. Mendelian Disorders
- Usually single-gene mutations

A. Autosomal recessive (AR) disorders

1. Inheritance pattern (Fig. 5-1)

   a. Individuals must be homozygous for the mutant recessive gene (aa) to express the disorder.

   b. Homozygotes are symptomatic early in life.

   c. Heterozygous individuals (Aa) are asymptomatic carriers.
   - The dominant gene (A) overrides the mutant recessive gene (a).

   d. Both parents must be heterozygous to transmit the disorder.
   - Example—Aa × Aa → AA, Aa, Aa, aa (25% without disorder; 50% asymptomatic carriers; 25% with disorder)

   > Cystic fibrosis (CF) is an AR disorder with a carrier rate of 1/25. To calculate the prevalence of CF in the population, the number of couples at risk of having a child with CF (1/25 × 1/25, or 1/625) is multiplied by the chance of having a child with CF (1/4). Prevalence of CF = 1/625 × 1/4, or 1/2500

2. AR protein defects (Table 5-1)

3. Inborn errors of metabolism (Table 5-2)

   a. Most metabolic disorders are due to an enzyme deficiency.

Most common type of mendelian disorder: autosomal recessive

AR inheritance: both parents must have mutant gene.

Most AR disorders involve enzyme deficiencies.

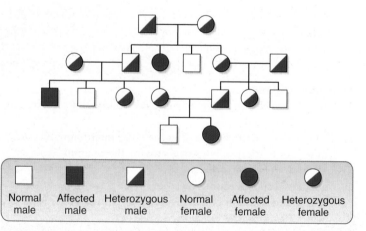

| Normal male | Affected male | Heterozygous male | Normal female | Affected female | Heterozygous female |

5-1: Pedigree of an autosomal recessive disorder. Both parents must have the mutant gene to transmit the disorder to their children. On average, 25% of the children of heterozygous parents are normal, 50% are asymptomatic heterozygous carriers, and 25% have the disorder.

TABLE 5-1: Protein Defects Associated with Selected Mendelian Disorders

Protein Type	Specific Protein	Disorder	Inheritance Pattern
Enzyme	C1 esterase inhibitor deficiency	Hereditary angioedema	Autosomal dominant
	Glucose-6-phosphate dehydrogenase	Glucose-6-phosphate dehydrogenase deficiency	X-linked recessive
Structural	Sickle hemoglobin	Sickle cell disease	Autosomal recessive
	Ankyrin	Hereditary spherocytosis	Autosomal dominant
	Dystrophin	Duchenne's muscular dystrophy	X-linked recessive
Transport	Cystic fibrosis transmembrane regulator	Cystic fibrosis	Autosomal recessive
Receptor	Low-density lipoprotein receptor	Familial hypercholesterolemia	Autosomal dominant
Growth regulating	Neurofibromin	Neurofibromatosis	Autosomal dominant
Hemostasis	Factor VIII	Hemophilia A	X-linked recessive

    b. Substrate and intermediates proximal to the enzyme block increase.
    c. Intermediates and the end product distal to the enzyme block decrease.

> Phenylketonuria (PKU) is characterized by a deficiency of phenylalanine hydroxylase, causing an increase in the substrate phenylalanine and a decrease in the product tyrosine. In individuals with PKU, phenylalanine is further metabolized into neurotoxic phenylketones and acids that produce mental retardation and urine with a musty odor.

PKU: ↑ phenylalanine, ↓ tyrosine

    d. Glycogenoses
      (1) Pathogenesis
        (a) Increase in glycogen synthesis (e.g., von Gierke's disease)
        (b) Inhibition of glycogenolysis (e.g., debranching enzyme deficiency)
        (c) Increase in normal or structurally abnormal glycogen
      (2) Clinical findings
        (a) Organ dysfunction (e.g., restrictive heart disease, Pompe's disease).
        (b) Fasting hypoglycemia
          • Decrease in gluconeogenesis (e.g., glucose-6-phosphatase deficiency, von Gierke's disease) or liver glycogenolysis (e.g., liver phosphorylase deficiency)
    e. Lysosomal storage diseases (Table 5-3)
      • Enzyme deficiencies lead to accumulation of undigested substrates (e.g., glycosaminoglycans, sphingolipids) in lysosomes.

Von Gierke's disease: glucose-6-phosphatase deficiency (gluconeogenic enzyme)

**TABLE 5-2:
Selected Inborn
Errors of
Metabolism**

Error of Metabolism	Deficient Enzyme	Accumulated Substrate(s)	Comments
Alkaptonuria	Homogentisate oxidase	Homogentisate	Black urine and cartilage, degenerative arthritis
Galactosemia	Galactose 1-phosphate-uridyltransferase (GALT)	Galactose 1-phosphate	Mental retardation, cirrhosis, hypoglycemia Avoid dairy products
Hereditary fructose intolerance	Aldolase B	Fructose 1-phosphate	Cirrhosis, hypoglycemia, renal disease Avoid fructose, sucrose, honey
Homocystinuria	Cystathionine synthase	Homocysteine and methionine	Mental retardation, vessel thrombosis
Maple syrup urine disease	Branched chain α-ketoacid dehydrogenase	Leucine, valine, isoleucine, and their ketoacids	Mental retardation, seizures, feeding problems, sweet-smelling urine
McArdle's disease	Muscle phosphorylase	Glycogen	Glycogenosis, muscle fatigue; no increase in lactic acid with exercise
Phenylketonuria (PKU)	Phenylalanine hydroxylase	Phenylalanine	Mental retardation, microcephaly, decreased tyrosine Restrict phenylalanine; avoid artificial sweeteners containing phenylalanine
Pompe's disease	α-1,4-Glucosidase (lysosomal enzyme)	Glycogen	Glycogenosis, cardiomegaly with early death
Von Gierke's disease	Glucose-6-phosphatase (gluconeogenic enzyme)	Glucose-6-phosphate	Glycogenosis, enlarged liver and kidneys, hypoglycemia (no increase in glucose with glucagon challenge)

Most common AR disorder: hemochromatosis

4. Other AR disorders
   • Hemochromatosis, 21-hydroxylase deficiency, Wilson's disease, thalassemia
B. **Autosomal dominant (AD) disorders**
   1. Inheritance pattern
      a. One dominant mutant gene (A) is required to express the disorder.
         (1) Heterozygotes (Aa) express the disorder.
         (2) Homozygotes (AA) are often spontaneously aborted.
         (3) Example—Aa × aa → Aa, Aa, aa, aa (50% with disorder; 50% without disorder)
      b. Some disorders arise by new mutations involving either an egg or a sperm.
   2. AD protein defects (see Table 5-1)
      • Enzyme deficiencies are relatively uncommon.

AD inheritance: heterozygotes with dominant mutant gene express disease

TABLE 5-3:
Selected Lysosomal
Storage Disorders

Disorder	Deficient Enzyme	Accumulated Substrate	Clinical Findings
Gaucher's disease (adult type)	Glucocerebrosidase	Glucocerebroside	Hepatosplenomegaly; fibrillar appearing macrophages in liver, spleen, and bone marrow
Hurler's syndrome	α-L-Iduronidase	Dermatan and heparan sulfate	Mental retardation, coarse facial features, corneal clouding, coronary artery disease X-linked recessive form (Hunter's syndrome) is milder
Niemann-Pick disease	Sphingomyelinase	Sphingomyelin	Mental retardation, hepatosplenomegaly, foamy macrophages
Tay-Sachs disease	Hexosaminidase	GM_2 ganglioside	Mental retardation, muscle weakness, cherry-red macula, blindness

3. Characteristics
   a. Delayed manifestations of disease
      (1) Symptoms and signs may *not* occur early in life.
      (2) Example—in adult polycystic kidney disease, cysts are *not* present at birth.
   b. Penetrance
      (1) Complete penetrance (Fig. 5-2A)
         • All individuals with the mutant gene express the disorder (e.g., familial polyposis).
      (2) Reduced penetrance (Fig. 5-2B)
         (a) Individuals with the mutant gene are phenotypically normal.
         (b) They transmit the disorder to their offspring (e.g., Marfan syndrome).
   c. Variable expressivity
      • All individuals with the mutant gene express the disorder but at different levels of severity.
4. Other AD disorders
   • Huntington's disease, osteogenesis imperfecta, achondroplasia, tuberous sclerosis

C. **X-linked recessive (XR) disorders**
   1. Inheritance pattern (Fig. 5-3)
      a. Males must have the mutant recessive gene on the X chromosome to express the disorder.
      b. Affected males (XY) transmit the mutant gene to all of their daughters.
         (1) Males are homozygous for the mutant gene.
         (2) Example—XY × XX → XX, XX, XY, XY
         (3) Daughters (XX) are usually asymptomatic carriers.

Reduced penetrance: individual with mutant gene does *not* express the disease

Most common AD disorder: von Willebrand disease

XR inheritance: asymptomatic female carrier transmits mutant gene to 50% of sons

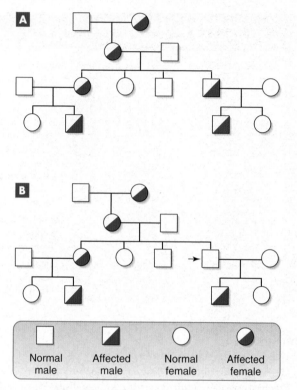

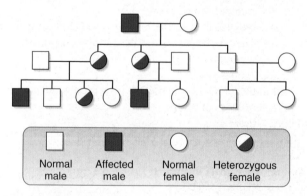

5-2: *Pedigrees showing complete and reduced penetrance in an autosomal dominant disorder. Complete penetrance (**A**) means that all individuals with the mutant gene express the disorder. Reduced penetrance (**B**) means that an individual has the mutant gene but does not express the disorder (arrow). The unaffected father has transmitted the disorder to his son.*

5-3: *Pedigree of an X-linked recessive disorder. The affected male transmits the mutant gene on the X chromosome to both of his daughters and none of his sons. Both daughters are asymptomatic heterozygous carriers of the mutant gene. The daughter with four children has transmitted the mutant gene to 50% of her sons.*

    c. Asymptomatic female carriers ($\underline{X}$ mutant gene) transmit the disorder to 50% of their male offspring.
- Example—$\underline{X}X \times XY \rightarrow \underline{X}X, XX, \underline{X}Y, XY$

    d. In rare cases, female carriers can be symptomatic.
      (1) Maternally derived X chromosomes (without the mutant gene) are preferentially inactivated.
- Only paternally derived X chromosomes with the mutant gene remain.

      (2) Offspring of a symptomatic male and asymptomatic female carrier
- Example—$\underline{X}X \times \underline{X}Y \rightarrow \underline{X}X, \underline{X}X, \underline{X}Y, XY$

    e. Some XR disorders may arise as new mutations.

2. XR protein defects (see Table 5-1)
- Enzymes are the most common type of protein affected in XR disorders.

3. Fragile X syndrome
    a. Trinucleotide repeat disorder
    b. Clinical findings
      (1) Mental retardation
        (a) Most common mendelian disorder that causes mental retardation
        (b) 50% of female carriers may develop mental retardation.
      (2) Phenotypic changes
- Long face, large mandible, everted ears

      (3) Macro-orchidism (enlarged testes) at puberty
    c. Diagnosis
      (1) DNA analysis to identify trinucleotide repeats (best test)
      (2) Fragile X chromosome study

> Most common X-linked disorder: fragile X syndrome

4. Lesch-Nyhan syndrome
    a. Deficiency of hypoxanthine-guanine phosphoribosyltransferase (HGPRT)
- Normally involved in salvaging the purines hypoxanthine and guanine

    b. Clinical findings
- Mental retardation, hyperuricemia, self-mutilation

5. Other XR disorders
- Testicular feminization, chronic granulomatous disease, Bruton's agammaglobulinemia

D. X-linked dominant (XD) disorders

1. Inheritance pattern
- Same as XR *except* the dominant mutant gene causes disease in males and females (Fig. 5-4)

2. Vitamin D–resistant rickets
    a. Defect in renal and gastrointestinal reabsorption of phosphate
    b. Causes defective bone mineralization (i.e., osteomalacia)

3. Alport's syndrome
- Hereditary glomerulonephritis with nerve deafness

> XD inheritance: female carriers are symptomatic

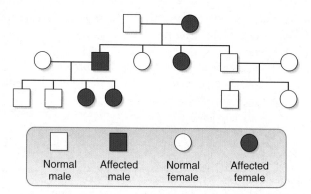

5-4: *Pedigree of an X-linked dominant disorder. In these rare disorders, female carriers and males with the mutant dominant gene express the disorder. The distribution is similar to that of X-linked recessive disorders, except that carrier females are symptomatic.*

III. Chromosomal Disorders

A. General considerations

1. Most human cells are diploid (46 chromosomes).
   a. Autosomes: 22 pairs
   b. Sex chromosomes (XX in females and XY in males): 1 pair
2. Gametes, the products of meiosis, are haploid (23 chromosomes).
3. Lyon hypothesis
   a. In females, one of the two X chromosomes is randomly inactivated.
      • Inactivation occurs in the embryonic period of development.
   b. The inactivated X chromosome is called a Barr body.
      (1) It is attached to the nuclear membrane of cells.
      (2) They are visible in squamous cells obtained by scraping the buccal mucosa.
   c. Normal females have one Barr body, and normal males have none.
   d. Inactivation accounts for the parental derivation of the X chromosomes in females.
      • ~50% of X chromosomes are paternal and ~50% are maternal.

B. Chromosomal alterations
   • Numeric or structural abnormalities of autosomes or sex chromosomes
1. Nondisjunction
   a. Unequal separation of chromosomes in the first phase of meiosis
   b. Results in 22 or 24 chromosomes in the egg or sperm
   c. Examples—Turner's syndrome (22 + 23 = 45 chromosomes), Down syndrome (24 + 23 = 47 chromosomes, trisomy)
2. Mosaicism
   a. Nondisjunction of chromosomes during mitotic division in the early embryonic period
   b. Two chromosomally different cell lines are derived from a single fertilized egg.
   c. Most often involves sex chromosomes (e.g., Turner's syndrome)

Number of Barr bodies = number of X chromosomes − 1

Nondisjunction: unequal separation of chromosomes in meiosis

Mosaicism: nondisjunction in mitosis

3. Translocation
   a. Transfer of chromosome parts between nonhomologous chromosomes
   b. Balanced translocation
      • Translocated fragment is functional.
   c. Robertsonian translocation
      • Balanced translocation between two acrocentric chromosomes (e.g., chromosomes 14 and 21)

> In a form of Down syndrome, the mother of an affected child has 45 (not 46) chromosomes because of a robertsonian translocation between the long arms of chromosomes 21 and 14, producing one long chromosome (14;21). The mother also has one chromosome 14 and one chromosome 21. The father has the normal 46 chromosomes. The affected child has 46 chromosomes with three functional 21 chromosomes including chromosome (14;21) and chromosome 21 from the mother and chromosome 14 and chromosome 21 from the father (Fig. 5-5).

4. Deletion
   a. Loss of a portion of a chromosome
   b. Cri du chat syndrome
      (1) Loss of the short arm of chromosome 5
      (2) Clinical findings
         • Mental retardation, cat-like cry, ventricular septal defect

Cri du chat syndrome: deletion short arm chromosome 5

C. **Disorders involving autosomes**
   1. Down syndrome

Mother

45 chromosomes

Father

46 chromosomes

**Down syndrome
46 chromosomes**

5-5: *Robertsonian translocation. See text for description.*

Down syndrome: most cases due to nondisjunction

a. Causes
   (1) Nondisjunction (95% of cases, trisomy 21)
   (2) Robertsonian translocation (4% of cases)
   (3) Mosaicism (1% of cases)
b. Risk factors
   (1) Increased maternal age is a risk factor.
   (2) Occurs in 1 in 25 live births in women over 45 years of age
c. Clinical findings
   (1) General

Most common genetic cause of mental retardation: Down syndrome

   (a) Most common genetic cause of mental retardation
   (b) Epicanthic folds, flat facial profile, macroglossia (Fig. 5-6A)
   (c) Simian crease (Fig. 5-6B)
   (2) Combined atrial and ventricular septal defects (cushion defects)
      • Major factor affecting survival in early childhood
   (3) Increased risk of Hirschsprung's disease and duodenal atresia
   (4) Increased risk of leukemia
      (a) Acute megakaryocytic leukemia (<3 years of age)
      (b) Acute lymphoblastic leukemia (>3 years of age)
   (5) Alzheimer's disease by 35 years of age in most cases
      • Major factor affecting survival in older individuals
   (6) Sterility in all males
   (7) Females have a 50% chance of having a child with Down syndrome.
2. Edwards' syndrome
   a. Trisomy 18
   b. Clinical findings
      (1) Mental retardation
      (2) Clenched hands with overlapping fingers
      (3) Ventricular septal defect (VSD)
      (4) Early death
3. Patau's syndrome
   a. Trisomy 13
   b. Clinical findings
      (1) Mental retardation
      (2) Cleft lip and palate

Advanced maternal age: increased risk for bearing offspring with trisomy syndromes

      (3) Polydactyly, VSD, cystic kidneys
      (4) Early death
D. **Disorders involving sex chromosomes**
   1. Turner's syndrome
      a. Causes
         (1) Nondisjunction
            • 45,X karyotype (~60% of cases)
         (2) Mosaicism
            • 45,X/46,XX karyotype (~40% of cases)

Turner's syndrome: 45,X karyotype

      b. Clinical and laboratory findings
         (1) Short stature
            (a) Cardinal finding

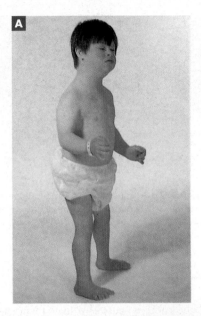

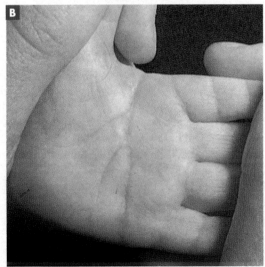

5-6: *Down syndrome. The facial profile (**A**) shows a short stature, small head with small nose and ears. The hand (**B**) shows a single palmar (simian) crease. (From Forbes C, Jackson W: Color Atlas and Text of Clinical Medicine, 2nd ed. St. Louis, Mosby, 2003, Figs. 7-168 and 7-172.)*

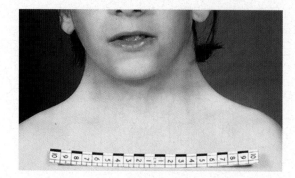

5-7: *Turner's syndrome is characterized by a webbed neck. Other findings include short stature, primary amenorrhea, and delayed secondary sex characteristics (e.g., underdeveloped breasts). (From Bouloux P-M: Self-Assessment Picture Tests: Medicine, vol. 1. St. Louis, Mosby, 1996, p 45.)*

Most common genetic cause of primary amenorrhea: Turner's syndrome

Turner's syndrome: "menopause before menarche"

        (b) Normal growth hormone and insulin-like growth factor
    (2) Lymphedema in hands and feet in infancy
       • Webbed neck is caused by dilated lymphatic channels (cystic hygroma) (Fig. 5-7).
    (3) Preductal coarctation and bicuspid aortic valve
    (4) Streak gonads
       (a) Ovaries replaced by fibrous stroma
       (b) Ovaries devoid of oocytes by 2 years of age
         • All patients with a 45X karyotype are infertile.
       (c) Increased risk for developing ovarian dysgerminoma
    (5) Primary amenorrhea with delayed sexual maturation
       (a) Decreased estradiol
       (b) Increased follicle-stimulating hormone (FSH) and luteinizing hormone (LH)
    (6) Normal intelligence, horseshoe kidney, hypothyroidism
    (7) No Barr bodies
  2. Klinefelter's syndrome
    a. Cause
      (1) Nondisjunction
      (2) XXY karyotype
    b. Clinical and laboratory findings (Fig. 5-8)
      (1) Female secondary sex characteristics at puberty
       (a) Persistent gynecomastia
       (b) Soft skin
       (c) Female hair distribution
      (2) Delayed sexual maturation (hypogonadism)
       (a) Testicular atrophy (decreased testicular volume)
       (b) Fibrosis of seminiferous tubules
         • Absence of spermatogenesis (azoospermia); loss of Sertoli cells
       (c) Leydig cell hyperplasia

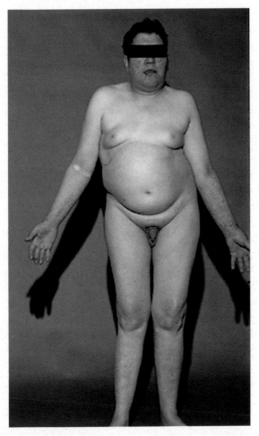

5-8: *Klinefelter's syndrome is characterized by female secondary sex characteristics, including gynecomastia (breast development) and a female distribution of pubic hair. The legs are disproportionately long. (From Bouloux P-M: Self-Assessment Picture Tests: Medicine, vol. 1. St. Louis, Mosby, 1996, p 82.)*

      (3) Disproportionately long legs, learning disabilities

      (4) Decreased inhibin (loss of Sertoli cells)

         (a) Causes increased FSH (loss of negative feedback with inhibin)

         (b) Increased FSH causes increased synthesis of aromatase in Leydig cells.

      (5) Decreased testosterone

         (a) Aromatase converts testosterone to estradiol; estradiol causes feminization.

         (b) Increased LH (loss of negative feedback with testosterone)

      (6) One Barr body

   3. XYY syndrome

     a. Caused by paternal nondisjunction

     b. Associated with aggressive (sometimes criminal) behavior

     c. Normal gonadal function

> Klinefelter's syndrome: ↓ testosterone and inhibin; ↑ LH and FSH, respectively

Polygenic disorders are more common than mendelian and chromosomal disorders.

IV. **Other Patterns of Inheritance**
A. **Multifactorial (polygenic) inheritance**
   1. Combination of multiple minor gene mutations plus environmental factors
   2. Examples of multifactorial inheritance
      a. Open neural tube defects
         • Associated with decreased maternal folate levels
      b. Type 2 diabetes mellitus
         • Associated with obesity, which down-regulates insulin receptor synthesis
B. **Mitochondrial DNA disorders (Fig. 5-9)**
   1. Function of mitochondrial DNA
      • Codes for enzymes involved in mitochondrial oxidative phosphorylation reactions
   2. Inheritance pattern
      a. Affected females transmit the mutant gene to all their children.
         • Ova contain mitochondria with the mutant gene.
      b. Affected males do *not* transmit the mutant gene to any of their children.
         • Sperm lose their mitochondria during fertilization.
   3. Examples—Leber's hereditary optic neuropathy, myoclonic epilepsy
C. **Genomic imprinting**
   1. Inheritance pattern
      a. Inheritance depends on whether the mutant gene is of maternal or paternal origin.
      b. Examples—Prader-Willi syndrome and Angelman syndrome
   2. Pathogenesis
      a. Normal changes in maternal chromosome 15 during gametogenesis
         (1) Prader-Willi gene is inactivated by methylation (imprinted).
         (2) Angelman gene is demethylated (activated).
      b. Normal changes in paternal chromosome 15 during gametogenesis
         (1) Prader-Willi gene is demethylated (activated).

Mitochondrial DNA disorders: associated with maternal inheritance

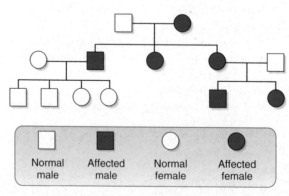

| Normal male | Affected male | Normal female | Affected female |

5-9: *Pedigree showing transmission of mitochondrial DNA. Affected females transmit the disorder to all their children, whereas affected males do not.*

        (2) Angelman gene is imprinted (inactivated).
    c. Microdeletion of the entire gene site on paternal chromosome 15
        (1) Causes Prader-Willi syndrome
        (2) Complete loss of Prader-Willi gene activity
            (a) Loss of activated Prader-Willi gene on paternal chromosome 15
            (b) Inactivated Prader-Willi gene on maternal chromosome 15
    d. Microdeletion of the entire gene site on maternal chromosome 15
        (1) Causes Angelman syndrome
        (2) Complete loss of Angelman gene activity
            (a) Loss of activated Angelman gene on maternal chromosome 15
            (b) Inactivated Angelman gene on paternal chromosome 15
3. Clinical findings in Prader-Willi syndrome (Fig. 5-10)
    a. Mental retardation, short stature, hypotonia at birth
    b. Obesity (tendency to overeat), hypogonadism
4. Clinical findings in Angelman syndrome (Fig. 5-11)
    a. Mental retardation
    b. Wide-based gait (resembles a marionette)
    c. Inappropriate laughter ("happy puppet" syndrome)

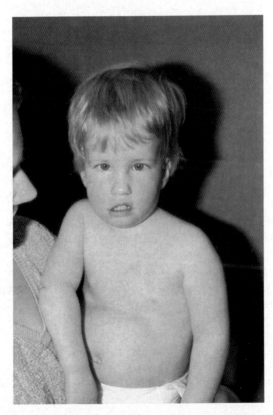

5-10: *Prader-Willi syndrome. The patient was hypotonic at birth. He is mentally retarded and has a tendency for overeating. (From Behrman RE, Kliegman RM, Jenson HB: Nelson Textbook of Pediatrics, 17th ed. Philadelphia, WB Saunders, 2004, Fig. 68-2B.)*

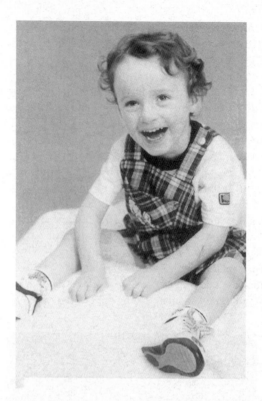

5-11: *Angelman syndrome. The child has frequent outbursts of laughing ("happy puppet" syndrome). (From Behrman RE, Kliegman RM, Jenson HB: Nelson Textbook of Pediatrics, 17th ed. Philadelphia, WB Saunders, 2004, Fig. 68-2C.)*

V. Disorders of Sex Differentiation
A. Normal sex differentiation
  1. Absence of the Y chromosome
     a. Germinal tissue differentiates into ovaries.
     b. Wolffian (mesonephric) duct structures undergo apoptosis.
  2. Presence of the Y chromosome
     a. Germinal tissue differentiates into testes.
     b. Müllerian inhibitory factor (MIF) causes müllerian tissue to undergo apoptosis.
        • MIF is synthesized in the Sertoli cells.
     c. Function of fetal testosterone
        (1) Develops the wolffian duct structures
        (2) Epididymis, seminal vesicles, vas deferens
     d. 5α-Reductase converts testosterone to dihydrotestosterone (DHT).
     e. Functions of fetal DHT
        (1) Develops the prostate gland
        (2) Develops the external male genitalia
           • Genitalia is phenotypically female before DHT is produced.

Y chromosome: determines the genetic sex of an individual

B. True hermaphrodite
  1. Fetus has both male and female gonads.
  2. Karyotype is usually 46,XX
C. Pseudohermaphrodite
  1. Phenotype and genotype do *not* match.
  2. Male pseudohermaphrodite
     a. Genotypic male (XY with testes)
     b. Phenotypic female
     c. Example—testicular feminization
  3. Female pseudohermaphrodite
     a. Genotypic female (XX with ovaries)
     b. Phenotypic male
     c. Example—virilization in adrenogenital syndrome
D. Testicular feminization (Fig. 5-12)
  1. XR disorder with a deficiency of androgen receptors
     • Fetal DHT and testosterone are unable to function without a receptor.
  2. Clinical and laboratory findings
     a. Testicles are present in the inguinal canal or abdominal cavity.
     b. Müllerian structures are absent because MIF is present.
        • Absence of fallopian tubes, uterus, cervix, upper vagina
     c. Male accessory structures are absent
        • *No* testosterone effect on the wolffian duct structures
     d. External genitalia remain female
        (1) *No* DHT effect
        (2) Vagina ends as a blind pouch.
     e. Hormone levels
        (1) Normal male levels of testosterone and DHT
        (2) Estrogen activity is unopposed, because estrogen receptors are present.
  3. Majority of patients are reared female.

VI. Congenital Anomalies
  • Defects present at birth that may or may not have a genetic basis.
A. Types of errors in morphogenesis
  1. Malformations
     a. Disturbances in the morphogenesis (development) of an organ
     b. Occur between the third and ninth weeks of embryogenesis
        • Most susceptible period is fourth to fifth weeks
     c. Causes
        • Multifactorial (e.g., drugs, infection)
     d. Examples—open neural tube defects, congenital heart disease, cleft lip/palate
  2. Deformations
     a. Extrinsic disturbances in fetal development
     b. Occur between the ninth week and term after fetal organs have developed

Testicular feminization:
most common
cause of male
pseudohermaphroditism

Testicular feminization:
deficiency of androgen
receptors

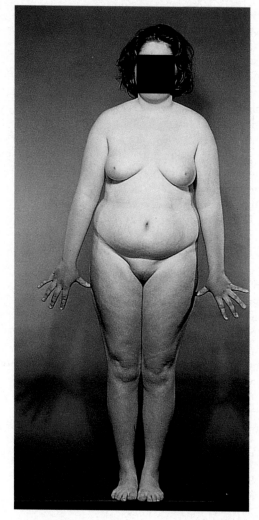

5-12: *Testicular feminization. The patient is genotypically male, but phenotypically female. The vagina ended as a blind pouch. (From Forbes C, Jackson W: Color Atlas and Text of Clinical Medicine, 2nd ed. St. Louis, Mosby, 2003, p 321, Fig. 7-55.)*

c. Most often due to restricted movement in uterine cavity
   • Examples—oligohydramnios, uterus with leiomyomas, twin pregnancies

> Oligohydramnios (decreased amniotic fluid) from decreased production of fetal urine (e.g., renal agenesis, cystic disease of the kidneys) restricts fetal movement in the uterine cavity. As a result, newborns have flat facial features (Potter's facies), underdevelopment of the chest wall, and clubfeet.

3. Agenesis
    a. Complete absence of an organ resulting from absence of the anlage (primordial tissue)
    b. Example—renal agenesis
4. Aplasia
    a. Anlage is present but *never* develops.
    b. Example—lung aplasia with tissue containing rudimentary ducts and connective tissue
5. Hypoplasia
    a. Anlage develops incompletely, but the tissue is histologically normal.
    b. Example—microcephaly
6. Atresia
    a. Incomplete formation of a lumen
    b. Example—duodenal atresia

B. Causes of congenital anomalies
1. Majority are unknown
2. Multifactorial
    • Combination of genetic and environmental factors
3. Environmental factors
    a. Maternal disorders
        (1) Diabetes mellitus
            (a) Increased risk of neural tube defects and congenital heart disease
            (b) Maternal hyperglycemia causes fetal macrosomia.
                • Hyperinsulinemia in the fetus increases muscle mass and stores of fat in the adipose tissue.
        (2) Systemic lupus erythematosus
            • Newborn may develop congenital heart block if the mother has anti-Ro antibodies.
        (3) Hypothyroidism
            • Newborn may develop cretinism.
    b. Drugs and chemicals (Table 5-4)
    c. Congenital infections (Table 5-5)
        (1) Newborn has an increase in cord blood IgM.
            • IgM normally is *not* synthesized in the fetus unless there is a congenital infection.

Most common pathogen causing a congenital infection: cytomegalovirus

Teratogen	Defect
Alcohol	Mental retardation, microcephaly, atrial septal defect
Cocaine	Microcephaly, renal agenesis, congenital heart disease
Diethylstilbestrol	Vaginal or cervical clear cell carcinoma, müllerian defects
Phenytoin	Nail and distal phalanx hypoplasia, cleft lip and/or palate
Retinoic acid	Craniofacial, central nervous system, and cardiovascular defects
Thalidomide	Amelia (absent limbs), phocomelia (seal-like limbs)
Tobacco	Intrauterine growth retardation, low birth weight
Valproate	Neural tube defects
Warfarin	Nasal hypoplasia, agenesis corpus callosum

**TABLE 5-4:
Teratogens Associated with Congenital Defects**

**TABLE 5-5:
Congenital
Infections
Associated with
Congenital Defects**

Infection	Transmission	Clinical Findings
Cytomegalovirus	Transplacental	Deafness, IUGR, CNS calcification (periventricular), microcephaly Culture urine (best fluid to culture); urine cytologic test shows intranuclear inclusions
Parvovirus B19	Transplacental	In utero hydrops fetalis
Herpes simplex type 2	Birth canal	IUGR, vesicular lesions
Rubella	Transplacental	Deafness, patent ductus arteriosus, cataract
Syphilis	Transplacental	Occurs after 20 weeks' gestation Hepatitis, saddle nose, blindness, peg teeth
Toxoplasmosis	Transplacental	Blindness, CNS calcification (basal ganglia) Pregnant woman should avoid cat litter
Varicella	Transplacental	Limb defects, mental retardation, blindness

CNS, central nervous system; IUGR, intrauterine growth retardation.

TORCH syndrome =
*toxoplasmosis, other
agents, rubella,
cytomegalovirus, herpes
simplex virus*

    (2) Vertical transmission; routes of transmission:
        (a) Transplacental (most common route)
        (b) Birth canal
        (c) Breast-feeding

C. Pathogenesis of congenital anomalies
    1. Timing of teratogenic insult
      a. Malformations occur during the embryonic period (between third and ninth weeks).
      b. Deformations occur during the fetal period (ninth week to term).
    2. Alterations during key steps in morphogenesis
      a. Mutations may occur in genes normally involved in morphogenesis.
        • Example—mutations of the *HOX* gene alters development of craniofacial structures.

> Pregnant women should *not* be treated for acne with retinoic acid. Retinoic acid disrupts the function of the *HOX* gene, leading to craniofacial, central nervous system, and cardiovascular defects.

      b. Alterations in cell proliferation, migration, and apoptosis

VII. Selected Perinatal and Infant Disorders
    A. Stillbirth
      1. Birth of a dead child
      2. Most often caused by an abruptio placentae
        • Premature separation of the placenta because of a retroplacental blood clot

Stillbirth: most often
caused by abruptio
placentae

    B. Spontaneous abortion
      1. Termination of a pregnancy before 20 weeks
      2. Caused by a fetal karyotypic abnormality
        • Usually trisomy 16 in ~50% of cases

Spontaneous abortion:
frequently caused by
trisomy 16

    3. Predisposing factors

      a. Advanced maternal age

      b. Infections (e.g., *Streptococcus agalactiae, Listeria monocytogenes*)

      c. Tobacco, alcohol use

C. Sudden infant death syndrome (SIDS)

  • Sudden and unexpected death of an infant before 1 year of age whose death remains unexplained after autopsy

    1. Epidemiology

      a. Most common cause of death of an infant younger than 1 year old in developed countries

      b. Most deaths occur between 2 and 4 months of age.

        • 90% occur in infants under 6 months

      c. Death usually occurs during sleep.

    2. Pathogenesis

      a. No single cause

      b. Maternal factors

        • Examples—smoking, young age

      c. Infant factors

        • Examples—prematurity, sleeping prone, neural developmental delay, inborn error of oxidation of fatty acids

    3. Autopsy findings

      • Nonspecific signs of tissue hypoxia are present.

      a. Thickened pulmonary arteries

      b. Petechiae on the pleura and epicardium

      c. Microscopic changes of hypoxia in the brainstem (e.g., arcuate nucleus)

D. Prematurity and intrauterine growth retardation (IUGR)

    1. Newborn classification based on weight and gestational age

      a. Appropriate for gestational age (AGA)

      b. Small for gestational age (SGA)

        • Highest mortality rate

      c. Large for gestational age (LGA)

        • Usually due to maternal diabetes mellitus

    2. Prematurity

      a. Gestational age less than 37 weeks

        • Usually weigh less than 2500 g

      b. Most common cause of neonatal death and morbidity

      c. Risk factors

        (1) Premature rupture of membranes

        (2) Chorioamnionitis (e.g., *Streptococcus agalactiae*)

        (3) Placental abnormalities

        (4) Twin pregnancies

      d. Complications

        (1) Respiratory distress syndrome (RDS, decreased surfactant)

        (2) Necrotizing enterocolitis (intestinal ischemia)

        (3) Intraventricular hemorrhage

> SIDS: majority of deaths occur before age 6 months

> LGA: most often due to maternal diabetes

> Prematurity: most common cause neonatal mortality/morbidity

3. IUGR usually occurs in SGA infants.
   a. Maternal factors
     (1) Most common cause of IUGR in SGA infants
     (2) Examples—preeclampsia, diabetes mellitus, drug addiction, alcoholism, smoking
   b. Fetal causes
     (1) Chromosomal disorders, congenital malformations, congenital infections
     (2) Symmetric growth retardation
       • Affects all organ systems equally
   c. Placental causes
     (1) Abruptio placentae, placental infarction
     (2) Asymmetric growth retardation
       • Example—the brain is spared relative to visceral organs such as the liver.

E. Neonatal period
  1. First 4 weeks of life
  2. Majority of deaths in childhood occur during this period.
  3. Common causes of death include RDS and congenital anomalies.

VIII. Diagnosis of Genetic and Developmental Disorders
  A. Amniocentesis
    • Used to identify prenatal genetic defects
  B. Ultrasound
    • Used to rule out neural tube defects
  C. Maternal triple marker screen
    1. α-Fetoprotein (AFP)
      a. Increased in neural tube defects
      b. Causally related to folate deficiency prior to conception.
    2. Human chorionic gonadotropin (hCG)
      • Levels vary with gestational age.
    3. Urine for unconjugated estriol
      • Excellent marker of fetal, placental, or maternal dysfunction
    4. Triple marker findings in Down syndrome
      a. AFP decreased
      b. hCG increased
      c. Urine estriol decreased
  D. Genetic analysis
    1. Chromosome karyotyping
      • Identifies numeric and structural abnormalities
    2. DNA polymerase chain reaction
      • Amplifies DNA fragments harboring abnormal gene loci
    3. Restriction fragment length polymorphism (RFLP)
      • Identifies abnormal gene when the exact site is unknown

Triple marker for Down syndrome: ↓ AFP, ↑ hCG, ↓ urine estriol

TABLE 5-6:
Age-Dependent
Changes

System	Description
Auditory	Presbycusis: sensorineural hearing loss, particularly at high frequency Otosclerosis: fusion of ear ossicles producing conductive hearing loss
Cardiovascular	Loss of elasticity in aorta (increases systolic pressure)
CNS	Cerebral atrophy with mild forgetfulness Impaired sleep patterns such as insomnia, early wakening Decreased dopaminergic synthesis: parkinsonian-like gait
Female reproductive	Breast and vulvar atrophy Decreased estrogen and progesterone: increased FSH and LH, respectively
Gastrointestinal	Decreased gastric acidity: predisposes to *Helicobacter pylori* infection Decreased colonic motility: constipation predisposing to diverticulosis
General	Increased body fat: decreased number insulin receptors (glucose intolerance)
Immune	Decreased skin response to antigens (called anergy)
Male reproductive	Prostate hyperplasia: predisposes to urinary retention Prostate cancer
Musculoskeletal	Osteoarthritis in weight-bearing joints
Renal	Decreased GFR: increased risk of drug toxicity from slow clearance of drugs
Respiratory	Mild obstructive pattern in pulmonary function tests: e.g., increased TLC Mild hypoxemia and increased A-a gradient
Skin	Decreased skin elasticity due to increased cross-bridging of collagen Senile purpura over the dorsum of the hands and lower legs
Visual	Cataracts: visual impairment, increased risk for falls Presbyopia: inability to focus on near objects

A-a, alveolar-arterial; CNS, central nervous system; FSH, follicle stimulating hormone; GFR, glomerular filtration rate; LH, luteinizing hormone; TLC, total lung capacity.

IX. Aging
A. Theories
1. Stochastic theory
   a. Cumulative injury to cell membranes and DNA due to free radical injury
   b. Increased cross-linking of proteins
      • Decreases elasticity
   c. Accumulation of errors in protein synthesis adversely affects cellular function.
2. Programmed
   • Apoptosis genes are programmed to kill cells at a set time.
B. Age-dependent changes
• Refers to changes that are inevitable with age (Table 5-6)
C. Age-related changes
• Refers to changes that have a greater incidence with age but are *not* inevitable (Table 5-7)

TABLE 5-7:
Age-Related
Changes

System	Description
Cardiovascular	Atherosclerosis: increased risk for coronary artery disease, peripheral vascular disease, strokes Aortic stenosis: most common valvular abnormality in the elderly Systolic hypertension: due to loss of aortic elasticity
CNS	Alzheimer's disease: most common cause dementia in people >65 years old Parkinson's disease Subdural hematomas: due to falls
Endocrine	Type 2 diabetes mellitus
Female reproductive	Increased incidence of cancers of the breast, endometrium, ovary
Gastrointestinal	Increased incidence of colorectal cancer
Immune	MGUS: most common cause of monoclonal gammopathy
Musculoskeletal	Osteoporosis: vertebral column in females and femoral head in males
Renal/lower urinary tract	Renovascular hypertension secondary to atherosclerosis Urinary incontinence
Respiratory	Pneumonia: usually *Streptococcus pneumoniae* Primary lung cancer: particularly in smokers
Skin	UVB-induced cancers: e.g., basal cell carcinoma (most common) Actinic (solar) keratosis: precursor for squamous cell carcinoma Pressure sores: pressure on capillaries is the most important risk factor
Visual	Macular degeneration: most common cause of blindness in the elderly

CNS, central nervous system; MGUS, monoclonal gammopathy of undetermined significance; UVB, ultraviolet light B.

Environmental Pathology

I. Chemical Injury
- The two leading causes of illness and death in the United States are tobacco and alcohol use.

A. Tobacco use
1. Tobacco is the leading cause of premature death in the United States.
2. The rate of cigarette smoking is increasing in females and decreasing in males.
3. Chemical components of tobacco
   a. Nicotine
   (1) Rapidly absorbed
   (2) Most addictive chemical in tobacco smoke
   (3) Cotinine is the most important metabolite of nicotine.
   - Screening test in blood or urine for detecting nicotine
   b. Polycyclic hydrocarbons are the primary carcinogens.
4. Smokeless tobacco (e.g., chewing tobacco)
   - Can cause nicotine addiction and cancer
5. Passive (secondhand) smoke inhalation
   a. Greatest impact on children
   (1) Increased risk of respiratory and middle ear infections
   (2) Exacerbates asthma
   b. Increased risk for lung cancer and coronary artery disease
6. Systemic effects associated with tobacco use (Table 6-1)
7. Beneficial effects of smoking cessation
   a. Risk for cardiovascular disease
   - Approaches nonsmoker after 15 years
   b. Risk for lung cancer
   - Approaches nonsmoker after 15 years
   c. Risk for stroke
   - Approaches nonsmoker after 5 to 15 years
   d. Other benefits
   (1) Reduced risk for cancers of the mouth, larynx, esophagus, pancreas, and urinary bladder
   (2) Improved pulmonary function regardless of severity of the disease
   (3) Reduced risk for pneumonia, influenza, and bronchitis

B. Alcohol abuse
1. Alcohol metabolism
   a. Absorption occurs in the stomach (25%)
   b. Metabolism occurs in the stomach and liver
   - Alcohol dehydrogenase is the rate-limiting enzyme.

Smoking: most important preventable cause of disease and death in United States

Cotinine: metabolite of nicotine; used for screening

Lung cancer: most common cancer associated with smoking

Nicotine patch: effective in treating ulcerative colitis

TABLE 6-1:
Systemic Effects
Associated with
Tobacco Use

System	Effects
Cardiovascular	Acute myocardial infarction (AMI) Sudden cardiac death Peripheral vascular disease Hypertension
Central nervous system	Strokes: intracerebral bleed, subarachnoid hemorrhage
Gastrointestinal	Oropharyngeal cancer: squamous cell carcinoma Upper, midesophageal cancer: squamous cell carcinoma Gastroesophageal reflux disease: decreases tone of lower esophageal sphincter Delayed healing of peptic ulcers Pancreatic cancer: adenocarcinoma
General	Low birth weight, fetal growth retardation Neutrophilic leukocytosis: decreased activation of neutrophil adhesion molecules Decreased concentration of ascorbic acid and β-carotenes
Genitourinary	Cervical cancer: squamous cell carcinoma Decreased testosterone in males Decreased estrogen in females Kidney cancer: renal cell carcinoma Urinary bladder cancer: transitional cell carcinoma
Integument	Increased facial wrinkling
Musculoskeletal	Osteoporosis: due to decreased estrogen in females and decreased testosterone in males
Respiratory	Laryngeal cancer: squamous cell carcinoma Chronic obstructive pulmonary disease: chronic bronchitis, emphysema Lung cancer: squamous cell carcinoma, small cell carcinoma, some types of adenocarcinoma
Special senses	Decreased sense of smell and taste Blindness: macular degeneration Cataracts

    c. Important products of alcohol metabolism
       (1) Reduced nicotinamide adenine dinucleotide (NADH)
          (a) Causes conversion of pyruvate to lactate
          (b) Causes conversion of acetoacetate to β-hydroxybutyrate
          (c) Causes conversion of dihydroxyacetone phosphate to glycerol 3-phosphate
       (2) Acetyl coenzyme A (acetyl CoA)
          (a) Used to synthesize fatty acids for triglyceride synthesis
          (b) Used to synthesize ketoacids
    d. Alcohol induction of the cytochrome P-450 enzyme system
      • Increases alcohol metabolism, which increases the tolerance for alcohol
    e. Legal blood alcohol limit for driving
      • Ranges from 80 to 100 mg/dL

System	Effects
Cardiovascular	Congestive (dilated) cardiomyopathy: due to thiamine deficiency Hypertension: vasopressor effects due to increase in catecholamines
Central nervous system (CNS)	CNS depressant: particularly cerebral cortex and limbic system Wernicke's syndrome: confusion, ataxia, nystagmus due to thiamine deficiency Korsakoff's psychosis: memory deficits due to thiamine deficiency Cerebellar atrophy: due to loss of Purkinje cells Cerebral atrophy: due to loss of neurons Central pontine myelinolysis: due to rapid intravenous fluid correction of hyponatremia in an alcoholic
Gastrointestinal	Oropharyngeal and upper to midesophageal cancer: squamous cell carcinoma Acute hemorrhagic gastritis Mallory-Weiss syndrome: tear of distal esophagus due to retching Boerhaave's syndrome: rupture of distal esophagus due to retching Esophageal varices: caused by portal vein hypertension in alcoholic cirrhosis Acute and chronic pancreatitis
General	Fetal alcohol syndrome: mental retardation, microcephaly, atrial septal defect
Genitourinary	Testicular atrophy: decreased testosterone, decreased spermatogenesis Increased risk for spontaneous abortion
Hematopoietic	Folate deficiency: decreased reabsorption in jejunum; macrocytic anemia Acquired sideroblastic anemia: microcytic anemia due to defect in heme synthesis Anemia chronic disease: most common anemia in alcoholics
Hepatobiliary	Fatty liver, alcoholic hepatitis, cirrhosis Hepatocellular carcinoma: preexisting cirrhosis
Integument	Porphyria cutanea tarda: photosensitive bullous skin lesions
Musculoskeletal	Rhabdomyolysis: direct alcohol effect on muscle
Peripheral nervous system	Peripheral neuropathy: due to thiamine deficiency

TABLE 6-2:
Systemic Effects Associated with Alcohol Abuse

2. Risk factors for alcohol-related disease
   a. Amount
   b. Duration
   c. Female sex
      (1) Decreased gastric alcohol dehydrogenase levels
         • Causes higher alcohol levels in women than in men, even after drinking the same amount of alcohol
      (2) Genetic susceptibility
3. Systemic effects associated with alcohol abuse (Table 6-2)
4. Laboratory findings in alcohol abuse
   a. Fasting hypoglycemia
      • Excess NADH causes pyruvate (substrate for gluconeogenesis) to convert to lactate.

Females: less gastric alcohol dehydrogenase than men

Alcohol abuse: most common cause of thiamine deficiency

b. Increased anion gap metabolic acidosis
   (1) Lactic acidosis
   (2) β-Hydroxybutyric ketoacidosis
       • Excess acetyl CoA is converted to β-hydroxybutyrate.
c. Other findings
   (1) Hyperuricemia (potential for developing gout)
       • Lactic acid and β-hydroxybutyric acid compete with uric acid for excretion in the proximal tubules.
   (2) Hypertriglyceridemia
       • Increased production of glycerol 3-phosphate, the key substrate for triglyceride synthesis in the liver
   (3) Serum aspartate aminotransferase (AST) greater than serum alanine aminotransferase (ALT) in liver disease
       • Alcohol is a mitochondrial toxin that causes release of AST, which is located in the mitochondria.
   (4) Increased serum γ-glutamyltransferase (GGT)
       • Alcohol induces hyperplasia of the smooth endoplasmic reticulum causing increased synthesis of GGT.

C. Other drugs of abuse
   • Sedatives, stimulants, hallucinogens (Table 6-3)
   1. CNS effects of long-term drug abuse
      a. Damage to neurotransmitter receptor sites
      b. Cerebral atrophy (e.g., alcohol)
   2. Complications of intravenous drug use (IVDU)
      a. Hepatitis B
      b. Human immunodeficiency virus (HIV)

↑ Anion gap metabolic acidosis in alcohol abuse: lactic acid, β-hydroxybutyric acid

Alcohol liver disease: AST > ALT; ↑ GGT

Hepatitis B: most common systemic complication of IVDU

TABLE 6-3:
Selected Drugs of Abuse and Their Effects

Drug	Description	Toxic Effects
Cocaine	Stimulant	Mydriasis, tachycardia, hypertension Associated risk of AMI, CNS infarction, perforation of nasal septum (intranasal use)
Heroin	Opiate	Miotic pupils, noncardiogenic pulmonary edema (frothing from mouth), focal segmental glomerulosclerosis (nephrotic syndrome) Granulomatous reactions in skin and lungs from material used to "cut" (dilute) drug
Marijuana (*Cannabis*)*	THC-containing psychoactive stimulant	Red conjunctiva, euphoria, delayed reaction time
MPTP	By-product of synthesis of meperidine	Irreversible Parkinson's disease: cytotoxic to neurons in nigrostriatal dopaminergic pathways

*Used medically to decrease nausea and vomiting associated with chemotherapy and to decrease intraocular pressure in glaucoma.
AMI, myocardial infarction; CNS, central nervous system; MPTP, 1-methyl-4-phenyl-1,2,3,6-tetrahydropyridine; THC, Δ^9-tetrahydrocannabinol.

    c. Infective endocarditis (tricuspid/aortic valves)
      • Caused by *Staphylococcus aureus*
    d. Tetanus
      • Complication of "skin popping"
  D. Adverse effects of therapeutic drug use (Table 6-4)
    1. Acetaminophen
      a. Conversion to free radicals in the liver
      b. May result in damage to the liver (e.g., fulminant hepatitis)
      c. May result in damage to the kidneys (e.g., renal papillary necrosis)

TABLE 6-4:
Adverse Reactions Associated with Therapeutic Drug Use

Reaction	Drug(s)
Blood Dyscrasias	
Aplastic anemia	Chloramphenicol, alkylating agents
Hemolytic anemia	Penicillin, methyldopa, quinidine
Macrocytic anemia	Methotrexate (most common), phenytoin, oral contraceptives, 5-fluorouracil
Platelet dysfunction	Aspirin, other NSAIDs
Thrombocytopenia	Heparin (most common), quinidine
Cardiac	
Congestive cardiomyopathy	Doxorubicin, daunorubicin
Central Nervous System	
Tinnitus, vertigo	Salicylates
Cutaneous	
Angioedema	ACE inhibitors
Maculopapular rash	Penicillin
Photosensitive rash	Tetracycline
Urticaria	Penicillin
Gastrointestinal	
Hemorrhagic gastritis	Iron, salicylates
Hepatic	
Cholestasis	Oral contraceptives, estrogen, anabolic steroids
Fatty change	Amiodarone, tetracycline, methotrexate
Hepatic adenoma	Oral contraceptives
Liver necrosis	Acetaminophen (most common), isoniazid, salicylates, halothane, iron
Pulmonary	
Asthma	Aspirin, other NSAIDs
Interstitial fibrosis	Bleomycin, busulfan, nitrofurantoin, methotrexate
Systemic	
Drug-induced lupus	Procainamide, hydralazine

ACE, angiotensin-converting enzyme; NSAID, nonsteroidal anti-inflammatory drug.

2. Aspirin (acetylsalicylic acid) overdose
   a. General symptoms
      - Tinnitus, vertigo, change in mental status (confusion, seizures), tachypnea
   b. Acid-base disorders
      (1) Respiratory alkalosis may occur initially (within 12–24 hours)
         (a) Due to direct stimulation of the respiratory center
         (b) Respiratory acidosis may occur as a late finding.
      (2) Shift to metabolic acidosis with an increased anion gap
         - Occurs more often in children
      (3) Mixed primary respiratory alkalosis and metabolic acidosis
         - Occurs more often in adults
   c. Hyperthermia
      (1) Salicylates damage the inner mitochondrial membrane.
      (2) Oxidative energy is released as heat, *not* as adenosine triphosphate.
   d. Hemorrhagic gastritis, fulminant hepatitis

3. Disorders associated with exogenous estrogen without progestin
   a. Cancer (adenocarcinoma)
      - Endometrium, breast
   b. Venous thromboembolism
      (1) Estrogen decreases synthesis of antithrombin III (ATIII).
         - ATIII normally neutralizes activated coagulation factors.
      (2) Estrogen increases synthesis of factors I (fibrinogen), V, and VIII.
   c. Intrahepatic cholestasis with jaundice
   d. Cardiovascular effects
      - Myocardial infarction (MI), stroke

4. Disorders associated with oral contraceptives
   - Contain estrogen and progestin
   a. Cancer
      (1) Breast (adenocarcinoma)
      (2) Cervix (squamous cell carcinoma)
   b. Venous thromboembolism
      - Similar pathogenesis to estrogen without progestin
   c. Folate deficiency
      - Decreases jejunal reabsorption of folate
   d. Hypertension
      - Due to increased synthesis of angiotensinogen
   e. Hepatic adenoma
      - Risk of intraperitoneal hemorrhage
   f. Intrahepatic cholestasis with jaundice
   g. Cholesterol gallstones
      - Estrogen increases cholesterol excretion in bile.

E. **Injuries caused by environmental chemicals (Table 6-5; Figs. 6-1 and 6-2)**

Both acetaminophen and aspirin cause fulminant hepatitis.

Oral contraceptives: ↓ risk for endometrial and ovarian cancer

Oral contraceptives: most common cause of hypertension in young women

TABLE 6-5:
Environmental Chemicals and Associated Toxic Effects

Chemical	Source	Toxic Effects
Arsenic	Pesticides, animal dips	Diarrhea, transverse bands in nails (Mee's lines), convulsions Squamous cell carcinoma of skin, liver angiosarcoma, lung cancer
Asbestos	Insulation, roofing material	Primary lung cancer, mesothelioma
Benzene	Solvent	Acute leukemia, aplastic anemia
Carbon monoxide	Automobile exhaust, house fires	Headache (first sign), cherry-red skin, coma Decreased oxygen saturation
Coral snake bite	Neurotoxin: binds to presynaptic nerve terminals and acetylcholine	Snake has "red on yellow" bands Toxic effects: mydriasis, paralysis, and respiratory failure
Crotaline bite	Venom cyto-hemo-neurotoxic	Rattlesnake, copperhead, water moccasin Toxic effects: local edema, shock, disseminated intravascular coagulation (DIC)
Cyanide	House fires	Seizures
Ethylene glycol	Antifreeze End product: oxalic acid	Increased anion gap metabolic acidosis Acute renal failure
Isopropyl alcohol	Rubbing alcohol End product: acetone	Deep coma
Latrodectus bite* (black widow spider)	Neurotoxin	Painful bite Muscle cramps/spasms: occur in thighs and abdomen and simulate an acute abdomen
Lead	Lead-based paint, batteries, metal casting	Microcytic anemia with coarse basophilic stippling, nephrotoxicity in proximal tubule
Loxosceles bite† (brown recluse spider)	Necrotoxin	Painless to mildly painful bite Painful reddish blister with blue-white halo followed by extensive skin necrosis
Mercury	Fish, insecticides	Diarrhea, constricted visual fields, nephrotoxicity in proximal tubule
Methanol	Window-washing fluid End product: formic acid	Increased anion gap metabolic acidosis Blindness due to optic atrophy
Organophosphates	Pesticides	Miotic pupils, paralysis Decreased serum and red blood cell cholinesterase levels
Polyvinyl chloride	Plastics industry	Liver angiosarcoma
Scorpion sting	Neurotoxin	Poisonous species in Southwestern deserts (*Centruroides* sp.) Toxic effects: initially has painful sting followed by numbness, hypertension, ascending motor paralysis leading to death; may cause acute pancreatitis

*See Figure 6-1.
†See Figure 6-2.

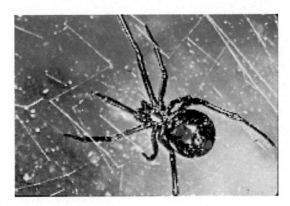

6-1: *Black widow spider. Note the glossy black color and the characteristic ventral red hourglass abdominal marking. (From Goldstein BG: Practical Dermatology, 2nd ed. St. Louis, Mosby, 1997, p 69, Fig. 6-11.)*

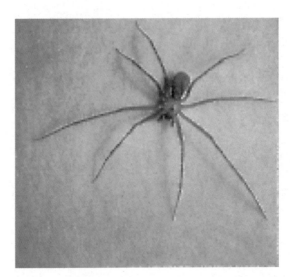

6-2: *Brown recluse spider. Note the yellow-brown body and violin-shaped dark brown marking on the dorsal surface of the spider. (From Goldstein BG: Practical Dermatology, 2nd ed. St. Louis, Mosby, 1997, p 69, Fig. 6-12.)*

II. Physical Injury
A. Mechanical injury
1. Types of skin wounds
   a. Contusion (bruise)
      - Blunt force injury to blood vessels with subsequent escape of blood into tissue
   b. Abrasion
      - Superficial excoriation of the epidermis
   c. Laceration

- Jagged tear with intact bridging blood vessels, nerves, and connective tissue
  - d. Incision
    - Wound with sharp margins with severed bridging blood vessels
- 2. Gunshot wounds
  - a. Contact wounds
    - (1) Stellate-shaped
    - (2) Contain soot and gunpowder (fouling)
  - b. Intermediate-range wounds
    - Powder tattooing (stippling) of the skin around the entrance site
  - c. Long-range wounds
    - *No* powder tattooing
  - d. Exit wounds
    - Typically larger and more irregular than entrance wounds
- 3. Motor vehicle collisions
  - a. Frequently cause mechanical injury
  - b. Frequently alcohol-related

B. Thermal injury
- 1. Burns
  - a. First-degree
    - (1) Painful partial-thickness burns (e.g., sunburn)
    - (2) Heal without scarring
  - b. Second-degree
    - (1) Painful partial-thickness burns
    - (2) Damage to entire epidermis
    - (3) Blister formation
    - (4) Usually heal without scarring
  - c. Third-degree
    - (1) Painless full-thickness burns
    - (2) Extensive necrosis of epidermis and adnexa
    - (3) Scarring is inevitable.
      - (a) Keloids (exaggerated scars) commonly occur.
      - (b) Potential for developing squamous cell carcinoma
    - (4) Healing of epithelial surface
      - Proliferation of residual epithelium located at burn margins and lining adnexal structures
  - d. Complications
    - (1) Infection
      - Sepsis due to *Pseudomonas aeruginosa* is the most common cause of death.
    - (2) Curling's ulcers (stomach)
- 2. Heat injuries (Table 6-6)
- 3. Frostbite
  - a. Pathogenesis
    - (1) Localized tissue injury caused by direct damage (e.g., ice crystallization in cells)
    - (2) Indirect damage (e.g., vasodilation, thrombosis)

Contact gunshot wound: fouling

Motor vehicle collisions: most common cause of accidental death in people ages 1 to 39 years

First- and second-degree burns: no permanent scarring

Most common cause of death in burn patients: sepsis caused by *Pseudomonas aeruginosa*

Heat stroke: >40°C (>104°F), anhidrosis (absence of sweating)

TABLE 6-6:
Heat Injuries*

Type of Injury	Body Temperature	Skin	Mental Status
Heat cramps	37.0°C (98.6°F)	Moist and cool	Normal
Heat exhaustion	>37.8°C (>100°F)	Sweating	Minimally altered
Heat stroke	>40°C (>104°F)	Dry (anhidrosis)	Impaired consciousness

*Heat injury is exacerbated by high humidity.

      b. Clinical findings
        (1) Loss of pain sensation
        (2) Waxy appearance

C. Electrical injury
  1. Produced by alternating current (AC) and direct current (DC)

> AC more dangerous than DC

    a. AC is more dangerous than DC.
    b. AC produces tetanic contractions
    c. DC produces a single shock
  2. Wet skin decreases resistance, which increases current.
  3. Dry skin increases resistance, which decreases current.
  4. Tissue damage increases with increased voltage and duration of exposure.
  5. Current moving from the left arm to the right leg
    a. Most dangerous route, because it affects the heart
    b. Death results from cardiorespiratory arrest.

D. Drowning
  1. Common cause of death in children from 1 to 14 years of age
  2. Terms
    a. Drowning refers to death by suffocation from immersion in liquid.
    b. Near drowning is defined as survival following asphyxia secondary to submersion.

> Most common drowning: Wet drowning

    c. Wet drowning
      (1) 90% of cases
      (2) Initial laryngospasm on contact with water followed by relaxation and aspiration of water
    d. Dry drowning is characterized by intense laryngospasm *without* aspiration.
  3. Pathophysiology
    a. Hypoxemia with damage to central nervous system, heart, kidneys
    b. Lung aspiration (fresh or salt water)
      (1) Damages type II pneumocytes, which decreases surfactant production
      (2) Diffuse alveolar damage
    c. Asphyxia in dry drowning
    d. Lung injury and hypoxemia in wet drowning
  4. Cold water drowning
    a. Activates diving reflex
      • Shunts blood from the periphery to the central core
    b. Hypothermia decreases metabolic demand.

E. High altitude injury
1. General
   a. O_2 concentration 21%
   b. Decreased barometric pressure
   c. Hypoxemic stimulus for respiratory alkalosis
      • Decrease in $Paco_2$ causes a corresponding increase in Pao_2.
   d. Respiratory alkalosis activates glycolysis
      (1) Increased synthesis of 2,3-bisphosphoglycerate
      (2) Right-shifts O_2-binding curve
         • Increases release of O_2 to tissue
2. Acute mountain sickness
   a. Usually occurs at above 8000 feet (2440 m) elevation
   b. Risk factors
      (1) Increased rate of ascent
      (2) Extreme altitude
   c. Clinical findings
      (1) Headache (most common)
      (2) Fatigue, dizziness, anorexia, insomnia
      (3) Acute pulmonary edema
         • Noncardiogenic (exudate)
      (4) Acute cerebral edema
         • Ataxia, stupor, coma
   d. Treatment
      • Immediate descent (if severe complications)

III. Radiation Injury
A. Ionizing radiation injury
   • Examples—x-rays, γ-rays
1. Pathophysiology
   a. Injury correlates with type of radiation, cumulative dose, and amount of surface area exposed.
   b. Direct or indirect DNA injury occurs via formation of hydroxyl free radicals.
2. Tissue susceptibility
   a. Most radiosensitive tissues (highest mitotic activity)
      (1) Lymphoid tissue (most sensitive)
      (2) Bone marrow
      (3) Mucosa of gastrointestinal tract, germinal tissue
   b. Least radiosensitive tissues
      (1) Bone (least sensitive)
      (2) Brain, muscle, skin
3. Radiation effects in different tissues
   a. Hematopoietic
      (1) Lymphopenia (first change)
      (2) Thrombocytopenia
      (3) Bone marrow hypoplasia

High altitude: O_2 concentration 21%, ↓ atmospheric pressure

Bone: least sensitive tissue to radiation

Total body radiation: lymphopenia first hematologic sign

b. Vascular
   (1) Thrombosis (early), fibrosis (late)
   (2) Ischemic damage
c. Epidermal
   (1) Acute effects are erythema, edema, blistering
   (2) Chronic effect is radiodermatitis
      • Potential for squamous cell carcinoma
d. Gastrointestinal
   (1) Acute effect is diarrhea.
   (2) Chronic effects are adhesions with potential for bowel obstruction.
4. Cancers caused by radiation
   a. Acute leukemia (most common)
   b. Papillary carcinoma of the thyroid
   c. Osteogenic sarcoma

B. Nonionizing radiation
1. Ultraviolet light B (UVB) is most damaging
   a. Pathogenesis
      (1) Pyrimidine dimers distort the DNA helix
      (2) Inactivation of the *TP53* suppressor gene
      (3) Activation of the *RAS* oncogene
   b. General effects
      (1) Sunburn
      (2) Actinic (solar) keratosis (Fig. 24-15)
         • Precursor of squamous cell carcinoma (2–5% of cases)
      (3) Corneal burns from skiing
   c. Cancers
      (1) Basal cell carcinoma (most common) (Fig. 8-8)
      (2) Squamous cell carcinoma, malignant melanoma (Fig. 8-9)
2. Effects of other types of radiation
   a. Laser radiation
      • Third-degree burns
   b. Microwave radiation
      • Skin burns, cataracts, sterility
   c. Infrared radiation
      • Skin burns, cataracts

Acute leukemia: most frequent type of cancer caused by radiation

UVB: increase in pyrimidine dimers distorts DNA helix

Basal cell carcinoma: most common UVB light–related skin cancer

7 CHAPTER

Nutritional Disorders

I. Nutrient and Energy Requirements in Humans
A. Recommended dietary allowance (RDA)
1. Optimal dietary intake of nutrients that under ordinary conditions will keep the general population in good health
2. Varies with sex, age, body weight, diet, and physiologic status
B. Daily energy expenditure (DEE)
1. Factors influencing DEE
   a. Basal metabolic rate (BMR)
   b. Thermic effect of food
   c. Physical activity
2. Basal metabolic rate (BMR)
   a. Accounts for ~60% of DEE
   b. Energy consumption involved in normal body functions
      • Examples—cardiac function, maintaining ion pumps
   c. Body weight is the most important factor determining BMR.
   d. Thyroid function alters the BMR.
      • BMR is increased or decreased in hyperthyroidism and hypothyroidism, respectively.
3. Thermic effect of foods
   • Energy used in digestion, absorption, and distribution of nutrients
4. Degree of physical activity
   • Varies with the level of physical activity

BMR: most important factor in determining daily energy expenditure

II. Dietary Fuels
A. Carbohydrates
1. Glucose
   a. Stored primarily as glycogen in liver and muscle
   b. RBCs use only glucose for energy.
   c. Complete oxidation produces 4 kcal/g.
2. Enzymatic digestion
   a. Begins in the mouth (amylase)
   b. Pancreatic amylase
      • In chronic pancreatitis, carbohydrates are *not* malabsorbed due to predigestion by salivary amylase.
   c. Brush border intestinal enzymes (disaccharidases)
      (1) Hydrolyze lactose, maltose, and sucrose
      (2) Disaccharidases produce glucose, galactose, and fructose.

Carbohydrate digestion: begins in the mouth

B. Proteins
1. Amino acids are substrates for gluconeogenesis

2. Digestion

    a. Begins in the stomach (pepsin and acid)

    b. Pancreatic proteases (e.g., trypsin) and peptidases release amino acids.

3. Complete oxidation produces 4 kcal/g.

C. Fats

1. Triglycerides

    a. Major dietary lipids

    b. Major source of energy for cells *except* RBCs and brain

2. Essential fatty acids

    a. Linolenic acid is cardioprotective.

    b. Linoleic acid is required for synthesis of arachidonic acid.

    c. Deficiency of essential fatty acids

       (1) Scaly dermatitis

       (2) Poor wound healing, hair loss

3. Digestion of dietary triglyceride

    a. Occurs primarily in the small intestine

       (1) Hydrolyzed by pancreatic lipase

       (2) Bile salts/acid required for reabsorption

       (3) Packaged into chylomicrons, which enter the blood

    b. Complete oxidation produces 9 kcal/g.

III. Protein-Energy Malnutrition (PEM)

    A. Kwashiorkor

      1. Pathogenesis

        a. Inadequate protein intake

        b. Adequate caloric intake consisting mainly of carbohydrates

        c. Protein in liver and other organs (i.e., visceral protein) is decreased.

        d. Muscle protein (i.e., somatic protein) is relatively unchanged.

      2. Clinical findings (Fig. 7-1, left)

        a. Pitting edema and ascites

          • Caused by hypoalbuminemia and loss of plasma oncotic pressure

        b. Fatty liver

          (1) Caused by decreased synthesis of apolipoproteins

          (2) Apolipoprotein B-100 is required for secretion and assembly of very low density lipoproteins (VLDLs) in the liver.

        c. Diarrhea

          • Caused by loss of the brush border enzymes and parasitic infections

        d. Anemia and defects in cell-mediated immunity (CMI)

    B. Marasmus

      1. Pathogenesis

        a. Dietary deficiency of both protein and calories

        b. Decrease in somatic protein

      2. Clinical findings (see Fig. 7-1, right)

        a. Extreme muscle wasting ("broomstick extremities")

          (1) Breakdown of muscle protein for energy

          (2) Loss of subcutaneous fat

         b. Growth retardation, anemia, defects in CMI

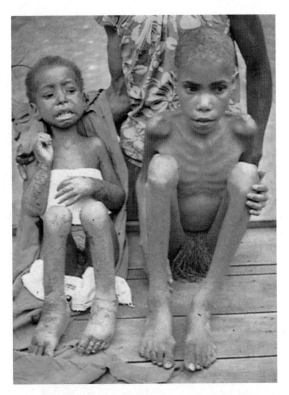

7-1: *Kwashiorkor and marasmus.* **Left,** *Child with kwashiorkor, showing dependent pitting edema involving the lower legs.* **Right,** *Child with marasmus, showing "broomstick" extremities with loss of muscle mass and subcutaneous tissue. (From Forbes C, Jackson W: Color Atlas and Text of Clinical Medicine, 2nd ed. St. Louis, Mosby, 2003, p 343, Fig. 7-138.)*

IV. Eating Disorders and Obesity
A. Anorexia nervosa
1. Pathogenesis
   a. Self-induced starvation leading to PEM (Fig. 7-2)
   b. Distorted body image
2. Clinical findings
   a. Secondary amenorrhea
      (1) Decreased gonadotropin-releasing hormone
         • Caused by loss of body fat and weight
      (2) Decreased serum gonadotropins produces hypoestrinism.
   b. Osteoporosis
      (1) Caused by hypoestrinism
      (2) Decreased osteoblastic activity and increased osteoclastic activity
   c. Increased lanugo (fine, downy hair)
   d. Increased hormones associated with stress (e.g., cortisol, growth hormone)
B. Bulimia nervosa
1. Pathogenesis
   • Binging with self-induced vomiting

Anorexia nervosa: distorted body image

Most common cause of death in anorexia nervosa: ventricular arrhythmia

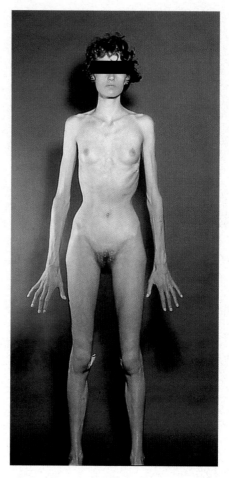

7-2: *Anorexia nervosa. Note the loss of muscle and subcutaneous tissue consistent with total calorie deprivation. (From Forbes C, Jackson W: Color Atlas and Text of Clinical Medicine, 2nd ed. St. Louis, Mosby, 2003, p 344, Fig. 7-141.)*

Vomiting in bulimia nervosa: produces hypokalemic metabolic alkalosis

Body mass index (BMI): weight (kg)/height (m^2)

2. Clinical findings
   a. Complications of vomiting
      (1) Acid injury to tooth enamel
      (2) Hypokalemia and metabolic alkalosis
   b. Ventricular arrhythmia is the most common cause of death.
C. Obesity
   1. Body mass index (BMI) $\geq 30\,\mathrm{kg/m^2}$ (normal: 18.5–24.9 kg/m^2)
      a. BMI = weight (kg)/height (m^2)
      b. Other factors than body weight
         (1) Excess fat in the waist and flanks is more important than an excess in the thighs and buttocks.
         (2) Excess visceral fat in the abdominal cavity has greater significance than excess subcutaneous fat.

2. Pathogenesis
    a. Genetic factors account for 50% to 80% of cases.
        • Examples—defects in the leptin gene, syndrome X (obesity, hypertension, diabetes)
    b. Acquired causes
        (1) Endocrine disorders—hypothyroidism, Cushing syndrome
        (2) Hypothalamic lesions, menopause
    c. Leptin
        (1) Hormone is secreted by adipose tissue that maintains energy balance.
        (2) Leptin increases when adipose stores are adequate.
            (a) Decreases food intake
            (b) Increases energy expenditure (stimulates β-oxidation of fatty acids)
        (3) Leptin decreases when adipose stores are inadequate.
            (a) Increases food intake
            (b) Decreases energy expenditure (inhibits β-oxidation of fatty acids)
        (4) Obesity may be due to several factors:
            (a) Resistance to leptin effects
            (b) Mutations resulting in inhibition of leptin release
3. Clinical findings (Table 7-1)

> Leptin gene: often defective in obesity

> ↑ VLDL causes ↓ HDL.

TABLE 7-1: Clinical Findings Associated with Obesity

Clinical Finding	Comments
Cancer	Increased incidence of estrogen-related cancers (e.g., endometrial, breast) because of increased aromatization of androgens to estrogens in adipose tissue
Cholelithiasis	Increased incidence of cholecystitis and cholesterol stones; bile is supersaturated with cholesterol
Diabetes mellitus, type 2	Increased adipose down-regulates insulin receptor synthesis Hyperinsulinemia increases adipose stores Weight reduction up-regulates insulin receptor synthesis
Hepatomegaly	Fatty change accompanied by liver cell injury and repair by fibrosis
Hypertension	Hyperinsulinemia increases sodium retention, leading to increase in plasma volume Left ventricular hypertrophy and stroke complicate hypertension
Hypertriglyceridemia	Hypertriglyceridemia decreases serum high-density lipoprotein levels, increasing risk of coronary artery disease
Increased low-density lipoprotein levels	Hypercholesterolemia predisposes to coronary artery disease
Obstructive sleep apnea	Weight of adipose tissue compresses upper airways causing respiratory acidosis and hypoxemia Potential for developing cor pulmonale (pulmonary hypertension and right ventricular hypertrophy)
Osteoarthritis	Degenerative arthritis in weight-bearing joints (e.g., femoral heads)

V. Fat-Soluble Vitamins

- Vitamins A, D, E, and K are fat soluble.

A. Vitamin A

1. Retinol
   a. Derived from dietary β-carotenes and retinol esters
   b. Main transport and storage form of vitamin A

   > An excess of β-carotenes in the diet causes the skin to turn yellow, but unlike in jaundice, the sclera remains white. β-Carotenes also have antioxidant activity (neutralize free radicals).

2. Retinal
   a. Product of the oxidation of retinol
   b. Component of the visual pigment rhodopsin
3. Functions of vitamin A
   a. Normal vision in reduced light
   b. Potentiating differentiation of mucus-secreting epithelium
   c. Stimulating the immune system
   d. Growth and reproduction
4. Clinical uses of vitamin A
   a. Treatment of acne (e.g., isotretinoin)
   b. Treatment of acute promyelocytic leukemia
5. Causes of deficiency
   a. Diets lacking sufficient yellow and green vegetables
   b. Fat malabsorption (e.g., celiac disease)
6. Causes of toxicity
   a. Consumption of polar bear liver
   b. Megadoses of vitamin A
   c. Treatment with isotretinoin
7. Clinical findings in vitamin A deficiency and toxicity (Table 7-2)

Night blindness: first sign of vitamin A deficiency

B. Vitamin D

1. Metabolism (Fig. 7-3)
   a. Preformed vitamin D in the diet consists of cholecalciferol (fish) and ergocalciferol (plants).
   b. Endogenous synthesis of vitamin D in the skin occurs by photoconversion of 7-dehydrocholesterol via sunlight.
   c. Reabsorption occurs in the small intestine.
   d. Liver hydroxylation to 25-hydroxyvitamin D (25-OH-D) occurs in the cytochrome P-450 system.
   e. Kidney hydroxylation by 1-α-hydroxylase produces 1,25-$(OH)_2$-D (active form of vitamin D).
   f. Vitamin D increases reabsorption of calcium and phosphorus from the intestine and calcium from the distal renal tubules.
2. Functions
   a. Maintenance of serum calcium and phosphorus
   b. Required for mineralization of epiphyseal cartilage and osteoid matrix
      (1) Receptor located on osteoblasts

TABLE 7-2:
Fat-Soluble Vitamins: Clinical Findings in Deficiency and Toxicity

Vitamin	Effects of Deficiency	Effects of Toxicity
A	Impaired night vision, blindness (squamous metaplasia of corneal epithelium) Follicular hyperkeratosis (loss of sebaceous gland function), pneumonia, growth retardation, renal calculi	Papilledema and seizures (due to an increase in intracranial pressure), hepatitis, bone pain (due to periosteal proliferation)
D	Pathologic fractures, excess osteoid, bow legs Children: rickets; craniotabes (soft skull bones); rachitic rosary (defective mineralization and overgrowth of epiphyseal cartilage in ribs) Adults: osteomalacia Continuous muscle contraction (tetany)	Hypercalcemia with metastatic calcification, renal calculi
E	Hemolytic anemia (damage to RBC membrane) Peripheral neuropathy, degeneration of posterior column (poor joint sensation) and spinocerebellar tract (ataxia)	Decreased synthesis of vitamin K–dependent procoagulant factors; synergistic effect with warfarin anticoagulation
K	Newborns: hemorrhagic disease of newborn (CNS bleeding, ecchymoses) Adults: gastrointestinal bleeding, ecchymoses; prolonged prothrombin time and partial thromboplastin time	Hemolytic anemia and jaundice in newborns if mother receives excess vitamin K

CNS, central nervous system.

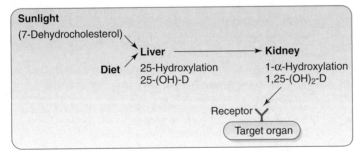

7-3: Vitamin D metabolism. See text for discussion.

    (2) Stimulates release of alkaline phosphatase
    (3) Alkaline phosphatase dephosphorylates pyrophosphate, which normally inhibits bone mineralization
  c. Stimulates macrophage stem cell conversion into osteoclasts
3. Causes of deficiency
  a. Renal failure
    • Decrease in 1-α-hydroxylation

Renal failure: most common cause of vitamin D deficiency

b. Inadequate exposure to sunlight
  - Decreased synthesis from 7-dehydrocholesterol
c. Fat malabsorption
  - Decreased reabsorption of vitamin D
d. Chronic liver disease
  - Decreased synthesis of 25-(OH)-D
e. Enzyme induction of the cytochrome P-450 enzyme system (e.g., alcohol)
  - Increased metabolism of precursors of 25-(OH)-D
4. Megadoses may cause toxicity.
5. Clinical findings in vitamin D deficiency and toxicity (see Table 7-2)

C. Vitamin E
1. Serves as an antioxidant
  a. Protects cell membranes from lipid peroxidation from free radicals
  b. Prevents oxidation of low-density lipoprotein
2. Deficiency is uncommon
  a. Fat malabsorption in children with cystic fibrosis
  b. Abetalipoproteinemia
3. Megadoses may cause toxicity.
4. Clinical findings in vitamin E deficiency and toxicity (see Table 7-2)

D. Vitamin K
1. Derived from endogenous bacteria and green vegetables
2. Activated by the liver microsomal enzyme epoxide reductase
  - Anticoagulant effect of coumarin derivatives results from the inhibition of epoxide reductase.
3. Function
  a. γ-Carboxylates glutamate residues in vitamin K–dependent procoagulants and anticoagulants (protein C and S)
    (1) Procoagulants include factors II (prothrombin), VII, IX, X
    (2) Procoagulants are nonfunctional.
  b. γ-Carboxylation allows vitamin K–dependent procoagulants to bind to calcium in fibrin clot formation.
4. Causes of deficiency
  a. Use of broad-spectrum antibiotics
    - Destroy bacterial synthesis of vitamin K
  b. Newborns
    (1) Lack bacterial colonization of the bowel
    (2) Must receive vitamin K at birth
      (a) Prevents hemorrhagic disease of the newborn
      (b) Breast milk is deficient in vitamin K.
  c. Coumarin derivatives/cirrhosis
    - Decreases epoxide reductase activation of vitamin K
  d. Fat malabsorption
    - Decreased intestinal reabsorption of vitamin K
5. Toxicity caused by excessive intake of vitamin K is uncommon.
6. Clinical findings in vitamin K deficiency and toxicity (see Table 7-2)

Vitamin E toxicity: decreased synthesis of vitamin K–dependent coagulation factors

Broad-spectrum antibiotics: most common cause of vitamin K deficiency in a hospital

Rat poison contains coumarin derivatives.

VI. Water-Soluble Vitamins

A. Thiamine (vitamin B$_1$)

1. Function
   a. Cofactor in biochemical reactions that produce adenosine triphosphate (ATP)
   b. Example—pyruvate dehydrogenase–catalyzed conversion of pyruvate to acetyl CoA
2. Causes of deficiency
   a. Chronic alcoholism (in the United States)
   b. Diet of nonenriched rice (in developing countries)
3. Clinical findings in thiamine deficiency (Table 7-3)
   - Signs and symptoms mainly result from ATP deficiency.

B. Riboflavin (vitamin B$_2$)

1. Active forms include flavin adenine dinucleotide (FAD) and flavin mononucleotide (FMN).
2. Deficiency is caused by severe malnourishment.
3. Clinical findings in riboflavin deficiency (see Table 7-3)

C. Niacin (vitamin B$_3$, nicotinic acid)

1. Functions
   a. Active forms of niacin
      (1) Oxidized nicotinamide adenine dinucleotide (NAD$^+$)
      (2) Oxidized nicotinamide adenine dinucleotide phosphate (NADP$^+$)

Chronic alcoholism: most common cause of thiamine deficiency in the United States

TABLE 7-3: Water-Soluble Vitamins: Clinical Findings in Deficiency

Vitamin	Effects of Deficiency
Thiamine (vitamin B$_1$)	Dry beriberi: peripheral neuropathy (demyelination) Wernicke's syndrome: ataxia, confusion, nystagmus, mamillary body hemorrhage Korsakoff's syndrome: antegrade and retrograde amnesia; demyelination in limbic system Wet beriberi: congestive cardiomyopathy with biventricular failure
Riboflavin (vitamin B$_2$)	Corneal neovascularization, glossitis, cheilosis (cracked lips), angular stomatitis (fissuring at angles of mouth)
Niacin (vitamin B$_3$)	Pellagra: diarrhea, dermatitis (hyperpigmentation in sun-exposed areas), dementia
Pyridoxine (vitamin B$_6$)	Sideroblastic anemia (microcytic anemia with ringed sideroblasts), convulsions, peripheral neuropathy
Cobalamin (vitamin B$_{12}$)	Megaloblastic anemia, neurologic disease (posterior column and lateral corticospinal tract demyelination), glossitis
Folic acid	Megaloblastic anemia, with *no* neurologic disease (unlike vitamin B$_{12}$), glossitis
Biotin	Dermatitis, alopecia, lactic acidosis
Ascorbic acid (vitamin C)	Weak capillaries and venules, skin ecchymoses, perifollicular hemorrhage (ring of hemorrhage around hair follicles), hemarthrosis, bleeding gums, anemia (combined iron and folate deficiency) Loosened teeth, glossitis, poor wound healing

b. NAD^+ and $NADP^+$ are cofactors in oxidation-reduction reactions.
2. Causes of deficiency (pellagra)
   a. Diets deficient in niacin
   b. Deficiency of tryptophan
      (1) Tryptophan is used to synthesize niacin
      (2) Causes of tryptophan deficiency
         (a) Diets deficient in tryptophan
         (b) Hartnup disease
            • Inborn error of metabolism with inability to reabsorb tryptophan in the small bowel and kidneys
         (c) Carcinoid syndrome
            • Tryptophan is used up in synthesizing serotonin.
3. Clinical findings in niacin deficiency (see Table 7-3)
4. Excessive intake of niacin
   a. Leads to flushing caused by vasodilation
      • Adverse effect of nicotinic acid, a lipid-lowering drug
   b. Intrahepatic cholestasis

D. Pyridoxine (vitamin B$_6$)
1. Functions
   • Required for transamination, heme synthesis, and neurotransmitter synthesis
2. Causes of deficiency
   a. Isoniazid (used in treating tuberculosis)
   b. Goat milk, chronic alcoholism
3. Clinical findings in pyridoxine deficiency (see Table 7-3)

E. Cobalamin (vitamin B$_{12}$) (see Chapter 11)
1. Present only in animal products (eggs, meat, dairy products)
2. Requires intrinsic factor for reabsorption in the terminal ileum
3. Functions
   a. DNA synthesis
   b. Propionate (odd-chain fatty acid) metabolism
4. Causes of deficiency
   a. Strict vegan diet
   b. Pernicious anemia
   c. Terminal ileal disease (e.g., Crohn's disease), bacterial overgrowth
5. Clinical findings in vitamin B$_{12}$ deficiency (see Table 7-3)

F. Folic acid (see Chapter 11)
1. Present in most foods
2. Function
   • DNA synthesis
3. Causes of deficiency
   a. Dietary deficiency
      • Elderly individuals, goat milk
   b. Drugs
      • Alcohol, methotrexate, phenytoin, oral contraceptives, trimethoprim, 5-fluorouracil
   c. Malabsorption, overutilization (e.g., pregnancy)

Corn-based diets: deficient in tryptophan and niacin

Three Ds of pellagra: dermatitis, diarrhea, dementia

Pernicious anemia: most common cause of vitamin B$_{12}$ deficiency

Alcohol excess: most common cause folate deficiency

4. Clinical findings in folic acid deficiency (see Table 7-3)
G. Biotin
  1. Function
     a. Cofactor in carboxylase reactions
     b. Example—pyruvate carboxylase–catalyzed conversion of pyruvate to oxaloacetate
  2. Causes of deficiency
     a. Eating raw eggs (avidin binds biotin)
     b. Taking antibiotics
  3. Clinical findings in biotin deficiency (see Table 7-3)
H. Ascorbic acid (vitamin C)
  1. Functions
     a. Hydroxylation of lysine and proline residues in collagen synthesis
        (1) Deficiency leads to collagen with reduced tensile strength.
        (2) Hydroxylation sites are anchors for cross-linking of tropocollagen.
     b. Antioxidant activity
        • Regenerates vitamin E and reduces oxidation of low-density lipoprotein
     c. Prevents nitrosylation
        (1) Inhibits amides from combining with nitrites present in food preservatives
        (2) Nitrosamines and nitrosamides are carcinogens implicated in stomach cancer.
     d. Reduces nonheme iron (+3 valence) from plants to the ferrous (+2 valence) state for reabsorption in the duodenum
        • Deficiency may produce iron deficiency (microcytic anemia).
     e. Keeps tetrahydrofolate (FH_4) in its reduced form
        • Deficiency may produce folate deficiency (macrocytic anemia).
     f. Cofactor in the conversion of dopamine to norepinephrine in catecholamine synthesis
  2. Causes of deficiency
     a. Diets lacking fruits and vegetables
     b. Cigarette smoking

Scurvy: deficiency of ascorbic acid

  3. Clinical findings in vitamin C deficiency (scurvy) (Fig. 7-4; see Table 7-3)
  4. Excess intake (hypervitaminosis C) may lead to the formation of renal calculi composed of uric acid.

VII. Trace Elements
  • Trace elements are micronutrients that are required in the normal diet.
  A. Zinc
    1. Functions
       a. Cofactor for metalloenzymes (e.g., collagenase in wound remodeling)
       b. Growth and spermatogenesis in children
    2. Causes of zinc deficiency
       a. Alcoholism, diabetes mellitus, chronic diarrhea
       b. Acrodermatitis enteropathica
          (1) Autosomal recessive disease

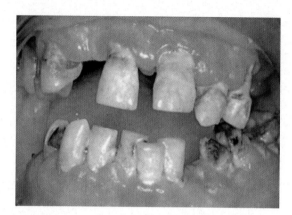

7-4: *Gums showing the effects of scurvy. The swelling and inflammation of the gingival papillae and the numerous caries are caused by poor oral hygiene. (From Forbes C, Jackson W: Color Atlas and Text of Clinical Medicine, 2nd ed. St. Louis, Mosby, 2003, p 361, Fig. 8-22.)*

TABLE 7-4:
Trace Metals:
Clinical Findings in
Deficiency

Trace Metal	Effects of Deficiency
Chromium	Metabolic: impaired glucose tolerance, peripheral neuropathy
Copper	Blood: microcytic anemia (cofactor in ferroxidase) Vessels: aortic dissection (weak elastic tissue) Metabolic: poor wound healing (cofactor in lysyl oxidase)
Fluoride	Teeth: dental caries
Iodide	Thyroid: thyroid enlargement (goiter), hypothyroidism
Selenium	Muscle: muscle pain and weakness, dilated (congestive) cardiomyopathy
Zinc	Metabolic: poor wound healing (cofactor in collagenase) Mouth: dysgeusia (cannot taste), anosmia (cannot smell), perioral rash Children: hypogonadism, growth retardation

Zinc deficiency: poor wound healing, dysgeusia, perioral rash

    (2) Dermatitis, growth retardation, decreased spermatogenesis, poor wound healing
  3. Clinical findings in zinc deficiency (Table 7-4)
 B. Copper
  1. Functions as a cofactor:
    a. Ferroxidase (binds iron to transferrin)
    b. Lysyl oxidase (cross-linking of collagen and elastic tissue)
    c. Tyrosinase (melanin synthesis)
  2. Copper deficiency
    • Most often due to total parenteral nutrition (TPN)
  3. Clinical findings in copper deficiency (see Table 7-4)
  4. Copper excess, Wilson's disease:
    a. Autosomal recessive disease
    b. Defect in eliminating copper into bile

      c. Defect in synthesizing ceruloplasmin (binding protein for copper)

      d. Chronic liver disease, Kayser-Fleischer ring in cornea, basal ganglia degeneration

C. Iodine

1. Function
   - Synthesis of thyroid hormone
2. Iodine deficiency
   - Most often due to inadequate intake of iodized table salt
3. Clinical findings in iodide deficiency (see Table 7-4)

Iodide deficiency: multinodular goiter

D. Chromium

1. Functions

   a. Component of glucose tolerance factor (maintains a normal glucose)

   b. Cofactor for insulin that facilitates binding of glucose to adipose and muscle
2. Chromium deficiency
   - Most often due to TPN
3. Clinical findings in chromium deficiency (see Table 7-4)

E. Selenium

1. Component of glutathione peroxidase
   - Antioxidant that converts peroxide to water using reduced glutathione (GSH)
2. Selenium deficiency
   - Most often due to TPN
3. Clinical findings in selenium deficiency (see Table 7-4)

F. Fluoride

1. Function
   - Component of calcium hydroxyapatite in bone and teeth
2. Fluoride deficiency
   - Most often due to inadequate intake of fluoridated water

MN: fluoride deficiency: dental caries

3. Fluoride excess

   a. Chalky deposits on the teeth

   b. Calcification of ligaments

   c. Increased risk for bone fractures
4. Clinical findings in fluoride deficiency (see Table 7-4)

Neoplasia

I. Nomenclature

  A. Benign tumors

   1. Suffix "oma" generally indicates a benign tumor.
   2. Benign tumors of epithelial origin
      a. Arise from ectoderm or endoderm
      b. Example—tubular adenoma (adenomatous polyp) arising from glands in the colon (Fig. 8-1)
   3. Benign tumors of connective tissue origin arise from mesoderm.
      • Example—lipoma from adipose (Fig. 8-2)
   4. Tumors that are usually benign
      a. Mixed tumors
         (1) Neoplastic cells have two different morphologic patterns but derive from the same germ cell layer.
         (2) Example—pleomorphic adenoma of the parotid gland
      b. Teratomas
         (1) Tumors that derive from more than one germ cell layer
            • Contain tissue derived from ectoderm, endoderm, and mesoderm (Fig. 8-3)
         (2) Sites
            • Ovaries, testes, anterior mediastinum, and pineal gland

  B. Malignant tumors (cancer)

   1. Carcinomas
      a. Derive from epithelial tissue—squamous, glandular, transitional
      b. Sites of squamous cell carcinoma (Fig. 8-4)
         • Oropharynx, larynx, upper/middle esophagus, lung, cervix, skin
      c. Sites of adenocarcinoma (glandular epithelium; Fig. 8-5)
         • Lung, distal esophagus to rectum, pancreas, liver, breast, endometrium, ovaries, kidneys, prostate
      d. Sites of transitional cell carcinoma
         • Urinary bladder, ureter, renal pelvis
   2. Sarcomas
      a. Derive from connective tissue
      b. Example—osteogenic sarcoma in bone (Fig. 8-6)

  C. Tumor-like conditions

   1. Hamartoma
      a. Non-neoplastic overgrowth of disorganized tissue indigenous to a particular site

Benign tumors: epithelial or connective tissue origin

Teratoma: derivatives from ectoderm, endoderm, mesoderm

Carcinomas: derive from squamous, glandular (adenocarcinoma), transitional epithelium

Sarcoma: derives from connective tissue

Hamartoma: non-neoplastic overgrowth of tissue

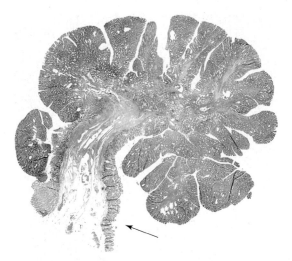

8-1: *Tubular adenoma (adenomatous polyp) of the colon showing a fibrovascular stalk (arrow) lined by normal colonic mucosa and a branching head surfaced by dysplastic (blue-staining) epithelial glands. (From Kumar V, Fausto N, Abbas A: Robbins and Cotran's Pathologic Basis of Disease, 7th ed. Philadelphia, WB Saunders, 2004, p 860, Fig. 17-57A.)*

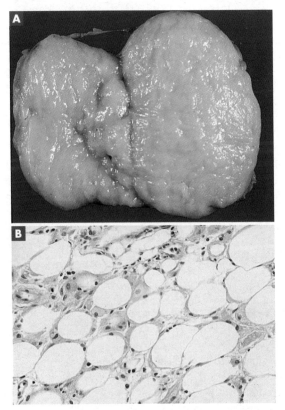

8-2: *Lipoma showing a well-circumscribed yellow tumor (**A**) containing benign adipose cells (**B**). (From Damjanov I: Pathology for the Health-Related Professions, 2nd ed. Philadelphia, WB Saunders, 2000, p 77, Fig. 4-7.)*

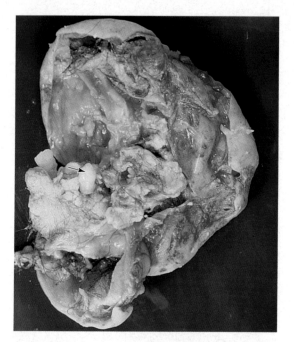

8-3: *Cystic teratoma of the ovary, showing the cystic nature of the tumor. Hair is present, and a tooth is visible (arrow). (From Damjanov I: Pathology for the Health-Related Professions, 2nd ed. Philadelphia, WB Saunders, 2000, p 79, Fig. 4-11.)*

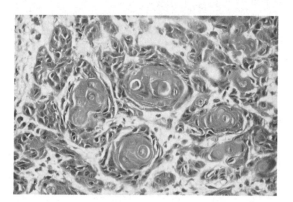

8-4: *Squamous cell carcinoma. The many well-differentiated foci of eosinophilic-staining neoplastic cells produce keratin in layers (keratin pearls; arrow). (From Forbes C, Jackson W: Color Atlas and Text of Clinical Medicine, 2nd ed. St. Louis, Mosby, 2003, p 211, Fig. 4-184.)*

      b. Examples—bronchial hamartoma (contains cartilage), Peutz-Jeghers polyp

    2. Choristoma (heterotopic rest)

      a. Non-neoplastic normal tissue in a foreign location

      b. Examples—pancreatic tissue in the stomach wall; gastric mucosa in Meckel diverticulum

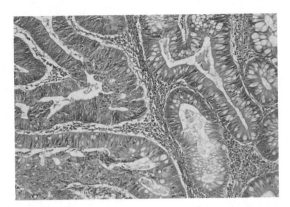

8-5: *Adenocarcinoma. Irregular glands infiltrate the stroma. The nuclei lining the gland lumens are cuboidal and contain nuclei with hyperchromatic nuclear chromatin. Many of the gland lumens contain secretory material. (From Damjanov I, Linder J: Pathology: A Color Atlas. St. Louis, Mosby, 2000, p 139, Fig. 7-59.)*

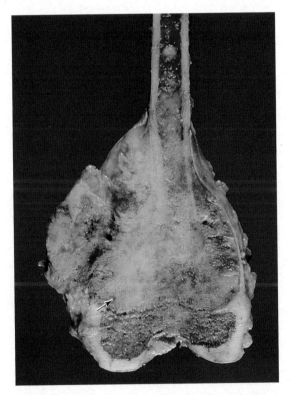

8-6: *Osteogenic sarcoma of the distal femur. The light-colored mass of tumor in the metaphysis abuts the epiphyseal plate (arrow) and has spread laterally out through the cortex and into the surrounding tissue. (From Damjanov I, Linder J: Pathology: A Color Atlas. St. Louis, Mosby, 2000, p 369, Fig. 17-35B.)*

II. Properties of Benign and Malignant Tumors

A. Components of benign and malignant tumors

1. Parenchyma
   - Neoplastic component that determines the tumor's biologic behavior
2. Stroma
   a. Non-neoplastic supportive tissue
   b. Most infiltrating carcinomas induce production of a dense, fibrous stroma

B. Differentiation

1. Benign tumors
   - Usually well-differentiated (resemble parent tissue)
2. Malignant tumors
   a. Well-differentiated or low grade
      (1) Resemble parent tissue
      (2) Example—produce keratin pearls or glandular lumens with secretions (see Figs. 8-4 and 8-5)
   b. Poorly differentiated, high grade, or anaplastic
      - No differentiating features
   c. Intermediate grade
      - Features are between low- and high-grade cancer.

Grade of cancer: Does the cancer resemble its parent tissue or not?

C. Nuclear features

1. Benign tumors
   a. Nuclear:cytoplasmic ratio is close to normal.
   b. Mitoses have normal mitotic spindles.
2. Malignant tumors
   a. Nuclear:cytoplasmic ratio is increased, and nucleoli are prominent.
   b. Mitoses have normal and atypical mitotic spindles.

D. Growth rate

1. Benign tumors usually have a slow growth rate.
2. Malignant tumors have a variable growth rate.
   a. Correlates with the degree of differentiation
   b. Anaplastic (high grade) cancers have an increased growth rate.
3. Thirty doubling times are required for a tumor to be clinically evident.
   - Equivalent to 10^9 cells, 1 g of tissue, volume of 1 mL

E. Monoclonality

1. Benign and malignant tumors derive from a single precursor cell.
2. Non-neoplastic proliferations derive from multiple cells (polyclonal).

The monoclonal origin of neoplasms has been shown by studying glucose-6-phosphate dehydrogenase (G6PD) isoenzymes A and B in selected neoplasms (e.g., leiomyoma of the uterus). All the neoplastic smooth muscle cells in uterine leiomyomas have either the A or the B G6PD isoenzyme. Non-neoplastic smooth muscle proliferations in the uterus (e.g., pregnant uterus) have some cells with the A isoenzyme and others with the B isoenzyme, indicating their polyclonal origin.

F. Telomerase activity
1. Telomerase function
   a. Preserves length of telomeres (sequences of nontranscribed DNA at the ends of chromosomes)
   b. Prevents gene loss after multiple cell divisions
2. Benign tumors have normal telomerase activity.
3. Malignant tumors have increased telomerase activity.
   - They do *not* lose genetic material after multiple cell divisions.

G. Local invasion
1. Benign tumors
   a. They do *not* invade.
   b. They are usually enclosed by a fibrous capsule.
      - Exception—uterine leiomyomas do not have a fibrous tissue capsule.
2. Malignant tumors invade tissue.
3. Some tissues resist invasion.
   - Examples—mature cartilage, elastic tissue in arteries
4. Sequence of invasion by malignant tumors
   a. Loss of intercellular adherence
      - E-cadherin (intercellular adhesion agent) is *not* produced.
   b. Cell invasion occurs.
      (1) Cell receptors attach to laminin (glycoprotein in the basement membrane).
      (2) Cells release type IV collagenase (metalloproteinase containing zinc).
         - Dissolves the basement membrane
      (3) Cell receptors attach to fibronectin in the extracellular matrix.
      (4) Cells produce cytokines (stimulate locomotion) and proteases (dissolve connective tissue).
      (5) Cells produce factors that stimulate angiogenesis.
         - Secrete vascular endothelial growth factor and basic fibroblast growth factor

> Basal cell carcinomas of the skin: invade tissue but do *not* metastasize

> Invasion: second most important criterion for malignancy

H. Metastasis
1. Benign tumors do *not* metastasize.
2. Malignant tumors metastasize.
3. Pathways of dissemination
   a. Lymphatic spread to lymph nodes
      - Usual mechanism of dissemination of carcinomas

   Regional lymph nodes are the first line of defense against the spread of a carcinoma. However, if the nodal architecture is destroyed, malignant cells enter the efferent lymphatics, which empty into the bloodstream. In the bloodstream, malignant cells metastasize to distant organ sites (e.g., liver, lungs, bone).

   b. Hematogenous spread
      (1) Usual mechanism of dissemination for sarcomas
      (2) Cells entering the portal vein metastasize to the liver.
      (3) Cells entering the vena cava metastasize to the lungs.

> Extranodal metastasis (e.g., liver) has greater prognostic significance than nodal metastasis.

Routes of metastasis: lymphatic, hematogenous, seeding of body cavities

Some carcinomas have both lymphatic and hematogenous spread. Renal cell carcinomas commonly invade the renal vein, where the tumor has the potential for extending into the vena cava and the right side of the heart. Hepatocellular carcinomas invade the portal and hepatic veins. Tumor obstruction of either vein produces portal hypertension, splenomegaly, and ascites.

  c. Seeding
   - Malignant cells exfoliate from a surface and implant and invade tissue in a body cavity.
   (1) Primary surface-derived ovarian cancers (e.g., serous cystadenocarcinoma) commonly seed the omentum.
   (2) Peripherally located lung cancers commonly seed the parietal and visceral pleura.
   (3) Glioblastoma multiforme commonly seeds the cerebrospinal fluid causing spread to the brain and spinal cord.
 4. Bone metastasis
  a. Vertebral column
   (1) Most common metastatic site in bone
   (2) Due to the Batson paravertebral venous plexus
    - It has connections with the vena cava and the vertebral bodies.
  b. Osteoblastic metastases
   (1) Radiodensities are seen on radiographs (e.g., prostate cancer).
   (2) Increased serum alkaline phosphatase indicates reactive bone formation.
  c. Osteolytic metastases
   (1) Radiolucencies are seen on radiographs (e.g., lung cancer).
   (2) Pathogenesis
    (a) Tumor may produce substances that activate osteoclasts.
     - Example—prostaglandin E_2, interleukin 1
    (b) Tumor produces parathyroid hormone (PTH)–related protein.
     - Examples—squamous cell carcinoma in the lung, renal cell carcinoma
   (3) Potential consequences of osteolytic metastases
    (a) Pathologic fractures
    (b) Hypercalcemia

Bone metastasis may be osteoblastic (radiodense) or osteolytic (radiolucent).

  d. Pain in bone metastasis is treated with local radiation therapy.
 5. Metastasis is often more common than a primary cancer.
  a. Lymph nodes (e.g., metastatic breast and lung cancer)
  b. Lungs (e.g., metastatic breast cancer)
  c. Liver (e.g., metastatic lung cancer) (Fig. 8-7)
  d. Bone (e.g., metastatic breast cancer)
  e. Brain (e.g., metastatic lung cancer)

III. Cancer Epidemiology
 A. Cancer incidence
  1. Cancers in children (in decreasing order)

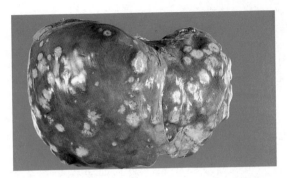

8-7: Metastasis to the liver. The liver contains multiple nodules that have a depressed central area ("umbilicated") and stellate-shaped borders. (From Damjanov I: Pathology for the Health-Related Professions, 2nd ed. Philadelphia, WB Saunders, 2000, p 303, Fig. 11-18.)

- Acute lymphoblastic leukemia, central nervous system tumors (e.g., cerebellar astrocytoma), Burkitt's lymphoma
    2. Cancers in men (in decreasing order)
        - Prostate, lung, colorectal
    3. Cancers in women (in decreasing order)
        - Breast, lung, colorectal
- **B. Cancer mortality rate**
    1. Cancer mortality rate in men (in decreasing order)
        - Lung, prostate, colorectal
    2. Cancer mortality rate in women (in decreasing order)
        - Lung, breast, colorectal

Most common cause of cancer death in adults: lung cancer

- **C. Cancer and heredity**
    1. Inherited predisposition to cancer accounts for <10% of all cancers.
    2. Categories of inherited cancers (Table 8-1)
        a. Autosomal dominant cancer syndromes
        b. Autosomal recessive disorders involving DNA repair
        c. Familial cancers
- **D. Cancer and geography**
    1. Worldwide
        - Malignant melanoma is increasing at the most rapid rate of all cancers.
    2. China
        - Nasopharyngeal carcinoma secondary to Epstein-Barr virus (EBV)
    3. Japan
        - Stomach adenocarcinoma due to smoked foods
    4. Southeast Asia
        - Hepatocellular carcinoma due to hepatitis B virus plus aflatoxins (produced by *Aspergillus*) in food
    5. Africa
        - Burkitt's lymphoma due to EBV and Kaposi sarcoma due to human herpesvirus 8
- **E. Acquired preneoplastic disorders (Table 8-2)**

Actinic (solar) keratosis: precursor of squamous cell carcinoma

TABLE 8-1:
Selected Inherited
Cancer Syndromes

Category	Cancer
Autosomal dominant cancer syndromes	Retinoblastoma: malignancy of eye in children; 40% are inherited; point mutation inactivates *RB* suppressor gene on chromosome 13; one gene inactivated in germ cells, remaining gene inactivated after birth (two-hit theory); predisposition for osteogenic sarcoma in adolescence Familial adenomatous polyposis: development of colorectal cancer from malignant transformation of polyps by age 50; inactivation of *APC* suppressor gene Li-Fraumeni syndrome: increased risk for sarcomas, leukemia, carcinomas (e.g., breast) before age 50; inactivation of *TP53* suppressor gene Hereditary nonpolyposis colon cancer (Lynch syndrome): increased risk for colorectal cancers *without* previous polyps; inactivation of DNA mismatch repair genes; cannot correct errors in nucleotide pairing; characteristic finding is alteration in microsatellite nucleotide sequences (normally do not change in cells) *BRCA1* and *BRCA2* genes: inactivation of genes increases risk for developing breast and ovarian cancer
Autosomal recessive syndromes with defects in DNA repair	Xeroderma pigmentosum: increased risk for developing skin cancers due to ultraviolet light (cross-links adjacent pyrimidine producing pyrimidine dimers); examples include basal cell carcinoma, squamous cell carcinoma Chromosome instability syndromes: chromosomes susceptible to damage by ionizing radiation and drugs; predisposition to cancers (e.g., leukemia, lymphoma); disorders include Fanconi anemia, ataxia telangiectasia, Bloom syndrome
Familial cancer syndromes	No defined pattern of inheritance, but cancers (e.g., breast, ovary, colon) develop with increased frequency in families; sometimes involves *BRCA1* and *BRCA2* genes

F. **Prevention modalities in cancer**
   1. Lifestyle modifications
      a. Stop smoking cigarettes—the most important factor (see Chapter 6)
      b. Increase fiber/decrease dietary saturated fat
         • Decreases risk for colorectal cancer
      c. Reduce alcohol intake (see Chapter 6)
      d. Reduce weight
         (1) Increased adipose tissue increases aromatase conversion of androgens to estrogen.
         (2) Increased estrogen increases risk for endometrial and breast cancer.
   2. Hepatitis B vaccination
      • Immunization decreases the risk for hepatocellular carcinoma due to hepatitis B–induced postnecrotic cirrhosis.
   3. Screening procedures
      a. Cervical Papanicolaou (Pap) smears

Cessation of smoking is most important factor in decreasing risk for cancer.

TABLE 8-2:
Acquired
Preneoplastic
Disorders*

Precursor Lesion	Cancer
Actinic (solar) keratosis	Squamous cell carcinoma
Atypical hyperplasia of ductal epithelium of breast	Adenocarcinoma
Chronic irritation at sinus orifice, third-degree burn scars	Squamous cell carcinoma
Chronic ulcerative colitis	Adenocarcinoma
Complete hydatidiform mole	Choriocarcinoma
Dysplastic nevus	Malignant melanoma
Endometrial hyperplasia	Adenocarcinoma
Glandular metaplasia of esophagus (Barrett's esophagus)	Adenocarcinoma
Glandular metaplasia of stomach (*Helicobacter pylori*)	Adenocarcinoma
Myelodysplastic syndrome	Acute leukemia
Regenerative nodules in cirrhosis	Adenocarcinoma
Scar tissue in lung	Adenocarcinoma
Squamous dysplasia of oropharynx, larynx, bronchus, cervix	Squamous cell carcinoma
Tubular adenoma of colon	Adenocarcinoma
Vaginal adenosis (diethylstilbestrol exposure)	Adenocarcinoma
Villous adenoma of rectum	Adenocarcinoma

*Metaplastic and hyperplastic cells become dysplastic *before* progressing to cancer.

(1) Decreases risk for cervical cancer

(2) Pap smear detects cervical dysplasia, which can be surgically removed.

b. Colonoscopy

- Detects and removes polyps that are precancerous

c. Mammography

- Detects nonpalpable breast masses

d. Prostate-specific antigen

(1) Detects prostate cancer

(2) Lacks specificity because it is increased in prostate hyperplasia

4. Treatment of conditions that predispose to cancer

a. Treatment of *Helicobacter pylori* infections

- Decreases risk for developing malignant lymphoma and adenocarcinoma of the stomach

b. Treatment of gastroesophageal reflux disease

- Decreases the risk for developing distal adenocarcinoma arising from Barrett's esophagus

IV. Carcinogenesis

- Cancer is a multistep process involving gene mutations, telomerase activation, angiogenesis, invasion, and metastasis.

A. Types of gene mutations

1. Point mutations are the most common type of mutation.

2. Balanced translocations

3. Other mutations

- Deletion, gene amplification (multiple copies of a gene), overexpression (increase in baseline gene activity)

Human papillomavirus immunization: decreases risk for cervical cancer

Treating *H. pylori* infection: reduces risk for developing gastric lymphoma and adenocarcinoma

Point mutations: most common type of mutation in cancer

TABLE 8-3:
Some Proto-oncogenes and Their Functions, Mutations, and Associated Cancers

Proto-oncogene	Function	Mutation	Cancer
ABL	Nonreceptor tyrosine kinase activity	Translocation t(9;22)	Chronic myelogenous leukemia (chromosome 22 is Philadelphia chromosome)
HER (ERBB2)	Receptor synthesis	Amplification	Breast carcinoma (marker of aggressiveness)
MYC	Nuclear transcription	Translocation t(8;14)	Burkitt's lymphoma
N-MYC	Nuclear transcription	Amplification	Neuroblastoma
RAS	Guanosine triphosphate signal transduction	Point mutation	Leukemia; lung, colon, pancreatic carcinomas
RET	Receptor synthesis	Point mutation	Multiple endocrine neoplasia IIa/IIb syndromes
SIS	Growth factor synthesis	Overexpression	Osteogenic sarcoma, astrocytoma

B. Genes involved in cancer

1. Proto-oncogenes
   a. Involved in normal growth and repair
   b. Proto-oncogene protein products
      - Growth factors, growth factor receptors, signal transducers, nuclear transcribers
   c. Mutations cause sustained activity of the genes (Table 8-3)
2. Suppressor genes (antioncogenes)
   a. Protect against unregulated cell growth
   b. Control G_1 to S phase of the cell cycle and nuclear transcription
   c. Mutations cause unregulated cell proliferation (Table 8-4).
3. Antiapoptosis genes; *BCL2* family of genes:
   a. Protein products prevent cytochrome *c* from leaving mitochondria.
      - Cytochrome *c* in the cytosol activates caspases initiating apoptosis.
   b. Mutation causes increased gene activity (e.g., overexpression), which prevents apoptosis; e.g., B-cell follicular lymphoma.
      (1) *BCL2* gene family (chromosome 18) produce gene products that prevent mitochondrial leakage of cytochrome *c* (signal for apoptosis).
      (2) Translocation t(14;18) causes overexpression of the BCL2 protein product.
         - Prevents apoptosis of B lymphocytes causing B-cell follicular lymphoma
4. Apoptosis genes
   a. Regulate programmed cell death
   b. Example—*BAX* apoptosis gene

Proto-oncogenes: involved in normal growth and repair

Suppressor genes: protect against unregulated cell growth

BCL2 gene family: antiapoptosis genes

BAX gene: apoptosis gene

TABLE 8-4:
**Some Tumor
Suppressor Genes,
Their Functions,
and Associated
Cancers**

Gene*	Function	Associated Cancers
APC	Prevents nuclear transcription (degrades catenin, an activator of nuclear transcription)	Familial polyposis (colorectal carcinoma)
BRCA1/BRCA2	Regulates DNA repair	Breast, ovary, prostate carcinomas
RB	Inhibits G_1 to S phase	Retinoblastoma, osteogenic sarcoma, breast carcinoma
TGF-β	Inhibits G_1 to S phase	Pancreatic and colorectal carcinomas
TP53	Inhibits G_1 to S phase Repairs DNA, activates BAX gene (initiates apoptosis)	Lung, colon, breast carcinomas Li-Fraumeni syndrome: breast carcinoma, brain tumors, leukemia, sarcomas
VHL	Regulates nuclear transcription	Von Hippel–Lindau syndrome: cerebellar hemangioblastoma, retinal angioma, renal cell carcinoma (bilateral), pheochromocytoma (bilateral)
WT1	Regulates nuclear transcription	Wilms' tumor

*APC, adenomatous polyposis coli; BRCA, breast cancer; RB, retinoblastoma; TGF-β, transforming growth factor β; VHL, von Hippel–Lindau; WT, Wilms' tumor.

    (1) Activated by a TP53 suppressor gene product if DNA damage is excessive
    (2) BAX protein product inactivates the BCL2 antiapoptosis gene.
    (3) Mutation inactivating TP53 suppressor gene renders the BAX gene inoperative, which prevents apoptosis.
  5. DNA repair genes (see Table 8-1 and Table 8-4)
    a. Examples of DNA repair
      (1) Mismatch repair genes produce proteins that correct errors in nucleotide pairing.
      (2) Nucleotide excision repair pathway excises pyrimidine dimers in ultraviolet light (UV)–damaged skin.
    b. Effect of mutations involving DNA repair genes
      • Allows cells with nonlethal damage to proliferate, which increases the risk for cancer

Repair genes: correct errors in nucleotide pairing; excise pyrimidine dimers

Enzymes involved in dimer excision: endonuclease, exonuclease, ligase

V. Carcinogenic Agents
  A. Chemical carcinogens (Table 8-5)
    1. Polycyclic hydrocarbons in tobacco smoke
      • Most common group of carcinogens in the United States
    2. Mechanisms
      a. Direct-acting carcinogens
        • Contain electron-deficient atoms that react with electron-rich atoms in DNA (e.g., alkylating agents)

TABLE 8-5: Chemical Carcinogens

Carcinogen	Associated Cancer
Aflatoxin (from *Aspergillus*)	Hepatocellular carcinoma in association with hepatitis B virus
Alcohol	Squamous cell carcinoma of oropharynx and upper/middle esophagus; pancreatic and hepatocellular carcinomas
Alkylating agents	Malignant lymphoma
Arsenic	Squamous cell carcinoma of skin, lung cancer, liver angiosarcoma
Asbestos	Bronchogenic carcinoma, pleural mesothelioma
Benzene	Acute leukemia
Beryllium	Bronchogenic carcinoma
Chromium	Bronchogenic carcinoma
Cyclophosphamide	Transitional cell carcinoma of urinary bladder
Diethylstilbestrol	Clear cell carcinoma of vagina
β-Naphthylamine (aniline dyes)	Transitional cell carcinoma of urinary bladder
Nickel	Bronchogenic carcinoma
Nitrosamines*	Stomach carcinoma
Oral contraceptives	Breast, cervical carcinomas
Polycyclic hydrocarbons	Squamous cell carcinoma: oral cavity, midesophagus, larynx, lung / Adenocarcinoma: distal esophagus, pancreas / Transitional cell carcinoma: urinary bladder, renal pelvis
Polyvinyl chloride	Liver angiosarcoma
Silica	Bronchogenic carcinoma

*Nitrosamines are produced when amines in food combine with sodium nitrite, a food preservative.

b. Indirect-acting carcinogens
- Activated by the liver cytochrome P-450 system (e.g., polycyclic hydrocarbons)
3. Sequence of chemical carcinogenesis
a. Initiation
- Irreversible mutation
b. Promotion
- Promoters (e.g., estrogen) stimulate mutated cells to enter the cell cycle.
c. Progression
(1) Development of tumor heterogeneity
(2) Examples—production of cells that invade or metastasize

B. Microbes
1. Viruses (Table 8-6)
2. Bacteria
- Examples—stomach cancer and low-grade malignant lymphoma due to *Helicobacter pylori*
3. Parasites
a. *Schistosoma hematobium*
- Squamous cell carcinoma of the urinary bladder
b. *Clonorchis sinensis* and *Opisthorchis viverrini*
- Cholangiocarcinoma of the bile ducts

> Tobacco is the agent most responsible for cancer and cancer deaths in the United States.

TABLE 8-6:
**Oncogenic RNA
and DNA Viruses**

Virus	Mechanism	Associated Cancer
RNA Viruses		
HCV	Produces postnecrotic cirrhosis	Hepatocellular carcinoma
HTLV-1	Activates *TAX* gene, stimulates polyclonal T-cell proliferation, inhibits *TP53* suppressor gene	T-cell leukemia and lymphoma
DNA Viruses		
EBV	Promotes polyclonal B-cell proliferation, which increases risk for t(8;14) translocation	Burkitt's lymphoma, CNS lymphoma in AIDS, mixed cellularity Hodgkin's lymphoma, nasopharyngeal carcinoma
HBV	Activates proto-oncogenes, inactivates *TP53* suppressor gene	Hepatocellular carcinoma
HHV-8	Acts via cytokines released from HIV and HSV	Kaposi sarcoma in AIDS
HPV types 16 and 18	Type 16: E6 gene product inhibits *TP53* suppressor gene Type 18: E7 gene product inhibits *RB* suppressor gene	Squamous cell carcinoma of vulva, vagina, cervix, anus (associated with anal intercourse)

CNS, central nervous system; EBV, Epstein-Barr virus; HBV, hepatitis B virus; HCV, hepatitis C virus; HHV, human herpesvirus; HPV, human papillomavirus; HSV, herpes simplex virus; HTLV, human T-cell lymphotropic virus.

C. Radiation
1. Ionizing radiation–induced cancers
   a. Mechanism
     • Hydroxyl free radical injury to DNA
   b. Examples
     (1) Acute or chronic myelogenous leukemia
       • Increased risk of leukemia in radiologists and individuals exposed to radiation in nuclear reactors
     (2) Papillary thyroid carcinoma
     (3) Lung, breast, and bone cancers
     (4) Liver angiosarcoma
       • Due to radioactive thorium dioxide used to visualize the arterial tree
2. UV light–induced cancers
   a. Mechanism
     • Formation of pyrimidine dimers, which distort DNA
   b. Basal cell carcinoma, squamous cell carcinoma, malignant melanoma (Figs. 8-8 and 8-9)

D. Physical injury
1. Squamous cell carcinoma may develop in third-degree burn scars.
2. Squamous cell carcinoma may develop at the orifices of chronically draining sinuses (e.g., chronic osteomyelitis).

Leukemia: most common cancer due to ionizing radiation

Basal cell carcinoma: most common cancer due to excessive UV light exposure

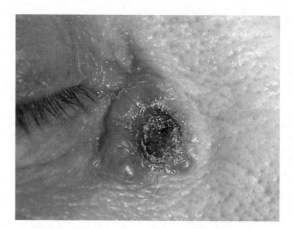

8-8: Basal cell carcinoma (invasive tumor that does not metastasize). There is an ulcerated nodular mass on the inner aspect of the nose. This is a particularly common site for ultraviolet light–induced cancers that arise from the basal cell layer of skin. (From Savin J, Hunter JA, Hepburn NC: Diagnosis in Color: Skin Signs in Clinical Medicine. London, Mosby-Wolfe, 1997, p 104, Fig. 4-27.)

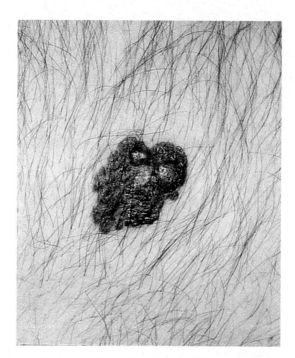

8-9: Malignant melanoma. The lesion on the patient's forearm is black, is multinodular, and has an irregular border with areas of pale-gray discoloration. Malignant melanomas arise from nevus cells, which are of neural crest origin. (From Damjanov I, Linder J: Pathology: A Color Atlas. St. Louis, Mosby, 2000, p 327, Fig. 15-57A.)

VI. Clinical Oncology

A. Host defense against cancer

1. Humoral immunity
   - Involves antibodies and complement
2. Type IV cellular immunity
   a. Most efficient mechanism for killing cancer cells
   b. Cytotoxic CD8 T cells
      - Recognize altered class I antigens on neoplastic cells and destroy them
3. Natural killer cells
   - Direct killing and indirect killing through type II hypersensitivity
4. Macrophages
   - Activated by γ-interferon

Cytotoxic CD8 T cells: most effective host defense against cancer

B. Grading and staging of cancer

1. Grading criteria
   a. Degree of differentiation (e.g., low, intermediate, or high grade)
   b. Nuclear features, invasiveness
2. Staging criteria
   a. Most important prognostic factor
   b. TNM system
      (1) Progresses from the least to the most important prognostic factor
      (2) T refers to tumor size
         - ≥ 2 cm correlates with metastatic ability.
      (3) N refers to whether lymph nodes are involved.
      (4) M refers to extranodal metastases (e.g., liver, lung).

C. Cancer effects on the host

1. Cachexia (wasting disease)
   a. Irreversible catabolic reaction
   b. Mechanism; tumor necrosis factor-α:
      (1) Secreted from host macrophages and cancer cells
      (2) Suppresses the appetite center
      (3) Increases β-oxidation of fatty acids
2. Anemia
   a. Anemia of chronic disease
   b. Iron deficiency
      - Due to gastrointestinal blood loss (e.g., colorectal cancer)
   c. Macrocytic anemia
      - Due to folate deficiency from rapid tumor growth
   d. Myelophthisic anemia
      (1) Anemia related to metastasis to bone
      (2) Immature hematopoietic elements in peripheral blood (i.e., leukoerythroblastic smear)
         (a) Nucleated RBCs, immature neutrophils (e.g., myeloblasts, metamyelocytes) in peripheral blood
         (b) Teardrop RBCs indicate myelofibrosis secondary to bone metastasis

Anemia of chronic disease: most common anemia in cancer

3. Hemostasis abnormalities
   a. Increased risk for vessel thrombosis
      (1) Due to thrombocytosis, increased synthesis of coagulation factors (e.g., fibrinogen, factors V and VIII)
      (2) Release of procoagulants from cancer cells (e.g., pancreatic carcinoma)
   b. Disseminated intravascular coagulation
      • Due to release of tissue thromboplastin from cancer cells

4. Fever
   a. Usually due to infection
   b. Example—gram-negative sepsis from *Escherichia coli* or *Pseudomonas aeruginosa*

5. Paraneoplastic syndromes
   a. Distant effects of a tumor that are unrelated to metastasis
      • May predate the onset of metastasis
   b. Occur in 10% to 15% of cancer patients
   c. Involve multiple organ systems and mimic metastatic disease (Table 8-7)
   d. May involve ectopic secretion of hormone (Table 8-8)

D. Tumor markers
1. Biologic markers (Table 8-9)
   • Include hormones, enzymes, oncofetal antigens, glycoproteins
2. Identify tumors
3. Estimate tumor burden
4. Detect recurrence

Gram-negative sepsis: most common cause of death in cancer

Hypercalcemia: most common paraneoplastic syndrome

TABLE 8-7: Paraneoplastic Syndromes

Syndrome	Associated Cancer	Comment
Acanthosis nigricans	Stomach carcinoma	Black, verrucoid-appearing lesion
Eaton-Lambert syndrome	Small cell carcinoma of lung	Myasthenia gravis–like symptoms (e.g., muscle weakness)
Hypertrophic osteoarthropathy	Bronchogenic carcinoma	Periosteal reaction of distal phalanx (often associated with clubbing of nail)
Nonbacterial thrombotic endocarditis	Mucus-secreting pancreatic and colorectal carcinomas	Sterile vegetations on mitral valve
Seborrheic keratosis	Stomach carcinoma	Sudden appearance of numerous pigmented seborrheic keratoses (Leser-Trélat sign)
Superficial migratory thrombophlebitis	Pancreatic carcinoma	Release of procoagulants (Trousseau's sign)

Disorder	Associated Cancer	Ectopic Hormone
Cushing syndrome	Small cell carcinoma of lung, medullary carcinoma of thyroid	ACTH
Gynecomastia	Choriocarcinoma (testis)	hCG
Hypercalcemia	Renal cell carcinoma, primary squamous cell carcinoma of lung, breast carcinoma	PTH-related protein
Hypocalcemia	Medullary carcinoma of thyroid	Calcitonin
Hypoglycemia	Hepatocellular carcinoma	Insulin-like factor
Hyponatremia	Small cell carcinoma of lung	Antidiuretic hormone
Secondary polycythemia	Renal cell and hepatocellular carcinomas	Erythropoietin

TABLE 8-8:
Paraneoplastic Syndrome Endocrinopathies

ACTH, adrenocorticotropic hormone; hCG, human chorionic gonadotropin; PTH, parathyroid hormone.

Tumor Marker	Associated Cancer
AFP	Hepatocellular carcinoma, yolk sac tumor (endodermal sinus tumor) of ovary or testis
Bence Jones protein	Multiple myeloma, Waldenström's macroglobulinemia (represent light chains in urine)
CA 15-3	Breast carcinoma
CA 19-9	Pancreatic carcinoma
CA 125	Surface-derived ovarian cancer (e.g., serous cystadenocarcinoma)
CEA	Colorectal and pancreatic carcinomas
PSA	Prostate carcinoma (also increased in prostate hyperplasia)

TABLE 8-9:
Tumor Markers and Associated Cancers

AFP, α-fetoprotein; CEA, carcinoembryonic antigen; PSA, prostate-specific antigen.

Vascular Disorders

I. Lipoprotein Disorders
  A. Lipoprotein fractions
    1. Chylomicron

Chylomicron: diet-derived triglyceride

      a. Transports diet-derived triglyceride in the blood
      b. Synthesized in intestinal epithelium
        • Requires apolipoprotein B-48 for assembly and secretion
      c. Absent during fasting
      d. Source of fatty acids and glycerol
        (1) Used to synthesize triglyceride in the liver and adipose
        (2) Hydrolysis by capillary lipoprotein lipase (CPL) leaves a chylomicron remnant.
    2. Very low-density lipoprotein (VLDL)
      a. Transports liver-synthesized triglyceride in the blood
        • Requires apolipoprotein B-100 for assembly and secretion

VLDL: liver-derived triglyceride

      b. Source of fatty acids and glycerol
        (1) Used to synthesize triglyceride in the adipose
        (2) Hydrolysis by CPL produces intermediate-density lipoprotein (IDL) and low-density lipoprotein (LDL)

Hypertriglyceridemia: causes turbidity in plasma

    3. Low-density lipoprotein (LDL)
      a. Transports cholesterol in the blood

LDL: transports cholesterol

      b. Calculated LDL = cholesterol − high-density lipoprotein − triglyceride/5
        • Presence of chylomicrons falsely lowers calculated LDL by increasing diet-derived triglyceride.
      c. Functions of cholesterol
        (1) Component of the cell membrane
        (2) Synthesis of vitamin D, adrenal cortex hormones, bile salts and acids
    4. High-density lipoprotein (HDL)
      a. "Good cholesterol"
        • Increased by exercise, wine, estrogen
      b. Synthesized by the liver and small intestine
      c. Functions of HDL

HDL: removes cholesterol from plaques for disposal in the liver

        (1) Source of apolipoproteins for other lipoprotein fractions
        (2) Removes cholesterol from atherosclerotic plaques
  B. Selected lipoprotein disorders
    1. Type II hyperlipoproteinemia
      a. Increase in serum LDL above 190 mg/dL (<130 mg/dL)
      b. Acquired causes

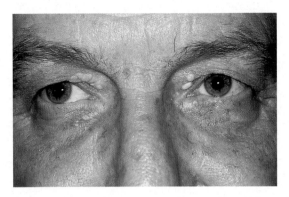

9-1: *Xanthelasma. Yellow, raised lesions are noted on the eyelids in both eyes. (From Forbes C, Jackson W: Color Atlas and Text of Clinical Medicine, 2nd ed. St. Louis, Mosby, 2003, p 340, Fig. 7-127.)*

      (1) Primary hypothyroidism
         • Decrease in LDL receptor synthesis
      (2) Nephrotic syndrome
         • Increase in LDL correlates with the degree of hypoalbuminemia

    c. Familial hypercholesterolemia
      (1) Autosomal dominant disorder
      (2) Deficiency of LDL receptors
      (3) Clinical findings
         (a) Premature coronary artery disease and stroke
         (b) Tendon xanthomas
            • Cholesterol deposit located over tendons (e.g., Achilles) and extensor surfaces of joints
         (c) Xanthelasma (Fig. 9-1)
            • Yellow, raised plaque on the eyelid

2. Type III hyperlipoproteinemia
    a. Familial dysbetalipoproteinemia ("remnant disease")
    b. Deficiency of apolipoprotein E
      (1) Decreased liver uptake of chylomicron remnants and IDL
      (2) Increase in serum cholesterol and triglyceride
    c. Clinical findings
      (1) Palmar xanthomas in flexor creases
      (2) Increased risk for coronary artery disease

3. Type IV hyperlipoproteinemia
    a. Increase in VLDL
      • Due to increase in synthesis or decrease in catabolism
    b. Acquired causes
      (1) Excess alcohol intake
      (2) Progesterone in oral contraceptives
      (3) Diabetes mellitus
    c. Familial hypertriglyceridemia
      (1) Autosomal dominant disorder

Type II hyperlipoproteinemia: ↑ LDL due to ↓ LDL receptors

Type III hyperlipoproteinemia: deficiency apoE; ↑ remnants

Type IV hyperlipoproteinemia: ↑ VLDL; most common lipid disorder

Type IV
hyperlipoproteinemia:
most common cause is
alcohol excess

      (2) Clinical findings

          (a) Eruptive xanthomas

             • Yellow, papular lesions

          (b) Increased risk for coronary artery and peripheral vascular disease

    4. Apolipoprotein B deficiency (abetalipoproteinemia)

      a. Autosomal recessive disorder

      b. Deficiency of apolipoprotein B-48 and B-100

          (1) Deficiency of chylomicrons, VLDL, and LDL

          (2) Decrease in serum cholesterol and triglyceride

      c. Clinical findings

          (1) Malabsorption

             (a) Chylomicrons accumulate in villi and prevent reabsorption of micelles.

             (b) Marked decrease in vitamin E

          (2) Ataxia, hemolytic anemia with thorny RBCs (acanthocytes)

II. Arteriosclerosis

  • Arteriosclerosis is thickening and loss of elasticity of arterial walls.

A. Medial calcification

    1. Dystrophic calcification in the wall of muscular arteries

      • Examples—calcification in uterine and radial arteries

    2. No clinical consequence unless associated with atherosclerosis

B. Atherosclerosis

    1. Pathogenesis

Atherosclerosis: due to
endothelial cell injury

      a. Endothelial cell damage of muscular and elastic arteries

      b. Causes of endothelial cell injury

        • Hypertension, smoking tobacco, homocysteine, LDL

      c. Cell response to endothelial injury

          (1) Macrophages and platelets adhere to damaged endothelium.

          (2) Released cytokines cause hyperplasia of medial smooth muscle cells.

          (3) Smooth muscle cells migrate to the tunica intima.

          (4) Cholesterol enters smooth muscle cells and macrophages (called foam cells).

          (5) Smooth muscle cells release cytokines that produce extracellular matrix.

            • Matrix components include collagen, proteoglycans, and elastin.

Fibrous cap:
pathognomonic lesion of
atherosclerosis

      d. Development of fibrous cap (plaque)

          (1) Components of fibrous cap

            • Smooth muscle, foam cells, inflammatory cells, extracellular matrix

C-reactive protein:
excellent marker of
disrupted fibrous plaques

          (2) Fibrous cap overlies a necrotic center.

            • Cellular debris, cholesterol crystals (slit-like spaces), foam cells

          (3) Disrupted plaques may extrude underlying necrotic material leading to vessel thrombosis (Fig. 9-2).

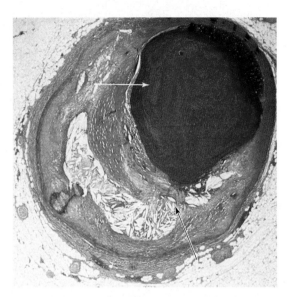

9-2: *Coronary artery thrombosis. The thrombus (white arrow) is red and occludes the vessel lumen. The fibrous cap stains blue and is disrupted (black arrow) allowing necrotic material (slit-like spaces containing cholesterol) to extrude into the lumen resulting in thrombus formation. (From Damjanov I, Linder J: Anderson's Pathology, 10th ed. St. Louis, Mosby, 1996, p 1320, Fig. 45-60.)*

> Serum C-reactive peptide is increased in patients with disrupted (inflammatory) plaques. Plaques may rupture and produce vessel thrombosis, which leads to acute myocardial infarction (MI). C-reactive protein may be a stronger predictor of cardiovascular events than LDL.

    (4) Fibrous plaque becomes dystrophically calcified and ulcerated.

2. Sites for atherosclerosis (descending order)
   a. Abdominal aorta
   b. Coronary artery
   c. Popliteal artery
   d. Internal carotid artery

Abdominal aorta: most common site for atherosclerosis

3. Complications of atherosclerosis
   a. Vessel weakness (e.g., abdominal aortic aneurysm)
   b. Vessel thrombosis
      (1) Acute MI (coronary artery)
      (2) Stroke (internal carotid artery, middle cerebral artery)
      (3) Small bowel infarction (superior mesenteric artery)
   c. Hypertension
      • Renal artery atherosclerosis may activate the renin-angiotensin-aldosterone system.
   d. Peripheral vascular disease
      (1) Increased risk of gangrene
      (2) Pain in the buttocks and when walking (claudication)

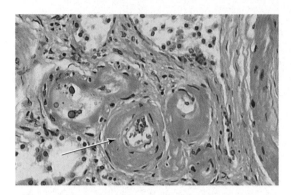

9-3: *Hyaline arteriolosclerosis. The arrow depicts eosinophilic material representing protein that has leaked through the basement membrane and deposited in the wall of an arteriole. Other neighboring arterioles demonstrate similar changes. (From Damjanov I, Linder J: Pathology: A Color Atlas. St. Louis, Mosby, 2000, p 32, Fig. 2-1A.)*

  e. Cerebral atrophy
    • Atherosclerosis involving circle of Willis vessels or internal carotid
      artery
C. Arteriolosclerosis
  • Hardening of arterioles
  1. Hyaline arteriolosclerosis
    a. Pathogenesis
      • Increased protein is deposited in the vessel wall and occludes the
        lumen (Fig. 9-3).
    b. Associated conditions
      (1) Diabetes mellitus
        (a) Due to nonenzymatic glycosylation of proteins in the
            basement membrane
        (b) Basement membrane leaks protein into the vessel wall.
      (2) Hypertension

Hyaline arteriolosclerosis: diabetes mellitus, hypertension

        • Increased intraluminal pressure pushes plasma proteins into the
          vessel wall.
  2. Hyperplastic arteriolosclerosis
    a. Pathogenesis
      (1) Renal arteriole effect caused by an acute increase in blood pressure.
        • Example—malignant hypertension
      (2) Smooth muscle cell hyperplasia and basement membrane
          duplication
    b. Arterioles have an "onion skin" appearance.

III. Vessel Aneurysms
  • Vessel aneurysms are due to weakening of the vessel wall, followed by dilation
    and a tendency to rupture.
A. Abdominal aortic aneurysm

Abdominal aortic aneurysm: most common aneurysm in men > 55 years of age

  1. Usually located below the renal artery orifices

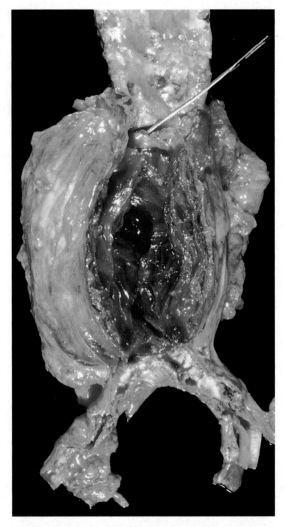

9-4: Abdominal aortic aneurysm. The aneurysmal dilation of the aorta is just above the bifurcation of the aorta. The probe is located at the rupture site. The lumen is filled with atherosclerotic debris and clot material. Ulcerated atheromatous plaques are proximal and distal to the aneurysm. (From Kumar V, Fausto N, Abbas A: Robbins and Cotran's Pathologic Basis of Disease, 7th ed. Philadelphia, WB Saunders, 2004, p 531, Fig. 11-19B.)

   2. Pathogenesis
      a. Atherosclerosis weakens vessel wall
        (1) Vessel wall stress increases with vessel diameter.
        (2) Lumen fills with atheromatous debris and blood clots (Fig. 9-4).
      b. Familial factors, structural defects in connective tissue
   3. Clinical findings
      a. Usually asymptomatic
      b. Rupture is the most common complication.

Rupture triad: left flank pain, hypotension, pulsatile mass

(1) Severe back pain is followed by hypotension from blood loss in the retroperitoneum.

(2) A pulsatile mass can be palpated.

B. Mycotic aneurysm

    1. Pathogenesis

       a. Vessel wall weakening due to an infection

       b. Fungi that invade vessels

         • *Aspergillus, Candida, Mucor*

       c. Bacteria that invade vessels

         • *Bacteroides fragilis, Pseudomonas aeruginosa, Salmonella* species

    2. Clinical findings

       a. Thrombosis with or without infarction

       b. Rupture

C. Berry aneurysm of cerebral arteries

    1. Pathogenesis

       a. Defect at the junction of communicating branches with main cerebral vessels

         • Vessel lacks an internal elastic lamina and smooth muscle.

       b. Risk factors for developing the aneurysm

         (1) Normal hemodynamic stress

         (2) Presence of hypertension of any cause

         (3) Coarctation of the aorta

       c. Rupture releases blood into the subarachnoid space

    2. Clinical findings

       a. Sudden onset of severe occipital headache

         • Described as the "worst headache I have ever had"

       b. Nuchal rigidity from irritation of the meninges

       c. Complications

         (1) Death may occur shortly after the bleed.

         (2) Rebleed, hydrocephalus, neurologic deficits

D. Syphilitic aneurysm

Aortic arch aneurysm: tertiary syphilis; vasculitis of vasa vasorum

    1. Complication of tertiary syphilis due to *Treponema pallidum*

       • Usually occurs in men 40 to 55 years of age

    2. Pathogenesis

       a. *T. pallidum* infects the vasa vasorum of the ascending and transverse portions of aortic arch.

         (1) Vasculitis is called endarteritis obliterans.

         (2) Characteristic plasma cell infiltrate is present in the vessel wall.

       b. Vessel ischemia of the medial tissue leads to dilation of the aorta and aortic valve ring.

    3. Clinical findings

       a. Aortic valve regurgitation

> Aortic regurgitation is a problem in closing the aortic valve. Because the aortic valve closes in diastole, the murmur occurs in early diastole as blood leaks back into the ventricle. The increase

in left ventricular end-diastolic volume results in an increase in stroke volume (increased systolic pressure). Blood rapidly draining back into the left ventricle produces a drop in the diastolic pressure. The wide pulse pressure (difference between the systolic and diastolic pressure) is manifested by a hyperdynamic circulation (e.g., pulsating uvula, bounding pulses).

  b. Brassy cough
   - Left recurrent laryngeal nerve is stretched by the aneurysm.

E. Aortic dissection
  1. Epidemiology
   a. Men with a mean age of 40 to 60 years with antecedent hypertension
    - Most common group
   b. Young patients with a connective tissue disorder
    - Examples—Marfan syndrome, Ehlers-Danlos syndrome (EDS)

Most common cause of death in Marfan syndrome and EDS: aortic dissection

   Marfan syndrome is an autosomal dominant disorder resulting in the production of weak elastic tissue due to a defect in synthesizing fibrillin. Cardiovascular abnormalities dominate. Dilation of the ascending aorta may progress to aortic dissection or aortic regurgitation. Mitral valve prolapse is the most common valvular defect and is often associated with conduction defects causing sudden death. Skeletal defects include eunuchoid proportions (lower body length > upper body length, arm span > height) and arachnodactyly (spider hands).

  2. Pathogenesis
   a. Cystic medial degeneration (CMD)
    (1) Elastic tissue fragmentation
    (2) Matrix material collects in areas of fragmentation in the tunica media
   b. Risk factors for CMD
    (1) Increase in wall stress
     - Hypertension, pregnancy (increased plasma volume), coarctation
    (2) Defects in connective tissue
     - Marfan syndrome (defect in elastic tissue), EDS (defect in collagen)
   c. Intimal tear
    (1) Due to hypertension or underlying structural weakness in the media
    (2) Usually occurs within 10 cm of the aortic valve
    (3) Blood dissects under arterial pressure through areas of weakness.
    (4) Blood dissects proximally and/or distally.
  3. Clinical findings
   a. Acute onset of severe retrosternal chest pain radiating to the back
   b. Aortic valve regurgitation
    (1) Due to aortic valve ring dilation
    (2) A radiograph or echocardiogram shows widening of the aortic valve root.

Aortic dissection: cardiac tamponade most common cause of death

    c. Loss of the upper extremity pulse
- Due to compression of the subclavian artery

    d. Rupture
- Usually into the pericardial sac, pleural cavity, or peritoneal cavity

IV. Venous System Disorders

A. Saphenous venous system
1. Superficial veins drain blood into the deep veins via penetrating branches.
2. Valves prevent reversal of blood flow into the superficial system.
3. Deep veins direct blood to the heart.

B. Varicose veins
1. Abnormally distended, lengthened, and tortuous veins
2. Locations
    a. Superficial saphenous veins (most common site)
    b. Distal esophagus (due to portal hypertension)
    c. Anorectal region (e.g., hemorrhoids)
    d. Left scrotal sac (e.g., varicocele)
3. Superficial varicosities; causes:
    a. Valve incompetence
- Exacerbated by pregnancy, prolonged standing, obesity, oral contraceptives, advanced age

    b. Familial tendency
    c. Secondary to deep venous thrombosis

C. Phlebothrombosis

Phlebothrombosis: stasis of blood flow most common cause

1. Thrombosis of a vein *without* inflammation
2. Causes
    a. Stasis of blood flow
    b. Hypercoagulability (e.g., antithrombin III deficiency)
3. Location
    a. Most often occurs in the deep vein of the calf
    b. Less common sites include portal vein, hepatic vein, dural sinuses
4. Clinical findings associated with deep vein thrombosis
    a. General findings
      (1) Swelling
      (2) Pain on dorsiflexion of foot and compression of calf
      (3) Pitting edema distal to the thrombosis
    b. Pulmonary thromboembolism
- Occurs when the thrombus extends into the femoral vein

Stasis dermatitis: sign of deep vein thrombosis

    c. Deep venous insufficiency
      (1) Stasis dermatitis
        (a) Orange discoloration (hemosiderin) around the ankles
        (b) Caused by rupture of the penetrating branches
      (2) Varicosities develop in the superficial system
- Due to retrograde blood flow into the superficial system

D. Thrombophlebitis
1. Pain and tenderness along the course of a superficial vein
2. Pathogenesis

a. Intravenous cannulation of veins
b. Infection (*Staphylococcus aureus*)
c. Carcinoma of the pancreatic head
   (1) Produces superficial migratory thrombophlebitis
   (2) Due to the release of thrombogenic substances by the cancer
3. Clinical findings
   a. Tender and palpable cord
   b. Erythema and edema of the overlying skin and subcutaneous tissue

E. Superior vena cava syndrome
1. Pathogenesis
   a. Extrinsic compression of the superior vena cava
   b. Due to a primary lung cancer (90% of cases)
      • Usually a small cell carcinoma of the lung
2. Clinical findings
   a. "Puffiness" and blue to purple discoloration of the face, arms, and shoulders
   b. Retinal hemorrhage, stroke

F. Thoracic outlet syndrome
1. Pathogenesis
   a. Compression of the neurovascular compartment in the neck
   b. Causes include cervical rib, spastic anterior scalene muscles, or positional change in the neck and arms
2. Clinical findings
   a. Vascular signs (e.g., arm "falls asleep" while person is sleeping)
   b. Nerve root signs (e.g., numbness, paresthesias)
   c. Positive Adson test
      • Pulse disappears when the arm is outstretched and the patient looks to the side of the outstretched arm.

Thoracic outlet syndrome: common among weight lifters

V. Lymphatic Disorders

A. Structure of lymphatic vessels
   • Lymphatic vessels have incomplete basement membranes, which predisposes them to infection and tumor invasion.

B. Acute lymphangitis
1. Inflammation of lymphatics ("red streak")
2. Usually due to cellulitis caused by *Streptococcus pyogenes*

C. Lymphedema
1. Collection of lymphatic fluid in interstitial tissue or body cavities
2. Obstructive lymphedema
   • Radiation damage following radical mastectomy
3. Turner's syndrome (see Chapter 5)
   a. Lymphedema of hands and feet in newborns caused by defective lymphatics
   b. Dilated lymphatic channels in the neck (cystic hygroma) produce webbed neck.
4. Chylous effusions (e.g., pleural cavity)
   a. Contain chylomicrons with triglyceride plus mature lymphocytes

Webbed neck: lymphatic abnormality

b. Damage to thoracic duct
  • Causes include malignant lymphoma, trauma

VI. Vascular Tumors and Tumor-like Conditions
A. Tumors
  • Most tumors derive from small vessels or arteriovenous anastomoses in glomus bodies.
B. Vessel tumors and tumor-like conditions (Table 9-1)

Capillary hemangiomas in newborns regress with age.

**TABLE 9-1:
Vascular Tumors and Tumor-like Conditions**

Tumor/Condition	Clinical Findings
Angiomyolipoma	Kidney hamartoma composed of blood vessels, muscle, and mature adipose tissue
	Association with tuberous sclerosis
Angiosarcoma	Liver angiosarcoma associated with exposure to polyvinyl chloride, arsenic, thorium dioxide
Bacillary angiomatosis	Benign capillary proliferation involving skin and visceral organs in AIDS patients
	Simulates Kaposi sarcoma in AIDS
	Caused by *Bartonella henselae*, a gram-negative bacillus
Capillary hemangioma	Facial lesion in newborns that regresses with age
Cavernous hemangioma	Most common benign tumor of liver and spleen
	May rupture if large
Cystic hygroma	Lymphangioma in the neck associated with Turner's syndrome
Glomus tumor	Derive from arteriovenous shunts in glomus bodies
	Painful red subungual nodule in a digit
Hereditary telangiectasia (AD)	Dilated vessels on skin and mucous membranes in mouth and gastrointestinal tract
	Chronic iron deficiency anemia
Kaposi sarcoma	Malignant tumor arising from endothelial cells or primitive mesenchymal cells
	Associated with human herpesvirus type 8
	Raised, red-purple discoloration that progresses from a flat lesion to a plaque to a nodule that ulcerates
	Common sites include skin, mouth, and gastrointestinal tract
Lymphangiosarcoma	Malignancy of lymphatic vessels
	Arises out of longstanding chronic lymphedema after modified radical mastectomy
Pyogenic granuloma	Vascular, red pedunculated mass that ulcerates and bleeds easily
	Post-traumatic or associated with pregnancy (relation to estrogen); usually regress postpartum
Spider telangiectasia	Arteriovenous fistula (disappears when compressed)
	Associated with hyperestrinism (e.g., cirrhosis, pregnancy)
Sturge-Weber syndrome	Nevus flammeus ("birthmark") on face in distribution of ophthalmic branch of cranial nerve V (trigeminal)
	Some cases show ipsilateral malformation of pia mater vessels overlying occipital and parietal lobes
Von Hippel–Lindau syndrome (AD)	Cavernous hemangiomas in cerebellum and retina
	Increased incidence of pheochromocytoma and bilateral renal cell carcinomas

AD, autosomal dominant.

VII. Vasculitic Disorders

- Inflammation of small vessels (arterioles, venules, capillaries), medium-sized vessels (muscular arteries), large vessels (elastic arteries), or combinations of these vessel types.

A. Pathogenesis

1. Type III hypersensitivity (immunocomplex)
   - Example—Henoch-Schönlein purpura
2. Type II hypersensitivity (antigen-antibody)
   - Example—Goodpasture syndrome (anti–basement membrane antibodies)
3. Antineutrophil cytoplasmic antibodies (ANCA)
   a. Activate neutrophils causing release of their enzymes and free radicals resulting in vessel damage
   b. c-ANCA type
      (1) Antibodies are directed against proteinase 3 in cytoplasmic granules.
      (2) Example—Wegener's granulomatosis
   c. p-ANCA type
      (1) Antibodies are directed against myeloperoxidase.
      (2) Examples—microscopic polyangiitis, Churg-Strauss syndrome
4. Direct invasion by all classes of microbial pathogens

B. Clinical findings

1. Small vessel vasculitis
   a. Called leukocytoclastic venulitis or hypersensitivity vasculitis
   b. Gross appearance
      (1) Skin overlying the vasculitis is hemorrhagic, raised, and painful to palpation (Fig. 9-5)
         - Called palpable purpura ("tumor" of acute inflammation)
      (2) Examples—Henoch-Schönlein purpura, microscopic polyangiitis

Small vessel vasculitis: palpable purpura

> Purpura due to thrombocytopenia or vessel instability (e.g., scurvy) is *not* palpable, because acute inflammation is *not* involved.

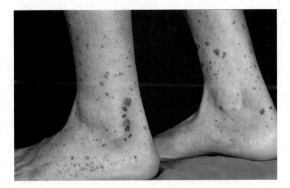

9-5: *Henoch-Schönlein purpura. Multiple erythematous, raised, palpable lesions around the ankles show areas of hemorrhage into the skin overlying areas of immunocomplex vasculitis involving small vessels. (From Bouloux P-M: Self-Assessment Picture Tests: Medicine, vol. 1. St. Louis, Mosby, 1996, p 38.)*

c. Microscopic appearance
  • Vessel is disrupted and contains a neutrophilic infiltrate associated with nuclear debris and fibrinoid necrosis.

2. Medium-sized vessel vasculitis
  a. Muscular artery vasculitis
  b. Presents with vessel thrombosis and infarction or aneurysms
  c. Examples—polyarteritis nodosa, Kawasaki disease
3. Large vessel vasculitis

  a. Elastic artery vasculitis
  b. Presents with loss of a pulse or stroke
  c. Examples—Takayasu arteritis, giant cell (temporal arteritis)
4. Summary table of vasculitides (Table 9-2)

VIII. Hypertension
  • Hypertension is defined as systolic blood pressure above 140 mm Hg and diastolic blood pressure above 90 mm Hg for a sustained period.

A. Pathophysiology of hypertension
1. Systolic blood pressure
  a. Correlates with stroke volume
  b. Determination of stroke volume:
    (1) Blood volume (equates with sodium homeostasis)
    (2) Force of contraction
    (3) Heart rate

2. Diastolic blood pressure
  a. Determination of diastolic blood pressure
    (1) Volume of blood in the arteries while the heart is filling in diastole
      • Depends on the vascular tone of the peripheral resistance arterioles
    (2) Elastic recoil of the aorta

  b. Role of the total peripheral resistance (TPR) arterioles
    (1) Abbreviated Poiseuille's equation
      • TPR = viscosity of blood/(radius of arteriole)^4
    (2) Vasodilation decreases TPR
      (a) Decreases diastolic blood pressure
      (b) Increases venous return to the heart

Vasodilators include nitric oxide, prostaglandins, histamine, β-blockers, and calcium-channel blockers.

    (3) Vasoconstriction increases TPR
      • Increases diastolic blood pressure

Factors that contract arteriole smooth muscle cells causing vasoconstriction include α-adrenergic stimuli, catecholamines, angiotensin II, vasopressin, and increased total body sodium.

TABLE 9-2:
Vasculitic Disorders: Elastic Artery, Muscular Artery, and Small Vessel Disease

Disorder	Vasculitis	Epidemiology/Etiology	Clinical/Laboratory Findings
Takayasu's arteritis ("pulseless disease")	Granulomatous large vessel vasculitis involving aortic arch vessels	Young Asian women and children	Absent upper extremity pulse Visual defects, stroke
Giant cell (temporal) arteritis	Granulomatous large vessel vasculitis involving superficial temporal and ophthalmic arteries; thrombi contain microabscesses	Adults > 50 years of age	Temporal headache, jaw claudication (pain when chewing) Blindness on ipsilateral side Polymyalgia rheumatica (muscle and joint pain; normal serum creatine kinase) Increased ESR
Polyarteritis nodosa	Necrotizing medium-sized vessel vasculitis involving renal, coronary, mesenteric arteries (spares pulmonary arteries)	Middle-aged men Association with HBsAg (30%)	Vessels at all stages of acute and chronic inflammation Focal vasculitis produces aneurysms (detected with angiography) Organ infarction in kidneys (renal failure), heart (acute MI), bowels (bloody diarrhea), skin (ischemic ulcer)
Kawasaki disease	Necrotizing medium-sized vessel vasculitis involving coronary arteries (e.g., thrombosis, aneurysms)	Children < 4 years of age	Desquamating rash, swelling of hands and feet, cervical adenopathy, oral erythema Abnormal ECG (e.g., acute MI) Corticosteroids contraindicated (danger of vessel rupture)
Thromboangiitis obliterans (Buerger's disease)	Medium-sized vessel vasculitis with digital vessel thrombosis	Men 25–50 years of age who smoke cigarettes	Foot claudication, Raynaud's phenomenon, ulceration, gangrene
Raynaud's disease	Medium-sized vessel vasculitis involving digital vessels in fingers and toes	Young women Exaggerated vasomotor response to cold or stress	Paroxysmal digital color changes (white-blue-red sequence) Ulceration and gangrene in chronic cases
Raynaud's phenomenon	Medium-sized vessel vasculitis involving digital vessels in fingers and toes	Adult men and women Secondary to other diseases (e.g., systemic sclerosis, CREST syndrome)	Systemic sclerosis and CREST syndrome: digital vasculitis with vessel fibrosis, dystrophic calcification, ulceration, gangrene
Wegener's granulomatosis	Necrotizing medium-sized and small vessel vasculitis involving upper respiratory tract, lung, renal vessels	Childhood to middle age	Necrotizing vasculitis in upper respiratory tract (nasopharynx, sinuses, trachea), lower respiratory tract (pulmonary vessels; infarction, pneumonia), kidneys (crescentic glomerulonephritis)

continued

TABLE 9-2:

Vasculitic Disorders: Elastic Artery, Muscular Artery, and Small Vessel Disease—cont'd

Disorder	Vasculitis	Epidemiology/Etiology	Clinical/Laboratory Findings
			Necrotizing granulomas in upper respiratory tract (saddle nose deformity), lungs c-ANCA antibodies (>90% of cases) Treatment: corticosteroids, cyclophosphamide
Microscopic polyangiitis	Small vessel vasculitis involving skin, lung, brain, GI tract, and postcapillary venules and glomerular capillaries	Children and adults Precipitated by drugs (e.g., penicillin), infections (e.g., streptococci), immune disorders (e.g., SLE)	Vessels at same stage of inflammation Palpable purpura, glomerulonephritis p-ANCA antibodies (>80% of cases)
Churg-Strauss syndrome	Small vessel vasculitis involving skin, lung, heart vessels	Children and adults	Allergic rhinitis, asthma p-ANCA antibodies (70% of cases), eosinophilia
Henoch-Schönlein purpura	Small vessel vasculitis involving skin, GI tract, renal, joint vessels	Children and young adults Most common vasculitis in children IgA immunocomplexes	Palpable purpura of buttocks and lower extremities Polyarthritis, glomerulonephritis, GI bleeding
Cryoglobulinemia	Small vessel vasculitis involving skin, GI tract, renal vessels	Adults Association with HCV, type I MPGN	Cryoglobulins: immunoglobulins that gel at cold temperatures Palpable purpura, acral cyanosis of nose and ears and Raynaud's phenomenon (reverses when in warm room)
Serum sickness	Small vessel vasculitis involving immunocomplex deposition in skin vessels	Children and adults Complication of treatment of rattlesnake envenomation with horse- or sheep-based antivenin	Fever, urticaria with vasculitis, arthralgia, GI pain with melena
Infectious vasculitis	Small vessel vasculitis involving skin vessels	Children and adults Involves all microbial pathogens	Rocky Mountain spotted fever: tick transmission of *Rickettsia rickettsiae;* organisms invade endothelial cells; petechiae on palms spread to trunk Disseminated meningococcemia due to *Neisseria meningitidis* Capillary thrombosis produces hemorrhage into skin and confluent ecchymoses

c-ANCA, cytoplasmic antineutrophil cytoplasmic antibodies; ECG, electrocardiogram; ESR, erythrocyte sedimentation rate; GI, gastrointestinal; HBsAg, hepatitis B surface antigen; HCV, hepatitis C virus; MI, myocardial infarction; MPGN, membranoproliferative glomerulonephritis; p-ANCA, perinuclear antineutrophil cytoplasmic antibodies; SLE, systemic lupus erythematosus.

3. Role of sodium in hypertension
   a. Excess sodium increases plasma volume
      • Increases stroke volume and systolic blood pressure
   b. Excess sodium produces vasoconstriction of TPR arterioles
      (1) Sodium enters arteriole smooth muscle cells and opens calcium channels, causing vasoconstriction.
      (2) Increases diastolic blood pressure

B. Essential hypertension
   1. Accounts for 95% of cases of hypertension
   2. Pathogenesis
      a. Genetic factors reduce renal sodium excretion.
      b. Unknown factors cause vasoconstriction of arterioles.
      c. Obesity, stress

Most common type of hypertension: essential hypertension

> Reduced renal sodium excretion is the primary mechanism of essential hypertension in black Americans and the elderly. Increased plasma volume suppresses renin release from the juxtaglomerular apparatus.

C. Secondary hypertension
   1. Accounts for 5% of cases of hypertension
   2. Renovascular hypertension
      a. Causes
         (1) Elderly men
            • Atherosclerotic plaque partially blocks blood flow at the renal artery orifice.
         (2) Young to middle-aged women
            • Fibromuscular hyperplasia occurs in multifocal areas of the renal artery.
      b. Pathogenesis
         (1) Decreased renal arterial blood flow activates the renin-angiotensin-aldosterone (RAA) system.
         (2) Angiotensin II vasoconstricts TPR arterioles.
         (3) Aldosterone increases sodium retention.
      c. Clinical findings
         (1) Severe, uncontrollable hypertension
         (2) Increased plasma renin activity (PRA)
         (3) Involved kidney has increased PRA in the renal vein.
         (4) Uninvolved kidney has decreased PRA.
            • Increased plasma volume due to aldosterone excess suppresses RAA system in normal kidney
         (5) Epigastric bruit
            • Sound is due to turbulence of blood flow through the narrow renal artery.
         (6) Angiography
            (a) Involved kidney shows diminished size (atrophy) and delayed emptying.

Renovascular hypertension: most common cause of secondary hypertension

Renovascular hypertension: activation of renin-angiotensin-aldosterone system

> (b) Renal artery has "beaded" appearance in fibromuscular hyperplasia.
>
> d. Other causes of secondary hypertension (Table 9-3)
>
> **D. Complications of hypertension (Table 9-4)**

**TABLE 9-3:
Causes of
Secondary
Hypertension**

System or Source	Description
Adrenal	Cushing syndrome: increased mineralocorticoids Pheochromocytoma: increased catecholamines Neuroblastoma: increased catecholamines 11-Hydroxylase deficiency: increased mineralocorticoids (i.e., deoxycorticosterone) Primary aldosteronism (Conn syndrome): increased aldosterone
Aorta	Postductal coarctation: activation of RAA system Elderly: systolic hypertension due to decreased elasticity of the aorta
CNS	Intracranial hypertension: release of catecholamines
Drugs	Oral contraceptive: increased synthesis of angiotensinogen; most common cause of hypertension in young women Cocaine: increased sympathetic activity
Parathyroid	Primary hyperparathyroidism: calcium increases peripheral resistance arteriole smooth muscle cell contraction
Pregnancy	Preeclampsia: increased angiotensin II
Renal	Renovascular disease: atherosclerosis (elderly men), fibromuscular hyperplasia (women) Renal parenchymal disease: e.g., diabetic nephropathy, adult polycystic kidney disease, glomerulonephritis
Thyroid	Graves' disease: systolic hypertension from increased cardiac contraction Hypothyroidism: diastolic hypertension due to retention of sodium

CNS, central nervous system; RAA, renin-angiotensin-aldosterone.

**TABLE 9-4:
Complications of
Hypertension**

System	Complications
Cardiovascular	Left ventricular hypertrophy: most common overall complication Acute myocardial infarction: most common cause of death Atherosclerosis
CNS	Intracerebral hematoma: due to rupture of Charcot-Bouchard aneurysms Berry aneurysm: rupture produces a subarachnoid hemorrhage Lacunar infarcts: small infarcts due to hyaline arteriolosclerosis
Renal	Benign nephrosclerosis: kidney disease of hypertension; due to hyaline arteriolosclerosis; atrophy of tubules and sclerosis of glomeruli; progresses to renal failure Malignant hypertension: rapid increase in blood pressure accompanied by renal failure and cerebral edema
Eyes	Hypertensive retinopathy: arteriovenous nicking, hemorrhage of retinal vessels, exudates (increased vessel permeability, retinal infarction), papilledema

Heart Disorders

I. Ventricular Hypertrophy

A. Pathogenesis of left and right ventricular hypertrophy

1. Sustained pressure increases wall stress.
   a. Causes duplication of sarcomeres
      (1) Duplication in parallel thickens muscle.
      (2) Duplication in series lengthens muscle.
   b. Sarcomeres are the contractile element of muscle.
2. Contraction against an increased resistance (afterload)
   a. Produces concentric thickening of the ventricular wall
      • New sarcomeres duplicate in parallel to the long axes of the cells.
   b. Causes of concentric left ventricular hypertrophy (LVH, see Fig. 1-4)
      (1) Essential hypertension (most common)
      (2) Aortic stenosis
   c. Causes of concentric right ventricular hypertrophy (RVH)
      (1) Pulmonary hypertension
      (2) Pulmonary artery stenosis
3. Volume overload (increased preload)
   a. Causes dilation and hypertrophy (eccentric hypertrophy) of ventricular wall
      (1) Frank-Starling mechanism causes increased force of contraction.
      (2) Sarcomeres duplicate in series and cell length and width are increased.
   b. Causes of eccentric hypertrophy of left ventricle
      (1) Mitral valve or aortic valve regurgitation
      (2) Left-to-right shunting of blood (e.g., ventricular septal defect)
         • Causes more blood to return to the left side of the heart
   c. Causes of eccentric hypertrophy of right ventricle
      • Tricuspid valve or pulmonary valve regurgitation

B. Consequences of ventricular hypertrophy

1. Left- or right-sided heart failure
2. Angina (primarily LVH)
3. S_4 heart sound
   a. Correlates with atrial contraction in late diastole
   b. Caused by blood entering a noncompliant ventricle

II. Congestive Heart Failure (CHF)

• The heart fails when it is unable to eject blood delivered to it by the venous system.

Wall stress increases sarcomere duplication.

Ventricular hypertrophy: due to increased afterload or increased preload

A. **Epidemiology**
1. Most common hospital admission diagnosis in elderly patients
2. Types of CHF
   a. Left-sided heart failure (most common type)
   b. Right-sided heart failure
   c. Biventricular heart failure (left- and right-sided heart failure)
   d. High-output heart failure
B. **Left-sided heart failure (LHF)**
1. Forward failure
   a. Left side of the heart cannot eject blood into the aorta
   b. Increase in left ventricular end-diastolic volume and pressure
   c. Backup of blood into the lungs causing pulmonary edema
2. Pathogenesis
   a. Decreased ventricular contraction (systolic dysfunction); causes:
      (1) Ischemia (most common cause)
      (2) Myocardial fibrosis, myocarditis, cardiomyopathy
   b. Noncompliant ventricle (diastolic dysfunction)
      (1) Restricted filling of the ventricle
      (2) Causes
          (a) Concentric LVH (most common cause)
          (b) Infiltration of muscle with amyloid, iron, or glycogen

> Systolic dysfunction is characterized by a low ejection fraction (EF) (<40%). The EF equals the stroke volume divided by the left ventricular end-diastolic volume. The normal value ranges from 55% to 80%. Diastolic dysfunction is characterized by normal to high EF (stiff ventricle) and an S_4 gallop due to increased resistance to filling in late diastole. There is an increase in left atrial pressure. The EF is normal.

   c. Increased workload
      • Due to increased afterload (resistance) or preload (volume)
3. Gross and microscopic findings
   a. Lungs are congested and exude a frothy pink transudate (edema).
   b. Alveolar macrophages contain hemosiderin ("heart failure" cells).
4. Clinical findings
   a. Dyspnea
      (1) Difficulty breathing
      (2) Patient cannot take a full inspiration
   b. Pulmonary edema
      (1) Bibasilar inspiratory crackles
      (2) Chest radiograph shows congestion in upper lobes and alveolar infiltrates
   c. Left-sided S_3 heart sound
      (1) Occurs in early diastole
          • Intensity of the heart sound increases with expiration.

Left-sided heart failure = forward failure → pulmonary edema

Systolic dysfunction: decreased ventricular contraction

Diastolic dysfunction: increased resistance to filling the ventricle

(2) Caused by blood entering a volume-overloaded left ventricle

(3) First cardiac finding in LHF

d. Mitral valve regurgitation

• Caused by stretching of the valve ring

> Mitral regurgitation is a problem in closing the mitral valve. The mitral valve normally closes in systole. Blood entering the left atrium during systole produces a pansystolic murmur that increases in intensity on expiration. The murmur is best heard at the apex.

e. Paroxysmal nocturnal dyspnea

(1) Choking sensation at night due to increased venous return to the failed left side of the heart

(2) Blood backs up into the lungs, producing pulmonary edema

(3) Relieved by standing or placing pillows under the head (pillow orthopnea)

• These maneuvers increase the effect of gravity on reducing venous return to the heart.

C. Right-sided heart failure (RHF)

1. Backward failure

a. Right side of the heart cannot pump blood from the venous system to the lungs.

b. Blood accumulates in the venous system.

2. Pathogenesis

a. Decreased contraction (e.g., right ventricular infarction)

b. Noncompliant right ventricle (e.g., RVH)

c. Increased afterload (left-sided heart failure most common cause)

d. Increased preload (e.g., tricuspid valve regurgitation)

3. Clinical findings

a. Prominence of jugular veins

• Due to increased venous hydrostatic pressure

b. Right-sided S_3 heart sound due to volume overload in the ventricle

• Increases in intensity with inspiration

c. Tricuspid valve regurgitation

• Caused by stretching of the valve ring

> Tricuspid regurgitation is a problem in closing the tricuspid valve. The tricuspid valve normally closes in systole. Blood entering the right atrium during systole produces a pansystolic murmur that increases in intensity on inspiration. The murmur is best heard along the left parasternal border.

d. Painful hepatomegaly

• Passive liver congestion due to backup of venous blood into the central veins

e. Dependent pitting edema and ascites

• Due to an increase in venous hydrostatic pressure

S_3 heart sound: first cardiac sign of LHF

Expiration: increases intensity for left-sided heart murmurs and abnormal heart sounds

Right-sided heart failure = backward failure → increase in venous hydrostatic pressure

Inspiration: increases intensity of right-sided heart murmurs and abnormal heart sounds

D. High-output heart failure
1. Definition
   • Form of heart failure in which cardiac output is increased compared with values for the normal resting state
2. Pathogenesis
   a. Increase in stroke volume
      • Example—hyperthyroidism
   b. Decrease in blood viscosity
      • Example—severe anemia
   c. Vasodilation of peripheral resistance arterioles
      • Examples—thiamine deficiency, early phase of endotoxic shock
   d. Arteriovenous fistula
      (1) Arteriovenous communications bypass the microcirculation
      (2) Increases venous return to the heart
      (3) Causes
         (a) Trauma from knife wound (most common cause)
         (b) Surgical shunt for hemodialysis

III. Ischemic Heart Disease
   • Imbalance between myocardial O_2 demand and supply from the coronary arteries
A. Coronary artery blood flow
1. Provides oxygen to cardiac muscle
   a. Coronary vessels fill in diastole.
   b. Tachycardia (>180 bpm) decreases filling time, leading to ischemia.
2. Left anterior descending (LAD) coronary artery
   a. Distribution
      (1) Anterior portion of the left ventricle
      (2) Anterior two thirds of the interventricular septum
   b. Accounts for 40% to 50% of coronary artery thromboses
3. Right coronary artery (RCA)
   a. Distribution
      (1) Posteroinferior part of the left ventricle
      (2) Posterior one third of the interventricular septum
      (3) Right ventricle
      (4) Posteromedial papillary muscle in left ventricle
      (5) Both atrioventricular and sinoatrial nodes
   b. Accounts for 30% to 40% of coronary artery thromboses
4. Left circumflex coronary artery
   a. Supplies the lateral wall of the left ventricle
   b. Accounts for 15% to 20% of coronary artery thromboses
B. Epidemiology
1. Major cause of death in the United States
   a. Ischemic heart disease is more common in men.
   b. Peaks in men after age 60 and in women after age 70
2. Types of ischemic heart disease
   a. Angina pectoris (most common type)

Tachycardia: decreases diastole and filling of coronary arteries

       b. Chronic ischemic heart disease

       c. Sudden cardiac death

       d. Myocardial infarction

  3. Risk factors

       a. Age

         • Men 45 years old and up, women 55 years old and up

       b. Family history of premature coronary artery disease or stroke

       c. Lipid abnormalities

         (1) Low-density lipoprotein above 160 mg/dL

         (2) High-density lipoprotein below 35 mg/dL

       d. Smoking tobacco, hypertension, diabetes mellitus

C. Angina pectoris

  1. Stable angina (most common variant)

       a. Causes

         (1) Atherosclerotic coronary artery disease (most common)

         (2) Aortic stenosis with concentric LVH

         (3) Hypertrophic cardiomyopathy

       b. Pathogenesis

         • Subendocardial ischemia due to decreased coronary artery blood flow

       c. Clinical findings

         (1) Exercise-induced substernal chest pain lasting 30 seconds to 30 minutes

         (2) Relieved by resting or nitroglycerin

         (3) Stress test shows ST-segment depression.

  2. Prinzmetal's angina

       a. Pathogenesis

         (1) Intermittent coronary artery vasospasm at rest

         (2) Vasoconstriction due to platelet thromboxane A_2 or increase in endothelin

       b. Clinical findings

         (1) Stress test shows ST-segment elevation (transmural ischemia).

         (2) Responds to nitroglycerin and calcium-channel blocker (vasodilator)

  3. Unstable angina

       a. Pathogenesis

         (1) Severe, fixed, multivessel atherosclerotic disease

         (2) Disrupted plaques with or without platelet nonocclusive thrombi

       b. Clinical findings

         (1) Frequent bouts of chest pain at rest or with minimal exertion

         (2) May progress to acute myocardial infarction (MI)

  4. Revascularization procedures

       a. Percutaneous transluminal coronary angioplasty (PTCA) and stenting

         (1) Balloon angioplasty dilates and ruptures the atheromatous plaque

           • Problem with restenosis

         (2) Intracoronary stents

           • Decrease the rate of restenosis

Angina pectoris: most common manifestation of coronary artery disease

Stable angina: subendocardial ischemia with ST-segment depression

Prinzmetal's angina: vasospasm with transmural ischemia and ST-segment elevation

(3) Most common early complication is a localized dissection with thrombosis

    b. Coronary artery bypass graft (CABG)

       (1) Used for multivessel coronary artery atherosclerosis

       (2) Internal mammary artery graft

         • Best graft patency after 10 years

       (3) Saphenous veins

         • "Arterialization" of the vessels, fibrosis, and occlusion common after 10 years

D. Chronic ischemic heart disease

  1. Progressive CHF resulting from long-term ischemic damage to myocardial tissue

  2. Replacement of myocardial tissue with noncontractile scar tissue

  3. Clinical findings

    a. Biventricular CHF

    b. Angina pectoris

    c. May develop dilated cardiomyopathy

E. Sudden cardiac death

  1. Unexpected death within 1 hour after onset of symptoms

  2. Diagnosis of exclusion after other causes are ruled out

  3. Pathogenesis

    a. Severe atherosclerotic coronary artery disease

    b. Disrupted fibrous plaques

    c. Absence of occlusive vessel thrombus (>80% of cases)

  4. Cause of death is ventricular fibrillation.

F. Myocardial infarction

  1. Pathogenesis

    a. Sequence:

       (1) Sudden disruption of an atheromatous plaque

       (2) Exposed subendothelial collagen or thrombogenic necrotic material

       (3) Platelet adhesion and eventual formation of a platelet thrombus

    b. Role of thromboxane A_2

       (1) Contributes to formation of the platelet thrombus

       (2) Causes vasospasm of the artery

  2. Less common causes of acute MI

    a. Vasculitis (e.g., polyarteritis nodosa, Kawasaki disease)

    b. Cocaine use

    c. Embolization of plaque material

    d. Thrombosis syndromes (e.g., antithrombin III deficiency, polycythemia)

  3. Types of myocardial infarction

    a. Transmural infarction (Q-wave infarction)

       (1) Involves the full thickness of the myocardium

       (2) New Q waves develop in an electrocardiogram (ECG).

    b. Subendocardial infarction (non–Q wave infarction)

       (1) Involves the inner third of the myocardium

       (2) Q waves are absent.

Rupture of disrupted plaque → platelet thrombus → acute MI

4. Reperfusion
   a. May follow thrombolytic therapy (e.g., tissue plasminogen activator)
   b. Early reperfusion salvages some injured but *not* necrotic myocytes.
      • Improves short- and long-term function and survival
   c. Reperfusion histologically alters irreversibly damaged cells.
      (1) Produces contraction band necrosis
      (2) Hypercontraction of myofibrils in dying cells due to the influx of Ca^{2+} and $O_2^{\cdot}$
5. Gross and microscopic findings of acute MI
   a. During 0 to 24 hours
      (1) No gross changes until 24 hours after MI
      (2) Coagulation necrosis without neutrophil infiltrate within 12 to 24 hours
   b. During 1 to 3 days
      (1) Pallor of infarcted myocardium
      (2) Myocyte nuclei and striations disappear.
      (3) Neutrophils lyse dead myocardial cells.
   c. During 3 to 7 days
      (1) Red granulation tissue surrounds area of infarction.
      (2) Macrophages begin removal of necrotic debris.
   d. During 7 to 10 days
      (1) Necrotic area is bright yellow (Fig. 10-1).
      (2) Granulation tissue and collagen formation are well developed.
   e. During 2 months
      • Infarcted tissue replaced by white, patchy, noncontractile scar tissue.
6. Clinical findings
   a. Sudden onset of severe retrosternal pain
      (1) Lasts more than 30 to 45 minutes
      (2) Not relieved by nitroglycerin

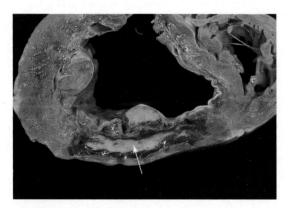

10-1: *Acute myocardial infarction (day 7) in the posterior wall of the left ventricle. The yellow area (arrow) is surrounded by a rim of dark, red granulation tissue. (From Damjanov I, Linder J: Pathology: A Color Atlas. St. Louis, Mosby, 2000, p 22, Fig. 1-47.)*

(3) Radiates down the left arm into the shoulders or into the jaw or epigastrium

(4) Associated with sweating (diaphoresis), anxiety, and hypotension

  b. "Silent" acute MIs

    (1) May occur in the elderly and in individuals with diabetes mellitus

    (2) Due to high pain threshold or problems with nervous system

7. Complications

  a. Arrhythmias

    (1) Ventricular premature contractions (most common)

    (2) Most common cause of death is ventricular fibrillation.

      • Frequently associated with cardiogenic shock

  b. Congestive heart failure

    • Usually occurs within the first 24 hours

  c. Rupture

    (1) Most commonly occurs between days 3 and 7 (range 1–10 days)

    (2) Anterior wall rupture

      (a) Causes cardiac tamponade

      (b) Associated with thrombosis of the LAD coronary artery

    (3) Posteromedial papillary muscle rupture or dysfunction

      (a) Associated with RCA thrombosis

      (b) Acute onset of mitral valve regurgitation and LHF

    (4) Interventricular septum rupture

      (a) Associated with LAD coronary artery thrombosis

      (b) Produces a left-to-right shunt causing RHF

  d. Mural thrombus

    (1) Most often associated with LAD coronary artery thrombosis

    (2) Danger of embolization

  e. Fibrinous pericarditis with or without effusion (Fig. 10-2)

    (1) Days 1 to 7 of transmural acute MI

      (a) Substernal chest pain relieved by leaning forward

      (b) Precordial friction rub is present.

        • Due to increased vessel permeability in the pericardium

    (2) Autoimmune pericarditis

      (a) Develops 6 to 8 weeks after an MI

      (b) Autoantibodies are directed against pericardial antigens.

      (c) Fever and precordial friction rub

  f. Ventricular aneurysm (Fig. 10-3)

    (1) Clinically recognized within 4 to 8 weeks

    (2) Precordial bulge during systole

      • Blood enters the aneurysm causing anterior chest wall movement.

    (3) Complications

      (a) CHF due to lack of contractile tissue

      (b) Danger of embolization of clot material

      (c) Rupture is uncommon.

  g. Right ventricular acute MI

    (1) Associated with RCA thrombosis

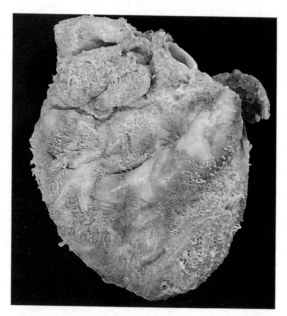

10-2: *Fibrinous pericarditis. The surface of the heart is covered by a shaggy, fibrinous exudate. (From Damjanov I, Linder J: Pathology: A Color Atlas. St. Louis, Mosby, 2000, p 25, Fig. 1-59.)*

      (2) Clinical findings
         • Hypotension, RHF, and preserved left ventricle function
  8. Laboratory diagnosis of acute MI (Fig. 10-4)
    a. Creatine kinase isoenzyme MB (CK-MB)
      (1) CK-MB appears within 4 to 8 hours; peaks at 24 hours; disappears within 1.5 to 3 days.
      (2) Reinfarction
         • Reappearance of CK-MB after 3 days
    b. Cardiac troponins I (cTnI) and T (cTnT)
      (1) Normally regulate calcium-mediated contraction
      (2) cTnI and cTnT appear within 3 to 6 hours; peak at 24 hours; disappear within 7 to 10 days.
      (3) Troponins are the gold standard for diagnosis of acute MI.
         • More specific for myocardial tissue than CK-MB and last longer
    c. Lactate dehydrogenase $(LDH)_{1-2}$ "flip"
      (1) Normally, LDH_2 is higher than LDH_1.
         • In acute MI, LDH_1 in cardiac muscle is released causing the "flip."
      (2) LDH_{1-2}
         • Appears within 10 hours; peaks at 2 to 3 days; disappears within 7 days
  9. Correlation of ECG changes with microscopic changes
    a. Inverted T waves
      • Correlate with areas of ischemia at the periphery of the infarct

Reinfarction: reappearance of CK-MB after 3 days

cTnI, cTnT: gold standard for diagnosis of acute MI

ECG findings in acute MI: inverted T waves, elevated ST segment, Q waves

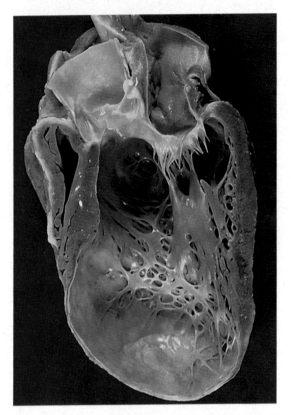

10-3: *Left ventricular aneurysm. The bulging aneurysm has a thin wall of scar tissue. (From Damjanov I, Linder J: Pathology: A Color Atlas. St. Louis, Mosby, 2000, p 24, Fig. 1-58.)*

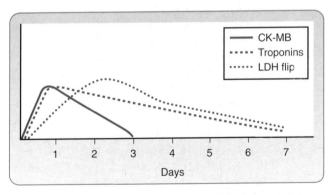

10-4: *Cardiac enzymes used in the diagnosis of an acute myocardial infarction. LDH, lactate dehydrogenase.*

b. Elevated ST segment
- Correlate with injured myocardial cells surrounding the area of necrosis
c. New Q waves
- Correlate with the area of coagulation necrosis

IV. Congenital Heart Disease
A. Fetal circulation
1. Chorionic villus in the placenta
   a. Fetus-derived
   b. Primary site for gas exchange in the fetus
   c. Chorionic villus vessels become the umbilical vein.
2. Umbilical vein
   - Vessel with the highest amount of oxygen (O_2) in the fetal circulation
3. Inferior vena cava blood drains into the right atrium.
   - Most blood is directly shunted into the left atrium through the foramen ovale.
4. Superior vena cava blood
   - Most blood is directed from the right atrium into the right ventricle.
5. Pulmonary artery blood
   a. Most blood is shunted through a patent ductus arteriosus into the aorta.
      - Kept open by prostaglandin E_2, a vasodilator
   b. Fetal pulmonary arteries
      (1) Hypertrophied from chronic vasoconstriction due to decreased P_{O_2}
      (2) Prevents blood from entering the pulmonary capillaries and left atrium
6. Descending aorta
   a. Blood flows toward the placenta via two umbilical arteries.
   b. These vessels have the lowest O_2 concentration.
7. Changes at birth
   a. Ductus arteriosus closes (becomes ligamentum arteriosum)
   b. Gas exchange occurs in the lungs.
   c. Foramen ovale closes.

B. Congenital heart disease
1. O_2 saturation (Sao_2) in shunts
   a. Left-sided to right-sided heart shunts
      - Increased Sao_2 from 75% to ~80% in affected chambers and vessels
   b. Right-sided to left-sided heart shunts
      - Decreased Sao_2 from 95% to ~80% in affected chambers and vessels
2. Left-sided to right-sided heart shunts
   a. Volume overload occurs in the right side of the heart; complications:
      (1) Pulmonary hypertension
      (2) RVH due to pulmonary hypertension
      (3) LVH due to excess blood originating from the right side of the heart
      (4) Reversal of the shunt

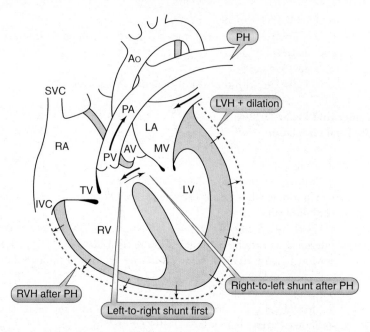

10-5: *Schematic of ventricular septal defect. Refer to the text for discussion. Ao, aorta; AV, aortic valve; IVC, inferior vena cava; LA, left atrium; LV, left ventricle; LVH, left ventricular hypertrophy; MV, mitral valve; PA, pulmonary artery; PH, pulmonary hypertension; PV, pulmonary valve; RA, right atrium; RV, right ventricle; RVH, right ventricular hypertrophy; SVC, superior vena cava; TV, tricuspid valve.*

(a) Occurs when pressure in right ventricle overrides left ventricular pressure
(b) Cyanosis (Eisenmenger syndrome) develops.

VSD: most common congenital heart disease in children

b. VSD (Fig. 10-5)
(1) Defect in the membranous interventricular septum
(2) Associated with cri du chat syndrome, trisomy 13, and trisomy 18
(3) Increased Sao_2 in right ventricle and pulmonary artery
(4) Most spontaneously close

ASD: most common congenital heart disease in adults

c. Atrial septal defect (ASD)
(1) Patent foramen ovale (most common type)
(2) Associated with fetal alcohol syndrome
(3) Increased Sao_2 in right atrium, right ventricle and pulmonary artery
(4) Congenital heart disease in children with Down syndrome
(a) Incomplete septum between the ventricles and the atria
(b) Abnormal tricuspid valve

d. Patent ductus arteriosus (PDA)
(1) Ductus arteriosus remains open.
(2) Associated with congenital rubella
(3) Increased Sao_2 in pulmonary artery
(4) Reversal of the shunt due to pulmonary hypertension

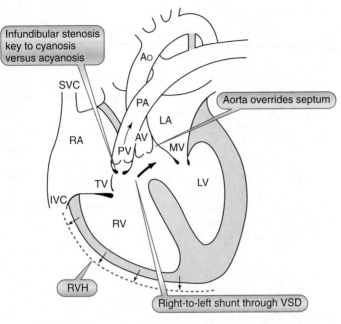

10-6: *Schematic of tetralogy of Fallot. Refer to the text for discussion. Ao, aorta; AV, aortic valve; IVC, inferior vena cava; LA, left atrium; LV, left ventricle; MV, mitral valve; PA, pulmonary artery; PV, pulmonary valve; RA, right atrium; RV, right ventricle; RVH, right ventricular hypertrophy; SVC, superior vena cava; TV, tricuspid valve; VSD, ventricular septal defect.*

(a) Unoxygenated blood enters the aorta below the subclavian artery
(b) Produces a pink upper body and cyanotic lower body
  (5) Machinery murmur is heard during systole and diastole.
3. Right-sided to left-sided heart shunts
  a. Cyanotic congenital heart disease
  b. Complications
    (1) Secondary polycythemia
      • Erythropoietin response due to decreased Sao_2
    (2) Infective endocarditis of damaged valves
      • Increased incidence of septic embolization and metastatic abscesses
  c. Tetralogy of Fallot
    (1) Most common cyanotic congenital heart disease (Fig. 10-6)
    (2) Defects
      (a) VSD
      (b) Infundibular or valvular pulmonary stenosis
      (c) RVH
      (d) Overriding aorta (least important)
    (3) Minimal pulmonary stenosis
      (a) Leads to oxygenation of blood in the lungs
      (b) Less right-to-left shunting through the VSD
      (c) Absence of cyanosis ($Sao_2 > 80\%$)

PDA: can be closed with indomethacin

(4) Severe pulmonic stenosis
    (a) Less oxygenation of blood in the lungs
    (b) Increased right-to-left shunting through the VSD
    (c) Cyanosis ($Sao_2 < 80\%$)
(5) Decreased Sao_2 in the left ventricle and aorta
(6) Cardioprotective shunts increase oxygenation
    (a) ASD steps up Sao_2 in the right atrium.
    (b) PDA shunts blood from the aorta to the pulmonary artery.
(7) Tet spells
    (a) Sudden increase in hypoxemia and cyanosis
    (b) Squatting increases systemic vascular resistance causing temporary reversal of the shunt.
    (c) Unoxygenated blood is forced into the pulmonary artery for oxygenation.

Tetralogy of Fallot: degree of pulmonary stenosis correlates with presence or absence of cyanosis

d. Complete transposition of the great vessels
  (1) Defects
    (a) Aorta arises from the right ventricle.
    (b) Pulmonary artery arises from the left ventricle.
    (c) Left and right atria are normal
  (2) Cardioprotective shunts
    (a) ASD steps up Sao_2 in the right atrium
      • Increases Sao_2 in the right ventricle for delivery to tissue via the aorta
    (b) VSD shunts blood into the left ventricle for oxygenation in the lungs via the pulmonary artery.
    (c) PDA shunts blood into the pulmonary artery for oxygenation in the lungs.
e. Other types of cyanotic congenital heart disease
  (1) Total anomalous pulmonary venous return
    • Pulmonary vein empties oxygenated blood into the right atrium.
  (2) Truncus arteriosus
    • Aorta and pulmonary artery share a common trunk and intermix blood.
  (3) Tricuspid atresia
    • Usually have an ASD with a right-to-left shunt
4. Coarctation of the aorta
  a. Infantile (preductal) coarctation
    (1) Constriction of aorta between the subclavian artery and ductus arteriosus
    (2) Associated with Turner's syndrome

Infantile coarctation: associated with Turner's syndrome

  b. Adult coarctation
    (1) Develops during adult life
    (2) Constriction of the aorta distal to the ligamentum arteriosum
      (a) Blood flow into the proximally located branch vessels is increased.

        (b) Blood flow below the constriction is decreased.

        (c) Produces a systolic murmur

        (d) Additional defect is a bicuspid aortic valve (50% of cases)

    (3) Clinical findings proximal to the constriction

        (a) Increased upper extremity blood pressure

        (b) Dilation of aorta and aortic valve ring (regurgitation)

          • Increased risk for developing an aortic dissection

        (c) Increased cerebral blood flow (increased risk for berry aneurysms)

    (4) Clinical findings distal to the constriction

        (a) Decreased blood pressure in the lower extremity

        (b) Leg claudication (pain in calf or buttocks when walking)

        (c) Decreased renal blood flow

          • Activates the renin-angiotensin-aldosterone system causing hypertension

    (5) Development of collateral circulation

        (a) Collaterals develop between intercostal arteries above and below the constriction.

        (b) Chest radiograph shows rib notching on the undersurface of ribs.

          • Due to increased blood flow through enlarged intercostal arteries

> Adult coarctation: disparity between upper and lower extremity blood pressure > 10 mm Hg

V. Acquired Valvular Heart Disease

A. Rheumatic fever

  1. Epidemiology

    a. Occurs at 5 to 15 years of age

    b. Develops 1 to 5 weeks after group A streptococcal pharyngitis

    c. Possible relapses may occur leading to chronic valvular disease

  2. Pathogenesis

    a. Immune-mediated disease that follows group A streptococcal infection

    b. Antibodies develop against group A streptococcal M proteins

      (1) Antibodies cross-react with similar proteins in human tissue

      (2) Type II hypersensitivity reaction

        • Cell-mediated immunity also involved

  3. Clinical findings

    a. Fibrinous pericarditis

      • Precordial chest pain with friction rub

    b. Myocarditis

      (1) Most common cause of death in acute disease

      (2) Aschoff bodies are present.

        • Central area of fibrinoid necrosis surrounded by Anitschkow cells (reactive histiocytes)

    c. Endocarditis

      (1) Most commonly involves the mitral valve (then aortic valve)

> Acute rheumatic fever: immune-mediated type II hypersensitivity reaction; cell-mediated immunity

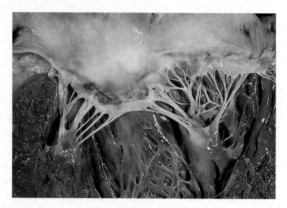

10-7: *Acute rheumatic fever. Uniform, verrucoid-appearing sterile vegetations appear along the line of closure of the mitral valve. (From Damjanov I, Linder J: Pathology: A Color Atlas. St. Louis, Mosby, 2000, p 13, Fig. 1-22.)*

(2) Sterile, verrucoid-appearing vegetations develop along the line of closure of the valve (Fig. 10-7).
  • Embolism is uncommon.
(3) Mitral valve regurgitation or aortic valve regurgitation
  • May result in CHF
(4) Recurrent infection of the mitral and aortic valves leads to mitral stenosis or aortic stenosis.
  d. Migratory polyarthritis
  (1) Most common initial presentation of acute rheumatic fever
  (2) Occurs in large joints (knees) and small joints (wrists)
  (3) *No* permanent joint damage
  e. Subcutaneous nodules occur on extensor surfaces.
  f. Erythema marginatum
  • Evanescent circular ring of erythema that develops around normal skin
  g. Sydenham's chorea
  (1) Reversible rapid, involuntary movements affecting all muscles
  (2) Late manifestation of acute rheumatic fever
4. Diagnosis of acute rheumatic fever
  a. Increased antistreptolysin O (ASO) titers
  b. Positive throat culture
  c. Leukocytosis, increased PR interval, increased C-reactive protein
B. Mitral stenosis
1. Etiology
  • Most often caused by recurrent attacks of rheumatic fever
2. Pathophysiology
  a. Narrowing of the mitral valve orifice (Fig. 10-8)
  b. Left atrium becomes dilated and hypertrophied
  • Due to increased work in filling the ventricle in diastole
3. Clinical findings
  a. Opening snap followed by mid-diastolic rumble

Rheumatic fever: mitral regurgitation in acute attack; mitral stenosis in chronic disease

Anti DNAase B also increased in acute rheumatic fever

Mitral stenosis: opening snap following by a mid-diastolic rumble

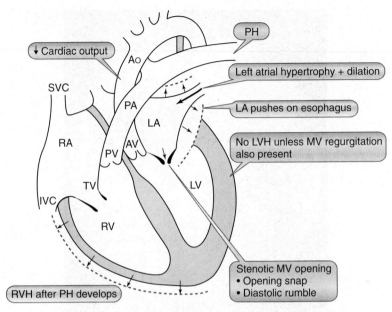

10-8: *Schematic of mitral stenosis. Refer to the text for discussion. Ao, aorta; AV, aortic valve; IVC, inferior vena cava; LA, left atrium; LV, left ventricle; LVH, left ventricular hypertrophy; MV, mitral valve; PA, pulmonary artery; PH, pulmonary hypertension; PV, pulmonary valve; RA, right atrium; RV, right ventricle; RVH, right ventricular hypertrophy; SVC, superior vena cava; TV, tricuspid valve.*

Mitral stenosis is a problem with opening the valve. The valve opens in diastole, and thus, the murmur occurs in diastole. Sudden opening of the thickened, nonpliable valve with left atrial contraction produces an opening snap followed by a rumble caused by rapid entry of blood into the left ventricle. The murmur is best heard at the apex.

b. Dyspnea and hemoptysis with rust-colored sputum (heart failure cells)
   • Due to pulmonary capillary congestion and hemorrhage into the alveoli
c. Atrial fibrillation
   (1) Due to left atrial dilation and hypertrophy
   (2) Intra-atrial thrombus develops due to stasis.
      • Danger of systemic embolization
d. Pulmonary venous hypertension
   (1) Due to chronic backup of atrial blood into the pulmonary vein
   (2) RVH eventually develops
e. Dysphagia for solids
   (1) Left atrium is the most posteriorly located chamber in the heart.
   (2) Dilation of the left atrium compresses the esophagus.

C. Mitral regurgitation
   1. Etiology
      a. Mitral valve prolapse (most common cause)

Atrial fibrillation: common in mitral stenosis

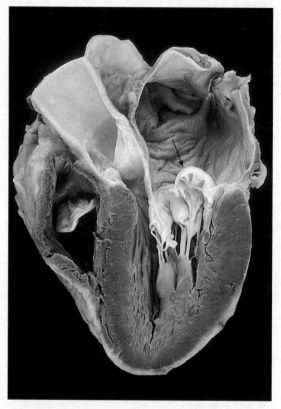

10-9: *Mitral valve prolapse. The arrow shows prolapse of the posterior mitral leaflet into the left atrium. (From Kumar V, Fausto N, Abbas A: Robbins and Cotran's Pathologic Basis of Disease, 7th ed. Philadelphia, WB Saunders, 2004, p 592, Fig. 12-23.)*

    b. Left-sided heart failure

    c. Infective endocarditis, rupture or dysfunction of the papillary muscle

  2. Pathophysiology

    a. Retrograde blood flow into the left atrium during systole

      • Due to an incompetent mitral valve or dilated mitral valve ring

    b. Volume overload in the left ventricle and left atrium leads to LHF.

  3. Clinical findings

    a. Pansystolic murmur with radiation to the axilla

    b. Dyspnea and cough from LHF

D. Mitral valve prolapse (MVP)

  1. Epidemiology

    a. Autosomal dominant inheritance in some cases

    b. More common in women

    c. Associated with Marfan and Ehlers-Danlos syndrome

  2. Pathophysiology

    a. Posterior bulging of the anterior and posterior leaflets into the left atrium during systole (Fig. 10-9)

Mitral valve prolapse: most common cause of mitral regurgitation

   b. Redundancy of valve tissue
      (1) Myxomatous degeneration of the mitral valve leaflets
      (2) Due to excess production of dermatan sulfate
3. Clinical findings
   a. Most patients are asymptomatic.
   b. Heart murmur
      (1) Mid-systolic click
         • Due to sudden restraint by the chordae of the prolapsed valve
      (2) Mid to late systolic regurgitant murmur follows the click.
      (3) Decreased preload causes the click and murmur to move closer to
         the S_1 heart sound; examples:
         (a) Anxiety
            • Increased heart rate decreases diastolic filling of left ventricle.
         (b) Standing
            • Decreases venous return to the right side of the heart
         (c) Valsalva maneuver (holding breath with epiglottis closed)
            • Positive intrathoracic pressure decreases venous return to
              the heart.
      (4) Increased preload causes the click and murmur to move closer to
         the S_2 heart sound; examples:
         (a) Reclining
            • Increases venous return to the right side of the heart
         (b) Squatting or sustained hand grip
            • Increases systemic vascular resistance, which impedes
              emptying of the left ventricle
   c. Palpitations, chest pain, rupture of chordae

E. Aortic stenosis
1. Etiology
   a. Dystrophic calcification of a normal aortic valve or bicuspid aortic
      valve
   b. Age-related sclerosis of the aortic valve
   c. Chronic rheumatic fever
2. Pathophysiology
   a. Obstruction to left ventricular outflow during systole (Fig. 10-10)
   b. Reduction in the aortic valve orifice area produces concentric LVH.
3. Clinical findings
   a. Systolic ejection murmur

> Aortic stenosis is a problem in opening the valve. Because the
> aortic valve opens in systole, the murmur occurs in systole. It is
> an ejection type of murmur with murmur intensity initially
> increasing and then decreasing (crescendo-decrescendo). It is
> best heard in the second right intercostal space and radiates into
> the carotid arteries. Decreasing preload lessens the volume the
> left ventricle must eject; therefore, murmur intensity decreases.
> Increasing preload increases the volume the left ventricle must
> eject; therefore, murmur intensity increases.

Mitral valve prolapse: myxomatous degeneration; excess dermatan sulfate

Aortic stenosis: most common cause calcification of normal or bicuspid valve

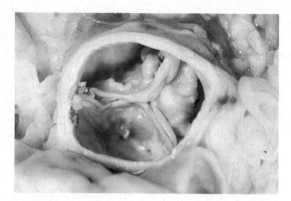

10-10: *Aortic stenosis. The superior view of the aortic valve shows severe aortic stenosis due to fibrocalcific involvement of all three valve cusps. (From Damjanov I, Linder J: Anderson's Pathology, 10th ed. St. Louis, Mosby, 1996, p 1268, Fig. 45-6A.)*

      b. Angina with exercise
        (1) Decreased blood flow through the stenotic valve leads to less filling of the coronary arteries during diastole.
        (2) Subendocardium of concentrically hypertrophied heart receives less blood.
      c. Syncope with exercise
        • Decreased blood flow through the stenotic valve leads to decreased blood flow to the brain.

> Aortic stenosis: most common valvular lesion causing syncope and angina with exercise

      d. Hemolytic anemia with schistocytes (see Chapter 11)

F. Aortic regurgitation
    1. Etiology
      a. Isolated aortic valve root dilation
      b. Infective endocarditis
        • Most common cause of acute aortic regurgitation

> Isolated aortic valve root dilation: most common cause of aortic regurgitation

      c. Long-standing essential hypertension
      d. Chronic rheumatic fever, aortic dissection, coarctation
    2. Pathophysiology
      a. Retrograde blood flow into the left ventricle
        (1) Due to an incompetent valve or dilated valve ring
        (2) Decreases diastolic pressure
          • Due to drop in arterial volume as blood flows back into the left ventricle
        (3) Volume overload of the left ventricle
          • Increases stroke volume (Frank-Starling mechanism)
      b. Increased pulse pressure (difference between systolic and diastolic pressure)
        • Produces hyperdynamic circulation (e.g., bounding pulses)
    3. Clinical findings
      a. Early diastolic murmur

Aortic regurgitation is a problem in closing the aortic valve. Because the valve closes in diastole, the murmur occurs in diastole. It is characterized by a high-pitched "blowing" early diastolic murmur immediately following the S_2 heart sound. It increases in intensity on expiration and is heard best along the left parasternal border.

    b. Bounding pulses (water hammer pulse), head nodding, pulsating uvula

    c. Austin Flint murmur

       (1) Regurgitant stream from incompetent aortic valve hits the anterior mitral valve leaflet producing a diastolic murmur

       (2) Presence of this murmur indicates the need for replacement of the valve.

Aortic regurgitation: early diastolic murmur; bounding pulses

G. Tricuspid regurgitation

  1. Etiology

    a. Right-sided heart failure

    b. Infective endocarditis in intravenous drug abuse

    c. Carcinoid heart disease

  2. Pathophysiology

    a. Retrograde blood flow into the right atrium during systole

       (1) Due to stretching of the valve ring or damage to the valve

       (2) Causes right ventricular overload and RHF

    b. Produces volume overload in the right atrium and right ventricle

  3. Clinical findings

    a. Pansystolic murmur that increases in intensity with inspiration

    b. Pulsating liver

      • Blood regurgitates into the venous system with systole.

H. Carcinoid heart disease

  1. Due to liver metastasis from a carcinoid tumor of small intestine (see Chapter 17)

  2. Serotonin causes fibrosis of the tricuspid valve and pulmonary valve.

    • Produces tricuspid valve regurgitation and pulmonary valve stenosis

I. Infective endocarditis (IE)

  1. Epidemiology

    a. Microbial pathogens

       (1) *Streptococcus viridans*

         • Most common overall cause of IE

       (2) *Staphylococcus aureus*

         • Most common cause of IE in intravenous (IV) drug abuse

       (3) *Staphylococcus epidermidis*

         • Most common cause of IE due to prosthetic devices

       (4) *Streptococcus bovis*

         • Most common cause of IE in ulcerative colitis or colorectal cancer

Streptococcus viridans: most common cause of infective endocarditis

  2. Valves involved in IE

    a. Mitral valve

      • Most common overall valve involved in IE

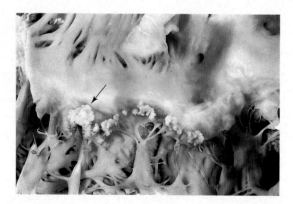

10-11: *Acute bacterial endocarditis. Large, friable, and irregular vegetation (arrow) is present on the margin of the mitral valve. Smaller vegetations are present along the line of closure of the valve. (From Damjanov I, Linder J: Pathology: A Color Atlas. St. Louis, Mosby, 2000, p 11, Fig. 1-16.)*

b. Tricuspid valve and aortic valve
- Most common valves involved in IE due to IV drug abuse

3. Pathogenesis
a. *Streptococcus viridans* infects previously damaged valves.
b. *Staphylococcus aureus* infects normal or previously damaged valves.

4. Pathology
a. Vegetations embolize producing abscesses and infarctions in distant organ sites (Fig. 10-11).
b. Valve destruction leads to regurgitation murmurs.

5. Clinical findings
a. Immunocomplex vasculitis
- Examples—splinter hemorrhages in nail beds, glomerulonephritis
b. Fever, splenomegaly, positive blood cultures

J. Libman-Sacks endocarditis
1. Associated with systemic lupus erythematosus (SLE)
2. Sterile vegetations are located over the mitral valve surface.
- Produces valve deformity and mitral regurgitation

K. Nonbacterial thrombotic endocarditis (marantic endocarditis)
1. Paraneoplastic syndrome (see Chapter 8)
2. Sterile, nondestructive vegetations on the mitral valve
- Procoagulant effect of circulating mucin from mucin-producing tumors of the colon and pancreas
3. Complications
a. Embolization
b. May be secondarily infected

VI. Myocardial and Pericardial Disorders
  A. Myocarditis
    1. Etiology
      a. Microbial pathogens
        (1) Coxsackievirus (most common cause)

Staphylococcus aureus: most common pathogen producing IE in IV drug abuse

Tricuspid valve regurgitation in intravenous drug abusers is due to infective endocarditis.

Libman-Sacks endocarditis: associated with SLE

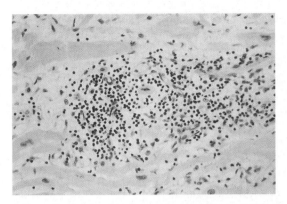

10-12: *Myocarditis. The biopsy shows a lymphocytic infiltrate with dissolution of myocardial fibers. (From Damjanov I, Linder J: Pathology: A Color Atlas. St. Louis, Mosby, 2000, p 15, Fig. 1-28.)*

(2) *Trypanosoma cruzi* (Chagas' disease)
  • Leishmanial forms infect cardiac muscle.
  b. Acute rheumatic fever, diphtheria toxin, drugs (e.g., doxorubicin), SLE
 2. Pathology
  a. Endocardial biopsy is sometimes performed if infection is suspected.
  b. A lymphocytic infiltrate is highly predictive of coxsackievirus (Fig. 10-12).
 3. Clinical findings
  a. Fever, chest pain, CHF
  b. Increased CK-MB and troponins

B. Pericarditis
 1. Etiology
  a. Similar to myocarditis
  b. Coxsackievirus most common overall cause
 2. Pathology
  a. Fibrinous type of pericardial exudate
   • Often accompanied by an effusion
  b. Dense scar tissue with dystrophic calcification may cause constrictive pericarditis.
 3. Clinical findings
  a. Precordial chest pain
   (1) Pain is relieved when leaning forward.
   (2) Pain increases with inspiration.
  b. Pericardial friction rub
   • Scratchy, three-component rub (systole, early, and late diastole)
  c. Pericardial effusion
   (1) Muffled heart sounds
    • Fluid surrounds the heart.
   (2) Hypotension associated with pulsus paradoxus
    • Drop in systolic blood pressure greater than 10 mm Hg during inspiration

Chagas disease: most common cause of CHF in Central/South America

Coxsackievirus: most common cause of myocarditis and pericarditis

A young woman with pericarditis and effusion most likely has SLE.

(3) Neck vein distention on inspiration
  - Blood cannot enter the right atrium and refluxes into the jugular vein (Kussmaul's sign).
(4) Chest radiograph shows a "water bottle" configuration.
  d. Constrictive pericarditis
    (1) Etiology
      (a) Tuberculosis is the most common cause worldwide.
      (b) Most cases in the United States are idiopathic.
    (2) Pathophysiology
      - Incomplete filling of the cardiac chambers due to thickening of the parietal pericardium
    (3) Pericardial knock
      - Due to the ventricles hitting the thickened parietal pericardium

VII. **Cardiomyopathy**
  A. **Definition**
    - Group of diseases that primarily involve the myocardium and produce myocardial dysfunction
  B. **Types of cardiomyopathy**
    1. Dilated (congestive)
    2. Hypertrophic
    3. Restrictive
  C. **Dilated cardiomyopathy**
    1. Epidemiology
      a. Most common cardiomyopathy
      b. Etiology
        (1) Idiopathic (most common)
        (2) Genetic causes (25–35%)
        (3) Myocarditis (see section VI)
        (4) Drugs (e.g., doxorubicin, cocaine)
        (5) Postpartum state, thiamine deficiency (alcoholism)
    2. Pathophysiology
      a. Decreased contractility with a decreased EF (<40%)
      b. Systolic dysfunction type of LHF
    3. Clinical findings
      a. Global enlargement of the heart
        (1) All chambers are dilated.
        (2) Echocardiography shows poor contractility.
      b. Biventricular CHF
      c. Bundle branch blocks and atrial and ventricular arrhythmias
  D. **Hypertrophic cardiomyopathy**
    1. Epidemiology
      a. Most common cause of sudden death in young individuals
      b. Familial form (autosomal dominant) in young individuals (majority of cases)
        - Due to mutations in heavy chain of β-myosin and in the troponins
      c. Sporadic form in elderly people

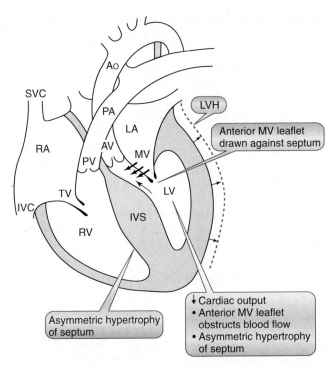

10-13: *Schematic of hypertrophic cardiomyopathy. Refer to the text for discussion. Ao, aorta; AV, aortic valve; IVC, inferior vena cava; IVS, interventricular septum; LA, left atrium; LV, left ventricle; LVH, left ventricular hypertrophy; MV, mitral valve; PA, pulmonary artery; PV, pulmonary valve; RA, right atrium; RV, right ventricle; SVC, superior vena cava; TV, tricuspid valve.*

    2. Pathophysiology
       a. Hypertrophy of the myocardium
         • Disproportionately greater thickening of the interventricular
           septum than of the free left ventricular wall
       b. Obstruction of blood flow is below the aortic valve
         • Anterior leaflet of the mitral valve is drawn against the
           asymmetrically hypertrophied septum as blood exits the left
           ventricle (Fig. 10-13).
       c. Aberrant myofibers and conduction system in the interventricular
         septum
         • Conduction disturbances are responsible for sudden death.
       d. Decreased diastolic filling
         • Muscle thickening restricts filling.
    3. Clinical findings
       a. Systolic ejection type murmur.
       b. Murmur intensity increases (obstruction worsens) with decreased
         preload
         • Examples—standing up, use of inotropic drugs (e.g., digitalis)

Hypertrophic cardiomyopathy: most common cause of sudden death in young individuals

       c. Murmur intensity decreases (obstruction lessens) with increased preload
- Examples—reclining, drugs decreasing cardiac contractility (e.g., β-blockers)

E. Restrictive cardiomyopathy

1. Etiology
   a. Tropical endomyocardial fibrosis
      - Most common cause worldwide
   b. Infiltrative diseases
      - Examples—Pompe's glycogenosis, amyloidosis, hemochromatosis
   c. Endocardial fibroelastosis in a child (thick fibroelastic tissue in the endocardium), sarcoidosis
2. Pathophysiology
   a. Decreased ventricular compliance
   b. Usually secondary to infiltrative disease of the myocardium
   c. Diastolic dysfunction type of LHF
3. Clinical findings
   - Arrhythmias (conduction defects), CHF

VIII. Tumors of the Heart

A. Epidemiology

1. Metastasis is more common than primary tumors
   - Example—extension of a primary lung cancer
2. Pericardium is the most common site for metastasis.
   - Leads to pericarditis and effusions
3. Primary tumors or tumor-like conditions
   - Cardiac myxoma, rhabdomyoma

B. Cardiac myxoma

1. Most common primary adult tumor
2. Pathology
   a. Benign primary mesenchymal tumor
   b. Approximately 90% arise from the left atrium
   c. Sessile or pedunculated
   d. "Ball-valve" effect blocks the mitral valve orifice
      - Blocks diastolic filling of the ventricle, simulating mitral valve stenosis
3. Clinical findings
   a. Nonspecific findings
      - Fever, fatigue, malaise, anemia
   b. Complications
      - Embolization, syncopal episodes (blocks mitral valve orifice)
4. Diagnosis
   - Transesophageal ultrasound (most useful study for viewing the left atrium)

C. Rhabdomyoma

1. Most common primary tumor of the heart in infants and children
   - Major association with tuberous sclerosis (see Chapter 25)
2. Hamartoma (non-neoplastic) arising from cardiac muscle

Myxomas occur in adults; rhabdomyomas occur in children.

Red Blood Cell Disorders

I. Erythropoiesis

- Erythropoiesis is the production of RBCs in the bone marrow and is dependent on the release of erythropoietin from the kidneys.

A. Erythropoiesis and erythropoietin (EPO)

1. Stimuli for EPO release
   - Hypoxemia, severe anemia, left-shifted O_2-binding curve (OBC), high altitude
2. Increased O_2 content suppresses EPO release (e.g., polycythemia vera).

> EPO increases the O_2-carrying capacity of blood by stimulating erythroid stem cells to divide. Epoetin alfa, a form of EPO produced by recombinant DNA technology, is frequently abused by athletes to increase their energy level. It also is used in the treatment of anemia associated with renal failure, chronic disease, and chemotherapy.

3. Other sources of EPO
   - Ectopic production by renal cell carcinoma and hepatocellular carcinoma
4. Peripheral blood markers of erythropoiesis
   a. Reticulocytes are newly released RBCs from the bone marrow.
   b. They are identified with supravital stains.
      - Detect thread-like RNA filaments in the cytoplasm (Fig. 11-1)
   c. In 24 hours, they become mature RBCs.

B. Reticulocyte count

1. Marker of effective erythropoiesis (bone marrow response to anemia)
2. Reported as a percentage (normal, <3%)
3. Percentage count is falsely increased in anemia.
   a. Initial percentage must be corrected for the degree of anemia.
   b. Corrected reticulocyte count = (actual Hct/45) × reticulocyte count, where 45 represents the normal hematocrit (Hct)
   c. Example
      (1) Hct 15%, reticulocyte count 18%
      (2) Corrected reticulocyte count is 6% (15/45 × 18% = 6%)
4. Corrected reticulocyte count at or above 3%
   a. Good bone marrow response to anemia (i.e., effective erythropoiesis)
   b. Examples—hemolytic anemia; after treatment of iron deficiency with iron
5. Corrected reticulocyte count below 3%
   a. Poor bone marrow response to anemia (i.e., ineffective erythropoiesis)
   b. Examples—untreated iron deficiency; aplastic anemia

Stimuli for EPO: hypoxemia, left-shifted OBC, high altitude

EPO is synthesized in the endothelial cells of peritubular capillaries.

Reticulocyte count: measure of effective erythropoiesis; corrected for the degree of anemia.

Corrected reticulocyte count: <3% ineffective erythropoiesis ≥3% effective erythropoiesis

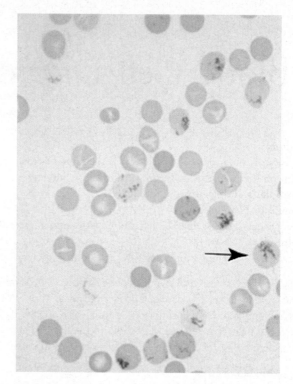

11-1: *Peripheral blood reticulocytes with supravital stain (new methylene blue). Red blood cells with thread-like material in the cytosol represent residual RNA filaments and protein (arrow). (From Hoffbrand AV: Color Atlas: Clinical Hematology, 3rd ed. St. Louis, Mosby, 2000, Fig. 1-43B.)*

C. **Extramedullary hematopoiesis (EMH)**
- RBC, white blood cell (WBC), and platelet production that occurs outside the bone marrow
1. Common sites of EMH are the liver and spleen.
2. Pathogenesis
   a. Intrinsic bone marrow disease (e.g., myelofibrosis)
   b. Accelerated erythropoiesis (e.g., severe hemolysis in sickle cell disease)
      (1) Expands the bone marrow cavity
      (2) Radiograph of the skull shows a "hair-on-end" appearance.
3. EMH produces hepatosplenomegaly.

EMH: most often occurs in the liver and spleen

> In the fetus, hematopoiesis (blood cell formation) begins in the yolk sac and subsequently moves to the liver and finally the bone marrow by the fifth to sixth months of gestation.

II. **Complete Blood Cell Count (CBC) and Other Studies**
   A. **Components of a CBC**
      1. Hemoglobin (Hb), Hct, RBC count
      2. RBC indices, RBC distribution width (RDW)

3. WBC count with a differential count, platelet count
4. Evaluation of the peripheral blood morphology

B. Hb, Hct, and RBC counts
1. Factors affecting the normal range (reference interval)
    a. Newborns
        (1) Newborns have higher normal ranges than do infants and children.
        (2) HbF ($2\alpha/2\gamma$ globin chains) shifts the OBC to the left causing the release of EPO.
            • EPO causes an increase in Hb, Hct, and RBC count.
        (3) After birth, the Hb drops from ~18.5 g/dL to 11 g/dL (physiologic anemia).

> Fetal RBCs containing HbF are destroyed by splenic macrophages over the ensuing 6 to 9 months. The unconjugated bilirubin derived from the initial destruction of fetal RBCs is responsible for physiologic jaundice of the newborn, which occurs ~3 days from birth.

        (4) HbF-containing cells are replaced by RBCs containing HbA (>97%), HbA_2 (<2.5%), and HbF (<1%).
    b. Sex of the patient
        • Men have higher normal ranges due to increased testosterone (stimulates erythropoiesis) and lack of cyclic bleeding.
    c. Pregnancy
        (1) Pregnant women have lower normal ranges than nonpregnant women.
        (2) There is an increase in plasma volume and RBC mass (i.e., more RBCs are produced).
            • Plasma volume is twice greater than RBC mass causing a slight decrease in Hb (dilutional effect).
2. Changes in thalassemia (i.e., a genetic globin chain disorder)
    a. Hb and Hct are decreased.
    b. RBC count is increased (unknown mechanism).
3. Anemia
    a. Decrease in Hb, Hct, or RBC concentration
    b. Sign of an underlying disease rather than of a specific diagnosis
    c. Clinical findings
        • Fatigue, dyspnea with exertion, inability to concentrate, dizziness

C. RBC indices
1. Mean corpuscular volume (MCV)
    a. Average volume of RBCs
    b. Used to classify anemia (Fig. 11-2)
        • Microcytic (<80 μm^3), normocytic (80–100 μm^3), macrocytic (>100 μm^3)
2. Mean corpuscular hemoglobin concentration (MCHC)
    a. Average Hb concentration in RBCs (Fig. 11-3)
    b. Decreased MCHC

Fetal Hb: left-shifts OBC causing an increase in Hb

Pregnancy: two times greater increase in plasma volume than RBC mass

Thalassemia: Hb, Hct decreased; RBC count increased

Anemia: O_2 saturation and arterial PO_2 are normal

MCV: useful for classification of anemias

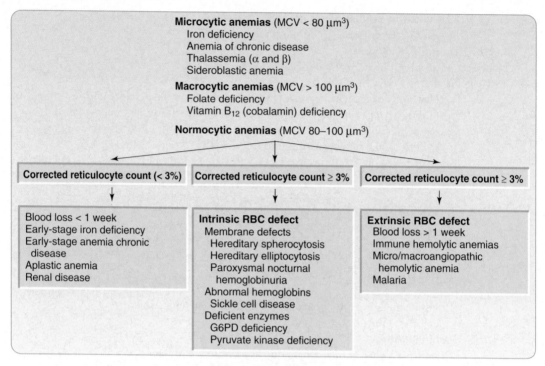

Microcytic anemias (MCV < 80 μm^3)
Iron deficiency
Anemia of chronic disease
Thalassemia (α and β)
Sideroblastic anemia

Macrocytic anemias (MCV > 100 μm^3)
Folate deficiency
Vitamin B$_{12}$ (cobalamin) deficiency

Normocytic anemias (MCV 80–100 μm^3)

Corrected reticulocyte count (< 3%)	**Corrected reticulocyte count ≥ 3%**	**Corrected reticulocyte count ≥ 3%**

Blood loss < 1 week
Early-stage iron deficiency
Early-stage anemia chronic
  disease
Aplastic anemia
Renal disease
	Intrinsic RBC defect
	  Membrane defects
	    Hereditary spherocytosis
	    Hereditary elliptocytosis
	    Paroxysmal nocturnal
	      hemoglobinuria
	  Abnormal hemoglobins
	    Sickle cell disease
	  Deficient enzymes
	    G6PD deficiency
	    Pyruvate kinase deficiency
		Extrinsic RBC defect
		  Blood loss > 1 week
		  Immune hemolytic anemias
		  Micro/macroangiopathic
		    hemolytic anemia
		  Malaria

11-2: *Classification of anemia using mean corpuscular volume (MCV). An intrinsic red blood cell (RBC) defect indicates a structural or biochemical flaw in the RBCs. An extrinsic RBC defect indicates that the RBCs are structurally normal, but that other factors cause the anemia. G6PD, glucose-6-phosphate dehydrogenase.*

(1) Correlates with decreased synthesis of Hb (e.g., microcytic anemias)
(2) Central area of pallor is greater than normal (called hypochromasia).

MCHC: decreased in microcytic anemias; increased in hereditary spherocytosis

  c. Increased MCHC
    (1) Correlates with the presence of spherical RBCs (e.g., hereditary spherocytosis)
    (2) There is no central area of pallor.

D. RDW
  1. Reflects variation in size of RBCs in the peripheral blood (anisocytosis)
  2. Increased if RBCs are *not* uniformly the same size
    • Example—mixture of microcytic and normocytic cells

Iron deficiency: ↑ RDW

  3. Iron deficiency
    • Only microcytic anemia with an increased RDW due to a mixture of normocytic and microcytic RBCs

E. Characteristics of mature RBCs
  1. Anaerobic glycolysis
    a. Main source of adenosine triphosphate (ATP)
    b. Lactic acid is the end product of RBC metabolism.

Mature RBC: anaerobic glycolysis

  2. Pentose phosphate pathway

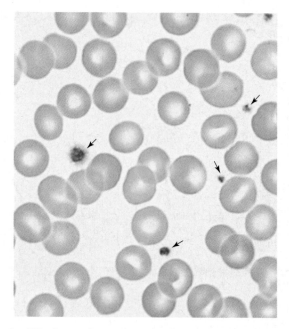

11-3: *Normal peripheral blood smear showing RBCs. The RBCs are uniform in size, and the central areas of pallor are slightly less than half the total diameter of an RBC. The four dark objects (arrows) outside the RBCs are platelets. (From Hoffbrand AV: Color Atlas: Clinical Hematology, 3rd ed. St. Louis, Mosby, 2000, p 22, Fig. 1-62.)*

      a. Synthesizes glutathione (GSH), an antioxidant that neutralizes hydrogen peroxide

      b. Hydrogen peroxide is a product of oxidative metabolism.

   3. Methemoglobin reductase pathway

      a. Methemoglobin (metHb) refers to heme iron that is oxidized (Fe^{3+}).

         • MetHb *cannot* bind O_2.

      b. Reductase system converts iron to ferrous (Fe^{2+}) so that the RBCs can bind O_2.

   4. Luebering-Rapaport pathway

      a. Synthesizes 2,3-bisphosphoglycerate (BPG)

      b. Required to right-shift the OBC (i.e., release O_2 to tissue)

   5. Mature RBCs lack mitochondria.

   6. Senescent RBCs

      a. Removed by splenic macrophages

      b. End product of heme degradation in macrophages is unconjugated bilirubin.

F. WBC count and differential

   1. 100-cell differential count subdivides leukocytes by percentage.

   2. Further classifies neutrophils as segmented or band neutrophils

G. Platelet count

   • Platelets are anucleate cells derived from cytoplasmic budding of megakaryocytes.

Unconjugated bilirubin: end product of heme degradation in macrophage

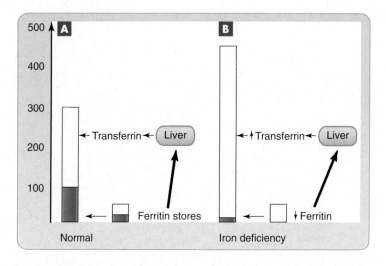

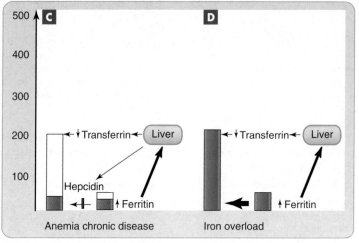

11-4: *Iron studies in normal people (**A**) and those with iron deficiency (**B**), anemia of chronic disease (**C**), and iron-overload diseases (**D**). See text for discussion.*

H. Iron studies (Fig. 11-4)

1. Serum ferritin

   a. Ferritin is the primary soluble iron storage protein.

   (1) Primary storage site is in the bone marrow macrophages.
   • See shaded area in the small box in Figure 11-4A

   (2) Serum levels correlate with ferritin stores in the macrophages.

   (3) Synthesis of ferritin in macrophages increases in inflammation.
   • Due to release of interleukin 1 and tumor necrosis factor-α

   b. Decreased serum ferritin
   • Diagnostic of iron deficiency (see Fig. 11-4B).

   c. Increased serum ferritin

        (1) Anemia of chronic disease (ACD) (see Fig. 11-4C)
        (2) Iron overload disease (see Fig. 11-4D)

    d. Hemosiderin
        (1) Insoluble degradation product of ferritin
        (2) Decreased and increased levels correlate with changes in ferritin stores

2. Serum iron
    a. Represents iron bound to transferrin, the binding protein of iron
        (1) Transferrin is synthesized in the liver.
        (2) Serum iron is the shaded area of the column in Figure 11-4A.
          • Note that the normal serum iron is $100\,\mu g/dL$.
    b. Decreased serum iron
        (1) Iron deficiency (see Fig. 11-4B)
        (2) ACD (see Fig. 11-4C).
    c. Increased serum iron
        • Iron overload diseases (see Fig. 11-4D)

3. Serum total iron binding capacity (TIBC)
    a. Serum TIBC correlates with the concentration of transferrin.
        (1) Height of the column in Figure 11-4A correlates with serum transferrin and TIBC
        (2) Note that the normal TIBC is $300\,\mu g/dL$.
    b. Relationship of transferrin synthesis with ferritin stores in macrophages
        (1) Decreased ferritin stores cause increased synthesis of transferrin (see Fig. 11-4B).
          • Increase in transferrin and TIBC is present in iron deficiency.
        (2) Increased ferritin stores causes decreased synthesis of transferrin (see Fig. 11-4C and D).
          • Decrease in transferrin and TIBC occurs in ACD (see Fig. 11-4C) and iron overload disease (see Fig. 11-4D).

4. Iron saturation (%)
    a. Represents the percentage of binding sites on transferrin occupied by iron
        (1) Iron saturation (%) = serum iron/TIBC $\times$ 100
        (2) In Figure 11-4A, the normal % saturation is $100/300 \times 100$ or 33%.
    b. Decreased percentage of iron saturation
        (1) Iron deficiency (see Fig. 11-4B)
        (2) ACD (see Fig. 11-4C)
    c. Increased percentage of iron saturation
        • Iron overload disease (see Fig. 11-4D)

I. Hb electrophoresis
    a. Primary use is to detect hemoglobinopathies.
        (1) Abnormality in globin chain structure (e.g., sickle cell disease)
        (2) Abnormality in globin chain synthesis (e.g., thalassemia)
    b. Types of normal Hb detected
        (1) HbA has $2\alpha/2\beta$ globin chains (97% in adults).
        (2) HbA_2 has $2\alpha/2\delta$ globin chains (2% in adults).
        (3) HbF has $2\alpha/2\gamma$ globin chains (1% in adults).

Margin notes:

Serum ferritin:
$\downarrow$ iron deficiency
$\uparrow$ ACD, iron overload disease

Serum iron:
$\downarrow$ iron deficiency, ACD
$\uparrow$ iron overload disease

$\downarrow$ TIBC = $\downarrow$ transferrin
$\uparrow$ TIBC = $\uparrow$ transferrin

$\downarrow$ Ferritin stores =
$\uparrow$ TIBC; iron deficiency
$\uparrow$ Ferritin stores =
$\downarrow$ TIBC; ACD, iron overload

$\downarrow$ % Saturation: iron deficiency, ACD
$\uparrow$ % Saturation: iron overload disease

HbA: $2\alpha/2\beta$
HbA_2: $2\alpha/2\delta$
HbF: $2\alpha/2\gamma$

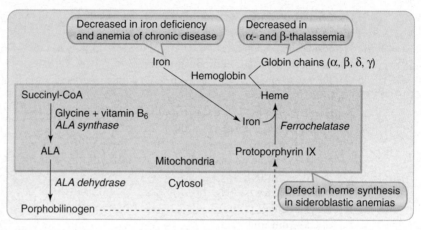

11-5: *Pathophysiology of microcytic anemias. ALA, aminolevulinic acid.*

III. Microcytic Anemias

A. Types of microcytic anemias

1. Iron deficiency (most common)
2. Anemia of chronic disease (ACD)
3. Thalassemia (α and β)
4. Sideroblastic anemias (least common)

B. Pathogenesis (Fig. 11-5)

1. Defects in the synthesis of Hb
   - Hb = heme + globin chains
2. Defects in the synthesis of heme (i.e., iron + protoporphyrin)
   - Iron deficiency, ACD, sideroblastic anemias
3. Defects in the synthesis of globin chains (i.e., α or β)
   - α-Thalassemia and β-thalassemia (thal)

C. Iron deficiency anemia

1. Epidemiology
   a. It is the most common anemia.
   b. Causes of iron deficiency (Table 11-1)
2. Pathogenesis
   - Decreased synthesis of heme (see Fig. 11-5)
3. Clinical and laboratory findings
   a. Plummer-Vinson syndrome
      (1) Caused by chronic iron deficiency
      (2) Esophageal web (dysphagia for solids but *not* liquids)
      (3) Achlorhydria (absent acid in the stomach)
      (4) Glossitis (inflammation of the tongue), spoon nails (koilonychia)
   b. Laboratory findings
      (1) Decreased MCV, serum iron, iron saturation (%), ferritin (<30 ng/mL)
      (2) Increased TIBC, RDW

Microcytic anemias: defects in the synthesis of Hb (heme + globin chains)

Iron deficiency: most often caused by bleeding

Iron deficiency: ↓ iron, % saturation, ferritin; ↑ TIBC, RDW

TABLE 11-1:
**Causes of Iron
Deficiency Anemia**

Classification	Causes	Discussion
Blood loss	Gastrointestinal loss	Meckel diverticulum (in older children) PUD (most common cause in men < 50 years old) Gastritis (e.g., NSAID) Hookworm infestation Polyps/colorectal cancer (most common cause in adults > 50 years old)
	Menorrhagia	Most common cause in women < 50 years old
Increased utilization	Pregnancy/lactation	Daily iron requirement is 3.4 mg during pregnancy and 2.5–3.0 mg during lactation
	Infants/children	Iron required for tissue growth and expansion of blood volume
Decreased intake	Infants/children	Most common cause of iron deficiency in young children
	Elderly	Restricted diets with little meat (lack of heme iron)
Decreased absorption	Celiac sprue	Absence of villous surface in the duodenum
Intravascular hemolysis	Microangiopathic hemolytic anemia PNH	Chronic loss of Hb in urine leads to iron deficiency

Hb, hemoglobin; NSAID, nonsteroidal anti-inflammatory drug; PNH, paroxysmal nocturnal hemoglobinuria; PUD, peptic ulcer disease.

> The stages of iron deficiency in sequence are as follows: absent iron stores; decreased serum ferritin; decreased serum iron, increased TIBC, decreased iron saturation (%); normocytic normochromic anemia; microcytic hypochromic anemia.

(3) Microcytic and normocytic cells with increased central area of pallor (Fig. 11-6)
(4) Thrombocytosis is a common finding in chronic iron deficiency.
(5) Leukocyte count is usually normal.
  • Eosinophilia occurs in hookworm infestations.

D. Anemia of chronic disease (ACD)
  1. Epidemiology
    a. Most common anemia in hospitalized patients
    b. Common causes
      (1) Chronic inflammation (e.g., rheumatoid arthritis, tuberculosis)
      (2) Alcoholism (most common anemia)
      (3) Malignancy (most common anemia)
  2. Pathogenesis
    a. Decreased synthesis of heme (Fig. 11-5)
    b. In some cases, there is a decrease renal production of EPO.
    c. Liver synthesis and release of hepcidin
      (1) Antimicrobial peptide

ACD: most common anemia in hospitalized patients

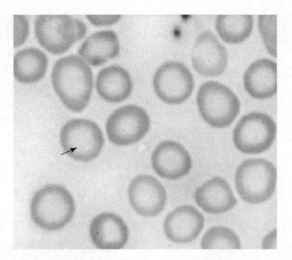

11-6: *Peripheral blood smear in iron deficiency anemia. The enlarged central area of pallor in the red blood cell (arrow) indicates a decrease in hemoglobin synthesis, which is characteristic of the microcytic anemias. The mean corpuscular hemoglobin concentration is decreased. (From Naeim F: Atlas of Bone Marrow and Blood Pathology. Philadelphia, WB Saunders, 2001, p. 27, Fig. 2-22A.)*

Hepcidin: ↑ macrophage iron stores

ACD: ↓ iron, TIBC, % saturation; ↑ ferritin

α-Thal: gene deletions

  (2) Acute phase reactant released by the liver in response to inflammation
  (3) Enters macrophages and prevents the release of iron to transferrin
  (4) Ferritin synthesis and iron stores increase in bone marrow macrophages
  3. Laboratory findings
    a. Decreased MCV, serum iron, TIBC, and iron saturation (%)
    b. Increased serum ferritin (>100 ng/mL)
E. **Thalassemia (thal; α and β)**
  1. Epidemiology
    a. Autosomal recessive disorders
    b. α-Thal is common in Southeast Asia and in black Americans.
    c. β-Thal is common in black Americans, Greeks, and Italians.
  2. Pathogenesis of α-thal
    a. Decrease in α-globin chain synthesis due to gene deletions (Fig. 11-5)
      • Four genes control α-globin chain synthesis.
    b. One gene deletion produces a silent carrier.
      • *Not* associated with anemia
    c. The combination of two gene deletions is called α-thal trait.
      (1) Mild anemia with an increased RBC count
      (2) Black American type
        • Associated with a loss of one gene on *each* chromosome (α/– α/–)
      (3) Asian type
        (a) Associated with a loss of both genes on the *same* chromosome (–/– α/α)
        (b) Increased risk for developing more severe types of α-thal

(4) Decreased MCV, Hb, and Hct

(5) Increased RBC count

(6) Normal RDW, serum ferritin, and Hb electrophoresis

> Hb electrophoresis is normal, because all Hb types require α-globin chains. The Hb concentration is decreased; however, the relative proportions of the normal Hbs remains the same.

(7) There is no treatment.

d. The combinations of three gene deletions is called HbH (four β-chains) disease.

  (1) Severe hemolytic anemia
   - Excess β-chain inclusions cause macrophage destruction of the RBCs.

  (2) Hb electrophoresis detects HbH.

e. The combination of four gene deletions is called Hb Bart (four γ-chains) disease.

  (1) Incompatible with life

  (2) Hb electrophoresis shows an increase in Hb Bart.

3. Pathogenesis of β-thal

 a. Decrease in β-globin chain synthesis (Fig. 11-5)

  (1) Mild anemia is most often due to DNA splicing defects.

  (2) Severe anemia is due to a nonsense mutation with formation of a stop codon.
   - Premature termination of β-globin chain synthesis or absent β-globin chain synthesis.

 b. Normal synthesis of α, δ, γ-globin chains.

> Normal β-globin chain synthesis is designated β; some β-globin chain synthesis is designated β^+; and, no β-globin chain synthesis is designated β^0.

 c. β-Thal minor (β/β^+)

  (1) Mild microcytic anemia

  (2) Mild protective effect against falciparum malaria
   - RBC life span is shorter than normal.

  (3) Decreased MCV, Hb, and Hct

  (4) Increased RBC count

  (5) Normal RDW and serum ferritin

  (6) Hb electrophoresis
   (a) Decreased HbA ($2\alpha/2\beta$)
   (b) Increased HbA_2 ($2\alpha/2\delta$) and HbF ($2\alpha/2\gamma$)

  (7) There is no treatment.

 d. β-Thal major (Cooley's anemia; β^0/β^0)

  (1) Severe hemolytic anemia
   (a) RBCs with α-chain inclusions are removed by macrophages in the spleen.
    - Causes an increase in unconjugated bilirubin

α-Thal trait: ↓ HbA, HbA_2, HbF (normal electrophoresis); ↑ RBC count

HbH: 4 β-chains

Hb Bart: 4 γ chains

β-Thal: mild—DNA splicing defect, severe—stop codon

β-Thal minor: ↓ HbA; ↑ RBC count, HbA_2, HbF

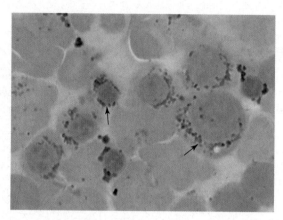

11-7: *Ringed sideroblasts in a bone marrow aspirate. Dark blue iron granules around the nucleus of developing normoblasts (arrows) represent iron trapped within mitochondria and indicate a defect in mitochondrial heme synthesis. (From Forbes C, Jackson W: Color Atlas and Text of Clinical Medicine, 2nd ed. St. Louis, Mosby, 2003, p 431, Fig. 10-27.)*

(b) RBCs with α-chain inclusions undergo apoptosis in the bone marrow (ineffective erythropoiesis).

(2) Extramedullary hematopoiesis

(3) Increased RDW and reticulocytes

(4) Hb electrophoresis

    (a) *No* synthesis of HbA

    (b) Increase in HbA_2 and HbF

(5) Long-term transfusion requirement

    • Danger of iron overload (called hemosiderosis)

F. **Sideroblastic anemia**

1. Epidemiology

    a. Chronic alcoholism (most common cause)

    b. Pyridoxine (vitamin B_6) deficiency

    c. Lead (Pb) poisoning

2. Pathogenesis

    a. Defect in heme synthesis within the mitochondria (Fig. 11-5)

    b. Iron accumulates in the mitochondria forming ringed sideroblasts (Fig. 11-7).

    c. Iron-overload type of anemia

       • Increase in iron stores in the bone marrow macrophages

3. Chronic alcoholism

    a. Alcohol is a mitochondrial toxin.

       • Damages heme biosynthetic pathways in the mitochondria

    b. Sideroblastic anemia occurs in ~30% of hospitalized chronic alcoholics.

4. Pyridoxine deficiency

    a. Vitamin B_6 is a cofactor for δ-aminolevulinic acid synthase.

       • Rate-limiting reaction of heme synthesis (Fig. 11-5)

    b. Most common cause of deficiency is isoniazid (INH) therapy.

       • INH is used in the treatment of tuberculosis.

Margin notes:

β-Thal major: no HbA; ↑ HbA_2, HbF

Sideroblastic anemia: defect in heme synthesis in the mitochondria; ringed sideroblasts

Sideroblastic anemia: alcohol most common cause

Pyridoxine deficiency: INH most common cause

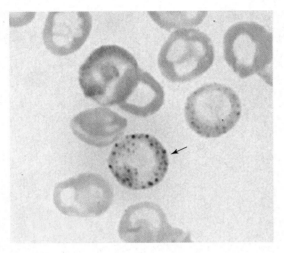

11-8: *Peripheral blood with coarse basophilic stippling of RBCs in lead poisoning. Note the mature RBC containing numerous dots representing ribosomes (arrow). Lead denatures ribonuclease; hence, the ribosomes persist in the cytoplasm. (From Naeim F: Atlas of Bone Marrow and Blood Pathology. Philadelphia, WB Saunders, 2001, p. 27, Fig. 2-22M.)*

5. Lead (Pb) poisoning
   a. Epidemiology
      (1) Pica (abnormal craving) for eating lead-based paint
         • Common cause of childhood lead poisoning in inner cities
      (2) Pottery painter
         • Pb-based paints are commonly used for decoration.
      (3) Working in a battery or ammunition factory
   b. Pb denatures enzymes:
      (1) Ferrochelatase (heme synthase)
         (a) Iron cannot bind with protoporphyrin to form heme.
         (b) Increase in protoporphyrin, which is proximal to the enzyme block
      (2) Aminolevulinic acid (ALA) dehydrase
         • Causes an increase in δ-ALA, which is proximal to the enzyme block
      (3) Ribonuclease
         (a) Ribosomes cannot be degraded and persist in the RBC.
         (b) Produces coarse basophilic stippling (Fig. 11-8)
   c. Clinical and laboratory findings
      (1) Abdominal colic with diarrhea
         • Pb is visible in the gastrointestinal tract on plain abdominal radiographs.
      (2) Encephalopathy in children
         • δ-ALA damages neurons, increases vessel permeability (cerebral edema), and causes demyelination.
      (3) Growth retardation in children

Pb poisoning: paint, batteries

Pb poisoning: coarse basophilic stippling

**TABLE 11-2:
Laboratory
Findings in
Microcytic Anemias**

Test	Iron Deficiency	Anemia of Chronic Disease	α-Thal/β-Thal Minor	Lead Poisoning
MCV	↓	↓	↓	↓
Serum iron	↓	↓	Normal	↑
TIBC	↑	↓	Normal	↓
Percent saturation	↓	↓	Normal	↑
Serum ferritin	↓	↑	Normal	↑
RDW	↑	Normal	Normal	Normal
RBC count	↓	↓	↑	↓
Hb electrophoresis	Normal	Normal	α-Thal trait normal β-Thal: ↓HbA, ↑HbA$_2$, ↑HbF	—
Ringed sideroblasts	None	None	None	Present
Coarse basophilic stippling	None	None	None	Present

Hb, hemoglobin; MCV, mean corpuscular volume; RDW, red blood cell distribution width; TIBC, total iron-binding capacity.

Pb poisoning: Pb deposits in epiphyses

(a) Pb deposits in the epiphysis of growing bone.
(b) Radiographs show increased density in the epiphyses.
(4) Peripheral neuropathy in adults
• Example—footdrop (peroneal nerve palsy)
(5) Nephrotoxic damage to proximal renal tubules

> Tubular damage by lead produces Fanconi's syndrome. The syndrome includes proximal renal tubular acidosis (loss of bicarbonate in urine), aminoaciduria, phosphaturia, and glucosuria.

(6) Increased whole blood and urine Pb levels
• Best screen and confirmatory test for Pb poisoning
6. Laboratory findings in sideroblastic anemias
a. Increased serum iron, iron saturation (%), and ferritin
b. Decreased MCV and TIBC
c. Ringed sideroblasts are present in a bone marrow aspirate.
7. Summary table of microcytic anemias (Table 11-2)

IV. **Macrocytic Anemias**
• Macrocytic anemias are most often caused by folate or vitamin B$_{12}$ deficiency.
A. **Vitamin B$_{12}$ metabolism**
1. Present in meat, eggs, and dairy products
2. Parietal cells synthesize intrinsic factor (IF) and hydrochloric acid.
3. Gastric acid converts pepsinogen to pepsin.
• Pepsin frees vitamin B$_{12}$ from ingested proteins.
4. Free vitamin B$_{12}$ is bound to R-binders synthesized in the salivary glands.

Vitamin B$_{12}$: present in animal products

TABLE 11-3:
Causes of Vitamin B_{12} Deficiency

Classification	Causes	Associated Factors
Decreased intake	Pure vegan diet	Breast-fed infants of pure vegans may develop deficiency
	Malnutrition	May occur in elderly patients
Malabsorption	↓ Intrinsic factor	Autoimmune destruction of parietal cells (i.e., pernicious anemia)
	↓ Gastric acid	Cannot activate pepsinogen to release vitamin B_{12}
	↓ Intestinal reabsorption	Crohn's disease or celiac disease involving terminal ileum (destruction of absorptive cells)
		Bacterial overgrowth (bacterial utilization of available vitamin B_{12})
		Fish tapeworm
		Chronic pancreatitis (cannot cleave off R-binder)
Increased utilization	Pregnancy/lactation	Deficiency is more likely in a pure vegan

    5. Pancreatic enzymes in the duodenum cleave off the R-binders.
      • Vitamin B_{12} binds to IF to form a complex.
    6. Vitamin B_{12}-IF complex is reabsorbed in the terminal ileum.
    7. Vitamin B_{12} binds to transcobalamin II and is secreted into plasma.
      • Delivered to metabolically active cells or stored in the liver (6–9 year supply).

B. Causes of vitamin B_{12} deficiency (Table 11-3)

C. Folate metabolism
    1. Present in green vegetables and animal proteins
      • In the form of polyglutamates
    2. Converted to monoglutamates by intestinal conjugase
      • Intestinal conjugase is inhibited by phenytoin.
    3. Monoglutamates are reabsorbed in the jejunum.
      a. Converted to methyltetrahydrofolate, the circulating form of folate
      b. Reabsorption is blocked by alcohol and oral contraceptives.
    4. There is only a 3- to 4-month supply of folate in the liver.

D. Causes of folate deficiency (Table 11-4)

E. Pathogenesis of macrocytic anemia in folate and vitamin B_{12} deficiency
    1. Impaired DNA synthesis
      a. Delayed nuclear maturation
        (1) Causes a block in cell division leading to large, nucleated hematopoietic cells
        (2) Enlarged cells are called megaloblasts.
      b. Affects all rapidly dividing cells
        • Examples—RBCs, leukocytes, platelets, intestinal epithelium
      c. Cellular RNA and protein synthesis continue unabated.
        • Cytoplasmic volume continues to expand.

Vitamin B_{12} deficiency: pernicious anemia most common cause

Intestinal conjugase: inhibited by phenytoin

Monoglutamate reabsorption: inhibited by alcohol and oral contraceptives

Folate deficiency: alcohol most common cause

TABLE 11-4:
Causes of Folate
Deficiency

Classification	Causes	Comment and Associated Factors
Decreased intake	Malnutrition Infants/elderly Chronic alcoholics Goat's milk	Decreased intake most common cause of folate deficiency
Malabsorption	Celiac disease Bacterial overgrowth	Deficiency usually occurs in association with other vitamin deficiencies (fat and water soluble)
Drug inhibition	5-Fluorouracil Methotrexate, trimethoprim-sulfa Phenytoin Oral contraceptives, alcohol	Inhibits thymidylate synthase Inhibit dihydrofolate reductase Inhibits intestinal conjugase Inhibit uptake of monoglutamate in jejunum Alcohol also inhibits the release of folate from the liver.
Increased utilization	Pregnancy/lactation Disseminated malignancy Severe hemolytic anemia	Increased utilization of folate in DNA synthesis

   2. Ineffective erythropoiesis
     a. Megaloblastic precursors outside the bone marrow sinusoids are phagocytosed by macrophages.
     b. Megaloblastic precursors undergo apoptosis causing pancytopenia.
       • Anemia, neutropenia, and thrombocytopenia
  F. **Vitamin B_{12} and folate in DNA synthesis (Fig. 11-9)**
    1. Vitamin B_{12} removes the methyl group from methyltetrahydrofolate (N^5-methyl-FH_4).
     a. Produces tetrahydrofolate (FH_4)
     b. Methyl-B_{12} transfers the methyl group to homocysteine to produce methionine.

↑ Homocysteine: folate (most common) and vitamin B_{12} deficiency

     c. Deficiency of folate or vitamin B_{12} increases plasma homocysteine.

> Folate deficiency is the most common cause of increased serum homocysteine levels in the United States. Homocysteine damages endothelial cells leading to vessel thrombosis.

    2. Thymidylate synthase converts deoxyuridine monophosphate (dUMP) to deoxythymidine monophosphate (dTMP).
      • Thymidylate synthase is inhibited by 5-fluorouracil.
    3. Dihydrofolate reductase converts dihydrofolate (FH_2) to FH_4.
      • Dihydrofolate reductase is inhibited by methotrexate and trimethoprim-sulfamethoxazole.
  G. **Vitamin B_{12} in odd-chain fatty acid metabolism**
    1. Propionyl CoA is converted to methylmalonyl CoA.
    2. Methylmalonyl CoA is converted to succinyl CoA.
      • Vitamin B_{12} is a cofactor for methylmalonyl CoA mutase.

Thymidylate synthase: inhibited by 5-fluorouracil

Dihydrofolate reductase: inhibited by methotrexate, trimethoprim

Vitamin B_{12}: odd chain fatty acid metabolism

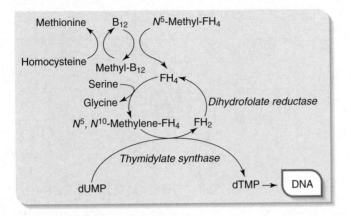

11-9: *Vitamin B$_{12}$ and folate in DNA metabolism. See text for discussion. dTMP, deoxythymidine monophosphate; dUMP, deoxyuridine monophosphate; FH$_2$, dihydrofolate; FH$_4$, tetrahydrofolate. (From Pelley J, Goljan EF: Rapid Review: Biochemistry. St. Louis, Mosby, 2004, Fig. 4-3.)*

3. Vitamin B$_{12}$ deficiency causes an increase in propionyl and methylmalonyl CoA and their corresponding acids.
   • Propionyl CoA replaces acetyl CoA in neuronal membranes resulting in demyelination.

H. Clinical findings in vitamin B$_{12}$ deficiency
   1. Findings in pernicious anemia
      a. Achlorhydria (lack of gastric acid) due to destruction of parietal cells
         (1) Maldigestion of food
         (2) Hypergastrinemia due to loss of acid inhibition of gastrin
      b. Antibodies associated with pernicious anemia
         (1) Antibodies directed against the proton pump in parietal cells
         (2) Antibodies that block binding of vitamin B$_{12}$ to IF
            • Most specific test for pernicious anemia
         (3) Antibodies that prevent binding of vitamin B$_{12}$-IF complexes to ileal receptors
      c. Antibody destruction of parietal cells causes chronic atrophic gastritis of the body and fundus.
         • Increased incidence of gastric adenocarcinoma
   2. Smooth, sore tongue with atrophy of papillae
   3. Neurologic disease
      a. Peripheral neuropathy with sensorimotor dysfunction
      b. Posterior column dysfunction
         • Decrease in vibratory sensation and proprioception (joint sense)
      c. Lateral corticospinal tract dysfunction with spasticity
      d. Dementia

I. Laboratory findings in vitamin B$_{12}$ deficiency
   1. Decreased serum vitamin B$_{12}$
   2. Increased serum homocysteine and methylmalonic acid (95% of cases)
   3. Peripheral blood findings

Macrocytic anemia + neurologic disease: vitamin B$_{12}$ deficiency

↑ Methylmalonic acid: most sensitive test for vitamin B$_{12}$ deficiency

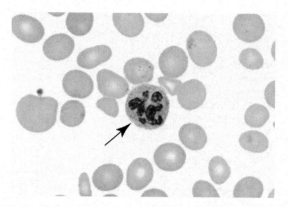

11-10: *Peripheral blood in megaloblastic anemia showing the hypersegmented neutrophil (arrow) with nine lobes. Neutrophils normally have less than five nuclear segments. Hypersegmented neutrophils are excellent markers of folate and vitamin B_{12} deficiency. The enlarged, egg-shaped red blood cells (macro-ovalocytes) characteristic of macrocytic anemias are associated with problems in DNA synthesis. (From Naeim F: Atlas of Bone Marrow and Blood Pathology. Philadelphia, WB Saunders, 2001, p. 180, Fig. 14-10B.)*

Hypersegmented neutrophil: marker for folate or vitamin B_{12} deficiency

a. Pancytopenia
b. Oval macrocytes
c. Hypersegmented neutrophils (Fig. 11-10)
  • More than five nuclear lobes
4. Bone marrow findings
  • Megaloblastic nucleated cells with primitive open (lacy) chromatin pattern
5. Schilling test localizes some of the causes of vitamin B_{12} deficiency
  (1) Utilizes oral administration of radioactive vitamin B_{12}
  (2) Reabsorption of radioactive vitamin B_{12}
    • Indicates dietary deficiency of vitamin B_{12} (e.g., pure vegan)
  (3) Reabsorption of radioactive vitamin B_{12} after administration of IF
    • Indicates pernicious anemia, where there is a lack of IF
  (4) Reabsorption of radioactive vitamin B_{12} after administration of antibiotics
    • Indicates bacterial overgrowth with destruction of vitamin B_{12}-IF complex
  (5) Reabsorption of radioactive B_{12} after administration of pancreatic extract
    • Indicates chronic pancreatitis with lack of enzymes to cleave off R-binder

Schilling test: defines the cause of vitamin B_{12} deficiency

J. **Clinical findings in folate deficiency**
  1. Similar to vitamin B_{12} deficiency with the *exception* of neurologic disease.
  2. Increased risk for open neural tube defects in the fetus
    • Due to decreased maternal intake of folate *prior* to conception

↓ Maternal intake folate: increased risk for open neural tube defect in newborn

K. **Laboratory findings in folate deficiency**
  1. Peripheral blood and bone marrow findings are similar to vitamin B_{12} deficiency.

Laboratory/Clinical Finding	Pernicious Anemia	Other Vitamin B₁₂ Deficiencies	Folate Deficiency
Achlorhydria	Present	Absent	Absent
Autoantibodies	Present	Absent	Absent
Chronic atrophic gastritis	Present	Absent	Absent
Gastric carcinoma risk	↑	None	None
Hypersegmented neutrophils	Present	Present	Present
Mean corpuscular volume	↑	↑	↑
Neurologic disease	Present	Present	None
Pancytopenia	Present	Present	Present
Plasma homocysteine	↑	↑	↑
Serum gastrin level	↑	Normal	Normal
Urine methylmalonic acid	↑	↑	Normal

TABLE 11-5: Clinical and Laboratory Findings in Vitamin B₁₂ and Folate Deficiencies

2. Decreased serum folate and RBC folate (best screening test)

> It is important to distinguish folate from vitamin B₁₂ deficiency. Pharmacologic doses of folate can correct the hematologic findings in both folate and vitamin B₁₂ deficiency; however, neurologic disease is *not* corrected.

RBC folate: best indicator of folate stores

L. Comparison table of vitamin B₁₂ and folate deficiency (Table 11-5)

V. Normocytic Anemias: Corrected Reticulocyte Count or Index Below 3%
- Anemias under this classification include acute blood loss, early iron deficiency or anemia of chronic disease (ACD), aplastic anemia, and chronic renal failure.

A. Acute blood loss
1. Epidemiology
   a. External blood loss (e.g., peptic ulcer)
      - May result in iron deficiency
   b. Internal blood loss (e.g., ruptured abdominal aortic aneurysm)
2. Clinical and laboratory findings (see Chapter 4)
3. Requires 5 to 7 days before a reticulocyte response is observed

Signs volume depletion: ↓ blood pressure, ↑ pulse

B. Early iron deficiency or ACD
1. Anemia is normocytic *before* it becomes microcytic.
   - ACD is microcytic in only 10% to 30% of cases.
2. Serum ferritin is most useful in distinguishing the two anemias.

C. Aplastic anemia
1. Causes (Table 11-6)
2. Pathogenesis
   a. Antigenic alteration of multipotent myeloid stem cells
      - Causes T-cell activation and release of cytokines that suppress stem cells
   b. Defective or deficient stem cells (acquired or hereditary)
3. Clinical findings
   a. Fever due to infection associated with neutropenia

Aplastic anemia: most cases idiopathic; drugs most common known cause

TABLE 11-6:
Causes of
Aplastic Anemia

Classification	Examples and Discussion
Idiopathic	Approximately 50–70% of cases are idiopathic
Drugs	Most common known cause of aplastic anemia Dose-related causes are usually reversible (e.g., alkylating agents) Idiosyncratic reactions are frequently irreversible (e.g., chloramphenicol)
Chemical agents	Toxic chemicals in industry and agriculture (e.g., benzene, insecticides–DDT, parathion)
Infection	May involve all hematopoietic cell lines (pancytopenia) or erythroid cell line alone (pure RBC aplasia) Examples—EBV; CMV; parvovirus; non-A, non-B hepatitis (most common)
Physical agents	Whole-body ionizing radiation (therapeutic or nuclear accident)
Miscellaneous	Thymoma (may be associated with pure RBC aplasia) Paroxysmal nocturnal hemoglobinuria

CMV, cytomegalovirus; EBV, Epstein-Barr virus; RBC, red blood cell.

    b. Bleeding due to thrombocytopenia
    c. Fatigue due to anemia
  4. Laboratory findings
    a. Pancytopenia
    b. Reticulocytopenia
    c. Hypocellular bone marrow
  5. Complete recovery occurs in less than 10% of cases.
D. Chronic renal failure (CRF)
  1. Pathogenesis
    • Decreased synthesis of EPO (most common cause)
  2. Laboratory findings
    a. Normocytic anemia
    b. Presence of burr cells (i.e., RBCs with an undulating membrane)
    c. Platelet dysfunction
      (1) Thrombocytopenia
      (2) Defect in platelet aggregation that is reversible with dialysis
        • Prolonged bleeding time

> Anemia CRF: ↓ EPO most common cause

VI. Normocytic Anemias: Corrected Reticulocyte Count at or Above 3%
  • Anemias include the hemolytic anemias due to defects within the RBC (intrinsic) or factors outside the RBC (extrinsic).
A. Pathogenesis of hemolytic anemias
  1. Intrinsic or extrinsic hemolytic anemias
    a. Intrinsic refers to a defect in the RBC causing the anemia.
      • Examples—membrane defects, abnormal Hb, enzyme deficiency
    b. Extrinsic refers to factors outside the RBC causing hemolysis.
      • Examples—stenotic aortic valve, immune destruction
  2. Mechanisms of hemolysis
    a. Extravascular hemolysis
      (1) RBC phagocytosis by macrophages in the spleen (most common site) and liver

(2) Reasons for phagocytosis
    (a) RBCs coated by IgG with or without C3b
    (b) Abnormally shaped RBCs (e.g., spherocytes, sickle cells)
(3) Increase in serum unconjugated bilirubin
    • End product of macrophage degradation of Hb
(4) Increased serum lactate dehydrogenase (LDH) from hemolyzed RBCs.

b. Intravascular hemolysis
  (1) Hemolysis occurs within blood vessels.
  (2) Causes of hemolysis
    (a) Enzyme deficiency (e.g., deficiency of glucose-6-phosphate dehydrogenase)
    (b) Complement destruction (e.g., IgM-mediated hemolysis)
    (c) Mechanical damage (e.g., calcific aortic valve stenosis)
  (3) Increased plasma and urine Hb
  (4) Hemosiderinuria
    • Renal tubules convert iron in Hb into hemosiderin.
  (5) Decreased serum haptoglobin

> Haptoglobin is an acute phase reactant that combines with Hb to form a complex that is phagocytosed and degraded by macrophages causing a decrease in serum haptoglobin. The amount of Hb in the complexes is so small that unconjugated bilirubin is *not* significantly increased.

  (6) Increased serum LDH from hemolyzed RBCs.

B. Hereditary spherocytosis
1. Pathogenesis
  a. Autosomal dominant disorder
  b. Intrinsic defect with extravascular hemolysis
  c. Membrane protein defect results in the loss of RBC membrane and spherocyte formation.
    (1) Mutation in ankyrin is the most common defect.
    (2) Mutation in band 2, spectrin (α and β), or band 3 account for other defects.
  d. Increased permeability of spherocytes to sodium
    • Due to membrane defect and dysfunctional Na^+/K^+-ATPase pump
2. Clinical findings
  a. Jaundice due to increased unconjugated bilirubin
  b. Increased incidence of calcium bilirubinate gallstones
    • Due to increased concentration of conjugated bilirubin in bile
  c. Splenomegaly
  d. Aplastic crisis
    • May occur in children especially after a viral infection (e.g., parvovirus)

Extravascular hemolysis: macrophage phagocytosis; unconjugated hyperbilirubinemia

Intravascular hemolysis: ↓ serum haptoglobin; hemoglobinuria

Hereditary spherocytosis: intrinsic defect, extravascular hemolysis

Hereditary spherocytosis: mutation in ankyrin in cell membrane

Aplastic crisis: parvovirus induced

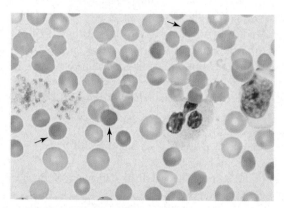

11-11: *Peripheral blood with spherocytes in hereditary spherocytosis. Numerous, round, dense red blood cells (RBCs) without central areas of pallor represent spherocytes (arrows). The mean corpuscular hemoglobin concentration is increased. (From Damjanov I, Linder J: Pathology: A Color Atlas. St. Louis, Mosby, 2000, p 75, Fig. 5-7.)*

3. Laboratory findings
   a. Normocytic anemia with spherocytosis (Fig. 11-11)
   b. Increased MCHC

Hereditary spherocytosis: ↑ RBC osmotic fragility

   c. Increased RBC osmotic fragility
      (1) Increased permeability of spherocytes to sodium and water
      (2) Spherocytes rupture in mildly hypotonic salt solutions.
4. Treatment is splenectomy
   • Spherocytes remain in the peripheral blood.

C. **Hereditary elliptocytosis**
   1. Pathogenesis
      a. Autosomal dominant disorder
      b. Defective spectrin and band 4.1
   2. Clinical findings
      a. Majority have no anemia or a mild hemolytic anemia
      b. Splenomegaly
   3. Laboratory findings

Hereditary elliptocytosis: >25% elliptocytes in peripheral blood

      a. Elliptocytes greater than 25% of RBCs in peripheral blood
      b. Increased osmotic fragility
   4. Treatment is splenectomy in symptomatic patients

D. **Paroxysmal nocturnal hemoglobinuria (PNH)**
   1. Pathogenesis
      a. Acquired membrane defect in multipotent myeloid stem cells

PNH: loss of anchor for DAF

         (1) Mutation causes loss of the anchor for decay accelerating factor (DAF).
         (2) Normally DAF neutralizes complement attached to RBCs, neutrophils, and platelets.
      b. Intravascular complement-mediated lysis of RBCs, neutrophils, and platelets

PNH: intrinsic defect, intravascular hemolysis

         • Occurs at night, because respiratory acidosis enhances complement attachment to these cells

2. Clinical findings
   a. Episodic hemoglobinuria
      - May cause iron deficiency
   b. Increased incidence of vessel thrombosis (e.g., hepatic vein)
      - Due to the release of aggregating agents from destroyed platelets
   c. Increased risk for developing acute myelogenous leukemia
3. Laboratory findings
   a. Screening test is the sucrose hemolysis test (sugar water test).
      - Sucrose enhances complement destruction of RBCs.
   b. Confirmatory test is the acidified serum test (Ham test).
      - Acidified serum activates the alternative pathway causing hemolysis.

   PNH: screen—sucrose hemolysis test; confirm—acidified serum test

   c. Peripheral blood findings
      (1) Normocytic anemia with pancytopenia
         - Microcytic if iron deficiency develops from hemoglobinuria
      (2) Decreased leukocyte alkaline phosphatase
   d. Decreased serum haptoglobin
   e. Increased serum/urine Hb

E. Sickle cell anemia
   1. Epidemiology
      a. Autosomal recessive disorder
      b. Most common hemoglobinopathy in black Americans
      c. Heterozygote condition (sickle cell trait, HbAS) has no anemia.
         - Present in 8% to 10% of black Americans
      d. Homozygous condition (HbSS) produces anemia.
      e. Protective against *Plasmodium falciparum* malaria
   2. Pathogenesis
      a. Predominantly extravascular hemolysis of sickle cells
      b. Missense point mutation

      Sickle cell anemia: intrinsic defect, extravascular hemolysis

         - Substitution of valine for glutamic acid at sixth position of β-globin chain
      c. Causes of sickling
         (1) HbS molecules aggregate and polymerize into long needle-like fibers
            - RBCs assume a sickle or boat-like shape (Fig. 11-12).
         (2) Sickle Hb (HbS) concentration greater than 60% is the most important factor for sickling.
            - HbS concentration is too low in HbAS to produce sickling in the peripheral blood.

      Sickling: ↑ HbS, ↑ deoxyHb

         (3) Increase in deoxyhemoglobin increases the risk for sickling.
            (a) Acidosis (causes O_2 release from RBCs)
            (b) Volume depletion (intracellular dehydration causes an increase in concentration of deoxyhemoglobin)
            (c) Hypoxemia (decrease in arterial PO_2 decreases O_2 saturation of Hb)
      d. Reversible and irreversible sickling
         (1) Initial sickling is reversible with administration of oxygen.

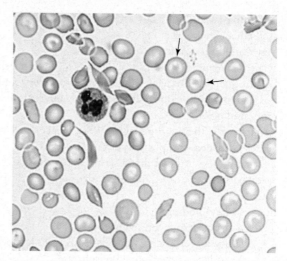

11-12: *Peripheral blood with sickle cells and target cells, showing the dense, boat-shaped sickle cells. Cells with a bull's-eye appearance are target cells (arrows), which have excess RBC membrane that bulges in the center of the cell. (From Hoffbrand AV: Color Atlas: Clinical Hematology, 3rd ed. St. Louis, Mosby, 2000, p 103, Fig. 5-85A.)*

Target cells: excess RBC membrane; sign of hemoglobinopathy or alcohol excess

Sickling: HbF prevents sickling

Dactylitis: most common presentation in infants

Acute chest syndrome: most common cause of death in adults

Howell-Jolly bodies: sign of splenic dysfunction

(2) Recurrent sickling causes irreversible sickling due to membrane damage.
(3) Irreversibly sickled cells have increased adherence to endothelial cells in the microcirculation.
- Microvascular occlusions (vaso-occlusive crises) produce ischemic damage.

e. HbF prevents sickling.
(1) Increased HbF at birth prevents sickling in HbSS for 5 to 6 months.
(2) Hydroxyurea increases the synthesis of HbF.

f. Key pathologic processes in HbSS
(1) Severe hemolytic anemia
(2) Vaso-occlusive crises

3. Clinical findings in HbSS
a. Dactylitis
- Painful swelling of hands and feet in infants (usually 6–9 months old) is due to bone infarcts.

b. Acute chest syndrome
(1) Vaso-occlusion of pulmonary capillaries
(2) Chest pain, lung infiltrates, hypoxemia
(3) Most common cause of death in adults

c. Aseptic necrosis of the femoral head

d. Autosplenectomy
(1) Spleen is enlarged but dysfunctional by 2 years of age.
- Nuclear remnants (Howell-Jolly bodies) appear in RBCs indicating loss of macrophage function (Fig. 11-13).

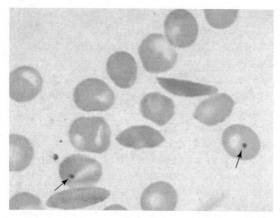

11-13: *Peripheral blood with sickle cells and Howell-Jolly bodies. The three dense boat-shaped sickle cells and the two cells containing a single dark, round inclusion (arrows) represent nuclear remnants. Howell-Jolly bodies in sickle cell disease indicate splenic dysfunction. (From Henry JB: Clinical Diagnosis and Management by Laboratory Methods, 20th ed. Philadelphia, WB Saunders, 2001, Fig. 26-2A.)*

      (2) Spleen is fibrosed and diminished in size in young adults.
   e. Increased susceptibility to infections
      (1) Due to dysfunctional spleen and impaired opsonization of encapsulated bacteria
      (2) Children are at risk for *Streptococcus pneumoniae* sepsis.
        • Most common cause of death in children
      (3) Increased incidence of osteomyelitis due to *Salmonella paratyphi*
   f. Aplastic crisis
      (1) Reticulocytopenia
      (2) Association with parvovirus
   g. Sequestration crisis
      (1) Rapid splenic enlargement with entrapment of RBCs causing hypovolemia
      (2) Reticulocytosis
   h. Increased risk for calcium bilirubinate gallstones
      • Due to increased conjugated bilirubin in bile from chronic hemolysis
  4. Renal findings in HbAS (also in HbSS)
   a. Sickling may occur in peritubular capillaries in the medulla.
      • Due to the low O_2 tension in the medulla
   b. Presents with microhematuria due to infarctions
   c. Renal papillary necrosis may occur.
      • Loss of concentration and dilution
  5. Laboratory findings
   a. Sickle cell screen
      • Sodium metabisulfite reduces O_2 tension, which induces sickling
   b. Hb electrophoresis
      (1) HbAS profile—HbA 55% to 60%, HbS 40% to 45%
      (2) HbSS profile—HbS 90% to 95%, HbF 5% to 10%, no HbA

Pathogens: *Streptococcus pneumoniae* sepsis, *Salmonella paratyphi* osteomyelitis

Sickle cell trait: no anemia; microhematuria

HbAS: HbA 55–60%, HbS 40–45%
HbSS: HbS 90–95%, HbF 5–10%, no HbA

c. Peripheral blood findings
  (1) Normal peripheral blood in HbAS
  (2) In HbSS, there are sickle cells and target cells.
d. Prenatal screening
  • Analysis of fetal DNA to detect the point mutation

F. **Glucose-6-phosphate dehydrogenase (G6PD) deficiency**

1. Epidemiology
   a. X-linked recessive disorder
   b. Subtypes of G6PD deficiency
     (1) Mediterranean variant in Greeks and Italians
     (2) Black American variant
   c. Protective against *Plasmodium falciparum* malaria

2. Pathogenesis
   a. Intrinsic defect with predominantly intravascular hemolysis
     • Mild component of extravascular hemolysis
   b. Decreased synthesis of NADPH and glutathione (GSH) in the pentose phosphate pathway
     (1) GSH normally neutralizes hydrogen peroxide, an oxidant product in RBC metabolism.
     (2) In G6PD deficiency, peroxide oxidizes Hb, which precipitates in the form of Heinz bodies.
       (a) Heinz bodies damage the RBC membranes causing intravascular hemolysis.
       (b) Heinz bodies removed from RBC membranes by splenic macrophages produce bite cells.
   c. Half-life of G6PD in the Mediterranean variant is markedly reduced.
     • Produces a severe, chronic hemolytic anemia
   d. Half-life of G6PD in the black American variant is moderately reduced.
     • Episodic type of hemolytic anemia after exposure to oxidant stresses.
   e. Oxidant stresses inducing hemolysis
     (1) Infection (most common)

Decrease in NADPH impairs neutrophils and monocyte killing of bacteria by the O_2-dependent myeloperoxidase system (see Chapter 2), which requires NADPH as a cofactor for NADPH oxidase.

     (2) Drugs
       • Examples—primaquine, chloroquine, dapsone, sulfonamides
     (3) Fava beans (mainly in Mediterranean variant)

3. Clinical findings
   • Sudden onset of back pain with hemoglobinuria 2 to 3 days after an oxidant stress

4. Laboratory findings
   a. Normocytic anemia
   b. Heinz bodies

G6PD deficiency: most common enzyme deficiency causing hemolysis

G6PD deficiency: intrinsic defect, primarily intravascular hemolysis

G6PD deficiency: oxidant damage with Heinz bodies and bite cells

(1) Identified with a supravital stain

(2) Best screen during active hemolysis

c. RBC enzyme analysis

- Confirmatory test *after* hemolysis has subsided

d. Peripheral blood findings

- Bite cells (macrophage removal of membrane)

G. **Pyruvate kinase (PK) deficiency**

1. Epidemiology

a. Autosomal recessive disease

b. Most common enzyme deficiency in the Embden-Meyerhof pathway

- PK normally converts phosphoenolpyruvate to pyruvate leading to a net gain of 2 ATP.

2. Pathogenesis

a. Intrinsic defect with extravascular hemolysis

b. Chronic lack of ATP causes membrane damage.

- Results in dehydration of the RBC (echinocytes)

3. Clinical findings

a. Hemolytic anemia with jaundice beginning at birth

b. Increase in 2,3-BPG synthesis proximal to enzyme block

- Right shift of OBC causes increased release of O_2, which offsets the clinical effects of the anemia.

4. Laboratory findings

a. Normocytic anemia

b. RBCs with thorny projections (echinocytes)

c. RBC enzyme assay is the confirmatory test.

H. **Immune hemolytic anemias**

- Group of extrinsic hemolytic anemias with extravascular or intravascular hemolysis.

1. Classification (Table 11-7)

a. Autoimmune

(1) Most common type of immune hemolytic anemia

(2) More common in women than men

- SLE is the most common cause of autoimmune hemolytic anemia (AIHA).

(3) 70% are warm type (IgG antibodies) of AIHA

(4) 30% are cold type (IgM antibodies) of AIHA

b. Drug-induced

c. Alloimmune (refer to Chapter 15)

2. Pathogenesis

a. IgG-mediated hemolysis

(1) RBCs coated by IgG are phagocytosed by splenic macrophages (extravascular hemolysis).

(2) Spherocytes are produced if a small portion of the membrane is removed.

b. Complement-mediated hemolysis

(1) RBCs coated by C3b alone are phagocytosed by liver macrophages (extravascular hemolysis).

Margin notes:

G6PD deficiency: active hemolysis screen with Heinz body prep

PK deficiency: intrinsic defect, extravascular hemolysis

PK deficiency: ↑ 2,3-BPG right-shifts OBC

Immune hemolytic anemia: autoimmune warm type most common cause

Drug-induced: drug adsorption (penicillin), immunocomplex (quinidine), autoantibody (methyldopa)

IgG-mediated: extravascular hemolysis; spherocytosis

TABLE 11-7:
Classification of
Immune Hemolytic
Anemias

Type of Immune Hemolytic Anemia	Examples
Autoimmune	
Warm antibodies (IgG)	Primary or idiopathic (no underlying cause)
	Secondary (e.g., SLE)
Cold antibodies (IgM)	Primary or idiopathic
	Secondary
	Mycoplasma pneumoniae (anti-I antibodies)
	Infectious mononucleosis (anti-i antibodies)
Drug-induced	Drug adsorption (e.g., penicillin): IgG antibody directed against the drug attached to the RBC membrane
	Immunocomplex (e.g., quinidine): drug-IgM immunocomplex deposits on the RBC causing intravascular hemolysis
	Autoantibody induction (e.g., α-methyldopa): drug alters Rh antigens on RBCs causing synthesis of autoantibodies against Rh antigens
Alloimmune	Hemolytic transfusion reaction (Chapter 15)
	ABO hemolytic disease of newborn (Chapter 15)
	Rh hemolytic disease of newborn (Chapter 15)

RBC, red blood cell; SLE, systemic lupus erythematosus.

Complement-mediated: intravascular or extravascular hemolysis

IgM-mediated: intravascular or extravascular hemolysis

    (2) RBCs coated by C5-C9 undergo intravascular hemolysis.
    (3) RBCs coated by IgG and C3b are phagocytosed by liver and splenic macrophages (e.g., SLE).
  c. IgM-mediated hemolysis
    • May be extravascular or intravascular depending on the degree of complement activation
3. Clinical findings
  a. Jaundice due to unconjugated hyperbilirubinemia
    • Occurs in extravascular types of hemolysis
  b. Hepatosplenomegaly
    • Due to work hyperplasia of splenic and liver macrophages
  c. Raynaud's phenomenon (see Chapter 9)
    • May occur in cold types of AIHA
4. Laboratory findings

DAT: most important marker of immune hemolytic anemia

  a. Positive direct antihuman globulin test (DAT; Coombs' test)
    • DAT detects RBCs sensitized with IgG and/or C3b.
  b. Positive indirect antihuman globulin test (indirect Coombs' test)
    • Detects antibodies in the serum (e.g., anti-D antibodies)
  c. Unconjugated hyperbilirubinemia in extravascular hemolysis is present.
  d. Hemoglobinuria, decreased serum haptoglobin in intravascular hemolysis
  e. Peripheral blood findings
    (1) Normocytic anemia
    (2) Spherocytosis due to macrophage removal of RBC membrane

TABLE 11-8:
Causes of
Micro- and
Macroangiopathic
Hemolytic Anemia

Types	Examples
Microangiopathic	
Platelet thrombi	Hemolytic uremic syndrome (see Chapter 14)
	Thrombotic thrombocytopenic purpura (see Chapter 14)
Fibrin thrombi	Disseminated intravascular coagulation (see Chapter 14)
	HELLP syndrome: H, hemolytic anemia; EL, elevated transaminases; LP, low platelets; associated with preeclampsia
Macroangiopathic	Aortic stenosis (most common cause)
	Prosthetic heart valves

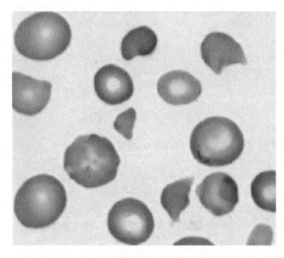

11-14: *Peripheral blood with schistocytes. The fragmented red blood cells (RBCs) with absence of central pallor, schistocytes, are produced when RBCs are mechanically injured by calcium deposits in an aortic valve, platelet thrombi, or fibrin clots in the microvasculature. (From Naeim F: Atlas of Bone Marrow and Blood Pathology. Philadelphia, WB Saunders, 2001, p. 27, Fig. 2-22D.)*

I. Micro- and macroangiopathic hemolytic anemias (MHA)

1. Causes (Table 11-8)
2. Pathogenesis
   a. Extrinsic defect with intravascular hemolysis
   b. Microangiopathic
      • Microcirculatory lesions cause RBC fragmentation (schistocytes; Fig. 11-14)
   c. Macroangiopathic
      • Hemolytic process caused by valvular defects (e.g., aortic stenosis)
3. Laboratory findings
   a. Normocytic anemia
      • Long-standing hemoglobinuria causes iron deficiency anemia.
   b. Decreased serum haptoglobin, hemoglobinuria
   c. Schistocytes in the peripheral blood

MHA: aortic stenosis most common cause

Schistocytes: sign of MHA

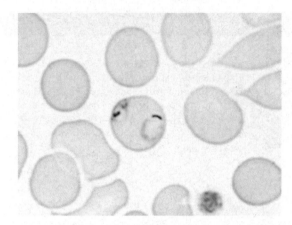

11-15: Plasmodium falciparum *ring forms in red blood cells (RBCs). This RBC has two ring forms. Multiple infestation of an RBC is characteristic of* P. falciparum *malaria. (From Hoffbrand AV: Color Atlas: Clinical Hematology, 3rd ed. St. Louis, Mosby, 2000, p 315, Fig. 18-4C.)*

J. Malaria
  1. Epidemiology
     • Female *Anopheles* mosquito transmits *Plasmodia* to humans.
  2. Pathogenesis
     a. Intraerythrocytic parasite causes intravascular hemolysis.
        • Correlates with fever spikes
     b. Extrinsic defect with predominantly intravascular hemolysis
        • Minor component of extravascular hemolysis
  3. Clinical findings
     a. Fever and splenomegaly
     b. *Plasmodium vivax*
        (1) Most common type
        (2) Tertian fever pattern (every 48 hours)
     c. *Plasmodium falciparum*
        (1) Most lethal type
        (2) Quotidian fever pattern (daily spikes with no pattern)
     d. *Plasmodium malariae*
        (1) Association with nephrotic syndrome
        (2) Quartan fever pattern (every 72 hours)
  4. Laboratory findings
     • Thin and thick smears identify organisms in RBCs (Fig. 11-15)
K. Summary table of normocytic anemias (Table 11-9)

Malaria: intravascular hemolysis correlates with fever spikes

TABLE 11-9:
Summary of
Normocytic
Anemias

Anemia	Pathogenesis	Discussion
Reticulocytosis < 3%		
Acute blood loss	Loss of whole blood	Initial Hb and Hct normal Signs of volume depletion
Early iron deficiency	Decreased iron stores	Normocytic *before* microcytic Iron studies abnormal
Early ACD	Iron trapped in macrophages by hepcidin	Normocytic *before* microcytic Iron studies abnormal
Aplastic anemia	Suppression or deficiency of multipotent myeloid stem cells	Pancytopenia Hypocellular marrow
Chronic renal failure	Deficiency of EPO	Presence of burr cells
Reticulocytosis ≥ 3%		
Hereditary spherocytosis	AD disorder Defect in ankyrin Extravascular hemolysis	Increased osmotic fragility Rx with splenectomy
Hereditary elliptocytosis	AD disorder Defect in spectrin and band 4.1 Extravascular hemolysis	Elliptocytes > 25%
Paroxysmal nocturnal hemoglobinuria	Loss of anchor for DAF in myeloid stem cell Complement destruction of hematopoietic cells Intravascular hemolysis	Pancytopenia Positive sugar water test (screen) and acidified serum test (confirmatory test)
Sickle cell anemia	AR disorder Valine substitution for glutamic acid β-globin chain Extravascular hemolysis	HbAS: HbA 55–60%; HbS 40–45% HbSS: HbS 90–95%; HbF 5–10%; no HbA
G6PD deficiency	XR disorder Deficiency GSH causes oxidant damage to Hb and RBC membrane Intravascular hemolysis	Heinz body preparation: screen during active hemolysis Enzyme assay: confirmatory test when hemolysis subsides
Pyruvate kinase deficiency	AR disease ↓ ATP synthesis Extravascular hemolysis	↑ 2,3-BPG right shifts OBC Dehydrated RBCs with thorny projections (echinocytes)
Acute blood loss	Loss of whole blood Reticulocytosis 5–7 days	↓ Hb, Hct, RBC count
Warm AIHA	IgG with or without C3b Extravascular hemolysis	Positive direct Coombs' test SLE most common cause
Cold AIHA	IgM with C3b Extravascular or intravascular hemolysis	Association with *Mycoplasma pneumoniae*; EBV

continued

**TABLE 11-9:
Summary of
Normocytic
Anemias—cont'd**

Anemia	Pathogenesis	Discussion
Drug-induced immune hemolytic anemia	Drug hapten: penicillin Extravascular hemolysis Immunocomplex: quinidine Intravascular hemolysis Autoantibody: methyldopa Extravascular hemolysis	Positive direct Coombs' test
Alloimmune hemolytic anemia	Antibodies against foreign RBC antigens Extravascular hemolysis	Hemolytic transfusion reaction ABO and Rh HDN Positive direct Coombs' test
Micro- and macroangiopathic hemolytic anemia	Mechanical destruction of RBCs with formation of schistocytes Intravascular hemolysis	Calcific aortic stenosis most common cause Chronic hemoglobinuria causes iron deficiency
Malaria	Transmitted by female *Anopheles* mosquito Intravascular hemolysis	Rupture of RBCs corresponds with fever

AD, autosomal dominant; AR, autosomal recessive; BPG, bisphosphoglycerate; DAF, decay accelerating factor; EBV, Epstein-Barr virus; EPO, erythropoietin; G6PD, glucose-6-phasphate dehydrogenase; GSH, glutathione; Hb, hemaglabin; HbAS, sickle cell trait; HbSS, Hct, hematocrit; sickle cell disease; OBC, oxygen binding curve; RBC, red blood cell; Rx, treatment; SLE, systemic lupus erythematosus; XR, X-linked recessive.

White Blood Cell Disorders

I. **Benign Qualitative White Blood Cell (WBC) Disorders**

   A. **Pathogenesis**

      1. Defects in leukocyte structure
         - Example—membrane fusion defect in Chédiak-Higashi syndrome (see Chapter 1)

      2. Defects in leukocyte function

         a. Leukocyte adhesion defect
            - Example—deficient selectin or CD11a/CD18 (see Chapter 2)

         b. Phagocytosis defect
            - Example—decreased opsonins in Bruton's agammaglobulinemia (see Chapter 2)

         c. Microbicidal defect
            - Example—deficiency of myeloperoxidase (see Chapter 2)

   B. **Clinical findings**

      1. Unusual pathogens (e.g., coagulase-negative *Staphylococcus*)
      2. Frequent infections and growth failure in children
      3. Lack of an inflammatory response (e.g., production of "cold" abscesses)
      4. Severe gingivitis

      > Job's syndrome is an autosomal recessive disorder of neutrophils, characterized by abnormal chemotaxis leading to "cold" soft tissue abscesses due to *Staphylococcus aureus*. Patients have red hair, a leonine face, chronic eczema, and increased IgE (hyperimmune E syndrome).

   C. **Unusual benign leukocyte reactions**

      1. Leukemoid reaction

         a. Absolute leukocyte count usually above 50,000/μL.
            - May involve neutrophils, lymphocytes, or eosinophils

         b. Etiology
            (1) Perforating appendicitis (neutrophils)
            (2) Whooping cough (lymphocytes)
            (3) Cutaneous larva migrans (eosinophils)

         c. Pathogenesis
            - Exaggerated response to infection

      2. Leukoerythroblastic reaction (Fig. 12-1)

         a. Immature bone marrow cells enter the peripheral blood

Qualitative WBC defects: defects in structure and function

Absolute count = % leukocytes × total WBC count

Leukemoid reaction: benign, exaggerated leukocyte response

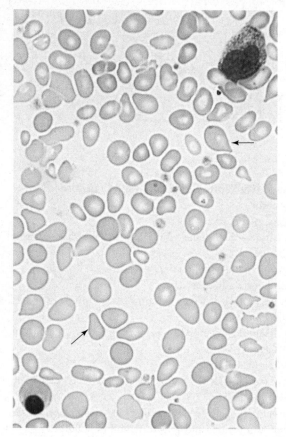

12-1: *Leukoerythroblastic reaction. Numerous bone marrow reticulocytes with a blue discoloration, a nucleated red blood cell (lower left corner), and a metamyelocyte (upper right corner). Many RBCs also have a teardrop configuration (arrows). (From Hoffbrand AV: Color Atlas: Clinical Hematology, 3rd ed. St. Louis, Mosby, 2000, p 251, Fig. 13-11A.)*

Leukoerythroblastic reaction in a woman over 50 years of age is usually due to metastatic breast cancer.

    b. Pathogenesis
       (1) Bone marrow infiltrative disease
       (2) Examples—fibrosis, metastatic breast cancer
    c. Peripheral blood findings
       (1) Myeloblasts, progranulocytes
       (2) Nucleated RBCs, tear drop RBCs

II. Benign Quantitative WBC Disorders
A. Disorders involving neutrophils
    1. Neutrophilic leukocytosis
      a. Absolute neutrophil count above 7000/μL
      b. Etiology
        (1) Infection (e.g., acute appendicitis)
        (2) Sterile inflammation with necrosis (e.g., acute myocardial infarction)

(3) Drugs (e.g., corticosteroids)
  c. Pathogenesis
    (1) Increased bone marrow production or release of neutrophils
    (2) Decreased activation of neutrophil adhesion molecules
      (a) Less neutrophils adhere to endothelial cells
      (b) Examples—corticosteroids, catecholamines, lithium
2. Neutropenia
  a. Absolute neutrophil count below 1500/μL
  b. Etiology
    (1) Aplastic anemia
    (2) Immune destruction
      • Example—systemic lupus erythematosus (SLE)
    (3) Septic shock
  c. Pathogenesis
    (1) Decreased production
    (2) Increased destruction (e.g., complement, macrophages)
    (3) Activation of neutrophil adhesion molecules (e.g., endotoxins)
      • Increase the number of neutrophils adhering to endothelium
B. Disorders involving eosinophils
  1. Eosinophilia
    a. Absolute eosinophil count over 700/μL
    b. Etiology
      (1) Type I hypersensitivity reaction
        • Examples—bronchial asthma, reaction to penicillin, hay fever
      (2) Invasive helminthic infection
        (a) Examples—strongyloidiasis, hookworm infection
        (b) Pinworms and adult ascariasis do *not* have eosinophilia (noninvasive).
      (3) Polyarteritis nodosa, Addison's disease (cortisol deficiency)
    c. Pathogenesis
      (1) Release of eosinophil chemotactic factor from mast cells (e.g., type I hypersensitivity)
      (2) No sequestering of eosinophils in lymph nodes (e.g., hypocortisolism)
  2. Eosinopenia
    a. Hypercortisolism (e.g., Cushing syndrome, corticosteroids)
    b. Corticosteroids sequester eosinophils in lymph nodes.
C. Disorders involving basophils; basophilia
  1. Absolute basophil count over 110/μL
  2. Etiology
    • Chronic myeloproliferative disorders (e.g., polycythemia vera)
D. Disorders involving lymphocytes
  1. Lymphocytosis
    a. Absolute lymphocyte count over 4000/μL in adults or over 8000/μL in children
    b. Etiology
      (1) Viral (e.g., mononucleosis) or bacterial (e.g., whooping cough)

Eosinophilia: type I hypersensitivity, invasive helminths, hypocortisolism

B cells have CD21 receptor sites for EBV.

Heterophile antibodies: IgM antibodies directed against horse, sheep, bovine RBCs

(2) Drugs (e.g., phenytoin)
(3) Graves' disease
  c. Pathogenesis
    (1) Increased production
    (2) Decreased entry into lymph nodes
      • Example—lymphocytosis-promoting factor produced by *Bordetella pertussis*
2. Atypical lymphocytosis
  a. Etiology
    (1) Infection
      • Examples—mononucleosis, viral hepatitis, cytomegalovirus infection, toxoplasmosis
    (2) Drugs (e.g., phenytoin)
  b. Pathogenesis
    (1) Antigenically stimulated lymphocytes
    (2) Prominent nucleoli and abundant blue cytoplasm
3. Infectious mononucleosis
  a. Caused by Epstein-Barr virus (EBV)
  b. Pathogenesis
    (1) Primarily transmitted by kissing
      • EBV initially replicates in the salivary glands and then disseminates.
    (2) EBV attaches to CD21 receptors on B cells.
      • Causes B-cell proliferation and increased synthesis of antibodies
    (3) Virus remains dormant in B cells.
      • Recurrences may occur.
  c. Clinical findings
    (1) Fatigue, tonsillitis
    (2) Hepatosplenomegaly, generalized lymphadenopathy
      • Danger of splenic rupture in contact sports
    (3) Rash develops if treated with ampicillin.
  d. Laboratory findings
    (1) Atypical lymphocytosis
      (a) Usually more than 20% of the total WBC count
      (b) Atypical lymphocytes are antigenically stimulated T cells (Fig. 12-2).
    (2) Positive heterophil antibody test
      • Detects IgM antibodies against horse (most common), sheep, and bovine RBCs
    (3) Positive antiviral capsid antigen test
      • Most sensitive test
    (4) Increased serum transaminases from hepatitis
      • Jaundice is rare.
4. Lymphopenia
  a. Absolute lymphocyte count below 1500/μL in adults or below 3000/μL in children
  b. Etiology

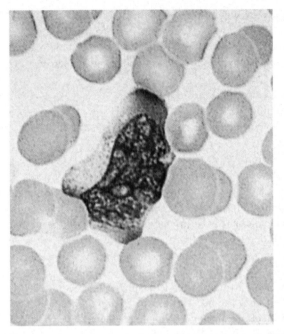

12-2: *Peripheral blood with atypical lymphocyte. The cell shows prominent nucleoli and coarse nuclear chromatin. The cytoplasm is abundant and is indented by adjacent red blood cells. (From Hoffbrand AV: Color Atlas: Clinical Hematology, 3rd ed. St. Louis, Mosby, 2000, p 128, Fig. 7-54B.)*

(1) Human immunodeficiency virus (HIV)

(2) Immunodeficiency

    (a) DiGeorge syndrome (T-cell deficiency)

    (b) Severe combined immunodeficiency (B- and T-cell deficiency)

(3) Immune destruction (e.g., SLE)

(4) Corticosteroids

(5) Radiation

    • Lymphocytes are the most sensitive cells to destruction by radiation.

  c. Pathogenesis

    (1) Increased destruction

      • Examples—lysis of CD4 helper T cells by the virus; apoptosis by corticosteroids; immune destruction

    (2) Decreased production

      • Example—radiation

    (3) Decreased release from lymph nodes

      • Example—corticosteroids

E. Disorders involving monocytes; monocytosis

  1. Absolute monocyte count over 800/μL

  2. Etiology

    a. Chronic infection (e.g., tuberculosis)

Lymphopenia in HIV: lysis of CD4 helper T cells by the virus

Corticosteroids produce neutrophilic leukocytosis, eosinopenia, and lymphopenia.

Monocytosis: chronic inflammation, malignancy

b. Autoimmune disease (e.g., rheumatoid arthritis)
c. Malignancy (e.g., carcinoma, malignant lymphoma)
3. Pathogenesis
- Response to chronic inflammation or malignancy

III. Leukemias (Acute and Chronic)

A. Epidemiology

1. Malignant diseases of bone marrow stem cells that may involve all cell lines
2. Risk factors
   a. Chromosomal abnormalities
      - Examples—Down syndrome, chromosome instability syndromes
   b. Ionizing radiation
   c. Chemicals (e.g., benzene)
   d. Alkylating agents (particularly busulfan)
3. Age ranges for common leukemias
   a. Newborn to 14 years old
      - Acute lymphoblastic leukemia (ALL)
   b. Persons 15 to 39 years old
      - Acute myelogenous leukemia (AML)
   c. Persons 40 to 60 years old
      (1) AML (>60% of cases)
      (2) Chronic myelogenous leukemia (~40% of cases)
   d. Persons over 60 years of age
      - Chronic lymphocytic leukemia (CLL)

Most common overall type of leukemia: CLL

B. Pathogenesis

1. Block in stem cell differentiation
   - Monoclonal proliferation of neoplastic leukocytes behind the block
2. Leukemic cells
   a. Replace the bone marrow
      - Replace normal hematopoietic cells
   b. Enter the peripheral blood
   c. Metastasize throughout the body

C. Clinical findings in acute leukemia

1. Abrupt onset of signs and symptoms
2. Fever (infection), bleeding (thrombocytopenia), fatigue (anemia)
3. Metastatic disease
   a. Hepatosplenomegaly
   b. Generalized lymphadenopathy
   c. Central nervous system (CNS) involvement (especially in ALL)
   d. Skin involvement (especially T-cell leukemias)
4. Bone pain and tenderness
   - Due to bone marrow expansion by leukemic cells

D. Laboratory findings in acute leukemia

1. Peripheral WBC count
   a. Below 10,000/μL (normal) to more than 100,000/μL
   b. Blast cells usually more than 20% (e.g., myeloblasts, lymphoblasts).

2. Normocytic to macrocytic anemia
   - Macrocytic if folate is depleted in production of leukemic cells
3. Thrombocytopenia (usually <100,000/μL)
4. Bone marrow findings
   - Hypercellular with more than 20% blasts (e.g., myeloblasts, lymphoblasts)

Most important test for diagnosing leukemia: bone marrow examination

E. **Clinical findings in chronic leukemia**
   a. Insidious onset
   b. Hepatosplenomegaly and generalized lymphadenopathy
F. **Laboratory findings in chronic leukemia**
   a. Peripheral WBC count
      (1) Similar to that of acute leukemia
      (2) Blast cells usually less than 10%
      (3) Evidence of maturation of cells
   b. Normocytic to macrocytic anemia
      - Macrocytic if folate is depleted in production of leukemic cells
   c. Thrombocytopenia (usually <100,000/μL)
      - *Exception* in CML, in which thrombocytosis occurs in 40% of cases

Acute versus chronic leukemia: bone marrow aspirate with blast count

   d. Bone marrow findings
      - Hypercellular with less than 10% blasts

IV. **Neoplastic Myeloid Disorders**
   A. **Overview**
      1. Myeloid disorders are neoplastic stem cell disorders.
         - May involve one or more stem cell lines
      2. Classification

Myeloid disorders: neoplastic stem cell disorders

         a. Chronic myeloproliferative disorders
         b. Myelodysplastic syndrome
         c. Acute myeloblastic leukemia
   B. **Chronic myeloproliferative disorders**
      1. Classification
         a. Polycythemia vera
         b. Chronic myelogenous leukemia
         c. Myeloid metaplasia with myelofibrosis
         d. Essential thrombocythemia
      2. General characteristics
         a. Splenomegaly
         b. Propensity for reactive bone marrow fibrosis ("spent phase")
         c. Propensity for transformation to acute leukemia
      3. Polycythemia (Fig. 12-3)
         a. Increased hemoglobin (Hb), hematocrit (Hct), and RBC count
         b. Plasma volume (PV) varies with the type of polycythemia.
         c. RBC count versus RBC mass
            (1) RBC count is the number of RBCs per μL of blood.
            (2) RBC mass is the total number of RBCs in the body in mL/kg.
            (3) RBC count is the ratio of RBC mass to plasma volume (PV).

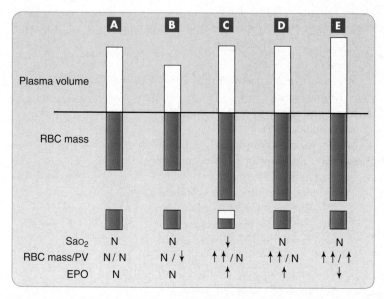

12-3: *Schematic showing RBC count, RBC mass, plasma volume (PV), erythropoietin (EPO) concentration, and O₂ saturation (SaO₂) in polycythemia and the normal (N) state: normal (**A**), relative polycythemia (**B**), appropriate absolute polycythemia (**C**), inappropriate absolute polycythemia due to ectopic production of EPO (**D**), polycythemia vera (**E**). See text for discussion.*

RBC count = RBC
mass/PV

Relative polycythemia:
↑ RBC count; ↓ PV;
normal RBC mass, SaO₂,
EPO

Appropriate absolute
polycythemia: ↑ RBC
mass, EPO; normal PV;
↓ SaO₂

- Figure 12-3A shows the normal relationship between RBC count, RBC mass, PV, erythropoietin (EPO), and O₂ saturation (SaO₂).
  d. Relative polycythemia (see Fig. 12-3B)
     (1) Increased RBC count due to a decrease in PV
        - Example—volume depletion from sweating
     (2) RBC mass is normal.
        - *No* increase in bone marrow production of RBCs
     (3) Erythropoietin (EPO) and SaO₂ are normal.
  e. Absolute polycythemia
     (1) Increase in bone marrow production of RBCs
        - Increased RBC count and RBC mass
     (2) Appropriate absolute polycythemia if there is a hypoxic stimulus for EPO release (see Fig. 12-3C)
        (a) Examples—primary lung disease, cyanotic congenital heart disease, living at high altitude
        (b) Decreased O₂ saturation (SaO₂)
        (c) Increased RBC count, RBC mass, EPO
        (d) Normal PV
     (3) Inappropriate absolute polycythemia if there is no hypoxic stimulus for EPO release
        (a) Polycythemia vera (see below)

Polycythemia	RBC Mass	Plasma Volume	SaO$_2$	EPO
Polycythemia vera	↑	↑	Normal	↓
Appropriate polycythemia (e.g., COPD, cyanotic congenital heart disease)	↑	Normal	↓	↑
Inappropriate polycythemia: ectopic EPO (e.g., renal disease)	↑	Normal	Normal	↑
Relative polycythemia (e.g., volume depletion)	Normal	↓	Normal	Normal

TABLE 12-1: Laboratory Findings in Polycythemias

COPD, chronic obstructive pulmonary disease; EPO, erythropoietin; SaO$_2$, oxygen saturation.

      (b) Ectopic secretion of EPO (e.g., renal cell carcinoma)
- Increased RBC count, RBC mass, EPO; normal PV and SaO$_2$ (see Fig. 12-3D)

4. Polycythemia vera (see Fig. 12-3E)
  a. Pathogenesis
    (1) Clonal expansion of the multipotent myeloid stem cell
    (2) Increase in RBCs, granulocytes (neutrophils, eosinophils, basophils), mast cells, and platelets
  b. Clinical findings
    (1) Splenomegaly
    (2) Thrombotic events due to hyperviscosity (e.g., hepatic vein thrombosis)
    (3) Signs of increased histamine (released from mast cells in the skin)
      (a) Ruddy face
      (b) Pruritus after bathing
      (c) Peptic ulcer disease (histamine stimulates production of gastric acid)
    (4) Gout
- Due to increased breakdown of nucleated cells with release of purines (converted to uric acid)
  c. Laboratory findings in polycythemia vera
    (1) Increased RBC mass and PV
- Only type of polycythemia with an increase in PV
    (2) Absolute leukocytosis (leukocytes >12,000/μL)
    (3) Thrombocytosis (platelets >400,000/μL)
    (4) Decreased EPO
      (a) Increased O$_2$ content inhibits EPO release.
      (b) Only type of polycythemia with decreased EPO
    (5) Normal SaO$_2$
    (6) Hypercellular bone marrow with fibrosis in later stages
  d. Summary table of the polycythemias (Table 12-1)
5. Chronic myelogenous leukemia (CML)

Inappropriate absolute polycythemia (ectopic secretion EPO): ↑ RBC mass, EPO; normal PV, SaO$_2$

Polycythemia vera: only type of polycythemia with ↑ PV and ↓ EPO

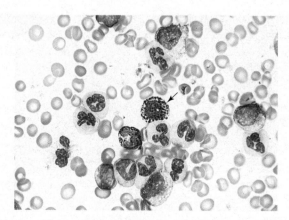

12-4: *Peripheral blood in chronic myelogenous leukemia. Marked leukocytosis shows neutrophils at different stages of development (segmented and band neutrophils, metamyelocytes and myelocytes). The cell in the center (arrow) depicts a basophil with dark granules in the cytosol and overlying the nucleus. Basophilia is prominent in chronic myeloproliferative diseases. (From Damjanov I, Linder J: Pathology: A Color Atlas. St. Louis, Mosby, 2000, p 80, Fig. 5-26.)*

a. Epidemiology
   (1) Usually occurs between 40 and 60 years of age
   (2) Risk factors
      • Exposure to ionizing radiation and benzene
b. Pathogenesis
   (1) Neoplastic clonal expansion of the pluripotential stem cell
      • This stem cell has the capacity to differentiate into a lymphoid or trilineage myeloid stem cell.
   (2) t9;22 translocation of *ABL* proto-oncogene
      • Proto-oncogene fuses with the break cluster region (BCR) on chromosome 22 *(BCR-ABL* fusion gene).

Philadelphia chromosome = chromosome 22

c. Clinical findings
   (1) Hepatosplenomegaly and generalized lymphadenopathy
      • Due to metastasis
   (2) Blast crisis
      (a) Usually occurs in ~5 years
      (b) Increase in numbers of myeloblasts or lymphoblasts
      (c) Myeloblasts do *not* contain Auer rods (see below)
d. Laboratory findings
   (1) Peripheral WBC count 50,000 to 200,000 cells/μL (Fig. 12-4)
      • Myeloid series in all stages of development
   (2) Normocytic to macrocytic anemia
      • Macrocytic if folate is depleted in the production of leukemic cells.
   (3) Platelet count
      • Thrombocytosis (40–50%), thrombocytopenia in the remainder of cases
   (4) Bone marrow findings

           (a) Myeloblasts less than 10%

           (b) Hypercellular

      (5) Positive Philadelphia chromosome (95% of cases)

           (a) It is *not* specific for CML and is present in other leukemias.

           (b) It is *not* lost during therapy unless α-interferon is used.

      (6) *BCR-ABL* fusion gene (100% of cases)

         • Fusion gene is the most sensitive and specific test for CML

      (7) Decreased leukocyte alkaline phosphatase (LAP)

         • LAP is absent in neoplastic granulocytes and present in benign granulocytes.

> *BCR-ABL* fusion gene: most sensitive and specific test for CML

6. Myelofibrosis and myeloid metaplasia

   a. Pathogenesis

     (1) Marrow fibrosis occurs earlier than in other types of myeloproliferative disease.

     (2) Neoplastic cells are produced in the spleen and other sites (extramedullary hematopoiesis, EMH).

   b. Clinical findings

     (1) Massive splenomegaly with portal hypertension

     (2) Splenic infarcts with left-sided pleural effusions

   c. Laboratory findings

     (1) Bone marrow fibrosis due to stimulation of fibroblasts

     (2) Peripheral WBC count 10,000 to 50,000 cells/μL

     (3) Normocytic anemia

       (a) Tear-drop cells (damaged RBCs)

       (b) Leukoerythroblastic reaction (see Fig. 12-1)

     (4) Platelet count is variable (increased or decreased).

> Myelofibrosis and myeloid metaplasia: EMH; marrow fibrosis

7. Essential thrombocythemia

   a. Pathogenesis

     (1) Neoplastic stem cell disorder with proliferation of megakaryocytes

     (2) Platelets are increased; however, they are nonfunctional.

   b. Clinical findings

     (1) Bleeding (usually gastrointestinal with concomitant iron deficiency)

     (2) Splenomegaly

   c. Laboratory findings

     (1) Thrombocytosis (platelets >600,000/μL)

      • Platelet morphology is abnormal.

     (2) Mild neutrophilic leukocytosis

     (3) Hypercellular bone marrow with abnormal megakaryocytes

C. Myelodysplastic syndrome

  1. Epidemiology

    • Usually occurs in men between 50 and 80 years old

  2. Pathogenesis

   a. Group of neoplastic stem cell disorders

    • Chromosomal abnormalities in 50% of cases (e.g., 5q$^-$, trisomy 8)

   b. Frequently progresses to acute myelogenous leukemia (AML; 30% of cases)

    • "Preleukemia"

TABLE 12-2: French-American-British Classification of Acute Myelogenous Leukemia (AML)

Class	Comments
M0: Minimally differentiated AML	No Auer rods
M1: AML without differentiation: 20%	Rare Auer rods
M2: AML with maturation	Most common type (30–40% of cases). Auer rods present 15–59-year-old age bracket
M3: Acute promyelocytic	Numerous Auer rods DIC is invariably present t(15;17) translocation Abnormal retinoic acid metabolism: high doses of vitamin A may induce remission by maturing cells
M4: Acute myelomonocytic	Auer rods uncommon
M5: Acute monocytic	No Auer rods Gum infiltration
M6: Acute erythroleukemia	Bizarre, multinucleated erythroblasts Myeloblasts present
M7: Acute megakaryocytic	Myelofibrosis in bone marrow Increased incidence in Down syndrome in children < 3 years old

DIC, disseminated intravascular coagulation.

3. Laboratory findings
   a. Severe pancytopenia
      (1) Normocytic to macrocytic anemia
         • Dimorphic RBC population (microcytic and macrocytic)
      (2) Leukoerythroblastic reaction
   b. Bone marrow findings
      (1) Ringed sideroblasts (nucleated RBCs with excess iron)
      (2) Myeloblasts less than 20% (if >20%, disease is progressing to AML)

D. **Acute myelogenous leukemia**
   1. Epidemiology
      a. Usually occurs between 15 and 59 years of age
      b. French-American-British (FAB) classification is used (Table 12-2).
   2. Cytogenetic abnormalities are common.
      • Example—t(15;17) in acute promyelocytic leukemia (M3)
   3. Clinical findings
      (1) Disseminated intravascular coagulation (DIC) is common.
         • Invariable in acute promyelocytic leukemia
      (2) Gum infiltration is common in acute monocytic leukemia (M5).
   4. Auer rods
      (1) Splinter-shaped to rod-shaped structures in the cytosol of myeloblasts
         • Auer rods are fused azurophilic granules (Fig. 12-5).
      (2) Only present in acute myelogenous leukemia (M2 and M3)
         • They are *not* present in myeloblasts in chronic myelogenous leukemia.

AML: Auer rods in the cytoplasm of myeloblasts

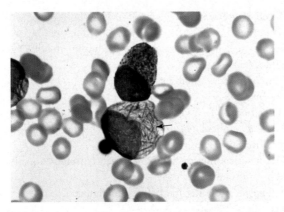

12-5: *Peripheral blood with promyelocyte filled with Auer rods in acute promyelocytic leukemia. The promyelocyte has numerous splinter-shaped inclusions in the cytoplasm (arrow) representing Auer rods. (From Damjanov I, Linder J: Pathology: A Color Atlas. St. Louis, Mosby, 2000, p 79, Fig. 5-21.)*

V. Lymphoid Leukemias
A. Acute lymphoblastic leukemia (ALL)
   1. Epidemiology
      a. Most common leukemia in children (newborn to 14 years of age)
      b. Subtypes
         (1) Early pre–B-cell ALL (80%)
         (2) Pre–B-, B-, and T-cell ALL
   2. Pathogenesis
      • Clonal lymphoid stem cell disease
   3. Early pre–B-cell ALL
      a. Positive marker studies for common ALL antigen (CALLA, CD10)
      b. Positive marker studies for terminal deoxynucleotidyl transferase (TdT)
      c. t(12;21) translocation offers a favorable prognosis.
      d. Greater than 90% achieve complete remission.
         • At least two thirds of patients can be considered cured.
   4. T-cell ALL
      • CD10 negative and TdT positive
   5. Clinical findings
      a. Metastatic sites similar to those of AML
      b. B-cell types
         • Commonly metastasize to the CNS and testicles
      c. T-cell type
         • Presents as anterior mediastinal mass or acute leukemia
   6. Laboratory findings
      a. Peripheral WBC count 10,000 to 100,000/µL
         • Over 20% lymphoblasts in peripheral blood
      b. Normocytic anemia with thrombocytopenia
      c. Bone marrow findings
         • Bone marrow often totally replaced by lymphoblasts

ALL: most common acute leukemia in children

ALL: CD10 and TdT positive

Adult T-cell leukemia:
association with HTLV-1

B. **Adult T-cell leukemia**
1. Epidemiology
   a. Malignant leukemia associated with human T-cell leukemia virus (HTLV-1)
   b. May present as a malignant lymphoma
2. Pathogenesis
   a. Activation of *TAX* gene, which inhibits the *TP53* suppressor gene
   b. Leads to monoclonal proliferation of neoplastic CD4 helper T cells
3. Clinical findings
   a. Hepatosplenomegaly and generalized lymphadenopathy
   b. Skin infiltration
      • Common finding in all T-cell malignancies
   c. Lytic bone lesions
      (1) Due to lymphoblast release of osteoclast-activating factor
      (2) Associated with hypercalcemia
4. Laboratory findings
   a. Peripheral WBC count 10,000 to 50,000/μL
      (1) Over 20% lymphoblasts
      (2) Positive CD4 marker study
      (3) Negative for TdT
   b. Normocytic anemia and thrombocytopenia
   c. Bone marrow findings
      • Replaced by CD4 lymphoblasts

C. **Chronic lymphocytic leukemia (CLL)**
CLL: most common cause
of generalized
lymphadenopathy in
individuals over 60 years
old
1. Epidemiology
   a. Occurs in individuals over 60 years old
   b. Most common overall leukemia
   c. Most common cause of generalized lymphadenopathy in the same age bracket
2. Pathogenesis
   • Neoplastic disorder of virgin B cells (B cells that cannot differentiate into plasma cells)
3. Clinical findings
   a. Generalized lymphadenopathy
   b. Metastatic sites similar to those of AML
   c. Increased incidence of immune hemolytic anemia
      • Both warm (IgG) and cold (IgM) types
4. Laboratory findings
   a. Peripheral WBC count 15,000 to 200,000/μL
      (1) Lymphoblasts less than 10%
      (2) Neutropenia
      (3) Numerous "smudge" cells (fragile leukemic cells) (Fig. 12-6)
   b. Normocytic anemia (50% of cases) and thrombocytopenia (40% of cases)
   c. Bone marrow findings: usually replaced by neoplastic B cells
   d. Hypogammaglobulinemia is common.

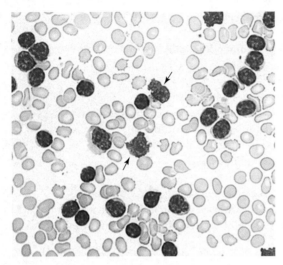

12-6: Peripheral blood in chronic lymphocytic leukemia. There are an increased number of lymphocytes with dense nuclear chromatin and scant cytoplasmic borders. The lymphocytes are extremely fragile and produce characteristic "smudge" cells (arrows) during preparation of a slide. (From Hoffbrand AV: Color Atlas: Clinical Hematology, 3rd ed. St. Louis, Mosby, 2000, p 179, Fig. 10-11.)

TABLE 12-3: Summary of Acute and Chronic Lymphoid Leukemias

Leukemia	Description
Acute lymphoblastic (Early pre-B type)	Most common leukemia in children Newborn to 14 years old CALLA (CD10) and TdT positive t(12;21) offers a good prognosis
Chronic lymphocytic	Virgin B cell leukemia Patients > 60 years old Most common cause of generalized lymphadenopathy in same age bracket Hypogammaglobulinemia
Adult T cell	HTLV-1 association Leukemic cells CD4 positive and TdT negative Skin infiltration Lytic bone lesions with hypercalcemia
Hairy cell	B cell leukemia Cytoplasmic projections TRAP stain positive Splenomegaly Absence of lymphadenopathy Pancytopenia Dramatic response to purine nucleosides

CALLA, common acute lymphoblastic leukemia antigen; HTLV, human T-cell leukemia; TdT, terminal deoxynucleotidyl transferase; TRAP, tartrate resistant acid phosphatase.

D. **Hairy cell leukemia**
   1. Type of B-cell leukemia
      - Most common in middle-aged men
   2. Clinical findings
      a. Splenomegaly (90% of cases)
      b. Absence of lymphadenopathy
         - Only leukemia *without* lymphadenopathy
      c. Hepatomegaly (20% of cases)
      d. Autoimmune vasculitis and arthritis
   3. Laboratory findings
      a. Pancytopenia
         - Leukemic cells have hair-like projections
      b. Positive tartrate-resistant acid phosphatase stain (TRAP)
E. **Summary table of the lymphoid leukemias (Table 12-3)**

Hairy cell leukemia:
positive TRAP stain

Lymphoid Tissue Disorders

I. Lymphadenopathy

  A. Locations of lymphoid tissue

    1. Locations
      a. Regional lymph nodes
      b. Tonsils and adenoids (Waldeyer's ring)
      c. Peyer's patches and appendix
      d. White pulp of the spleen

    2. B cells
      a. Germinal follicles in lymph nodes
      b. Peripheral areas of spleen white pulp
> B cells: germinal follicles

    3. T cells
      a. Paracortex (parafollicular) in lymph nodes
      b. Periarteriolar sheath in spleen
      c. Thymus
> T cells: paracortex

    4. Histiocytes
      a. Sinuses in lymph nodes
      b. Skin (Langerhan's cells)

    5. Locations of lymphoid disorders (Fig. 13-1)
> Histiocytes: sinuses

  B. Lymphadenopathy

    1. Epidemiology
      a. Age
        (1) Patients younger than 30 years old
          • Nodal enlargement is usually benign disease (~80% of cases).
        (2) Patients older than 30 years old
          • Nodal enlargement is usually malignant disease (~60% of cases).
      b. Causes
        (1) Reactive lymphadenitis
          • Hyperplasia of B cells, T cells, or histiocytes
        (2) Infiltrative disease
          • Examples—metastasis (most common), malignant lymphoma

    2. Clinical findings
      a. Painful nodes imply inflammation (e.g., infection)
        (1) Localized
> Painful lymphadenopathy: inflammation

          (a) Drain sites of infection (e.g., tonsillitis)
          (b) Most common sites are the anterior cervical nodes and inguinal nodes.

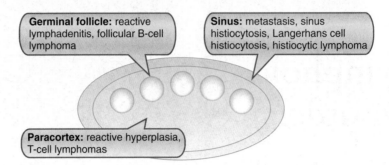

Germinal follicle: reactive lymphadenitis, follicular B-cell lymphoma

Sinus: metastasis, sinus histiocytosis, Langerhans cell histiocytosis, histiocytic lymphoma

Paracortex: reactive hyperplasia, T-cell lymphomas

13-1: Sites of pathologic processes in lymph nodes. Some lymphoid disorders initially localize in the germinal follicles, where B cells are located; others localize in the paracortex, where T cells are located. Mixed B- and T-cell reactions also may occur. Histiocytic disorders involve the sinuses.

(2) Generalized
    (a) Systemic disease
    (b) Examples—infectious mononucleosis, systemic lupus erythematosus (SLE)

b. Painless nodes imply a malignancy.

Painless lymphadenopathy: metastasis or primary malignant lymphoma

  (1) Lymph nodes are indurated and often fixed to surrounding tissue.
  (2) Localized
    (a) Nodes draining a primary cancer site (e.g., axillary nodes in breast cancer)
    (b) Hodgkin's lymphoma
  (3) Generalized
    (a) Metastasis in leukemia
    (b) Follicular B-cell lymphoma

c. Key nodal groups involved in primary or metastatic cancer
  (1) Submental
    • Metastatic squamous cell carcinoma in the floor of the mouth
  (2) Cervical
    (a) Metastatic head and neck tumors (e.g., larynx; thyroid, nasopharynx)
    (b) Hodgkin's lymphoma
  (3) Left-sided supraclavicular (Virchow's nodes)
    • Metastatic abdominal cancers (e.g., stomach; pancreas)

Left supraclavicular node metastasis: stomach or pancreatic carcinoma

  (4) Right-sided supraclavicular
    (a) Metastatic lung and esophageal cancers
    (b) Hodgkin's lymphoma
  (5) Axillary
    • Metastatic breast cancer
  (6) Hilar
    • Metastatic lung cancer
  (7) Mediastinal
    (a) Metastatic lung cancer
    (b) Hodgkin's lymphoma (particularly nodular sclerosing type)
    (c) T-cell lymphoblastic lymphoma

(8) Para-aortic
    (a) Metastatic testicular cancer
       • Testicles migrate to the scrotum from an abdominal location.
    (b) Burkitt's lymphoma
(9) Inguinal
    • Metastatic vulvar and penis cancers

C. Types of reactive lymphadenitis

1. Follicular hyperplasia
    a. B-cell antigenic response
       (1) Germinal follicles are sharply demarcated from the paracortex.
       (2) Cells are in different stages of development.
    b. Examples
       (1) Early stages of human immunodeficiency virus (HIV) infection
       (2) Rheumatoid arthritis and SLE

> Follicular hyperplasia: prominent germinal follicles

2. Paracortical hyperplasia
    a. T-cell antigenic response
    b. Dermatopathic lymphadenitis
       (1) Nodes draining chronic dermatitis (e.g., psoriasis)
       (2) Nodes contain macrophages with phagocytosis of melanin pigment.
         • Simulates metastatic malignant melanoma
    c. Phenytoin, viral infections
3. Mixed B- and T-cell hyperplasia; cat-scratch disease
    a. Granulomatous microabscesses in regional lymph nodes (e.g., axillary, cervical)
    b. Due to *Bartonella henselae*

> Cat-scratch disease: due to *Bartonella henselae*

4. Sinus histiocytosis
    a. Benign histiocytic response in lymph nodes draining a tumor.
    b. Favorable sign in the axillary nodes in breast cancer.

II. Non-Hodgkin's Lymphomas (NHL)

A. Epidemiology

1. Account for ~60% of adult lymphomas
    • Over 80% are of B-cell origin and derive from the germinal follicle.

> NHL: most common malignant lymphoma

2. Childhood lymphomas
    a. NHL accounts for 60% of cases.
       • Usually T-cell lymphoblastic lymphoma or Burkitt's lymphoma
    b. Generally more aggressive than adult lymphomas
3. Risk factors for NHL
    a. Viruses
       (1) Epstein-Barr virus (EBV)
         (a) Burkitt's lymphoma
         (b) Diffuse large B-cell lymphoma
       (2) Human T-cell leukemia virus type I
         • Adult T-cell lymphoma or leukemia

> Epstein-Barr virus: Burkitt's lymphoma

H. pylori: malignant
lymphoma of stomach

    b. *Helicobacter pylori*
      • Malignant lymphoma derives from mucosa-associated lymphoid
        tissue in the stomach.
    c. Autoimmune disease
      (1) Sjögren's syndrome
        • Predisposes to salivary gland and gastrointestinal lymphomas
      (2) Hashimoto's thyroiditis
        • Predisposes to thyroid malignant lymphoma
    d. Immunodeficiency syndromes
      (1) Chromosome instability syndromes (e.g., Bloom syndrome)
      (2) Acquired immunodeficiency syndrome (AIDS)
    e. Immunosuppressive therapy
      • Recipients of organ or bone marrow transplants
    f. High-dose radiation
      • Treatment of Hodgkin's lymphoma

B. Pathogenesis
  1. Mutation produces a block at a specific stage in development of B or T
    cells.
  2. Example—accumulation of small cleaved B cells in follicular lymphoma

C. B-cell lymphomas (Table 13-1)

D. T-cell lymphomas
  1. Precursor T-cell lymphoblastic leukemia/lymphoma
    a. Precursor T-cell lymphoma accounts for 40% of childhood
      lymphomas.
      (1) Primarily involves the anterior mediastinum and cervical nodes
      (2) Bone marrow and central nervous system involvement is common.
    b. Precursor T-cell lymphoblastic leukemia
      • Leukemic variant of this lymphoma
  2. Mycosis fungoides and Sézary syndrome

Mycosis fungoides:
neoplasm of CD4 T_H
cells; skin involvement

    a. Epidemiology
      (1) Both conditions involve neoplastic peripheral CD4 T_H cells.
      (2) Usually involves adults 40 to 60 years of age
    b. Mycosis fungoides
      (1) Begins in skin (rash to plaque to nodular masses)
        • Progresses to lymph nodes, lung, liver, and spleen
      (2) Groups of neoplastic cells in the epidermis are called Pautrier's
        microabscesses.
    c. Sézary syndrome
      (1) Mycosis fungoides with a leukemic phase
      (2) Circulating cells are called Sézary cells (prominent nuclear cleft).

III. Hodgkin's Lymphoma
  A. Epidemiology
    1. Accounts for ~40% of adult lymphomas
    2. Age and sex
      a. Slightly more common in men
        • *Exception*—nodular sclerosing type is more common in women

TABLE 13-1:
Common Types
of B-Cell
Non-Hodgkin's
Lymphoma

Type	Epidemiology	Description/ Immunophenotype	Clinical Findings
Burkitt's lymphoma	30% of children with non-Hodgkin's lymphoma (NHL)	EBV relationship with t(8;14) "Starry sky" appearance with neoplastic B cells (dark of night) and macrophages (stars)	American type: GI tract, para-aortic nodes African type: jaw Bone marrow involvement Leukemic phase common
Diffuse large B-cell lymphoma	50% of adults with NHL; elderly and childhood populations	Derives from germinal center	Localized disease with extranodal involvement: GI tract, brain (EBV association with AIDS)
Extranodal marginal zone lymphoma	Association with *Helicobacter pylori* gastritis	Derives from MALT	Low-grade malignant lymphoma of the stomach
Follicular lymphoma	40% of adults with NHL; elderly patients	Derives from germinal center t(14;18) causing overexpression of *BCL2* antiapoptosis gene	Generalized lymphadenopathy Bone marrow involvement
Small lymphocytic lymphoma (SLL)	Patients usually >60 years of age	Neoplasm of small, mature B lymphocytes SLL if confined to lymph nodes CLL if leukemic phase is present	Generalized lymphadenopathy

CLL, chronic lymphocytic leukemia; EBV, Epstein-Barr virus; GI, gastrointestinal; MALT, mucosa-associated lymphoid tissue.

    b. More common in adults than children
    c. More common in whites than black Americans
  3. Bimodal age distribution
    a. First large peak in the third decade
    b. Second smaller peak in individuals older than 45 to 50 years of age
    c. Involves younger age bracket than NHL
  4. EBV association
    • EBV is identified in more than 50% of cases of mixed cellularity Hodgkin's lymphoma.
  5. Defects in cellular immunity
    • Defects in cutaneous anergy to common antigens (anergy)

EBV: association with mixed cellularity Hodgkin's lymphoma

TABLE 13-2: Some Types of Hodgkin's Lymphoma

Type	Epidemiology	Clinical Findings
Lymphocyte predominant	5% of cases Occurs mainly in males	Asymptomatic young male with cervical or supraclavicular nodal enlargement Difficult to find classic RS cells L and H variants present
Mixed cellularity	30% of cases Men > 50 years of age Strong Epstein-Barr virus association	RS cells numerous ↑ Eosinophils, plasma cells, histiocytes
Nodular sclerosing	60% of cases Occurs mainly in females	Usually involves anterior mediastinal nodes and either cervical or supraclavicular nodes RS cells infrequent Lacunar cells present Collagen separates nodular areas

RS, Reed-Sternberg.

Nodular sclerosing Hodgkin's lymphoma: most common type of Hodgkin's lymphoma

Reed-Sternberg cell: neoplastic cell of Hodgkin's lymphoma

6. Classification (Table 13-2)
   a. Lymphocyte predominant
   b. Nodular sclerosing (most common type)
   c. Mixed cellularity
   d. Lymphocyte depletion (not discussed)

B. Pathogenesis
1. Reed-Sternberg (RS) cells
   a. Neoplastic cell of Hodgkin's lymphoma
      (1) In most cases, it is a transformed germinal center B cell.
      (2) CD15, CD30 positive
   b. Classic RS cell
      • Two mirror image nuclei, each with an eosinophilic nucleolus surrounded by a clear halo (Fig. 13-2)
   c. RS variants
      (1) L and H variant
         (a) Large, pale staining, multilobed cell ("popcorn cell")
         (b) Present in lymphocyte predominant type
      (2) Lacunar cells
         (a) Pale cell with multilobed nucleus containing many small nucleoli
         (b) Cell lies within a clear space in formalin-fixed tissue
         (c) Present in nodular sclerosing type
2. Diagnosis of Hodgkin's lymphoma
   a. Presence of a classic RS cell
   b. Presence of RS variant cells in a background of reactive cells
      • Reactive cells include eosinophils, plasma cells, histiocytes.

C. Pathology findings
1. Involves localized groups of nodes and has contiguous spread

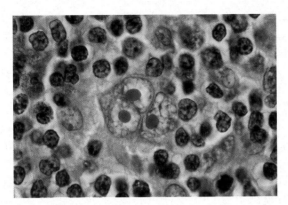

13-2: *Classic Reed-Sternberg (RS) cell. The large, multilobed cell with prominent nucleoli is surrounded by a halo of clear nucleoplasm. Classic RS cells are more easily found in mixed-cellularity Hodgkin's lymphoma than in lymphocyte-predominant and nodular-sclerosing Hodgkin's lymphoma. (From Damjanov I, Linder J: Anderson's Pathology, 10th ed. St. Louis, Mosby, 1996, p 1145, Fig. 42-47A.)*

      a. Often involves cervical or supraclavicular nodes
      b. Cut section has a bulging "fish-flesh" appearance
    2. Differences from NHL
      • Less commonly involves Waldeyer's ring, mesenteric nodes, and extranodal sites

D. Clinical findings and prognosis
    1. Constitutional signs
      a. Fever, unexplained weight loss, night sweats
      b. Pruritus
      c. Pel-Ebstein fever (uncommon variant of fever)
        • Alternating bouts of fever followed by remissions
    2. Hematologic findings
      a. Normocytic anemia
      b. Painless enlargement of single groups of lymph nodes
        • Usually cervical, supraclavicular, or anterior mediastinal nodes
    3. Main factors determining prognosis
      a. Clinical stage is more important than the type of Hodgkin's.
      b. Majority have lymphadenopathy above the diaphragm (stage I and II).
        • Usually involves supraclavicular nodes and anterior mediastinal nodes
    4. Increased risk for second malignancies
      a. Acute myelogenous leukemia or NHL
      b. Complication of treatment with radiation and alkylating agents

IV. Langerhans Cell Histiocytoses (Histiocytosis X)
  A. Epidemiology
    1. Langerhans histiocytes
      a. CD1 positive
      b. Contain Birbeck granules (tennis racket appearance)
        • Visible only with electron microscopy

Nodular sclerosing Hodgkin's lymphoma: anterior mediastinal mass + singe group of nodes above diaphragm

Histiocytes: CD1 positive; contain Birbeck granules

    2. Primarily occurs in children and young adults

    3. Classification

       a. Letterer-Siwe disease

       b. Hand-Schüller-Christian disease

       c. Eosinophilic granuloma

B. Letterer-Siwe disease

    1. Malignant histiocytosis

    2. Epidemiology

      • Occurs in infants and children younger than 2 years old

    3. Clinical findings

       a. Diffuse eczematous rash

       b. Multiple organ involvement

       c. Cystic defects in the skull, pelvis, and long bones

       d. Rapidly fatal

C. Hand-Schüller-Christian disease

    1. Malignant histiocytosis

    2. Epidemiology

      • Mainly affects children

    3. Clinical findings

       a. General

         (1) Fever

Malignant histiocytoses:
skin involvement is
common

         (2) Localized rash on scalp and in ear canals

       b. Classic triad due to infiltrative disease

         (1) Cystic skull defects

         (2) Diabetes insipidus due to invasion of posterior pituitary

         (3) Exophthalmos from infiltration of the orbit

       c. Intermediate prognosis

D. Eosinophilic granulomas

    1. Benign histiocytosis

    2. Epidemiology

      • Occurs in adolescents and young adults

Eosinophilic granuloma:
benign histiocytosis;
pathologic fractures

    3. Clinical findings

       a. Unifocal lytic lesions in bone (skull, ribs, and femur)

       b. Bone pain and pathologic fractures are common

V. Mast Cell Disorders

  A. Overview

    1. Presentation

       a. Localized—urticaria pigmentosum, solitary mastocytoma

       b. Systemic—systemic mastocytosis

    2. Signs and symptoms relate to mast cell release of histamine

      • Pruritus and swelling of tissue

  B. Urticaria pigmentosum

    1. Skin lesions

       a. Multiple oval, red-brown, nonscaling macules (flat lesions) or papules

       b. Scratching results in erythematous swelling of the lesions and pruritus.

         • Called Darier's sign

c. Dermatographism
- Dermal edema occurs when apparently normal skin is stroked with a pointed object.

d. Lesions remain hyperpigmented when they regress.

e. Skin biopsy
  (1) Mast cells have metachromatic granules.
  (2) Granules stain positive with toluidine blue and Giemsa stain.

2. Pruritus and flushing may be triggered by foods, alcohol, drugs (e.g., codeine)

Mast cell disease: pruritus, swelling, hyperpigmentation

VI. Plasmas Cell Dyscrasias

A. Overview

1. Monoclonal B-cell disorders
   a. Increase in a single immunoglobulin
   b. Increase in the corresponding light chain

2. Immunoglobulin is detected as a monoclonal spike (M component) on serum protein electrophoresis.

Plasma cell dyscrasia: monoclonal spike

3. Clinical significance of M components
   a. Most commonly due to an increase in IgG
      - Other plasma cell clones are suppressed.
   b. Bence Jones (BJ) protein
      (1) Refers to κ or λ light chains excreted in urine
      (2) Associated with a plasma cell malignancy
   c. Immunoelectrophoresis or immunofixation
      - Techniques that identify the immunoglobulin and light chain in serum and light chains in urine

Bence Jones protein: light chains in the urine

B. Multiple myeloma

1. Epidemiology
   a. More common in black Americans than in whites
   b. Rare under 40 years of age
   c. Increased risk with radiation exposure
   d. M-spike occurs in 80% to 90% of cases
      (1) Usually IgG κ followed by IgA and pure light chain myeloma
      (2) Urine BJ protein is positive in 60% to 80% of cases.

2. Pathologic findings
   a. Sheets of malignant plasma cells are present in a bone marrow aspirate (Fig. 13-3).
   b. Plasma cells account for over 10% of cells in the aspirate.

3. Skeletal system findings
   a. Bone pain
      (1) Due to "punched out" lytic lesions (Fig. 13-4)
      (2) Vertebra is the most common site.
      (3) Other sites include ribs, skull, pelvis
      (4) Commonly presents with pathologic fractures
   b. Hypercalcemia (25% of cases)

4. Renal findings
   a. Renal failure (30–50% of cases)

Bone findings: lytic lesions, pathologic fractures, hypercalcemia

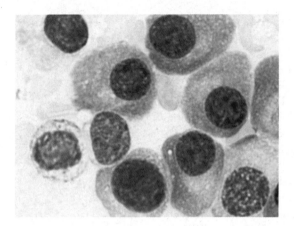

13-3: *Malignant plasma cells in multiple myeloma. The majority of malignant plasma cells show a gray-blue cytoplasm, peripherally located nuclei, and perinuclear clearing. (From Hoffbrand AV: Color Atlas: Clinical Hematology, 3rd ed. St. Louis, Mosby, 2000, p 233, Fig. 12-4B.)*

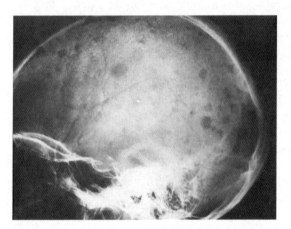

13-4: *Radiograph of a skull showing multiple "punched out" lytic lesions in multiple myeloma. When these lesions are located in other areas, such as the ribs, pathologic fractures frequently occur. (From Damjanov I, Linder J: Anderson's Pathology, 10th ed. St. Louis, Mosby, 1996, p 1105, Fig. 41-61.)*

BJ renal disease: proteinaceous casts with multinucleated giant cell reaction

    b. Myeloma kidney has different presentations
        (1) Proteinaceous tubular casts
            (a) Composed of BJ protein
            (b) BJ protein damages tubular epithelium
            (c) Intratubular multinucleated giant cell reaction
        (2) Nephrocalcinosis
            (a) Metastatic calcification of tubular basement membranes in the collecting ducts
            (b) Most common cause of acute renal failure in multiple myeloma
        (3) Metastatic disease to interstitial tissue

(4) Primary amyloidosis
    (a) Light chains are converted into amyloid (Chapter 3).
    (b) Produces a nephrotic syndrome
5. Hematologic findings
  a. Normocytic anemia with rouleaux
  b. Increased erythrocyte sedimentation rate
  c. Prolonged bleeding time
    • Due to a defect in platelet aggregation
6. Radiculopathy from bone compression and vertebral fractures
7. Recurrent infections are the most common cause of death.
8. Prognosis
    • Median survival is 6 months without treatment.

C. Other plasma cell dyscrasias (Table 13-3)

MGUS: most common monoclonal gammopathy

TABLE 13-3: Additional Plasma Cell Dyscrasias

Type	Discussion
MGUS	Most common monoclonal gammopathy Small IgG M spike in elderly patients Plasma cells < 3% in bone marrow No BJ protein
Solitary skeletal plasmacytoma	Bone sites: vertebra, ribs, pelvis Slight increase in monoclonal protein No plasmablasts in bone marrow No BJ protein 75% develop multiple myeloma
Extramedullary plasmacytoma	Sites: upper respiratory tract (nasopharynx, sinuses, larynx) Slight increase in monoclonal protein Absence of malignant plasma cells in the bone marrow Absence of BJ protein Small percentage may develop multiple myeloma
Lymphoplasmacytic lymphoma (Waldenström's macroglobulinemia)	Neoplastic lymphoplasmacytoid B cells Elderly male-dominant disease M spike with IgM BJ protein is present Generalized lymphadenopathy (not present in myeloma) Anemia and bone marrow (no lytic lesions like myeloma), liver, and spleen involvement Hyperviscosity syndrome due to increased IgM: retinal hemorrhages, strokes, platelet aggregation defects Median survival 5 years
Heavy-chain diseases	M protein heavy chain *without* light chains Absence of BJ protein α-Heavy-chain disease: neoplastic infiltration of the jejunum, leading to malabsorption or localized upper respiratory tract disease γ-Heavy-chain disease: presents as a lymphoma μ-Heavy-chain disease: often associated with chronic lymphocytic leukemia or lymphoma

BJ, Bence Jones; MGUS, monoclonal gammopathy of undetermined significance.

VII. Spleen Disorders
  A. Clinical anatomy and physiology
  1. Red pulp
     • Contains the cords of Billroth with fixed macrophages and sinusoids
  2. White pulp
     • Contains B and T cells
  3. Important functions of the spleen
     a. Blood filtration; macrophages remove:
        (1) Hematopoietic elements (e.g., old red blood cells)
        (2) Intraerythrocytic parasites (e.g., malaria)
        (3) Encapsulated bacteria (e.g., *Streptococcus pneumoniae*)
     b. Antigen trapping and processing in macrophages
     c. Reservoir for one third of the peripheral blood platelet pool
     d. Site for extramedullary hematopoiesis (Chapter 11)
  B. Splenomegaly
  1. Causes of splenomegaly
     a. Reactive hyperplasia of white pulp
        (1) Autoimmune disorders
           • Examples—SLE, immune thrombocytopenia and anemia
        (2) Infectious mononucleosis
           • Due to antigenic stimulation of T cells
        (3) Parasitic infections
           • Malaria is the most common cause of splenomegaly in developing countries.
     b. Infiltrative diseases in white pulp
        • Examples—metastatic NHL, primary amyloidosis
     c. Infiltrative diseases of macrophages in red pulp; lysosomal storage diseases:
        (1) Gaucher disease
           (a) Deficiency of glucocerebrosidase
              • Lysosomal accumulation of glucocerebrosides
           (b) Macrophages have a fibrillary appearance (Fig. 13-5).
        (2) Niemann-Pick disease
           (a) Deficiency of sphingomyelinase
              • Lysosomal accumulation of sphingomyelin
           (b) Macrophages have soap bubble appearance (Fig. 13-6).
     d. Infiltrative diseases of the red and white pulp
        • Examples—acute and chronic myelogenous and lymphoid leukemias
     e. Phagocytic hyperplasia in the red pulp
        • Example—extravascular hemolytic anemia in hereditary spherocytosis
     f. Extramedullary hematopoiesis in the sinusoids
        • Example—myelofibrosis and myeloid metaplasia
     g. Vascular congestion in the sinusoids
        • Example—portal hypertension in cirrhosis
  2. Clinical findings
     a. Left upper quadrant pain

Malaria: most common cause splenomegaly in developing countries

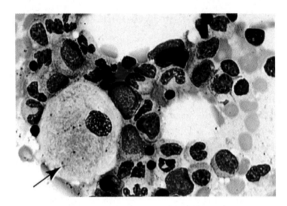

13-5: *Gaucher disease. Note the fibrillary appearance of the cytoplasm in the macrophages. (From Naeim F: Atlas of Bone Marrow and Blood Pathology. Philadelphia, WB Saunders, 2001, p. 157, Fig. 11-14B.)*

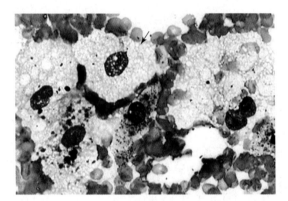

13-6: *Niemann-Pick disease. Note the soap bubble appearance of the cytoplasm in the macrophages (arrow). (From Naeim F: Atlas of Bone Marrow and Blood Pathology. Philadelphia, WB Saunders, 2001, p. 159, Fig. 11-17B.)*

- • May be associated with splenic infarctions causing friction rubs and a left-sided pleural effusion
  - b. Hypersplenism (see below)
- **C. Portal hypertension in cirrhosis**
  1. Gross findings
     - • Spleen is often surfaced by a thickened ("sugar-coated") capsule from perisplenitis.
  2. Microscopic findings
     - • Calcium and iron concretions called Gamna-Gandy bodies are present in collagen.
- **D. Hypersplenism**
  1. Definition
     - a. Exaggeration of normal splenic function
     - b. Red blood cells (RBCs), white blood cells (WBCs), and platelets, either singly or in combination, are sequestered and destroyed.

Hypersplenism: destruction of hematopoietic cells

2. Portal hypertension associated with cirrhosis is the most common cause.
3. Clinical findings
   a. Splenomegaly
   b. Peripheral blood cytopenias
      • Anemia, thrombocytopenia, neutropenia alone or in combination
   c. Compensatory reactive bone marrow hyperplasia
      • Attempt by the marrow to replace lost cells
   d. Correction of cytopenias with splenectomy

E. **Splenic dysfunction and splenectomy**
   1. Splenic dysfunction
      a. Presence of Howell-Jolly bodies (nuclear remnants) in peripheral blood RBCs
      b. Predisposition to infections
         (1) Infections include septicemia, peritonitis
         (2) Mechanism
            (a) Concentration of IgM drops leading to a decrease in complement system activation
            (b) Reduction in C3b, an opsonizing agent, leads to infection.
         (3) Pathogens commonly involved
            (a) *Streptococcus pneumoniae*
               • Other pathogens include *Hemophilus influenzae* and *Salmonella paratyphi*.
            (b) Immunization helps prevent infectious complications.
   2. Splenectomy
      a. Increases the risk for infections
      b. Hematologic findings
         (1) Nucleated RBCs
         (2) Howell-Jolly bodies
         (3) Target cells (excess membrane cannot be removed)
         (4) Thrombocytosis
            • Platelets normally sequestered in the spleen are now circulating.

Splenic dysfunction: ↑ risk for *Streptococcus pneumoniae* sepsis

14 CHAPTER

Hemostasis Disorders

I. Normal Hemostasis and Hemostasis Testing
- Prevention of blood loss while maintaining maximal perfusion requires the interaction of the blood vessels, platelets, coagulation factors, and fibrinolytic agents.

A. Normal anticoagulation in small blood vessels
- Small blood vessels include capillaries, venules, arterioles.
    1. Heparin-like molecules
        a. Enhance antithrombin III (ATIII) activity
        b. Neutralize activated serine protease coagulation factors
            - Factors XII, XI, IX, and X; thrombin (activated prothrombin)
    2. Prostaglandin (PG) I_2 (prostacyclin)
        a. Synthesized by intact endothelial cells
        b. PGH_2 is converted by prostacyclin synthase to PGI_2.
        c. Vasodilator and inhibits platelet aggregation
        d. Aspirin does *not* inhibit synthesis of PGI_2 by endothelial cells.
    3. Protein C and S
        a. Vitamin K–dependent factors
        b. Inactivate factors V and VIII
        c. Enhance fibrinolysis
    4. Tissue plasminogen activator (tPA)
        a. Synthesized by endothelial cells
        b. Activates plasminogen to release plasmin
        c. Plasmin degrades coagulation factors and lyses fibrin clots (thrombi).

B. Procoagulants released in small vessel injury
    1. Thromboxane A_2 (TXA_2)
        a. Synthesized by platelets
            (1) PGH_2 is converted into TXA_2 by thromboxane synthase.
            (2) Aspirin *irreversibly* inhibits platelet cyclooxygenase.
                - Prevents formation of PGH_2, the precursor for TXA_2
            (3) Other nonsteroidal anti-inflammatory drugs *reversibly* inhibit platelet cyclooxygenase.
        b. Functions of TXA_2 in hemostasis
            - Vasoconstrictor, enhances platelet aggregation
    2. Von Willebrand factor (vWF)
        a. Synthesized by endothelial cells and megakaryocytes
            (1) Synthesized in Weibel-Palade bodies in endothelial cells
            (2) Platelets carry vWF in their α-granules.
        b. Functions of vWF
            (1) Platelet adhesion molecule

Heparin: enhances ATIII

PGI_2: vasodilator, inhibits platelet aggregation

Proteins C and S: inactivate factors V and VIII, enhance fibrinolysis

tPA: activates plasminogen to release plasmin

TXA_2: vasoconstrictor; enhances platelet aggregation

(a) Binds platelets to exposed collagen
(b) Platelets have glycoprotein (Gp)Ib receptors for vWF.
(2) Complexes with factor VIII:C in the circulation
(a) VIII:vWF complexes prevent degradation of factor VIII:C (procoagulant factor).
(b) Decrease in vWF secondarily decreases VIII:C activity.

> Factor VIII:C is synthesized in the liver. When VIII:C is activated by thrombin, it dissociates from the VIII:vWF complex and performs its procoagulant function in the intrinsic coagulation cascade system.

vWF: platelet adhesion; prevents degradation of VIII:C

3. Tissue thromboplastin (factor III)
   a. Noncirculating ubiquitous substance
      • Released from injured tissue
   b. Activates factor VII in the extrinsic coagulation system
4. Extrinsic and intrinsic coagulation systems (see below)

Tissue thromboplastin: activates factor VII in extrinsic coagulation system

C. Platelet structure and function
1. Derivation
   a. Cytoplasmic fragmentation of megakaryocytes
   b. Approximately 1000 to 3000 platelets are produced per megakaryocyte.
2. Locations
   a. Peripheral blood (live for ~9–10 days)
   b. Approximately one third of the total platelet pool is stored in the spleen.
3. Platelet receptors
   a. Glycoprotein receptors for vWF are designated GpIb.
   b. Glycoprotein receptors for fibrinogen are designated GpIIb:IIIa.
      (1) Ticlopidine and clopidogrel
         (a) Inhibit ADP-induced expression of platelet GpIIb:IIIa receptors
         (b) Prevent fibrinogen binding and platelet aggregation
      (2) Abciximab
         • Monoclonal antibody that is directed against the GpIIb:IIIa receptor

Platelet receptors: GpIb (binds to vWF) GpIIb/IIIa (binds to fibrinogen)

4. Platelet factor 3 (PF$_3$)
   a. Located on the platelet membrane
   b. Phospholipid substrate required for the clotting sequence
5. Platelet structure
   a. Contractile element
      (1) Called thrombosthenin
      (2) Helps in clot retraction
   b. Dense bodies contain:
      (1) Adenosine diphosphate (ADP), an aggregating agent
      (2) Calcium, a binding agent for vitamin K–dependent factors
   c. α-Granules contain:
      (1) vWF, fibrinogen

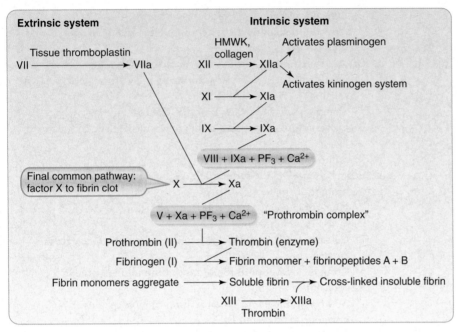

Extrinsic system

Intrinsic system

VII $\xrightarrow{\text{Tissue thromboplastin}}$ VIIa

XII $\xrightarrow{\text{HMWK, collagen}}$ XIIa $\xrightarrow{\text{Activates plasminogen}}$

XIIa $\xrightarrow{\text{Activates kininogen system}}$

XI $\longrightarrow$ XIa

IX $\longrightarrow$ IXa

VIII + IXa + PF$_3$ + Ca^{2+}

Final common pathway: factor X to fibrin clot $\rightarrow$ X $\longrightarrow$ Xa

V + Xa + PF$_3$ + Ca^{2+} "Prothrombin complex"

Prothrombin (II) $\longrightarrow$ Thrombin (enzyme)

Fibrinogen (I) $\longrightarrow$ Fibrin monomer + fibrinopeptides A + B

Fibrin monomers aggregate $\longrightarrow$ Soluble fibrin $\longrightarrow$ Cross-linked insoluble fibrin

XIII $\longrightarrow$ XIIIa
Thrombin

14-1: *Coagulation cascade. Both the extrinsic and intrinsic coagulation systems use the final common pathway for the formation of a fibrin clot. a, activated; HMWK, high-molecular-weight kininogen; PF3, platelet factor 3.*

    (2) Platelet factor 4 (PF4)
      • Heparin neutralizing factor
  6. Platelet function
    a. Fill gaps between endothelial cells in small vessels
      (1) Prevents leakage of RBCs into the interstitium
      (2) Platelet dysfunction causes leakage of RBCs, producing petechia.
    b. Formation of the hemostatic plug in small vessel injury
    c. Platelet-derived growth factor stimulates smooth muscle hyperplasia.
      • Important in the pathogenesis of atherosclerosis
D. Coagulation system (Fig. 14-1)
  1. Coagulation cascade
    a. Extrinsic system (factor VII)
    b. Intrinsic system (factors XII, XI, IX, VIII)
  2. Extrinsic system
    a. Factor VII is activated (factor VIIa) by tissue thromboplastin.
    b. Factor VIIa activates factor X in the final common pathway.
  3. Intrinsic system
    a. Factor XII (Hageman factor) is activated by:
      (1) Exposed subendothelial collagen
      (2) High-molecular-weight kininogen (HMWK)
    b. Functions of factor XIIa
      (1) Activates factor XI

Important platelet storage proteins: vWF, fibrinogen

Extrinsic system: factor VII

Intrinsic system: factors XII, XI, IX, VIII

(2) Activates plasminogen (produces plasmin)

(3) Activates the kininogen system (produces kallikrein and bradykinin)

c. Factor XIa activates factor IX to form factor IXa

    (1) Four-component complex is formed (IXa, VIII, platelet factor 3, calcium)

    (2) Complex activates factor X in the final common pathway.

    (3) Calcium binds factor IXa, a vitamin K–dependent coagulation factor.

4. Final common pathway

    a. Includes factors X, V, prothrombin (II), and fibrinogen (I)

    b. Prothrombin complex

        (1) Four-component system consisting of factor Xa, factor V, platelet factor 3, and calcium

        (2) Calcium binds factor Xa, a vitamin K–dependent coagulation factor.

        (3) Complex cleaves prothrombin into thrombin (enzyme).

    c. Functions of thrombin

        (1) Acts on fibrinogen to produce fibrin monomers plus fibrinopeptides A and B

        (2) Activates fibrin stabilizing factor XIII

            (a) Factor XIIIa converts soluble fibrin monomers to insoluble fibrin.

            (b) Enhances protein-protein cross-linking to strengthen the fibrin clot

        (3) Activates VIII:C in the intrinsic system

5. Vitamin K–dependent factors

    a. Factors II, VII, IX, X, protein C, and protein S

    b. Synthesized in the liver as nonfunctional precursor proteins

    c. Function of vitamin K

        (1) Vitamin K is activated in the liver by epoxide reductase.

          • Majority of vitamin K is synthesized by colonic bacteria.

        (2) Activated vitamin K γ-carboxylates each factor.

          • Carboxylated factors can bind to calcium and PF3 in the cascade sequence.

Margin notes:

Final common pathway: factors X, V, II, I

Factor XIII: cross-links insoluble fibrin monomers

Vitamin K: activated in the liver by epoxide reductase

Calcium: binds γ-carboxylated vitamin K–dependent factors

Warfarin: inhibits epoxide reductase; vitamin K is nonfunctional

---

> Warfarin is an anticoagulant that inhibits epoxide reductase, which prevents any further γ-carboxylation of the vitamin K–dependent coagulation factors. However, full anticoagulation does *not* immediately occur, because previously γ-carboxylated factors are still present. Prothrombin has the longest half-life; therefore, full anticoagulation requires at least 3 to 4 days before all functional prothrombin has disappeared. This explains why patients are initially placed on both heparin and warfarin, because heparin immediately anticoagulates the patient by enhancing ATIII activity.

6. Certain coagulation factors are consumed in the formation of a fibrin clot.
   - Consumed factors are fibrinogen (I), factor V, factor VIII, and prothrombin (II)

   > When blood is drawn into a clot tube (no anticoagulant is added), a fibrin clot is formed. When the tube is spun down in a centrifuge, the supranate is called serum, which, unlike plasma, is missing fibrinogen, prothrombin (II), factor V, and factor VIII.

E. Fibrinolytic system
  1. Activation
     a. tPA activates plasminogen to release the enzyme plasmin.
        - Alteplase and reteplase are recombinant forms of tPA used in thrombolytic therapy.
     b. Other activators of plasminogen
        (1) Factor XIIa
        (2) Streptokinase (derived from streptococci)
        (3) Anistreplase (complex of streptokinase and plasminogen)
        (4) Urokinase (derived from human urine)
     c. Aminocaproic acid
        - Competitively blocks plasminogen activation, thereby inhibiting fibrinolysis
  2. Functions of plasmin
     a. Cleaves insoluble fibrin monomers and fibrinogen into fibrin(ogen) degradation products (FDPs)
        - Fragments of cross-linked insoluble fibrin monomers are called D-dimers.
     b. Degrades factors V and VIII
     c. α_2-Antiplasmin (synthesized in the liver) inactivates plasmin.

D-Dimers: cross-linked fibrin monomers

F. Small vessel hemostasis response to injury (Fig. 14-2)
  1. Sequence involves vascular, platelet, coagulation, and fibrinolytic phases.
  2. Vascular phase
     a. Transient vasoconstriction occurs directly after injury.
     b. Factor VII (extrinsic system) is activated by tissue thromboplastin.
     c. Exposed collagen activates factor XII (intrinsic system).
  3. Platelet phase
     a. Platelet adhesion
        - Platelet GpIb receptors adhere to exposed vWF in damaged endothelial cells.
     b. Platelet release reaction
        - Release of adenosine diphosphate (ADP) causes platelet aggregation in the lumens of injured vessels.
     c. Platelet synthesis and release of TXA_2
        (1) Vessels constrict (reduce blood flow).
        (2) Platelet aggregation is further enhanced.
     d. Temporary platelet plug stops bleeding.

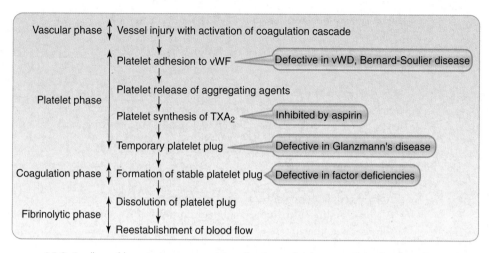

14-2: *Small vessel hemostasis response to injury. See the text for discussion. TXA$_2$, thromboxane A$_2$; vWD, von Willebrand disease; vWF, von Willebrand factor.*

Platelet sequence: adhesion, release reaction, synthesis TXA$_2$, temporary plug

    (1) Aggregated platelets have fibrinogen attached to their GpIIb-IIIa receptors.

    (2) It is an unstable plug that can easily be dislodged.

  4. Coagulation phase

    a. Thrombin is produced by localized activation of the coagulation cascade.

      • Occurs in the vascular phase

    b. Fibrinogen attached to GpIIb/IIIa receptors is converted to insoluble fibrin monomers.

    c. Stable platelet plug is formed.

  5. Fibrinolytic phase

    a. Plasmin cleaves the insoluble fibrin monomers holding the platelet plug together.

    b. Blood flow is reestablished.

G. Platelet tests

  1. Platelet count

    a. Normal count is 150,000 to 400,000 cells/μL.

    b. A normal count does *not* guarantee normal platelet function.

  2. Bleeding time

Bleeding time: test of platelet function to formation of temporary plug

    a. Evaluates platelet function up to the formation of the temporary platelet plug

      • Normal reference interval is 2 to 7 minutes.

    b. Disorders causing a prolonged bleeding time are listed in Table 14-1.

  3. Platelet aggregation test

    a. Evaluates platelet aggregation in response to aggregating reagents

    b. Aggregating agents include ADP, epinephrine, collagen, and ristocetin.

  4. Tests for vWF

    a. Ristocetin cofactor assay

TABLE 14-1:
Causes of
Prolonged Bleeding
Time

Cause	Nature of Defect	Comments
Aspirin or NSAIDs	Platelet aggregation defect Inhibition of platelet COX, which ultimately inhibits synthesis of TXA$_2$	Normal platelet count
Bernard-Soulier syndrome	Platelet adhesion defect Autosomal recessive disease Absent GpIb platelet receptors for vWF	Thrombocytopenia, giant platelets Lifelong bleeding problem
Glanzmann's disease	Platelet aggregation defect Autosomal recessive disease Absent GpIIb-IIIa fibrinogen receptors Absent thrombosthenin	Lifelong bleeding problem
Renal failure	Platelet aggregation defect Inhibition of platelet phospholipid by toxic products	Reversed with dialysis and desmopressin acetate
Scurvy	Vascular defect Caused by vitamin C deficiency Defective collagen resulting from poor cross-linking	May cause ecchymoses and hemarthroses
Thrombocytopenia	Decreased platelet number	Increased bleeding time when platelet count < 90,000 cells/μL
Von Willebrand disease	Platelet adhesion defect Autosomal dominant disorder Absent or defective vWF Decreased VIII:C	Combined platelet and coagulation factor disorder

COX, cyclooxygenase; NSAID, nonsteroidal anti-inflammatory drug; TXA$_2$, thromboxane A$_2$; vWF, von Willebrand factor.

    (1) Evaluates vWF function
    (2) Abnormal assay
        (a) Classic von Willebrand disease (deficiency of vWF)
        (b) Bernard-Soulier disease (absent GpIb receptor)
  b. vWF antigen assay
    (1) Measures the quantity of vWF regardless of function
    (2) Decreased in classic von Willebrand disease

H. Coagulation tests (Fig. 14-3)
  1. Prothrombin time (PT)
    a. Evaluates the extrinsic system down to formation of the fibrin clot
      • Factors evaluated include VII, X, V, II, and I
    b. Normal reference interval for PT is 11 to 15 seconds.
      • Only prolonged when a factor level is 30% to 40% of normal
    c. International normalized ratio (INR)
      (1) Standardizes the PT for use in warfarin therapy

Ristocetin cofactor assay: test of vWF function

PT: evaluates factors VII, X, V, II, and I

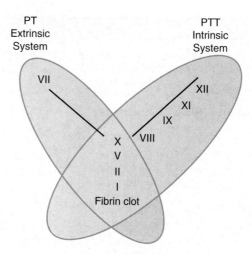

14-3: *Prothrombin time (PT) and partial thromboplastin time (PTT). See the text for discussion.*

        (2) Results are the same regardless of the reagents used to perform the test.

    d. Uses of PT

        (1) Follow patients who are taking warfarin for anticoagulation

        (2) Evaluate liver synthetic function

          • Increased PT indicates severe liver dysfunction.

        (3) Detect factor VII deficiency

 2. Partial thromboplastin time (PTT)

    a. Evaluates the intrinsic system down to formation of a fibrin clot

      • Factors evaluated include XII, XI, IX, VIII, X, V, II, and I.

    b. Normal reference interval for PTT is 25 to 40 seconds.

      • Only prolonged when a factor level is 30% to 40% of normal

    c. Uses of PTT

        (1) Follow heparin therapy

          (a) Heparin enhances ATIII activity.

          (b) PTT is *not* required to follow low-molecular-weight heparin therapy.

        (2) Detect factor deficiencies in the intrinsic system

> Whether the patient is anticoagulated with heparin or warfarin, both the PT and PTT are prolonged, because both inhibit factors in the final common pathway. Experience has shown that the PT performs better in monitoring warfarin, while the PTT performs better in monitoring heparin.

I. Fibrinolytic system tests

 1. Fibrin(ogen) degradation products (FDPs)

    • Detects fragments associated with plasmin degradation of fibrinogen or insoluble fibrin in fibrin clots

---

Margin notes:

PTT: evaluates factors XII, XI, IX, VIII, X, V, II, I

FDPs: increased with lysis of fibrinogen or fibrin in fibrin thrombi

2. D-Dimer assay
   a. Only detects cross-linked insoluble fibrin monomers in a fibrin clot
   b. Does *not* detect fibrinogen degradation products (not cross-linked)
   c. Most specific test for evidence of degradation of a fibrin clot (thrombus); examples:
      (1) Thrombolytic therapy for coronary artery thrombosis
         • Thrombus is composed of platelets held together by fibrin (see Chapter 4)
      (2) Screening test for pulmonary thromboembolism
         • Thrombus is composed of RBCs, platelets, white blood cells (WBCs) held together by fibrin (see Chapter 4)
      (3) Screening test for disseminated intravascular coagulation (DIC)
         • Thrombus is composed of RBCs, platelets, and WBCs held together by fibrin (see Section III).

D-Dimer assay: specific for lysis of fibrin thrombi (clots)

II. Platelet Disorders
A. Classification of platelet disorders
   1. Quantitative platelet disorders
      a. Thrombocytopenia
      b. Thrombocytosis
   2. Qualitative (functional) platelet disorders
B. Pathogenesis
   1. Thrombocytopenia (Table 14-2)
      • Decreased number of platelets
      a. Decreased production
         • Examples—aplastic anemia, leukemia
      b. Increased destruction
         (1) Immune
            • Examples—idiopathic thrombocytopenic purpura, drugs
         (2) Nonimmune
            • Examples—thrombotic thrombocytopenic purpura, DIC
      c. Sequestration in the spleen
         • Hypersplenism in portal hypertension

Acute ITP: most common cause of thrombocytopenia in children

   2. Thrombocytosis
      • Increased platelet count
      a. Primary thrombocytosis
         • Examples—essential thrombocythemia, polycythemia vera
      b. Secondary (reactive) thrombocytosis
         • Examples—chronic iron deficiency, infections, splenectomy, malignancy
   3. Qualitative platelet disorders
      • Acquired (e.g., aspirin) or hereditary (e.g., Glanzmann's disease)

Aspirin: most common cause of a qualitative platelet defect

C. Clinical findings associated with platelet dysfunction
   1. Epistaxis (nosebleeds) is the most common symptom.
   2. Petechia and multiple small ecchymoses (purpura)
      a. Petechia are pinpoint areas of hemorrhage in subcutaneous tissue (Fig. 14-4).

TABLE 14-2:
Disorders
Producing
Thrombocytopenia

Disorder	Pathogenesis	Comments
Acute idiopathic thrombocytopenic purpura (ITP)	IgG antibodies directed against GpIIb:IIIa receptors (type II hypersensitivity reaction) Macrophages phagocytose platelets	Most common childhood cause of thrombocytopenia Abrupt onset after an upper respiratory tract infection Absence of lymphadenopathy and splenomegaly Responds to corticosteroids
Chronic idiopathic thrombocytopenic purpura	IgG antibodies directed against GpIIb:IIIa receptors (type II hypersensitivity reaction)	Most common cause of thrombocytopenia in adults Newborn infants may have transient thrombocytopenia due to transplacental passage of IgG antibodies Secondary causes: SLE, HIV
Heparin-induced thrombocytopenia	Type II variant: macrophage removal of platelets surfaced by IgG antibody directed against heparin attached to PF_4 (type II hypersensitivity)	Occurs 5–14 days after heparin treatment Must discontinue heparin Release of PF_4 after platelet destruction may cause vessel thrombosis
HIV thrombocytopenia	Similar to ITP	Most common hematologic abnormality in HIV (not AIDS-defining condition)
Thrombotic thrombocytopenic purpura (TTP)	Acquired or genetic deficiency in vWF-cleaving metalloprotease in endothelial cells Excess of vWF increases platelet adhesion to areas of endothelial injury at arteriole-capillary junctions Platelets consumed in the formation of thrombi causes thrombocytopenia Enhanced by factors that damage endothelial cells (e.g., ticlopidine, hypertension)	Occurs in adult females Clinical pentad: fever, thrombocytopenia, renal failure, microangiopathic hemolytic anemia with schistocytes (damage by platelet thrombi), CNS deficits Treated with plasmapheresis Mortality rate is 10–20%
Hemolytic uremic syndrome (HUS)	Endothelial damage at arteriole-capillary junction caused by Shiga-like toxin of 0157:H7 serotype of *Escherichia coli* Organisms proliferate in undercooked beef	Primarily occurs in children Clinical findings similar to TTP CNS findings are less frequent Mortality rate 3–5%

CNS, central nervous system; DIC, disseminated intravascular coagulation; PF_4, platelet factor 4; SLE, systemic lupus erythematosus; vWF, von Willebrand factor.

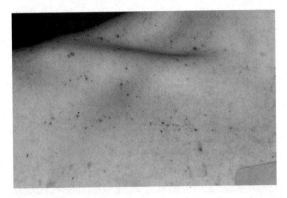

14-4: *Petechiae in idiopathic thrombocytopenic purpura showing pinpoint hemorrhages, a sign of platelet dysfunction, in the skin over the thorax and shoulders. When touched, petechiae do not blanch with pressure. (From Forbes C, Jackson W: Color Atlas and Text of Clinical Medicine, 2nd ed. St. Louis, Mosby, 2003, Fig. 10-10.)*

- RBCs leak through gaps in the endothelium of venules and capillaries.
  b. Ecchymoses are the size of a quarter.

> Ecchymoses (purpura) can be caused by a variety of disorders unrelated to platelet dysfunction. Palpable purpura (purpura that can be felt) is a sign of a small vessel vasculitis (Chapter 9). Because vasculitis is a type of acute inflammation, the lesions are palpable due to increased vessel permeability and *not* a platelet disorder. Senile purpura is a normal finding in elderly patients and is due to vessel instability (Fig. 14-5). Ecchymoses develop in areas of trauma (e.g., back of the hands, shins).

3. Bleeding from superficial scratches
   - No temporary platelet plug is present to stop bleeding from injury to small vessels.
4. Other findings
   a. Menorrhagia, hematuria
   b. Bleeding from tooth extraction sites
   c. Gastrointestinal and intracranial bleeding

III. Coagulation Disorders
A. Classification of coagulation disorders
1. Acquired
   - Single or multiple coagulation factor deficiencies
2. Hereditary
   - Usually a single coagulation factor deficiency

B. Pathogenesis
1. Decreased production
   - Examples—hemophilia A, cirrhosis

Coagulation disorders: most are due to decreased production of a coagulation factor

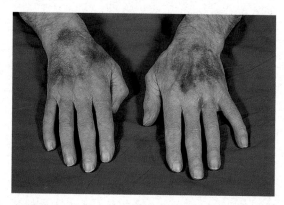

14-5: *Senile purpura showing the large, irregular areas of hemorrhage on the backs of both hands. This benign condition primarily occurs in body areas that are frequently traumatized. It is due to the normal vessel instability that is associated with aging. (From Forbes C, Jackson W: Color Atlas and Text of Clinical Medicine, 2nd ed. St. Louis, Mosby, 2003, Fig. 10-112.)*

    2. Pathologic inhibition
       • Example—acquired circulating antibodies (inhibitors) against coagulation factors
    3. Excessive consumption
       • Example—disseminated intravascular coagulation

C. Clinical findings in coagulation disorders
    1. Late rebleeding after surgery or wisdom tooth extraction
      a. Temporary platelet plug is the only mechanical block preventing bleeding.
      b. Lack of thrombin prevents formation of a stable platelet plug held together by fibrin.
    2. Findings in severe factor deficiencies
      a. Hemarthroses
      b. Retroperitoneal and deep muscular bleeding
    3. Findings similar to platelet disorders
      a. Ecchymoses, epistaxis
      b. Menorrhagia, hematuria
      c. Bleeding from tooth extraction sites
      d. Gastrointestinal and intracranial bleeding

D. Hemophilia A
    1. Epidemiology
      a. X-linked recessive
        (1) Females are asymptomatic carriers.
        (2) Females transmit the abnormal X chromosome to 50% of their sons.
      b. Absent family history of hemophilia
        • Most likely due to a new mutation (30% of cases)
      c. Female carriers with symptomatic disease
        (1) Due to inactivation of more maternal than paternal X chromosomes

Hemophilia A: X-linked recessive

(2) Females become "homozygous" for the abnormal X chromosome
2. Pathogenesis
   • Decreased synthesis of factor VIII:C in the intrinsic system
3. Clinical findings in hemophilia A
   a. Signs and symptoms correlate with the level of factor VIII:C activity
      • Activity below 1% correlates with severe disease (e.g., spontaneous hemarthroses).
   b. Bleeding problems may occur in newborns (10–15% of cases).
      • Excessive bleeding may occur after circumcision or umbilical cord separation.

> Hemophilia B (Christmas disease) is an X-linked recessive disorder involving a deficiency of factor IX. It is clinically indistinguishable from hemophilia A.

   c. Laboratory findings in hemophilia A
      (1) Increased PTT and a normal PT
      (2) Decreased factor VIII:C activity
      (3) Decreased factor VIII:antigen (VIII:Ag)
         • Factor VIII protein
      (4) Detection of female carriers
         • DNA techniques are most sensitive.
4. Treatment of hemophilia A
   a. Mild cases respond to desmopressin acetate
      • Increases VIII:C activity
   b. Severe cases require infusion of recombinant factor VIII
      • *No* risk for HIV

Hemophilia A: ↓ VIII:C, VIII:Ag; ↑ PTT

E. Classic von Willebrand disease (vWD)
1. Epidemiology
   a. Autosomal dominant disorder
   b. Most common hereditary coagulation disorder
2. Pathogenesis
   • Decreased vWF and factor VIII:C activity
3. Clinical findings in vWD
   a. Menorrhagia, epistaxis, easy bruisability
   b. Association with angiodysplasia of the right colon (see Chapter 17)
4. Laboratory findings in vWD
   a. Increased PTT and a normal PT
   b. Increased bleeding time
      • Due a platelet adhesion defect
   c. Abnormal ristocetin cofactor assay
   d. Decreased vWF antigen
   e. Decreased VIII:Ag and VIII:C activity
5. Treatment of vWD
   a. Desmopressin acetate (increases vWF and VIII:C activity)
   b. Oral contraceptive (estrogen has a similar action as desmopressin)

vWD: most common hereditary coagulation disorder

vWD: combined platelet and coagulation factor disorder

vWD: ↑ PTT, bleeding time

E. Circulating anticoagulants (inhibitors)

1. Pathogenesis
   a. Coagulation factor is destroyed by antibodies.
   b. Most common type is antibodies against factor VIII:C (e.g., post-partum).
2. Clinical findings
   - Similar to those with coagulation factor deficiencies due to decreased production
3. Laboratory findings
   a. Prolonged PT and/or PTT, depending on the factor deficiency
      - Does *not* differentiate immune destruction versus decreased production
   b. Mixing studies
      - Normal plasma is mixed with patient plasma in a test tube.
      (1) *No* correction of PT and/or PTT indicates immune destruction.
      (2) Correction of PT and/or PTT indicates decreased production.

Circulating anticoagulant: PT and PTT *not* corrected with mixing study

F. Vitamin K deficiency

1. Function of vitamin K
   - γ-Carboxylates vitamin K–dependent factors II, VII, IX, X and proteins C and S
2. Causes of vitamin K deficiency
   a. Decreased synthesis of vitamin K by colonic bacteria
      (1) Newborns lack bacterial colonization of the bowel.
         (a) Vitamin K levels normally decrease between days 2 and 5.
         (b) Danger of severe bleeding (e.g., intracerebral hemorrhage)
         (c) Newborns require an intramuscular injection of vitamin K at birth.
            - Breast milk contains very little vitamin K.
      (2) Prolonged treatment with antibiotics
         (a) Antibiotics sterilize the bowel causing decreased production of vitamin K.
         (b) Most common cause of vitamin K deficiency in a hospitalized patient
   b. Decreased small bowel reabsorption of vitamin K
      (1) Malabsorption of fat causes malabsorption of fat-soluble vitamins.
      (2) Example—celiac disease
   c. Decreased activation of vitamin K by epoxide reductase in the liver
      (1) Warfarin inhibits epoxide reductase.
         (a) Vitamin K–dependent factors are nonfunctional.
         (b) Rat poison contains warfarin.
         (c) Children may have exposure to warfarin from elders living in the household.
      (2) Cirrhosis
         (a) Decreased activation of vitamin K and synthesis of vitamin K–dependent coagulation factors
         (b) Prolonged PT is *not* corrected with intramuscular injection of vitamin K.

Vitamin K deficiency in hospitalized patient: due to antibiotic therapy

Cirrhosis: ↓ synthesis of vitamin K–dependent factors, ↓ activation of vitamin K

3. Clinical findings of vitamin K deficiency
   a. Gastrointestinal bleeding
   b. Bleeding into subcutaneous tissue
   c. Bleeding at the time of circumcision
   d. Intracranial hemorrhage
4. Treatment of vitamin K deficiency
   a. If bleeding is *not* severe, treatment is an intramuscular injection of vitamin K.
      • Corrects bleeding in a few hours
   b. If bleeding is severe, treatment is with fresh frozen plasma.
      (1) Immediate correction
      (2) Vitamin K–dependent factors are γ-carboxylated.

G. Hemostasis disorders in liver disease
   1. Pathogenesis
      a. Decreased synthesis of coagulation factors
         (1) Multiple coagulation factor deficiencies
         (2) Decreased γ-carboxylation of vitamin K–dependent factors
      b. Decreased synthesis of anticoagulants
         • Examples—ATIII, proteins C and S
      c. Decreased synthesis of fibrinolytic agents (e.g., plasminogen)
      d. Decreased clearance of FDPs and D-dimers
         • Interfere with platelet aggregation and polymerization of fibrin
      e. Decreased clearance of tPA and decreased synthesis of α_2-antiplasmin
         • May produce primary fibrinolysis (see section IV)

Cirrhosis: multiple hemostasis abnormalities

   2. Laboratory findings in liver disease
      a. Increased PT and PTT
      b. Increased FDPs and D-dimers
      c. Increased bleeding time

H. Disseminated intravascular coagulation (DIC)
   1. Causes of DIC
      a. Sepsis
         • Common pathogens include *E. coli* (most common) and *Neisseria meningitidis*

Sepsis: most common cause of DIC

      b. Disseminated malignancy
         (1) Acute promyelocytic leukemia
         (2) Pancreatic cancer with release of procoagulants in mucin
      c. Other causes
         • Crush injuries, rattlesnake envenomation, amniotic fluid embolism
   2. Pathogenesis
      a. Activation of the coagulation cascade
         • Due to release of tissue thromboplastin and/or endothelial cell injury
      b. Fibrin thrombi develop in the microcirculation.
         (1) Thrombi obstruct blood flow.
         (2) Thrombi consume coagulation factors (I, II, V, VIII) and trap platelets.

DIC: consumption of coagulation factors

      c. Activation of the fibrinolytic system
         • Secondary fibrinolysis due to activation of plasminogen by factor XII

3. Clinical findings in DIC
   a. Thrombohemorrhagic disorder
      (1) Ischemia from occlusive fibrin thrombi
      (2) Bleeding from anticoagulation
         • Factors I, II, V, and VIII are consumed in the fibrin thrombi
   b. Shock due to blood loss
   c. Diffuse oozing of blood from all breaks in the skin and mucous membranes
   d. Petechiae and ecchymoses
4. Laboratory findings in DIC
   a. Coagulation abnormalities
      (1) Increased PT and PTT
      (2) Decreased fibrinogen
   b. Platelet abnormalities
      (1) Thrombocytopenia
      (2) Increased bleeding time
   c. Fibrinolysis abnormalities
      • Presence of FDPs and D-dimers
   d. Normocytic anemia with schistocytes and reticulocytosis
      • RBCs are damaged by fibrin thrombi (microangiopathic hemolytic anemia).
5. Treatment
   a. Treating the underlying disease is most important.
   b. Transfuse blood components
      (1) Fresh frozen plasma for multiple coagulation factor deficiencies
      (2) Packed RBCs for anemia
      (3) Platelet concentrates for thrombocytopenia

IV. Fibrinolytic Disorders
A. Primary fibrinolysis
1. Causes
   a. Open heart surgery
      • Cardiopulmonary bypass causes a decrease in α_2-antiplasmin and increase in tPA.
   b. Radical prostatectomy
      • Causes increased release of urokinase
   c. Diffuse liver disease
      • Causes a decrease in the synthesis of α_2-antiplasmin
2. Pathogenesis
   a. FDPs interfere with platelet aggregation.
   b. Plasmin degrades coagulation factors causing multiple factor deficiencies.
3. Clinical findings
   • Severe bleeding
4. Laboratory findings
   a. Increased PT and PTT
      • Due to multiple factor deficiencies

   b. Increased bleeding time
      • Due to interference with platelet aggregation
   c. Positive test for FDPs
   d. Negative D-dimer assay
      • *No* fibrin thrombi are present.
   e. Normal platelet count
B. Secondary fibrinolysis
   1. Compensatory reaction in the presence of intravascular coagulation
   2. Increase in both FDPs and D-dimers

V. Summary of Laboratory Test Results in Hemostasis Disorders (Table 14-3)

VI. Thrombosis Syndromes
   A. Acquired thrombosis syndromes
      1. Antiphospholipid syndrome (APLS)
         a. Epidemiology
            • Associations include SLE and HIV
         b. Pathogenesis
            (1) Presence of antiphospholipid antibodies (APAs)
               • Directed against phospholipids bound to plasma proteins
            (2) APAs include anticardiolipin antibody and lupus anticoagulant.
               • Anticardiolipin antibody reacts with the cardiolipin reagent in
                 the rapid plasma reagin test for syphilis.
         c. Clinical findings in APLS
            (1) Produce arterial and venous thrombosis syndromes
            (2) Repeated abortions due to thrombosis of placental bed vessels
            (3) Strokes, thromboembolism
      2. Other acquired causes of thrombosis
         a. Postoperative state with stasis of blood flow
         b. Malignancy
            (1) Increase in coagulation factors
            (2) Thrombocytosis
            (3) Release of procoagulants from tumors, particularly pancreatic
                cancers

Anticardiolipin antibody: produces a false-positive syphilis serologic test

TABLE 14-3: Laboratory Findings in Common Hemostasis Disorders

Disorder or Condition	Platelet Count	Bleeding Time	PT	PTT
Thrombocytopenia ITP, TTP, HUS	↓	↑	Normal	Normal
Von Willebrand disease	Normal	↑	Normal	↑
Hemophilia A	Normal	Normal	Normal	↑
DIC	↓	↑	↑	↑
Primary fibrinolysis	Normal	↑	↑	↑
Aspirin or NSAID use	Normal	↑	Normal	Normal
Warfarin or heparin use	Normal	Normal	↑	↑

DIC, disseminated intravascular coagulation; HUS; hemolytic uremic syndrome; ITP, idiopathic thrombocytopenic purpura; NSAID, nonsteroidal antiinflammatory drug; PT, prothrombin time; PTT, partial thromboplastin time; TTP, thrombotic thrombocytopenic purpura.

   c. Folate or vitamin B_{12} deficiency
      • Due to increased plasma homocysteine levels
   d. Oral contraceptives
      • Estrogen increases the synthesis of coagulation factors and decreases ATIII
   e. Hyperviscosity
      (1) Polycythemia syndromes
      (2) Waldenström's macroglobulinemia
B. Hereditary thrombosis syndromes
   1. Epidemiology
      a. Autosomal dominant syndromes
      b. Deep venous thrombosis and pulmonary emboli occur at an early age.
      c. Venous thromboses often occur in unusual places.
         • Examples—hepatic vein, dural sinus
   2. Factor V_{Leiden}
      a. Most common hereditary thrombosis syndrome.
      b. Mutant form of factor V *cannot* be degraded by protein C and protein S.
   3. Antithrombin III (ATIII) deficiency
      a. Functions of ATIII
         (1) Activity is enhanced by heparin.
         (2) Neutralizes activated serine proteases (e.g., factors XII, XI, IX, X, thrombin)
      b. *No* prolongation of PTT after injecting a standard dose of heparin
      c. Treatment
         (1) Infuse a greater dose of heparin than normal
            • PTT eventually increases due to enhancement of whatever ATIII is present.
         (2) Send the patient home on warfarin.
   4. Proteins C and S deficiency
      a. Pathogenesis
         • Cannot inactivate factors V and VIII
      b. Treatment
         (1) Begin with heparin and a very low dose of warfarin to reduce the risk for developing hemorrhagic skin necrosis.
         (2) Send the patient home on warfarin.

Factor V_{Leiden}: most common hereditary thrombosis syndrome

Hemorrhagic skin necrosis: associated with warfarin therapy in protein C deficiency

There is a potential for heterozygote carriers of protein C deficiency to develop hemorrhagic skin necrosis when placed on warfarin. Heterozygote carriers have ~50% protein C activity. Protein C has a short half-life (~6 hours). When patients are placed on warfarin, protein C activity falls to zero activity in 6 hours, causing a hypercoagulable state due to increased activity of factors V and VIII. This causes cutaneous vessel thrombosis and concomitant skin necrosis.

Blood Banking and Transfusion Disorders

I. ABO Blood Group Antigens

A. Definition of ABO blood group antigens
- They are glycoproteins attached to the RBC surface.

B. Blood group O characteristics
1. Most common blood group
   - *No* blood group antigens are present on the RBC membrane.
2. Natural antibodies (isohemagglutinins) in serum
   a. Anti-A-IgM, anti-B-IgM
   b. Most people have anti-AB-IgG antibodies.

> Blood group antibodies are natural antibodies that are synthesized in Peyer's patches. A and B antigens that are normally present in food are trapped by specialized epithelial cells called M cells that overlie Peyer's patches. M cells have close proximity to B lymphocytes lying within the epithelium. M cells transport the A and B antigens to these lymphocytes, resulting in the development of natural antibodies against the antigens. Natural antibodies develop against antigens that are *not* present on the RBC, which explains why blood group O patients have antibodies against both A and B antigens.

3. Increased incidence of duodenal ulcers

C. Blood group A characteristics
1. Anti-B-IgM antibodies
2. Increased incidence of gastric carcinoma

D. Blood group B characteristics
- Anti-A-IgM antibodies

E. Blood group AB characteristics
1. Least common blood group
2. *No* natural antibodies

F. Newborns
1. Do *not* have natural antibodies at birth
2. IgG antibodies are of maternal origin.
   - IgG antibodies cross the placenta.

G. Elderly people
- Frequently lose their natural antibodies

Blood group O: most common blood group

Group O: anti-A-IgM, anti-B-IgM, anti-AB-IgG
Group A: anti-B-IgM
Group B: anti-A-IgM
Group AB: no antibodies

Newborns: lack natural antibodies

Elderly people: frequently lose natural antibodies

	Forward Type		Back Type	
Blood group	Anti-A	Anti-B	A RBCs	B RBCs
O	−	−	+	+
A	+	−	−	+
B	−	+	+	−
AB	+	+	−	−

15-1: Forward and back type to identify ABO blood groups. Forward type identifies the blood group antigen by reacting anti-A and anti-B against patient RBCs. Back type identifies the natural antibodies in the patient serum by reacting A RBCs and B RBCs against the patient serum. Refer to the text for discussion of the blood groups and their natural antibodies.

Elderly patients may *not* have a hemolytic transfusion reaction if they are transfused with the wrong blood group because they frequently lose their natural antibodies.

H. Paternity issues in newborns
  1. Blood group AB parents *cannot* have an O child.
  2. Blood group O parents *cannot* have an AB, A, or B child.
  3. Blood group A and B parents can have O children if both have AO and BO phenotypes.

Forward typing: identifies blood group antigen

I. Determining the ABO group (Fig. 15-1)
  1. Forward type
    a. Identifies the blood group antigen
      • Patient RBCs are added to test tubes that contain either anti-A or anti-B test serum.
    b. Example—blood group A RBCs
      • Agglutination reaction with anti-A test serum but *not* with anti-B test serum

Back typing: identifies natural antibodies

  2. Back type
    a. Identifies the natural antibodies
      • Patient serum is added to test tubes containing either A or B test RBCs.
    b. Example—blood group A serum
      • Patient anti-B-IgM antibodies agglutinate B test RBCs but *not* A test RBCs.

II. Rh and Non-Rh Antigen Systems
  A. Rh antigen system
    1. It has three adjoining gene loci.
      a. Locus coding for D antigen (no d antigen)
      b. Locus coding for C and c antigen
      c. Locus coding for E and e antigen

Five Rh antigens: D, C, c, E, e

    2. Autosomal codominant inheritance
      a. One of the sets of three Rh antigens from each parent is transmitted to each child.

(1) Example—child with CDe from the father and cde from the mother
  • Note that the child lacks E antigen.
(2) Absence of D antigen on a chromosome is designated d even though the antigen does *not* exist.
  b. Possible Rh antigen profiles
    (1) DD, Dd, or dd
    (2) CC, Cc, or cc
    (3) EE, Ee, or ee
3. An individual who is Rh positive is D antigen positive.
  a. Approximately 85% of the population has D antigen.
  b. Individuals lacking D antigen are considered Rh negative.
4. Rh phenotype of an individual
  a. RBCs are reacted with test antisera against each of the Rh antigens.
  b. Example—Rh phenotype that is positive for C, c, D, and E antigens but negative for e antigen (phenotype is CcDE)

B. Alloimmunization
1. Production of an antibody against a foreign antigen *not* present on an individual's RBCs
  a. Patient exposure to Rh antigen he is lacking (e.g., D antigen)
  b. Patient exposure to non-Rh antigen she is lacking (e.g., Kell antigen)
  c. These antibodies are called atypical antibodies.
    • The individual is considered sensitized if atypical antibodies are present.
2. Significance of atypical antibodies
  a. May produce a hemolytic transfusion reaction (HTR)
    (1) Occurs when blood containing the foreign antigen is infused into an individual
    (2) Example—individual with anti-Kell antibodies is exposed to Kell antigen positive RBCs.
    (3) IgG antibodies are more likely to produce an HTR than IgM antibodies.
      • IgG antibodies react best in warm temperatures, but IgM antibodies react best in cold temperatures.
  b. Transfusion requirements in an individual with atypical antibodies
    (1) Individual must receive blood that is negative for the foreign antigen.
    (2) Example—individual with anti-Kell antibodies must receive Kell antigen negative blood.

C. Clinically important non-Rh antigens
1. Duffy (Fy) antigens
  a. Fy antigens are the binding site for infestation of RBCs by *Plasmodium vivax.*
  b. Majority of black Americans lack the Fy antigen.
    • Offers protection against contracting *P. vivax* malaria
2. I and i antigen systems
  a. IgM antibodies (cold agglutinins) may develop against I or i antigen.

Rh positive: D antigen positive

Alloimmunization: antibodies develop against foreign antigens

Individual with an atypical antibody must receive blood lacking the antigen.

Fy antigen negative RBCs: protection against *P. vivax* malaria

    b. Increased risk for developing a cold autoimmune hemolytic anemia (see Chapter 11)
      (1) Anti-i hemolytic anemia may occur in infectious mononucleosis.
      (2) Anti-I hemolytic anemia may occur in *Mycoplasma pneumoniae* infections.

III. Blood Transfusion Therapy
A. Blood donors
1. Autologous transfusion
   a. Process of collection, storage, and reinfusion of the individual's own blood
   b. Safest form of transfusion

Autologous transfusion: safest transfusion

2. Tests performed on donor blood
   a. Group (ABO) and type (Rh)
   b. Antibody screen (indirect Coombs' test)
    • Detects atypical antibodies (e.g., anti-D, anti-Kell)
   c. Screening tests for infectious disease
    • Examples—syphilis, hepatitis B and C, HIV-1 and 2, HTLV-1

CMV: most common pathogen transmitted by transfusion

> There is a risk for transmitting infection when transfusing blood because there is an incubation period before specific antibodies are developed against the pathogen. The risk for developing an infection per unit of blood for different pathogens is as follows: 1:3300 for hepatitis C; 1:200,000 for hepatitis B; and, 1:2,000,000 for HIV. The most common infectious agent transmitted by blood transfusion is cytomegalovirus (CMV), which is present in donor lymphocytes.

B. Patient crossmatch
1. Components of a standard crossmatch
   a. ABO group and Rh type
   b. Antibody screen for atypical antibodies
   c. Direct Coombs' test to identify atypical IgG antibodies on patient RBCs
   d. Major crossmatch
2. Major crossmatch
   a. Purpose of a major crossmatch
    • Detect atypical antibodies that are directed against foreign antigens on donor RBCs

A negative antibody screen ensures that a major crossmatch will be compatible.

   b. Patient serum is mixed with a sample of RBCs from a donor unit.
    (1) Each unit of donor blood must have a separate crossmatch.
    (2) Lack of RBC agglutination or hemolysis indicates a compatible crossmatch.

> Patients with a negative antibody screen should have a compatible crossmatch. However, a compatible crossmatch does *not* guarantee that the recipient will not develop atypical antibodies, a transfusion reaction, or an infection.

TABLE 15-1:
Blood Components

Component	Discussion
Packed RBCs	Purpose: increase O_2 transport to tissues Packed RBCs have less volume and a higher Hct than whole blood Each unit of packed RBCs should raise the Hb by 1 g/dL and the Hct by 3%; lack of an increment implies a hemolytic transfusion reaction or blood loss in the patient *Yersinia enterocolitica*, a pathogen that thrives on iron, is the most common contaminant of stored blood
Platelets	Purpose: stop medically significant bleeding related to thrombocytopenia or qualitative platelet defects (e.g., aspirin) Platelets have HLA antigens and ABO antigens on their surface; however, they lack Rh antigens Each unit of platelets should raise the platelet count by 5000–10,000 cells/μL
Fresh frozen plasma	Purpose: treatment of multiple coagulation deficiencies (e.g., DIC; cirrhosis) or treatment of warfarin over-anticoagulation if bleeding is life-threatening
Cryoprecipitate	Purpose: treatment of coagulation factor deficiencies involving fibrinogen and factor VIII (e.g., DIC) Cryoprecipitate contains fibrinogen, factor VIII, and factor XIII Desmopressin acetate is used instead of cryoprecipitate in treating mild hemophilia A and von Willebrand disease

DIC, disseminated intravascular coagulation; Hct, hematocrit; Hb, hemoglobin.

3. Use of blood group O packed RBCs for transfusion
   a. Can be transfused into any patient, regardless of the blood group
      (1) Blood group O RBCs lack A and B antigens.
      (2) Blood group O individuals are considered universal donors.
   b. Blood group O individuals can receive only O blood.
      • Anti-A-IgM and anti-B-IgM will hemolyze transfused A, B, or AB RBCs.
4. Blood group AB individuals can be transfused with blood from any blood group.
   a. They lack natural antibodies.
   b. They are considered universal recipients.

Blood group O individuals: universal donors

Blood group AB individuals: universal recipients

Before blood is transfused into newborns or patients with T-cell deficiencies, it must be irradiated to kill donor lymphocytes. This prevents the patient from developing a graft-versus-host reaction (see Chapter 3) or a CMV infection.

C. **Blood component therapy (Table 15-1)**
D. **Transfusion reactions**
   1. Allergic reactions
      a. Most common transfusion reaction
      b. Type I IgE-mediated hypersensitivity reaction against proteins in the donor blood

Allergic transfusion reaction: IgE-mediated

c. Clinical findings
  (1) Urticaria with pruritus
  (2) Fever, tachycardia, wheezing
  (3) Potential for anaphylactic shock
  (4) Mild cases are treated with antihistamines.

> Individuals who are deficient in IgA and who have antibodies directed against IgA from previous exposure to a blood product may develop a severe anaphylactic reaction. IgA deficient individuals must receive blood or blood products that lack IgA.

2. Febrile reaction
  a. Pathogenesis
    (1) Recipient has anti–human leukocyte antigen (HLA) antibodies directed against foreign HLA antigens on donor leukocytes.
      • There are *no* HLA antigens on RBCs.
    (2) Type II hypersensitivity reaction
  b. Clinical findings
    (1) Fever, chills, headache, and flushing
    (2) Treated with antipyretics

Febrile transfusion reaction: anti-HLA antibodies against donor leukocytes

> Anti-HLA antibodies develop when individuals are exposed to foreign HLA antigens (e.g., previous blood transfusion or organ transplant). Women commonly have these reactions owing to pregnancy, when there is an increased risk for exposure to fetal blood during delivery or after a spontaneous abortion.

3. Acute hemolytic transfusion reaction (HTR)
  a. May be intravascular or extravascular hemolytic reactions (see Chapter 11)
  b. Intravascular hemolysis
    (1) ABO blood group incompatibility
    (2) Example—group B patient receives group A donor blood.
      • Anti A-IgM attaches to A positive donor RBCs producing intravascular hemolysis.
    (3) Type II hypersensitivity reaction
  c. Extravascular hemolysis
    (1) An atypical antibody reacts with a foreign antigen on donor RBCs.
      • Macrophage phagocytosis and destruction of donor RBCs coated by the atypical antibody
    (2) Jaundice commonly occurs.
      • Unconjugated bilirubin is the end product of macrophage degradation of Hb.
    (3) Type II hypersensitivity reaction

Acute HTRs are due to blood group incompatibility or presence of an atypical antibody.

> Individuals who have been infused with blood in the past may have been exposed to a foreign blood group antigen and developed atypical antibodies that are no longer circulating;

> therefore, the pretransfusion antibody screen is negative. However, memory B cells are present and reexposure to the foreign antigen causes them to produce antibodies, resulting in an extravascular hemolytic anemia. This reaction may occur within hours to 3 to 10 days after the transfusion.

    d. Clinical findings
        (1) Fever, back pain, hypotension
        (2) Disseminated intravascular coagulation, oliguria (renal failure)
    e. Laboratory findings
        (1) Positive direct Coombs' test
           • IgG antibody and/or C3b is coating donor RBCs.
        (2) Positive indirect Coombs' test
           • Atypical antibody is present in serum.
        (3) *No* significant increase in Hb over pretransfusion levels.
        (4) Hemoglobinuria (sign of intravascular hemolysis)
        (5) Jaundice (sign of extravascular hemolysis)

IV. Hemolytic disease of the newborn (HDN)

    • HDN results from the transplacental passage of maternal IgG antibodies (e.g., anti-D antibodies, anti-AB antibodies in O mothers) resulting in an extravascular hemolytic anemia in the fetus.

A. ABO HDN

    1. Epidemiology
        a. Most common HDN
           • Present in 20% to 25% of all pregnancies
        b. Mothers are blood group O and the fetus is either blood group A or B.

ABO HDN: most common HDN

    2. Pathogenesis
        a. Blood group O individuals have anti-AB-IgG antibodies.
           (1) IgG antibodies cross the placenta and attach to fetal A or B RBCs.
           (2) Fetal splenic macrophages phagocytose RBCs, causing anemia.
           (3) Unconjugated bilirubin from extravascular hemolysis is disposed of in the mother's liver.
        b. May affect the firstborn or any future pregnancy if ABO incompatibility exists

ABO HDN: mother group O, fetus blood group A or B

    3. Clinical and laboratory findings
        a. Jaundice develops within the first 24 hours after birth.
           (1) ABO HDN is the most common cause of jaundice in this period.
              • Newborn liver cannot handle the excess bilirubin load.
           (2) Risk for kernicterus is very small (see below).
        b. Anemia
           (1) Mild normocytic anemia or no anemia at all
           (2) Exchange transfusions are rarely indicated.
        c. Positive direct Coombs' test on fetal cord blood RBCs
           • Due to anti-AB-IgG antibodies coating fetal A or B RBCs
        d. Spherocytes are present in the cord blood peripheral smear.
           • Due to macrophage removal of a portion of the RBC membrane

ABO HDN: positive direct Coombs' test on fetal RBCs

Rh HDN: mother Rh
negative, fetus Rh
positive

B. Rh HDN

1. Pathogenesis
   a. Mother is Rh (D antigen) negative and the fetus is Rh positive.
   b. Mother is exposed to fetal Rh positive blood (fetomaternal bleed).
      • Occurs during the last trimester or during childbirth itself
   c. Cytotrophoblast is absent during the last trimester.
      • Increases the risk for a fetomaternal bleed
   d. Mother develops anti-D-IgG antibodies when exposed to fetal Rh positive cells.
      • First Rh incompatible pregnancy does *not* affect the firstborn.
   e. Subsequent Rh incompatible pregnancies result in extravascular hemolytic anemia in the fetus.
      (1) Anti-D-IgG antibodies cross the placenta and attach to fetal Rh positive RBCs.
      (2) Fetal splenic macrophages phagocytose RBCs, causing severe anemia.
         (a) Fetus may develop high-output cardiac failure leading to hydrops fetalis and death.
         (b) Hydrops fetalis is a combined left- and right-sided heart failure with ascites and edema.
         (c) Extramedullary hematopoiesis is present in the liver and spleen.
         (d) Unconjugated bilirubin is conjugated in the mother's liver.

2. Prevention of Rh HDN in Rh negative mothers without anti-D

Prevention of Rh HDN:
Rh immune globulin
(anti-D globulin)

   a. Receive anti-D globulin (Rh immune globulin) during the 28th week of pregnancy
   b. Anti-D globulin does *not* cross the placenta.
   c. Anti-D globulin protects the mother from sensitization to fetal Rh positive cells that may enter her circulation during the last trimester.
   d. Anti-D globulin lasts ~3 months in the mother's blood.
   e. Additional anti-D globulin is given to the mother after delivery if the baby is Rh positive.

   > Special tests are performed on the mother's blood that detect fetal RBCs in her blood. The amount of fetal blood is quantified so that the appropriate amount of anti-D globulin is given to the mother. Anti-D globulin masks the antigenic sites on the fetal RBCs or destroys the fetal RBCs so that the mother does not host an antibody response against the D antigen. If the patient develops anti-D antibodies, there is no indication for giving the globulin either during or after delivery, because its main purpose is to prevent sensitization.

3. Clinical and laboratory findings
   a. Degree of anemia is more severe than with ABO HDN.
   b. Jaundice develops shortly after birth.
      (1) Level of unconjugated bilirubin is much higher than with ABO HDN.

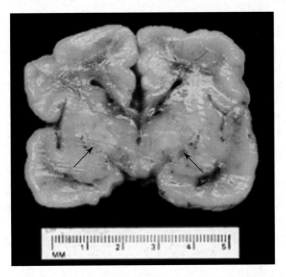

15-2: *Cross section of the brain of a newborn with kernicterus. Arrows depict yellow bilirubin pigment deposited in the basal ganglia. Bilirubin is toxic to neurons and produces long-term neurologic sequelae. (From Kumar V, Fausto N, Abbas A: Robbins and Cotran's Pathologic Basis of Disease, 7th ed. Philadelphia, WB Saunders, 2004, p 487, Fig. 10-16.)*

- Most of the unconjugated bilirubin is *not* bound by albumin and circulates free in the blood.
(2) Increased risk for kernicterus
  - The free, unbound lipid soluble unconjugated bilirubin poses the greatest risk for bilirubin entry into the brain (Fig. 15-2).

> Kernicterus refers to deposition of free (not bound to albumin) lipid-soluble unconjugated bilirubin in the basal ganglia owing to an incompletely formed blood-brain barrier. Bilirubin damages neurons in the brain, causing severe dysfunction.

c. Positive direct and indirect Coombs' tests on fetal cord blood
d. Spherocytes are *not* present in cord blood.
  - Macrophages phagocytose the entire RBC.
e. Exchange transfusions are required.
  (1) Newborn's blood is removed and replaced with fresh blood.
  (2) Transfusion corrects anemia and removes antibodies and unconjugated bilirubin.

> ABO incompatibility protects the mother from developing Rh sensitization. For example, in a mother who is O negative and carrying a fetus who is A positive, any A positive fetal RBCs entering her circulation will be destroyed by maternal anti-A-IgM antibodies, thereby preventing sensitization.

Kernicterus: free unconjugated bilirubin deposits in basal ganglia

ABO incompatibility: protects mother from Rh sensitization

Blue fluorescent light: converts bilirubin in skin to water-soluble dipyrrole

C. Use of blue fluorescent light
1. Used as a treatment of jaundice in the newborn
2. Unconjugated bilirubin in the skin absorbs light energy from blue fluorescent light.
3. Photoisomerization converts unconjugated bilirubin to a nontoxic water-soluble dipyrrole (called lumirubin).
   • Lumirubin is excreted in bile or urine.

16 CHAPTER

Upper and Lower Respiratory Disorders

I. **Signs and Symptoms of Respiratory Disease (Table 16-1)**

II. **Pulmonary Function Tests**
  A. **Calculation of the alveolar-arterial (A-a) gradient**
    1. A-a gradient is the difference between the alveolar Po_2 (PAo_2) and arterial Po_2 (Pao_2).
      a. A-a gradient is normally due to a mismatch between ventilation and perfusion in the lungs.
        • Example—An A-a gradient exists when perfusion is greater than ventilation in the lower lobes.
      b. It is useful in differentiating causes of hypoxemia (decreased Pao_2).
        (1) Hypoxemia due to pulmonary causes increases A-a gradient.
        (2) Hypoxemia due to extrapulmonary causes has a normal A-a gradient.
    2. Calculation of the A-a gradient
      a. $PAo_2 = \% \ O_2 \ (713) -$ arterial $Pco_2/0.8$
        • % O_2 is the percentage of O_2 the patient is breathing; 713 is the atmospheric pressure (760 mm Hg) minus the water vapor pressure (47 mm Hg); and 0.8 is the respiratory quotient.
      b. Example using normal values
        (1) Normal $PAo_2 = 0.21 \ (713) - 40/0.8 = 100$ mm Hg
        (2) Normal $Pao_2 = 95$ mm Hg
        (3) Normal A-a gradient = 100 mm Hg − 95 mm Hg = 5 mm Hg
        (4) Medically significant A-a gradient ≥ 30 mm Hg
    3. Causes of hypoxemia with an increased A-a gradient
      a. Ventilation defect
        (1) Impaired O_2 delivery to the alveoli for gas exchange
        (2) Example—airway collapse due to the respiratory distress syndrome
      b. Perfusion defect
        (1) Decreased or absent blood flow to the alveoli
        (2) Example—pulmonary embolus
      c. Diffusion defect
        (1) O_2 cannot diffuse through the alveolar-capillary interface.
        (2) Example—interstitial fibrosis, pulmonary edema

↑ A-a gradient: hypoxemia of pulmonary origin

Normal A-a gradient: hypoxemia of extrapulmonary origin

$PAo_2 = \% \ O_2 \ (713) -$ arterial $Pco_2/0.8$

TABLE 16-1:
Common Symptoms of Respiratory Disease

Symptom	Causes and Discussion
Dyspnea	Difficulty with breathing Due to stimulation of J receptors causing decrease in full inspiration Causes of dyspnea Decreased compliance (e.g., interstitial fibrosis) Increased airway resistance (e.g., chronic bronchitis) Chest bellows disease (e.g., obesity, kyphoscoliosis) Interstitial inflammation/fluid accumulation (e.g., left-sided heart failure)
Cough	Cough with a normal chest x-ray Postnasal discharge is the most common cause Nocturnal cough GERD: due to acid reflux in tracheobronchial tree at night Bronchial asthma: due to bronchoconstriction Productive cough Chronic bronchitis: due to smoking cigarettes Typical bacterial pneumonia Bronchiectasis Drugs causing cough ACE inhibitors: inhibit degradation of bradykinin, causing mucosal swelling and irritation in tracheobronchial tree Aspirin: causes an increase in LT C-D-E$_4$ (bronchoconstrictors)
Hemoptysis	Coughing up blood-tinged sputum Mechanisms Parenchymal necrosis Bronchial and/or pulmonary vessel damage Causes Chronic bronchitis (most common cause) Pneumonia, bronchogenic carcinoma TB, bronchiectasis, aspergilloma (fungus living in a cavitary lesion)

ACE, angiotensin-converting enzyme; GERD, gastroesophageal reflux disease; LT, leukotriene; TB, tuberculosis.

    d. Right-to-left cardiac shunt
      • Example—tetralogy of Fallot

> Calculate the A-a gradient in a patient breathing 0.30 O_2 who has a Pco_2 of 80 mm Hg and Pao_2 of 40 mm Hg. PAo_2 = 0.30 (713) − 80/0.8 = 114 mm Hg. A-a gradient = 114 − 40 = 74 mm Hg, which is medically significant and indicates one or more of the above-mentioned lung disorders or a right-to-left shunt in the heart.

  4. Causes of hypoxemia with a normal A-a gradient
    a. Depression of the respiratory center in the medulla
      • Examples—barbiturates, brain injury
    b. Upper airway obstruction
      (1) Café coronary (food blocking airway)
      (2) Epiglottitis due to *Hemophilus influenzae*
      (3) Croup due to parainfluenza virus (narrows the trachea)

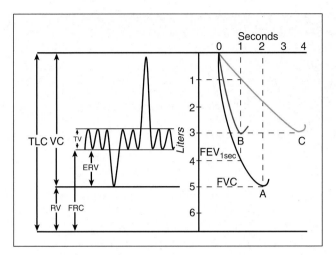

16-1: Spirometry showing normal lung volumes and capacities and forced expiratory volume at 1 second (FEV$_{1 sec}$) and forced vital capacity (FVC) findings in a normal person (A), a person with restrictive lung disease (B), and a person with obstructive lung disease (C). ERV, expiratory reserve volume; FRC, functional residual capacity; RV, residual volume; TLC, total lung capacity; TV, tidal volume; VC, vital capacity. (From Goljan EF: Star Series: Pathology. Philadelphia, WB Saunders, 1998, p 229, Fig. 11-1.)

    c. Chest bellows (muscles of respiration) dysfunction
      (1) Paralyzed diaphragm
      (2) Amyotrophic lateral sclerosis with degeneration of anterior horn cells

> Calculate the A-a gradient in a patient breathing room air who has a Pco$_2$ of 80 mm Hg and Pao$_2$ of 40 mm Hg. PAo$_2$ = 0.21 (713) − 80/0.8 = 50 mm Hg. A-a gradient = 50 − 40 = 10 mm Hg, which is *not* medically significant and indicates an extrapulmonary cause of hypoxemia.

B. Spirometry (Fig. 16-1)
   • Useful in distinguishing restrictive from obstructive lung disease
  1. Volumes and capacities that are *not* directly measured by spirometry
    a. Functional residual capacity (FRC)
      • Total amount of air in the lungs at the end of a normal expiration
    b. Total lung capacity (TLC)
      • Total amount of air in a fully expanded lung
    c. Residual volume (RV)
      • Volume of air left over in the lung after maximal expiration
  2. Tidal volume (TV)
    • Volume of air that enters or leaves the lungs during normal quiet respiration
  3. Forced vital capacity (FVC), forced expiratory volume in 1 second (FEV$_{1 sec}$), and FEV$_{1 sec}$/FVC

TABLE 16-2:
Comparison of Pulmonary Function Tests in Restrictive and Obstructive Lung Disease

Parameter	Restrictive Disease	Obstructive Disease
Total lung capacity	Decreased	Increased
Residual volume	Decreased	Increased
FEV_{1sec}	Decreased	Decreased
FVC	Decreased	Decreased
FEV_{1sec}/FVC	Normal to increased	Decreased
PaO_2	Decreased	Decreased
A-a gradient	Increased	Increased

A-a, alveolar-arterial; FEV, forced expiratory volume; FVC, forced vital capacity.

    a. FVC is the total amount of air expelled after a maximal inspiration
- Normal FVC is 5 L (see Fig. 16-1A).

    b. Forced expiratory volume in 1 second ($FEV_{1 sec}$)
      (1) Amount of air expelled from the lungs in 1 second after a maximal inspiration
      (2) Normal $FEV_{1 sec}$ is 4 L (see Fig. 16-1A).

    c. Ratio of $FEV_{1 sec}$/FVC is normally 80%.
- Normal ratio is 4 L/5 L, or 80%.

4. Expiratory reserve volume (ERV)
    a. It refers to the amount of air forcibly expelled at the end of a normal expiration.
    b. It is commonly used to calculate residual volume (FRC − ERV = RV).

5. Comparison of pulmonary function tests in restrictive and obstructive lung disease (Table 16-2)

III. Upper Airway Disorders

A. Choanal atresia
1. Unilateral or bilateral bony septum between the nose and the pharynx
2. Newborn turns cyanotic when breast-feeding.
- Crying causes the child to "pink up" again.

B. Nasal polyps
1. Nasal polyps are non-neoplastic tumefactions.
- Develop as a response to chronic inflammation
2. Allergic polyps
    a. Most common polyp
    b. Most often seen in adults with a history of IgE-mediated allergies
3. Nasal polyps associated with aspirin and other nonsteroidal drugs
    a. Epidemiology
- Most often occur in women with chronic pain syndromes
    b. Pathogenesis
      (1) Drugs block cyclooxygenase leaving the lipoxygenase pathway open.
      (2) Leukotrienes (LT) C-D-E_4 are increased, causing bronchoconstriction.
    c. Clinical triad—nonsteroidal drugs, asthma, and nasal polyps
4. Nasal polyps are often associated with cystic fibrosis.

Choanal atresia: newborn cannot breathe through the nose

Allergic polyp: most common polyp

Nasal polyps in child: order a sweat test to rule out cystic fibrosis

C. Obstructive sleep apnea (OSA)
  1. Epidemiology
     a. Excessive snoring with intervals of breath cessation (called apnea)
     b. Causes
        (1) Obesity (very common)
           • Pharyngeal muscles collapse due to the weight of tissue in the neck.
        (2) Tonsillar hypertrophy, nasal septum deviation
  2. Pathogenesis
     • Airway obstruction causes CO_2 retention, leading to hypoxemia.
  3. Clinical findings
     a. Excessive snoring with episodes of apnea
     b. Daytime somnolence often simulating narcolepsy
  4. Laboratory findings
     a. Decreased Po_2 and O_2 saturation during apneic episodes
     b. Increase in arterial Pco_2 (respiratory acidosis)
  5. Complications
     a. Pulmonary hypertension (PH) leading to right ventricular hypertrophy
        • Called cor pulmonale (see section VII)
     b. Secondary polycythemia
        • Due to a hypoxemic stimulus for erythropoietin release
  6. Polysomnography
     • Confirmatory test that documents periods of apnea during sleep
  7. Treatment
     a. Nasal continuous positive airway pressure (CPAP)
     b. Surgical correction of any obstructive lesions, weight loss

D. Sinusitis
  1. Epidemiology
     a. Maxillary sinus is most often involved in adults.
     b. Ethmoid sinus is most often involved in children.
     c. Causes
        (1) Upper respiratory infections (e.g., virus, bacteria)
        (2) Deviated nasal septum, allergic rhinitis, barotrauma, smoking cigarettes
     d. Pathogens causing sinusitis
        (1) *Streptococcus pneumoniae* (most common)
        (2) Rhinoviruses, anaerobes (chronic sinusitis)
        (3) Systemic fungi (e.g., *Mucor* or *Aspergillus* species)
           • Diabetics commonly have sinusitis due to *Mucor* species.
  2. Pathogenesis
     • Blockage of drainage into the nasal cavity
  3. Clinical findings
     a. Fever, nasal congestion, pain over sinuses
     b. Computed tomography (CT) scan is the most sensitive test.

E. Nasopharyngeal carcinoma
  1. Epidemiology
     a. Most common malignant tumor of the nasopharynx

OSA: apnea causes respiratory acidosis and hypoxemia

OSA: risk for developing cor pulmonale

Upper respiratory infections: most common cause of sinusitis

Streptococcus pneumoniae: most common pathogen causing sinusitis

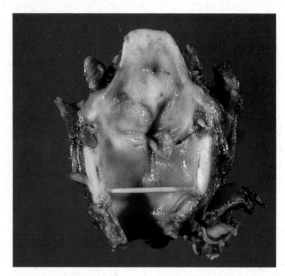

16-2: *Laryngeal squamous cell carcinoma involving the right vocal cord (arrow). (From Damjanov I, Linder J: Pathology: A Color Atlas. St. Louis, Mosby, 2000, p 47, Fig. 3-16.)*

b. Male dominant

c. Increased incidence in the Chinese and African populations

2. Pathogenesis

• Causal relationship with Epstein-Barr virus (EBV)

3. Pathologic findings

a. Squamous cell carcinoma or undifferentiated cancer

b. Metastasizes to cervical lymph nodes

F. Laryngeal carcinoma

1. Epidemiology and pathogenesis

a. More common in men than in women

b. Risk factors

(1) Cigarette smoking (most common cause)

(2) Alcohol (synergistic effect with smoking)

(3) Squamous papillomas and papillomatosis

• Human papillomavirus type 6 and 11 association

c. Majority are located on the true vocal cords (Fig. 16-2).

2. Majority are keratinizing squamous cell carcinomas.

3. Clinical findings

• Persistent hoarseness often associated with cervical lymphadenopathy

IV. Atelectasis

• Loss of lung volume due to inadequate expansion of the airspaces (collapse)

A. Resorption atelectasis

1. Pathogenesis

a. Airway obstruction prevents air from reaching the alveoli.

• Obstruction occurs in bronchi, segmental bronchi, or terminal bronchioles.

Nasopharyngeal carcinoma: association with EBV

Laryngeal carcinoma: cigarette smoking is the most common cause

    b. Causes of obstruction

      (1) Mucus or mucopurulent plug after surgery

      (2) Aspiration of foreign material

      (3) Centrally located bronchogenic carcinoma

    c. Cause of alveolar collapse

      • Lack of air and distal resorption of preexisting air through the pores of Kohn in the alveolar walls

    d. Collapse may involve all or part of a lung.

  2. Clinical findings

    a. Fever and dyspnea

      • Both usually occur within 24 to 36 hours of collapse.

    b. Absent breath sounds and vocal vibratory sensation (tactile fremitus)

    c. Ipsilateral elevation of the diaphragm and tracheal deviation

      • Collapsed lung gives up space, causing the preceding findings.

    d. Collapsed lung does *not* expand on inspiration (inspiratory lag).

B. Compression atelectasis

  1. Air or fluid in the pleural cavity under increased pressure collapses small airways beneath the pleura.

  2. Examples

    a. Tension pneumothorax (air compresses lung)

    b. Pleural effusion (fluid compresses lung)

  3. Trachea deviates to the contralateral side.

C. Atelectasis due to loss of surfactant

  1. Surfactant

    a. Synthesized by type II pneumocytes

      (1) Stored in lamellar bodies (Fig. 16-3)

      (2) Synthesis begins in 28th week of gestation.

    b. Phosphatidylcholine (lecithin) is the major component.

    c. Synthesis is increased by cortisol and thyroxine.

    d. Synthesis is decreased by insulin.

    e. Surfactant reduces surface tension in the small airways.

      • Prevents collapse on expiration, when collapsing pressure is greatest

  2. Respiratory distress syndrome (RDS) in newborns

    a. Pathogenesis

      (1) Decreased surfactant in the fetal lungs; causes:

        (a) Prematurity

        (b) Maternal diabetes

          • Fetal hyperglycemia increases insulin release.

        (c) Cesarean section

          • Lack of stress-induced increase in cortisol from a vaginal delivery

> Women who have to deliver their babies prematurely receive glucocorticoids in order to increase fetal surfactant synthesis thereby reducing the potential for developing RDS. Good maternal glycemic control decreases the risk for RDS.

Resorption atelectasis: most common cause of fever 24 to 36 hours after surgery

Compression atelectasis: air under pressure or fluid in pleural cavity

Surfactant: synthesized in type II pneumocytes

Surfactant: cortisol increases synthesis, insulin inhibits synthesis

RDS: due to a decrease in surfactant

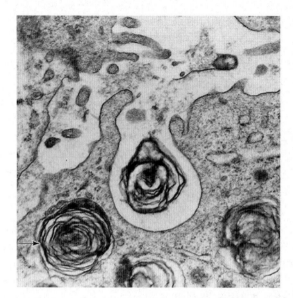

16-3: *Electron micrograph of a type II pneumocyte showing lamellar body (arrow) containing surfactant. (From Corrin B: Pathology of the Lungs. London, Churchill Livingstone, 1999, p 15, Fig. 1-26.)*

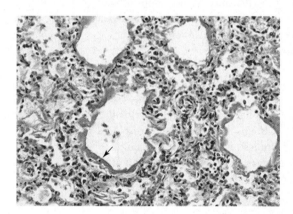

16-4: *Neonatal respiratory distress syndrome. Some of the dilated respiratory bronchioles and alveolar ducts are lined with a fibrin-rich membrane (hyaline membrane) (arrow). The subjacent alveoli are collapsed. (From Damjanov I: Pathology for the Health-Related Professions, 2nd ed. Philadelphia, WB Saunders, 2000, p 128, Fig. 5-25.)*

      (2) Widespread atelectasis results in massive intrapulmonary shunting.
         • Perfusion without ventilation
    b. Collapsed alveoli are lined by hyaline membranes (Fig. 16-4).
      • Derived from proteins leaking out of damaged pulmonary vessels
    c. Clinical findings
      (1) Respiratory difficulty begins within a few hours after birth.
      (2) Infants develop hypoxemia and respiratory acidosis.

(3) Chest radiograph shows a "ground glass" appearance.

d. Complications

(1) Superoxide free radical damage from O_2 therapy
- May result in blindness and permanent damage to small airways (bronchopulmonary dysplasia)

(2) Intraventricular hemorrhage

(3) Patent ductus arteriosus (due to persistent hypoxemia)

(4) Necrotizing enterocolitis
- Intestinal ischemia allows entry of gut bacteria into the intestinal wall.

(5) Hypoglycemia in newborn
- Excess insulin decreases serum glucose producing seizures and damage to neurons.

RDS O_2 complications: blindness, bronchopulmonary dysplasia

Hypoglycemia in newborn: due to excess insulin in response to fetal hyperglycemia

V. Acute Lung Injury

A. Pulmonary edema

1. Edema due to alterations in Starling pressure (transudate)

a. Increased hydrostatic pressure in pulmonary capillaries
- Left-sided heart failure, volume overload, mitral stenosis

b. Decreased oncotic pressure
- Nephrotic syndrome, cirrhosis

2. Edema due to microvascular or alveolar injury (exudate)

a. Infections (e.g., sepsis, pneumonia)

b. Aspiration (e.g., drowning, gastric contents)

c. Drugs (e.g., heroin), shock, massive trauma

d. High altitude

Left-sided heart failure: most common cause of pulmonary edema

B. Acute respiratory distress syndrome (ARDS)

- Noncardiogenic pulmonary edema resulting from acute alveolar-capillary damage.

1. Epidemiology

a. Due to direct injury to the lungs or systemic diseases

b. Risk factors for ARDS

(1) Gram-negative sepsis (40% of cases)

(2) Gastric aspiration (30% of cases)

(3) Severe trauma with shock (10% of cases)

(4) Diffuse pulmonary infections, heroin, smoke inhalation

2. Pathogenesis

a. Acute damage to alveolar capillary walls and epithelial cells

b. Alveolar macrophages and other cells release cytokines.

(1) Cytokines are chemotactic to neutrophils.

(2) Neutrophils transmigrate into the alveoli through pulmonary capillaries.

(3) Capillary damage causes leakage of a protein-rich exudate producing hyaline membranes.

(4) Neutrophils damage type I and II pneumocytes.
- Decrease in surfactant causes atelectasis with intrapulmonary shunting.

ARDS: acute alveolar-capillary damage; sepsis most common cause

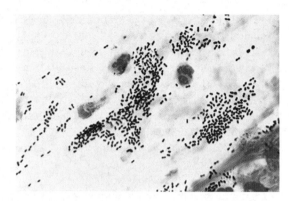

16-5: *Gram stain of* Streptococcus pneumoniae. *The sputum stain shows numerous lancet-shaped diplococci with the tapered ends pointing to each other. A few neutrophils contain phagocytosed bacteria. (From Henry JB: Clinical Diagnosis and Management by Laboratory Methods, 20th ed. Philadelphia, WB Saunders, 2001, Plate 50-1.)*

      c. Late findings
        (1) Repair by type II pneumocytes
        (2) Progressive interstitial fibrosis (restrictive lung disease)
    3. Clinical findings
      a. Dyspnea with severe hypoxemia *not* responsive to O_2 therapy
      b. Acute respiratory acidosis
    4. Poor prognosis (~60% mortality rate)

VI. Pulmonary Infections
  A. Pneumonia
    1. Epidemiology
      a. Classified as community-acquired or nosocomial (hospital-acquired)
      b. Community-acquired pneumonia is further subdivided into typical or atypical.
    2. Typical community-acquired pneumonia
      a. Epidemiology
        (1) Majority are caused by bacterial pathogens.
        (2) Most often due to *Streptococcus pneumoniae* (Fig. 16-5)
      b. Pathogenesis
        (1) Inhalation of aerosol from an infected patient
        (2) Aspiration of nasopharyngeal flora while sleeping
      c. Bronchopneumonia
        (1) Begins as an acute bronchitis and spreads locally into the lungs
        (2) Usually involves the lower lobes or right middle lobe
        (3) Lung has patchy areas of consolidation (Fig. 16-6).
          • Microabscesses are present in the areas of consolidation.
      d. Lobar pneumonia
        • Complete or almost complete consolidation of a lobe of lung
      e. Complications

Streptococcus pneumoniae: most common cause of typical community-acquired pneumonia

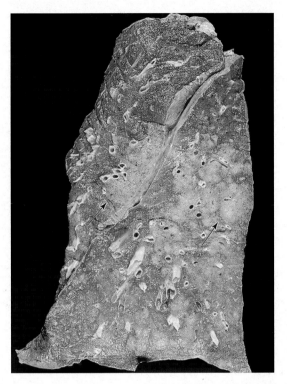

16-6: *Bronchopneumonia showing patchy areas of consolidation (arrows) representing collections of neutrophils in the alveoli and bronchi. (From Kumar V, Fausto N, Abbas A: Robbins and Cotran's Pathologic Basis of Disease, 7th ed. Philadelphia, WB Saunders, 2004, p 749, Fig. 15-33.)*

       (1) Lung abscesses, empyema (pus in the pleural cavity)
       (2) Sepsis
   f. Clinical findings
       (1) Sudden onset of high fever with productive cough
       (2) Signs of consolidation (alveolar exudate)
          (a) Dullness to percussion
          (b) Increased vocal tactile fremitus
             • Sound is transmitted well through alveolar consolidations.
          (c) Inspiratory crackles (air moving through exudate in the alveoli)
       (3) Chest radiograph (gold standard screen)
          • Patchy infiltrates (bronchopneumonia) or lobar consolidation
       (4) Laboratory findings
          (a) Positive Gram stain
          (b) Neutrophilic leukocytosis
  3. Atypical community-acquired pneumonia
   a. Epidemiology
       (1) Usually caused by *Mycoplasma pneumoniae*

Typical pneumonia: signs of consolidation (alveolar exudate)

Chest radiograph: gold standard for diagnosing pneumonia

Mycoplasma pneumoniae: most common cause of atypical pneumonia

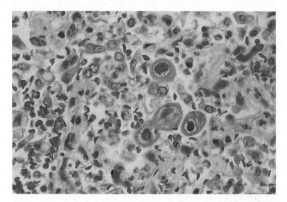

16-7: *Cytomegalovirus. The enlarged nuclei of many of the type I pneumocytes contain large inclusions (basophilic staining with hematoxylin and eosin stain) surrounded by a clear halo. (From Damjanov I, Linder J: Pathology: A Color Atlas. St. Louis, Mosby, 2000, p 56, Fig. 4-24.)*

      (2) Other pathogens
        (a) *Chlamydia pneumoniae* (TWAR agent)
        (b) Viruses (respiratory syncytial virus, influenzavirus, adenovirus)
        (c) *Chlamydia trachomatis* (newborns)
    b. Pathogenesis
      • Contracted by inhalation (droplet infection)

Atypical pneumonia: interstitial pneumonia

    c. Patchy interstitial pneumonia
      (1) Mononuclear infiltrate
      (2) Alveolar spaces usually free of exudate
    d. Clinical findings
      (1) Insidious onset, low-grade fever, nonproductive cough
      (2) Flu-like symptoms
        • Pharyngitis, laryngitis, myalgias, headache
      (3) *No* signs of consolidation
  4. Nosocomial pneumonia
    a. Epidemiology; risk factors
      (1) Severe underlying disease
      (2) Antibiotic therapy, immunosuppression
      (3) Respirators (most common source of infection)

Pseudomonas aeruginosa: nosocomial pneumonia; contracted from respirators

    b. Pathogens
      (1) Gram-negative bacteria
        • *Pseudomonas aeruginosa* (respirators), *Escherichia coli*
      (2) Gram-positive bacteria (e.g., *Staphylococcus aureus*)
  5. Pneumonia in immunocompromised hosts
    a. Complication of AIDS and bone marrow transplantation
    b. Common opportunistic infections:
      (1) Cytomegalovirus (Fig. 16-7)

Pneumocystis jiroveci: most common pathogen causing pneumonia

      (2) *Pneumocystis jiroveci* (Fig. 16-8)
        • Trimethoprim-sulfamethoxazole is used for prophylaxis and treatment.
      (3) *Aspergillus fumigatus* (Fig. 16-9)

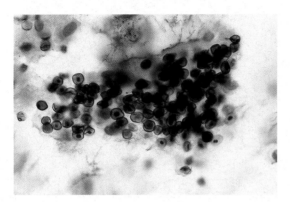

16-8: Pneumocystis jiroveci *pneumonia. This silver-impregnated cytologic smear prepared from bronchial washings in an HIV-positive patient contains numerous* P. jiroveci *cysts. Some cysts look like crushed ping-pong balls. (From Damjanov I, Linder J: Pathology: A Color Atlas. St. Louis, Mosby, 2000, p 56, Fig. 4-22B.)*

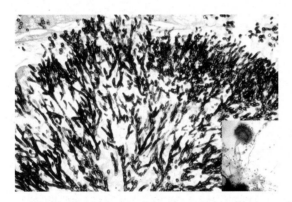

16-9: *Lung biopsy stained with Gomori methenamine-silver showing septated hyphae and fruiting body (inset) of Aspergillus fumigatus. (From Kumar V, Fausto N, Abbas A: Robbins and Cotran's Pathologic Basis of Disease, 7th ed. Philadelphia, WB Saunders, 2004, p 400, Fig. 8-49B.)*

6. Tuberculosis (TB)
    a. Epidemiology and pathophysiology
        (1) Contracted by inhalation of *Mycobacterium tuberculosis*
        (2) Characteristics
            • Strict aerobe, acid-fast (due to mycolic acid in cell wall) (Fig. 16-10)
        (3) Screening
            (a) Purified protein derivative (PPD) intradermal skin test
            (b) Does *not* distinguish active from inactive disease
    b. Primary TB
        (1) Subpleural location
            • Upper part of the lower lobes or lower part of the upper lobes
        (2) Usually resolves
            (a) Produces a calcified granuloma or area of scar tissue
            (b) May be a nidus for secondary TB

PPD: does *not* distinguish active from inactive TB

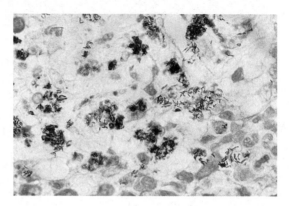

16-10: *Acid-fast stain of a lung biopsy in a patient with reactivation tuberculosis due to Mycobacterium tuberculosis. Large numbers of red-staining, acid-fast bacilli are present. (From Hoffbrand AV: Color Atlas: Clinical Hematology, 3rd ed. St. Louis, Mosby, 2000, p 136, Fig. 7-85B.)*

c. Secondary (reactivation) TB
   (1) Due to reactivation of a previous primary TB site
   (2) Involves one or both apices in upper lobes
      • Ventilation (oxygenation) is greatest in the upper lobes.

(margin note) Reactivation TB: upper lobe cavitary lesion(s)

   (3) Cavitary lesion due to release of cytokines from memory T cells
d. Clinical findings
   • Fever, drenching night sweats, weight loss
e. Complications
   (1) Miliary spread in lungs due to invasion into the bronchus or lymphatics
   (2) Miliary spread to extrapulmonary sites

(margin note) Kidneys: most common extrapulmonary site in TB

      (a) Due to invasion of pulmonary vein tributaries
      (b) Kidney is the most common extrapulmonary site.
   (3) Massive hemoptysis, bronchiectasis, scar carcinoma
   (4) Granulomatous hepatitis, spread to vertebra (Pott's disease)
7. *Mycobacterium avium-intracellulare* complex (MAC)
   a. Atypical mycobacterium
   b. Most common TB in AIDS (often disseminates)
      • Occurs when CD4 T_H count falls below 50 cells/μL
8. Systemic fungal infections (Fig. 16-11)
   a. Contracted from inhalation of the pathogen
   b. Produce a granulomatous inflammatory reaction with or without caseation
9. Summaries of respiratory microbial pathogens (Table 16-3)
B. Lung abscess
1. Causes of lung abscesses

(margin note) Lung abscesses: most often due to aspiration of oropharyngeal material

   a. Most often due to aspiration of oropharyngeal material (e.g., tonsillar material)

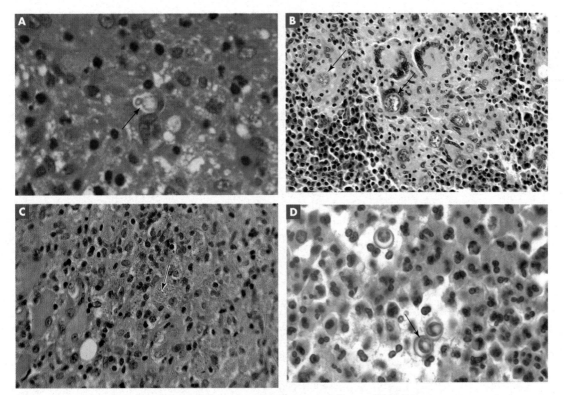

16-11: *Common systemic fungal infections. The yeast form of* Cryptococcus neoformans *(A) produces a narrow-based bud (arrow).* Coccidioides immitis *(B) has spherules containing endospores (arrows). Multinucleated giant cells are also present.* Histoplasma capsulatum *(C) has yeast forms (arrows) phagocytosed by macrophages.* Blastomyces dermatidis *(D) has yeast forms with broad-based buds (arrow). The yeasts also contain nuclei. (Part A from Corrin B: Pathology of the Lungs. London, Churchill Livingstone, 1999, p 215, Fig. 5-4-23A; Parts B and D from Kumar V, Fausto N, Abbas A: Robbins and Cotran's Pathologic Basis of Disease, 7th ed. Philadelphia, WB Saunders, 2004, pp 755 and 756, Figs. 15-39A and 15–40, respectively; Part C from Hoffbrand AV: Color Atlas: Clinical Hematology, 3rd ed. St. Louis, Mosby, 2000, p 303, Fig. 17-29.)*

       (1) Aerobic and anaerobic streptococci and *Staphylococci, Prevotella, Fusobacterium*

       (2) Occurs in patients with depressed cough reflexes (e.g., after anesthesia)

    b. Complication of bacterial pneumonia (e.g., *Staphylococcus aureus, Klebsiella*)

    c. Septic embolism (e.g., infective endocarditis)

    d. Obstructive lung neoplasia

       • From 10% to 15% of abscesses are behind a bronchus obstructed by cancer.

  2. Gross findings

    a. Vary in size and location

TABLE 16-3:
Summary of
Respiratory
Microbial
Pathogens

Pathogen	Discussion
Viruses	
Rhinovirus	Most common cause of the common cold Transmitted by hand to eye-nose contact
RSV	Most common viral cause of atypical pneumonia and bronchiolitis (wheezing) in children Occurs in late fall and winter
Parainfluenza	Most common cause of croup (laryngotracheobronchitis) in infants Inspiratory stridor (upper airway obstruction) due to submucosal edema in trachea Anterior x-ray of neck shows "steeple sign," representing mucosal edema in the trachea (site of obstruction)
CMV	Common pneumonia in immunocompromised hosts (e.g., bone marrow transplants, AIDS) Enlarged alveolar macrophages/pneumocytes, contain basophilic intranuclear inclusions surrounded by a halo (see Fig. 16-7)
Influenzavirus	Type A viruses are most often involved Hemagglutinins bind virus to cell receptors in the nasal passages Neuraminidase dissolves mucus and facilitates release of viral particles Influenza A pneumonia may be complicated by a superimposed bacterial pneumonia (usually *Staphylococcus aureus*)
Rubeola	Fever, cough, conjunctivitis, and excessive nasal mucus production Koplik spots in the mouth precede onset of the rash Warthin-Finkeldey multinucleated giant cells are a characteristic finding
SARS	Infects lower respiratory tract and then spreads systemically to produce severe respiratory infection First transmitted to humans through contact with masked palm civets (China) and then from human-to-human contact through respiratory secretions (e.g., hospitals, families) Diagnose with viral detection by PCR or detection of antibodies
Chlamydia	
C. pneumoniae	Second most common cause of atypical pneumonia
C. trachomatis	Newborn pneumonia (passage through birth canal) Afebrile, staccato cough (choppy cough), conjunctivitis, wheezing
Rickettsia	
Coxiella burnetii	Only rickettsia transmitted *without* a vector Contracted by dairy farmers, veterinarians Associated with the birthing process of infected sheep, cattle, and goats, and handling of milk or excrement Atypical pneumonia, myocarditis, granulomatous hepatitis
Mycoplasma	
M. pneumoniae	Most common cause of atypical pneumonia Common in adolescents and military recruits (closed spaces) Insidious onset with low-grade fever Complications: bullous myringitis, cold autoimmune hemolytic anemia due to anti-I-IgM antibodies Cold agglutinins in blood
Bacteria	
Streptococcus pneumoniae	Gram-positive lancet-shaped diplococcus Most common cause of typical community acquired pneumonia Rapid onset, productive cough, signs of consolidation

TABLE 16-3:
Summary of
Respiratory
Microbial
Pathogens—cont'd

Pathogen	Discussion
Bacteria— cont'd	
Staphylococcus aureus	Gram-positive coccus in clumps Yellow sputum Commonly superimposed on influenza pneumonia and measles pneumonia Major lung pathogen in cystic fibrosis and intravenous drug abusers Hemorrhagic pulmonary edema, abscess formation, and tension pneumatocysts (intrapleural blebs), which may rupture and produce a tension pneumothorax
Corynebacterium diphtheriae	Gram-positive rod Toxin inhibits protein synthesis by ADP-ribosylation of elongation factor 2 involved in protein synthesis; toxin also impairs β-oxidation of fatty acids in the heart Toxin-induced pseudomembranous inflammation produces shaggy gray membranes in the oropharynx and trachea
Haemophilus influenzae	Gram-negative rod Common cause of sinusitis, otitis media, conjunctivitis (pink eye) Inspiratory stridor may be due to acute epiglottitis; swelling of epiglottis produces "thumbprint sign" on lateral x-ray of the neck Most common bacterial cause of acute exacerbation of COPD
Moraxella catarrhalis	Gram-negative diplococcus Common cause of typical pneumonia, especially in the elderly Second most common pathogen causing acute exacerbation of COPD Common cause of chronic bronchitis, sinusitis, otitis media
Pseudomonas aeruginosa	Gram-negative rod Green sputum (pyocyanin) Water-loving bacteria most often transmitted by respirators Most common cause of nosocomial pneumonia and death due to pneumonia in cystic fibrosis; pneumonia often associated with infarction due to vessel invasion
Klebsiella pneumoniae	Gram-negative fat rod surrounded by a mucoid capsule Most common gram-negative organism causing lobar pneumonia and typical pneumonia in elderly patients in nursing homes Common cause of pneumonia in alcoholics; however, *S. pneumoniae* is still the most common pneumonia Pneumonia associated with blood-tinged, thick, mucoid sputum; lobar consolidation and abscess formation are common
Legionella pneumophila	Gram-negative rod (requires IF stain or Dieterle silver stain to identify in tissue); antigens can also be detected in urine Water-loving bacteria (water coolers; mists in produce section of grocery stores; outdoor restaurants in summer; rain forests in zoos) Pneumonia associated with high fever, dry cough, flu-like symptoms May produce tubulointerstitial disease with destruction of the juxtaglomerular apparatus leading to hyporeninemic hypoaldosteronism (type IV renal tubular acidosis—hyponatremia, hyperkalemia, metabolic acidosis)
Systemic Fungi	
Cryptococcus neoformans (Fig. 16-11A)	Budding yeast with narrow-based buds; surrounded by a thick capsule Found in pigeon excreta (around buildings, outside office windows, under bridges) Most common opportunistic fungal infection Primary lung disease (40%): granulomatous inflammation with caseation

TABLE 16-3: Summary of Respiratory Microbial Pathogens—cont'd

Pathogen	Discussion
Systemic Fungi—cont'd	
Aspergillus fumigatus (Fig. 16-9)	Fruiting body and narrow-angled (<45 degrees), branching septate hyphae Aspergilloma: fungus ball (visible on x-ray) that develops in a preexisting cavity in the lung (e.g., old TB site); cause of massive hemoptysis Allergic bronchopulmonary aspergillosis: type I and type III hypersensitivity reactions; IgE levels increased; eosinophilia; intense inflammation of airways and mucus plugs in terminal bronchioles; repeated attacks may lead to bronchiectasis and interstitial lung disease Vessel invader with hemorrhagic infarctions and a necrotizing bronchopneumonia
Mucor species	Wide-angled hyphae (>45 degrees) without septa Clinical settings: diabetes, immunosuppressed patients Vessel invader and produces hemorrhagic infarcts in the lung Invades the frontal lobes in patients with diabetic ketoacidosis (rhinocerebral mucormycosis)
Coccidioides immitis (Fig. 16-11B)	Spherules with endospores in tissues; contracted by inhaling arthrospores in dust while living or passing through arid desert areas in the southwestern United States ("valley fever"); increased after earthquakes (increased dust) Flu-like symptoms and erythema nodosum (painful nodules on lower legs; inflammation of subcutaneous fat) Granulomatous inflammation with caseous necrosis
Histoplasma capsulatum (Fig. 16-11C)	Most common systemic fungal infection; endemic in Ohio and central Mississippi River valleys; inhalation of microconidia in dust contaminated with excreta from bats (increased incidence in cave explorers, spelunkers), starlings, or chickens (common in chicken farmers) Granulomatous inflammation with caseous necrosis Yeast forms are present in macrophages Simulates TB lung disease; produces coin lesions, consolidations, miliary spread, and cavitation Marked dystrophic calcification of granulomas; most common cause of multiple calcifications in the spleen
Blastomyces dermatitidis (Fig. 16-11D)	Yeasts have broad-based buds and nuclei; occurs in Great Lakes region and central and southeastern United States; male-dominant disease Produces skin and lung disease; skin lesions simulate squamous cell carcinoma Granulomatous inflammation with caseous necrosis
*Pneumocystis jiroveci** (Fig. 16-8)	Cysts and trophozoites present; cysts attach to type I pneumocytes Primarily an opportunistic infection; occurs when CD4 T_H count < 200 Most common initial AIDS-defining infection Patients develop fever, dyspnea, and severe hypoxemia; diffuse intra-alveolar foamy exudates with cup-shaped cysts best visualized with silver or Giemsa stains; chest x-ray shows diffuse alveolar and interstitial infiltrates Rx: TMP/SMX given prophylactically when CD4 counts < 200 cells/µL

*Recent nomenclature change from *P. carinii*.
ADP, adenosine diphosphate; CMV, cytomegalovirus; COPD, chronic obstructive pulmonary disease; IF, immunofluorescence; PCR, polymerase chain reaction; RSV, respiratory syncytial virus; SARS, severe acute respiratory syndrome; TB, tuberculosis; TMP/SMX, trimethoprim-sulfamethoxazole.

BOX 16-1

ASPIRATION SITES IN THE LUNGS

Foreign material localizes to different portions of the lung, depending on the position of the patient. In the standing or sitting position, material localizes in the posterobasal segment of the right lower lobe; in the supine position, the superior segment of the right lower lobe; and in the right-sided position, the right middle lobe or the posterior segment of the right upper lobe. The most common aspiration site is the superior segment of the right lower lobe.

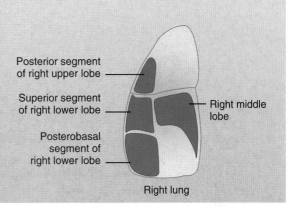

Posterior segment of right upper lobe

Superior segment of right lower lobe

Right middle lobe

Posterobasal segment of right lower lobe

Right lung

b. Those due to aspiration are primarily located on the right side (Box 16-1).

3. Clinical findings
    a. Spiking fever with productive cough (foul-smelling sputum)
    b. Chest radiograph shows cavitation with an air-fluid level.

VII. Vascular Lung Lesions
  A. Pulmonary thromboembolism
    1. Epidemiology and pathogenesis
        a. Source
            • Majority (95%) originate in the femoral vein
        b. Risk factors for thromboembolism (see Chapter 4)
            • Stasis of blood flow (e.g., prolonged bed rest), hypercoagulable states
        c. Size of the embolus determines pulmonary vessel that is occluded.
            (1) Large emboli occlude the major vessels (saddle embolus) (Fig. 16-12).
            (2) Small emboli occlude medium-sized and small pulmonary arteries.
        d. Potential consequences of pulmonary artery occlusion
            (1) Increase in pulmonary artery pressure
            (2) Decrease blood flow to pulmonary parenchyma
                • May cause hemorrhagic infarction.

> In a patient with normal bronchial artery blood flow (originates from thoracic aorta and intercostal arteries) and ventilation, a pulmonary embolus produces a hemorrhagic infarction in ~10% of cases. However, if the patient has

Superior segment, right lower lobe: most common site for aspiration

Source of pulmonary thromboemboli: femoral veins

Bronchial arteries: protect lungs from infarction

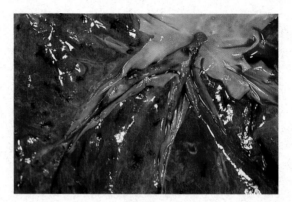

16-12: *Saddle embolus occluding the main branches of the pulmonary artery. (From Damjanov I, Linder J: Pathology: A Color Atlas. St. Louis, Mosby, 2000, p 57, Fig. 4-26.)*

decreased bronchial artery blood flow (e.g., decreased cardiac output), or previously underventilated lung (e.g., obstructive lung disease), then occlusion of the pulmonary vessel will likely result in a hemorrhagic infarction, which significantly increases risk of morbidity and death.

2. Red-blue, raised, wedge-shaped area that extends to the pleural surface (see Fig. 1-10)
   a. Pleural surface has a fibrinous exudate (produces a pleural friction rub).
      • Hemorrhagic pleural effusion may also occur.
   b. Majority are located in the lower lobes.
      • Perfusion is greater than ventilation in the lower lobes.
3. Clinical findings
   a. Saddle embolus
      (1) Sudden increase in pulmonary artery pressure
      (2) Produces acute right ventricular strain and sudden death
   b. Pulmonary infarction
      (1) Sudden onset of dyspnea and tachypnea
      (2) Fever
      (3) Pleuritic chest pain (pain on inspiration), friction rub, effusion
4. Laboratory findings with a pulmonary infarction
   a. Respiratory alkalosis (arterial $P_{CO_2} < 33\,mm\,Hg$)
   b. Pa_{O_2} less than $80\,mm\,Hg$ (90% of cases)
   c. Increase in A-a gradient (100% of cases)
   d. Abnormal perfusion radionuclide scan
      (1) Ventilation scan is normal, but the perfusion scan is abnormal.
      (2) Pulmonary angiogram is gold standard confirmatory test.
   e. Positive D-dimers (see Chapter 14)

B. Pulmonary hypertension (PH)
   1. Epidemiology and pathogenesis

Pulmonary infarction: dyspnea and tachypnea most common symptom and sign

Pulmonary infarction: normal ventilation scan, abnormal perfusion scan

a. Primary PH
   (1) Primary type is more common in women.
   (2) Vascular hyperreactivity with proliferation of smooth muscle
b. Secondary PH
   (1) Endothelial cell dysfunction
      • Loss of vasodilators (e.g., nitric oxide), increase in vasoconstrictors (e.g., endothelin)
   (2) Hypoxemia and/or respiratory acidosis stimulate vasoconstriction of pulmonary arteries.
      • Causes smooth muscle hyperplasia and hypertrophy
   (3) Causes

   Main cause of secondary PH: respiratory acidosis and/or hypoxemia

      (a) Chronic hypoxemia (e.g., chronic lung disease)
      (b) Chronic respiratory acidosis (e.g., chronic bronchitis)
      (c) Loss of pulmonary vasculature (e.g., emphysema)
         • Increases workload for remaining vessels
      (d) Left-to-right cardiac shunts (see Chapter 10)
      (e) Mitral stenosis
         • Backup of blood into the pulmonary veins
2. Pathologic findings
   a. Atherosclerosis of main elastic pulmonary arteries
      • Due to increased pressure on the endothelium leading to injury
   b. Proliferation of myointimal cells and smooth muscle cells
3. Clinical findings
   a. Progressive dyspnea and chest pain with exertion
   b. Chest radiograph shows tapering of the pulmonary arteries
   c. Accentuated P_2 (sign of PH)
   d. Left parasternal heave (sign of right ventricular hypertrophy, RVH)
      • PH imposes an increased afterload on the right ventricle.
   e. Right-sided heart failure due to cor pulmonale
4. Cor pulmonale
   • Combination of PH and right RVH leading to right-sided heart failure
C. **Goodpasture syndrome (see Chapter 19)**
   • Pulmonary hemorrhage with hemoptysis often precedes renal failure.

VIII. **Restrictive Lung Diseases**
   • These disorders are characterized by reduced total lung capacity in the presence of a normal or reduced expiratory flow rate.
A. **Causes of restrictive disease**
   1. Chest wall disorders in the presence of normal lungs
      • Examples—kyphoscoliosis, pleural disease (e.g., mesothelioma), obesity
   2. Acute or chronic interstitial lung diseases
      a. Acute interstitial disease (e.g., ARDS, see section V)
      b. Chronic interstitial disease
         (1) Fibrosing disorders (e.g., pneumoconiosis)
         (2) Granulomatous disease (e.g., sarcoidosis)

B. Pathogenesis of interstitial fibrosis
1. Earliest manifestation is an alveolitis.
   - Leukocytes release cytokines, which stimulate fibrosis.
2. Effects of interstitial fibrosis
   a. Decreases lung compliance
      (1) Decreased expansion of the lung parenchyma during inspiration
      (2) Damage to type I/II alveolar cells and endothelial cells
         - Functional loss of alveolar and capillary units
   b. Increases lung elasticity
      - Recoil of the lung on expiration is increased.
3. Clinical and laboratory findings in all restrictive lung diseases
   a. Dry cough and exertional dyspnea
   b. Late inspiratory crackles in lower lung fields
   c. Potential for cor pulmonale
   d. Pulmonary function test findings and arterial blood gases
      (1) All volumes and capacities are equally decreased.
      (2) Decreased $FEV_{1\,sec}$ (see Fig. 16-1B)
         - Example—3 L (normal 4 L)
      (3) Decreased FVC (see Fig. 16-1B)
         - Often the same value as $FEV_{1\,sec}$ (3 L) due to increased lung elasticity
      (4) Increased ratio of $FEV_{1\,sec}/FVC$
         - Example—3/3 = 100% (normal is 80%)
      (5) Respiratory alkalosis (arterial $P_{CO_2} < 33\,mm\,Hg$)
      (6) Decreased Pa_{O_2}
   e. Chest radiograph findings
      - Diffuse bilateral reticulonodular infiltrates

C. Pneumoconioses
1. Epidemiology
   a. Inhalation of mineral dust into the lungs leading to interstitial fibrosis
      (1) Mineral dust includes coal dust, silica, asbestos, and beryllium.
      (2) Accounts for ~25% of cases of chronic interstitial lung disease
   b. Particle size determines site of lung deposition
      (1) 1- to 5-μm particles
         - Reach the bifurcation of the respiratory bronchioles and alveolar ducts
      (2) Smaller than 0.5-μm particles
         - Reach the alveoli and are phagocytosed by alveolar macrophages
   c. Coal dust is the least fibrogenic particle.
   d. Silica, asbestos, and beryllium are very fibrogenic.
2. Coal worker's pneumoconiosis (CWP)
   a. Sources of coal dust (anthracotic pigment)
      - Coal mines, large urban centers, tobacco smoke
   b. Pulmonary anthracosis
      (1) Usually asymptomatic

Restrictive lung disease: ↓ compliance, ↑ elasticity

Restrictive lung disease: ↓ volumes/capacities, normal to ↑ $FEV_{1\,sec}/FVC$ ratio

Pneumoconiosis: inhalation of mineral dust

        (2) Anthracotic pigment in interstitial tissue and hilar nodes
- Alveolar macrophages with anthracotic pigment are called "dust cells."

   c. Simple CWP

        (1) Fibrotic opacities are smaller than 1 cm in upper lobes and upper portions of lower lobes.

        (2) Coal deposits adjacent to respiratory bronchioles produce centrilobular emphysema (see section IX).

   d. Complicated CWP (progressive massive fibrosis)

        (1) Fibrotic opacities larger than −1 to 2 cm with or without necrotic centers

        (2) Crippling lung disease ("black lung" disease)

        (3) *No* increased incidence of TB or primary lung cancer

        (4) Cor pulmonale may occur.

        (5) Caplan syndrome may occur.
- CWP plus large cavitating rheumatoid nodules in the lungs

> Complicated CWP: black lung disease

3. Silicosis

   a. Epidemiology

        (1) Most common occupational disease in the world

        (2) Quartz (crystalline silicone dioxide) is most often implicated
- Sources: foundries (casting metal), sandblasting, working in mines

   b. Pathogenesis

        (1) Quartz is highly fibrogenic and deposits in the upper lungs.

        (2) Quartz activates and is cytolytic to alveolar macrophages.
- Macrophages release cytokines that stimulate fibrogenesis.

   c. Chronic exposure

        (1) Nodular opacities in the lungs

            (a) Concentric layers of collagen with or without central cavitation

            (b) Quartz polarizes in the nodules.

        (2) "Egg-shell" calcification in hilar nodes
- Rim of dystrophic calcification in the nodes

> Silicosis: opacities contain collagen and quartz

   d. Complications

        (1) Cor pulmonale, Caplan syndrome

        (2) Increased risk for developing lung cancer and TB

4. Asbestos-related disease

   a. Geometric forms of asbestos

        (1) Serpentine

            (a) Curly and flexible fibers (e.g., chrysotile)

            (b) Produces interstitial fibrosis and lung cancer

        (2) Amphibole

            (a) Straight and rigid (e.g., crocidolite)

            (b) Produces interstitial fibrosis, lung cancer, mesothelioma

        (3) Deposition sites
- Respiratory bronchioles, alveolar ducts, alveoli

> Asbestos fibers deposit in the respiratory unit.

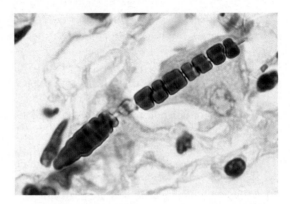

16-13: *Asbestos body. The straight, golden-brown, beaded asbestos body represents an asbestos fiber coated by iron and protein. (From Damjanov I, Linder J: Pathology: A Color Atlas. St. Louis, Mosby, 2000, p 65, Fig. 4-51B.)*

b. Sources
   (1) Insulation around pipes in old naval ships
   (2) Roofing material used over 20 years ago
   (3) Demolition of old buildings

c. Appearance in tissue
   (1) Fibers are coated by iron and protein (called ferruginous bodies)
      • Macrophages phagocytose and coat the fibers with ferritin.
   (2) Golden, beaded appearance in sputum or in distal, small airways (Fig. 16-13)

d. Asbestos-related disease
   (1) Benign pleural plaques
      (a) Calcified plaques on the pleura and dome of the diaphragm
      (b) They are *not* a precursor lesion for a mesothelioma.
   (2) Diffuse interstitial fibrosis with or without pleural effusions
   (3) Primary bronchogenic carcinoma
      (a) Risk further increases if the patient smokes cigarettes.
      (b) Occurs ~20 years after first exposure.
   (4) Malignant mesothelioma of pleura
      (a) *No* etiologic relationship with smoking
      (b) Arises from the serosal cells lining the pleura
      (c) Encases and locally invades the subpleural lung tissue (Fig. 16-14)
      (d) Occurs ~25 to 40 years after first exposure
   (5) *No* increased risk for TB

e. Complications
   • Cor pulmonale, Caplan syndrome

5. Berylliosis
   a. Exposure in the nuclear and aerospace industry
   b. Diffuse interstitial fibrosis with noncaseating granulomas
   c. Increased risk for cor pulmonale and primary lung cancer

Benign pleural plaques: most common lesions

Bronchogenic carcinoma: most common asbestos-related cancer

Malignant mesothelioma: arises from serosa of pleura; encases the lung

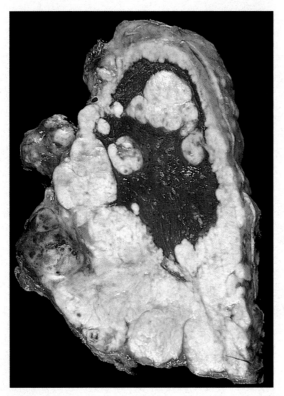

16-14: *Malignant mesothelioma encases the lung and invades locally into the lung parenchyma. (From Kumar V, Fausto N, Abbas A: Robbins and Cotran's Pathologic Basis of Disease, 7th ed. Philadelphia, WB Saunders, 2004, p 768, Fig. 15-48.)*

D. Sarcoidosis
- Multisystem granulomatous disease of unknown etiology
1. Epidemiology
    a. Accounts for ~25% of cases of chronic interstitial lung disease
    b. Common in black Americans and nonsmokers
2. Pathogenesis
    a. Disorder in immune regulation
    b. CD4 T_H cells interact with an unknown antigen.
        - Releases cytokines causing formation of noncaseating granulomas
    c. Diagnosis of exclusion
        - Must rule out other granulomatous diseases
3. Lung disease
    a. Primary target organ
        (1) Granulomas located in the interstitium and mediastinal and hilar nodes
        (2) Granulomas contain multinucleated giant cells (Fig. 16-15).
            - Contain laminated calcium concretions (Schaumann bodies) and stellate inclusions (called asteroid bodies)
    b. Dyspnea is the most common symptom.

Sarcoidosis: most common noninfectious granulomatous disease of the lungs

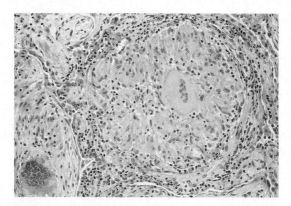

16-15: *Sarcoid granuloma showing pink-staining epithelioid cells and foreign body type of multinucleated giant cells. (From Kumar V, Fausto N, Abbas A: Robbins and Cotran's Pathologic Basis of Disease, 7th ed. Philadelphia, WB Saunders, 2004, p 738, Fig. 15-23.)*

4. Skin lesions
   a. Nodular lesions containing granulomas
   b. Violaceous rash occurs on the nose and cheeks (called lupus pernio).
   c. Erythema nodosum
      (1) Painful nodules on lower extremities
      (2) Inflammation of subcutaneous fat
5. Eye lesions; produces uveitis:
   • Blurry vision, glaucoma, and corneal opacities
6. Liver lesions
   • Granulomatous hepatitis
7. Other multisystem findings
   a. Enlarged salivary and lacrimal glands
   b. Diabetes insipidus (hypothalamic and/or posterior pituitary disease)
   c. Granulomas in the bone marrow and spleen
8. Laboratory findings
   a. Increased angiotensin-converting enzyme (ACE)
      • Good marker of disease activity and response to corticosteroid therapy
   b. Hypercalcemia (5% of cases)
      • Increased synthesis of 1-α-hydroxylase in granulomas (hypervitaminosis D)
   c. Other findings
      (1) Polyclonal gammopathy
      (2) Cutaneous anergy to common skin antigens (e.g., *Candida*)
         • Due to consumption of CD4 T_H cells in granulomas and loss of cells in alveolar secretions
9. Chest radiograph
   a. Enlarged hilar and mediastinal lymph nodes (called "potato nodes")
   b. Reticulonodular densities throughout the lung parenchyma

Sarcoidosis: most common noninfectious granulomatous disease of the liver

10. Prognosis
    a. Progressive disease or intermittent disease with periods of activity and remissions
    b. Between 10% and 15% develop severe interstitial fibrosis, leading to cor pulmonale and death.

E. Idiopathic pulmonary fibrosis

1. Epidemiology
   a. Accounts for ~15% of cases of chronic interstitial lung disease
   b. More common in males than in females
   c. Usually occurs in individuals over 40 to 70 years old
2. Pathogenesis
   a. Repeated cycles of alveolitis triggered by an unknown agent
   b. Release of cytokines produces interstitial fibrosis
3. Alveolar fibrosis leads to proximal dilation of the small airways.
   • Lung has a honeycomb appearance.

F. Collagen vascular diseases

1. Account for ~10% of cases of chronic interstitial lung disease
2. Systemic sclerosis (see Chapter 3)
   • Most common cause of death is lung disease.
3. Systemic lupus erythematosus (SLE)
   a. Interstitial lung disease occurs in 50% of patients.
   b. Pleuritis with pleural effusions

> Any unexplained pleural effusion in a young woman is SLE until proved otherwise. Pleural fluid contains an inflammatory infiltrate (exudate), and LE cells (neutrophils with phagocytosed DNA) are sometimes present. One of the key criteria for diagnosing SLE is the presence of serositis, pleuritis with a pleural effusion being an example of this type of inflammation.

4. Rheumatoid arthritis (RA)
   a. Rheumatoid nodules in lungs plus a pneumoconiosis is called Caplan syndrome.
   b. Pulmonary findings in RA
      (1) Interstitial fibrosis with or without intrapulmonary rheumatoid nodules
      (2) Pleuritis with pleural effusions

G. Hypersensitivity pneumonitis

1. Extrinsic allergic alveolitis associated with exposure to a *known* inhaled antigen
   • Does *not* involve IgE antibodies (type I hypersensitivity) or have eosinophilia
2. Farmer's lung
   a. Exposure to *Saccharopolyspora rectivirgula* (thermophilic actinomycetes bacteria) in moldy hay
   b. First exposure
      • Patient develops precipitating IgG antibodies (present in serum)
   c. Second exposure

Farmer's lung: antigen is thermophilic actinomyces in moldy hay

(1) Antibodies combine with inhaled allergens to form immune complexes.
  • Type III hypersensitivity reaction
(2) Immunocomplexes produce an inflammatory reaction in lung tissue.
  d. Chronic exposure
    • Additional component of granulomatous inflammation (type IV hypersensitivity)
3. Silo filler's disease
  a. Inhalation of gases (oxides of nitrogen) from plant material
  b. Causes an immediate hypersensitivity reaction associated with dyspnea
4. Byssinosis
  a. Epidemiology
    (1) Occurs in workers in textile factories
    (2) Contact with cotton, linen, hemp products
  b. Clinical findings
    (1) Develop dyspnea on exposure to cotton, linen, or hemp products
    (2) Workers feel better over the weekend (no exposure to antigens)
      • Depression occurs when returning to work on Monday ("Monday morning blues")

H. Drugs associated with interstitial fibrosis
1. Amiodarone
2. Bleomycin and busulfan
3. Cyclophosphamide
4. Methotrexate and methysergide
5. Nitrosourea and nitrofurantoin

I. Radiation-induced lung disease
1. Acute pneumonitis may occur 1 to 6 months after therapy.
2. Clinical findings
  • Fever, dyspnea, pleural effusions, and radiologic infiltrates
3. Some patients develop chronic radiation pneumonitis.

IX. Obstructive Lung Disease
  • Obstruction to airflow out of the lungs
A. Emphysema
1. Permanent enlargement of all or part of the respiratory unit
  • Respiratory bronchioles, alveolar ducts, alveoli
2. Epidemiology
  a. Causes
    (1) Cigarette smoking is the most common cause.
    (2) α_1-Antitrypsin (AAT) deficiency
  b. Types of emphysema associated with smoking or loss of AAT
    (1) Centriacinar (centrilobular) emphysema
    (2) Panacinar emphysema
3. Pathogenesis
  a. Increased compliance and decreased elasticity

Silo filler's disease: inhalation of gases (oxides of nitrogen)

Byssinosis: contact with cotton, linen, hemp products

Emphysema: targets the respiratory unit

Cigarette smoking: most common cause of emphysema

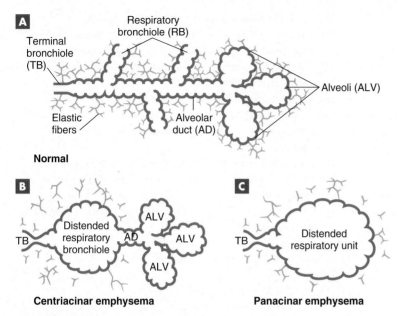

16-16: Types of emphysema. **A,** The schematic shows a normal distal airway, including a terminal bronchiole (TB) leading into the respiratory unit consisting of a respiratory bronchiole (RB), alveolar duct (AD), and alveoli (ALV). Elastic fibers apply radial traction to keep these airways open. **B,** Centriacinar emphysema is characterized by trapping of air in the respiratory bronchioles. Note how the elastic fibers of the distal TB are destroyed causing obstruction to airflow. This causes the trapped air to distend the RBs, whose elastic tissue support is destroyed. **C,** Panacinar emphysema is characterized by trapping of air in the entire respiratory unit behind the collapsed TB.

(1) Imbalance between elastase and antielastases (e.g., α_1-antitrypsin, AAT)

(2) Imbalance between oxidants (free radicals) and antioxidants (e.g., glutathione)

(3) Elastase and oxidants derive from neutrophils and macrophages.

(4) Net effect of the preceding is destruction of elastic tissue.

b. Cigarette smoke is chemotactic to neutrophils and macrophages.

- They accumulate in the respiratory unit and release free radicals and elastases.

c. Free radicals in cigarette smoke inactivate AAT and antioxidants.

- Produces a functional AAT deficiency

d. Normal function of elastic tissue

(1) Fibers attach to the outside wall of the small airways (Fig. 16-16A).

(2) Fibers apply radial traction to keep the airway lumens open.

e. Destruction of elastic tissue causes loss of radial traction.

- Small airways collapse, particularly on expiration.

f. Sites of elastic tissue destruction in emphysema

(1) Distal terminal bronchiole at its junction with the respiratory bronchiole (RB)

(2) All or part of the respiratory unit

Emphysema:
↑ compliance,
↓ elasticity

g. Site of obstruction and air trapping in emphysema
   (1) During expiration, the distal terminal bronchioles collapse preventing egress of air out of the respiratory unit.
   (2) Trapped air distends parts of the respiratory unit that have lost their elastic tissue support.
4. Centriacinar (centrilobular) emphysema (see Fig. 16-16B)
   a. Epidemiology
      • Most common type of emphysema in smokers
   b. Pathogenesis
      (1) Primarily involves the apical segments of the upper lobes
      (2) Distal terminal bronchioles and the RBs are the sites of elastic tissue destruction.
      (3) Air trapped behind the collapsed distal terminal bronchioles distends the RBs.
         • The trapped air increases RV and TLC.
5. Panacinar emphysema (see Fig. 16-16C)
   a. Epidemiology
      (1) Associated with AAT deficiency
         • Genetic or acquired causes (cigarette smoke inactivates AAT)
      (2) Genetic type of AAT deficiency
         (a) Autosomal dominant disorder
         (b) MM phenotype is normal.
            • Normal amounts of AAT are synthesized in the liver.
         (c) ZZ phenotype has decreased synthesis of AAT by the liver.
      (3) Emphysema develops at an early age in the genetic type.
   b. Pathogenesis
      (1) Primarily affects the lower lobes
      (2) Distal terminal bronchioles and all parts of the respiratory units are the sites of elastic tissue destruction.
      (3) Air trapped behind the collapsed terminal bronchioles distends the entire respiratory unit.
   c. Laboratory finding
      • Absent α_1-globulin peak in a serum protein electrophoresis
6. Clinical findings in centriacinar and panacinar emphysema
   a. Progressive dyspnea and hyperventilation
      (1) Dyspnea is severe and occurs early in the disease.
      (2) Sometimes patients are called "pink puffers."
   b. Centriacinar type frequently coexists with chronic bronchitis.
   c. Breath sounds are diminished due to hyperinflation.
   d. Cor pulmonale is uncommon.
7. Chest radiograph (Fig. 16-17)
   a. Hyperlucent lung fields
   b. Increased anteroposterior diameter
   c. Vertically oriented heart
   d. Depressed diaphragms due to hyperinflated lungs
8. Pulmonary function tests and arterial blood gases
   a. Increased TLC due to an increase in RV

Centriacinar emphysema: destruction of the distal terminal bronchioles and RB

Panacinar emphysema: targets distal terminal bronchioles and the entire respiratory unit

Emphysema: pink puffers

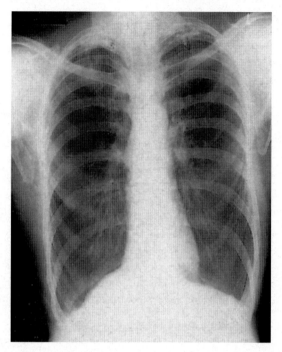

16-17: *Chest radiograph in emphysema showing a vertically oriented heart and depressed diaphragm. (From Forbes C, Jackson W: Color Atlas and Text of Clinical Medicine, 2nd ed. St. Louis, Mosby, 2003, p 186, Fig. 4-94.)*

  b. Decreased $FEV_{1\,sec}$ (e.g., 1 L versus 4 L; see Fig. 16-1C)
  c. Decreased FVC (e.g., 3 L versus 5 L; see Fig. 16-1C)
    • Decreased $FEV_{1\,sec}$/FVC ratio (e.g., 1/3 = 33%)
  d. Decreased Pao_2 develops late in the disease.
    • Destruction of the capillary bed matches destruction of the respiratory unit
  e. Normal to decreased arterial Pco_2 (respiratory alkalosis)
 9. Other types of emphysema unrelated to smoking or AAT deficiency
  a. Paraseptal emphysema
    (1) Localized disease in a subpleural location
      • Primarily targets the alveolar ducts and alveoli
    (2) Does *not* produce obstructive airway disease
    (3) Increased incidence of spontaneous pneumothorax
      • Due to rupture of subpleural blebs
  b. Irregular emphysema
    (1) Localized disease is associated with scar tissue.
    (2) Does *not* produce obstructive airway disease
B. Chronic bronchitis
 1. Epidemiology
  a. Productive cough for at least 3 months for 2 consecutive years

Paraseptal emphysema: risk for spontaneous pneumothorax

Irregular emphysema: scar emphysema

Smoking cigarettes: most common cause of chronic bronchitis

b. Causes
   (1) Smoking cigarettes
   (2) Cystic fibrosis
2. Pathogenesis
   a. Hypersecretion of mucus in bronchi
   b. Obstruction to airflow in the terminal bronchioles
      • Airflow obstruction is proximal to the obstruction in emphysema.
   c. Irreversible fibrosis of terminal bronchioles

> Turbulent airflow in the bronchi is converted to laminar airflow in the terminal (nonrespiratory) bronchioles. The terminal bronchioles undergo parallel branching, which reduces airflow resistance and spreads air out over a large cross-sectional area. Small airway disease associated with expiratory wheezing is due to narrowing of the terminal bronchioles by mucus plugs, inflammation, and fibrosis. Mucus plugs located in a proximal terminal bronchiole prevent the exodus of a large amount of CO_2 arising from the distally located airways producing respiratory acidosis.

   d. Changes in the bronchi
      (1) Hypersecretion of submucosal mucus-secreting glands in trachea and bronchi
         • Primarily responsible for sputum overproduction
      (2) Acute inflammation (neutrophils) often superimposed on chronic inflammation
      (3) Loss of ciliated epithelium and presence of squamous metaplasia
   e. Changes in the terminal bronchioles
      (1) Mucus plugs in lumens (block the exodus of CO_2)
      (2) Goblet cell metaplasia
      (3) Hypertrophy of mucous-secreting glands
      (4) Chronic inflammation and fibrosis narrowing the lumen
3. Clinical findings

Chronic bronchitis: productive cough at least 3 months for 2 consecutive years

Chronic bronchitis: blue bloaters

   a. Productive cough
   b. Dyspnea occurs late in the disease.
   c. Cyanosis of skin and mucous membranes
      (1) Decreased O_2 saturation from hypoxemia (see Chapter 1)
      (2) Patients are called "blue bloaters."
   d. Tend to be stocky or obese
   e. Expiratory wheezing and sibilant rhonchi
   f. Cor pulmonale is commonly present.
4. Chest radiograph
   a. Large, horizontally oriented heart
   b. Increased bronchial markings
5. Pulmonary function tests and arterial blood gases

Chronic bronchitis: chronic respiratory acidosis and hypoxemia

   a. Less increase in TLC and RV than emphysema
   b. Chronic respiratory acidosis

Parameter	Emphysema	Chronic Bronchitis
PaO_2	Decreased	Decreased
$PaCO_2$	Normal to decreased	Increased
pH	Normal to increased	Decreased
Cyanosis	Absent	Present
Habitus	Thin	Stocky
Cor pulmonale	Rare	Common
Onset of hypoxemia	Late	Early
Onset of dyspnea	Early	Late

**TABLE 16-4:
Comparison of
Emphysema and
Chronic Bronchitis**

      (1) Arterial PCO_2 greater than 45 mm Hg
      (2) Bicarbonate greater than 30 mEq/L
   c. Moderate to severe hypoxemia early in the disease
  6. Summary of findings in chronic bronchitis and emphysema (Table 16-4)

C. Asthma
  1. Epidemiology
    a. Episodic and reversible airway disease
    b. Primarily targets the bronchi and terminal bronchioles
    c. Most common chronic respiratory disease in children
    d. Extrinsic and intrinsic types
  2. Extrinsic asthma
    a. Pathogenesis
      (1) Type I hypersensitivity reaction with exposure to extrinsic
         allergens
        • Typically develops in children with an atopic family history to
          allergies
      (2) Initial sensitization to an inhaled allergen
        (a) Stimulate induction of subset 2 helper T cells (CD4 T_H2)
           that release interleukin (IL) 4 and IL-5
        (b) IL-4 stimulates isotype switching to IgE production.
        (c) IL-5 stimulates production and activation of eosinophils.
      (3) Inhaled antigens cross-link IgE antibodies on mast cells on
         mucosal surfaces.
        (a) Release of histamine and other preformed mediators
        (b) Functions of mediators
         • Stimulate bronchoconstriction, mucus production, influx
          of leukocytes
      (4) Late phase reaction (4–8 hours later)
        (a) Eotaxin is produced.
         • Chemotactic for eosinophils and activates eosinophils
        (b) Eosinophils release major basic protein and cationic protein.
         • Damage epithelial cells and produce airway constriction
    b. Other mediators involved
      (1) LTC-D-E_4 cause prolonged bronchoconstriction.
      (2) Acetylcholine causes airway muscle contraction.

Asthma: episodic and
reversible airway disease

Extrinsic asthma: type I
hypersensitivity reaction

IL-4: isotype switching to
IgE production
IL-5: production and
activation of eosinophils

c. Histologic changes in bronchi
   (1) Thickening of the basement membrane
   (2) Edema and a mixed inflammatory infiltrate
   (3) Hypertrophy of submucosal glands
   (4) Hypertrophy/hyperplasia of smooth muscle cells
d. Histologic changes in the terminal bronchioles
   (1) Formation of spiral-shaped mucus plugs
      (a) Contain shed epithelial cells called Curschmann spirals·
      (b) Pathologic effect of major basic protein and cationic protein
   (2) Crystalline granules in eosinophils coalesce to form Charcot-Leyden crystals.
   (3) Patchy loss of epithelial cells, goblet cell metaplasia
   (4) Thick basement membrane
   (5) Smooth muscle cell hypertrophy and hyperplasia
e. Clinical findings
   (1) Episodic expiratory wheezing (inspiratory as well when severe)
   (2) Nocturnal cough
   (3) Increased anteroposterior diameter
      • Due to air trapping and increase in residual volume

Bronchial asthma: initially present with respiratory alkalosis

f. Laboratory findings
   (1) Initially develop respiratory alkalosis
      (a) Patients work hard at expelling air through inflamed airways.
      (b) May progress into respiratory acidosis if bronchospasm is *not* relieved
         • Respiratory acidosis is an indication for intubation and mechanical ventilation.
   (2) Eosinophilia, positive skin tests for allergens
g. Treatment of mild disease
   • Metered-dose inhaler with a β_2-agonist (e.g., albuterol)
h. Treatment of more advanced disease
   (1) Metered low-dose inhaler with corticosteroids
   (2) Use of leukotriene inhibitors
3. Intrinsic asthma
   a. Nonimmune
   b. Causes
      (1) Virus-induced respiratory infection
         • Examples—rhinovirus, parainfluenza virus, respiratory syncytial virus
      (2) Air pollutants

> Ozone (O_3) is an air pollutant that derives from interactions of O_2 with oxides of nitrogen and sulfur, and hydrocarbons. It forms highly reactive free radicals in the airways that cause inflammation and irritation, often precipitating asthma.

      (3) Aspirin or nonsteroidal drug sensitivity (see section III)
      (4) Stress, exercise, cigarette smoke

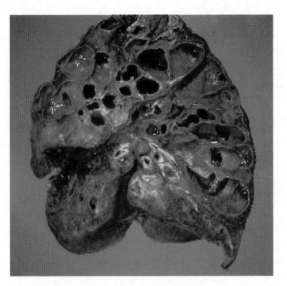

16-18: *Bronchiectasis showing dilated airways filled with pus. (From Corrin B: Pathology of the Lungs. London, Churchill Livingstone, 1999, p 85, Fig. 3-5.)*

D. Bronchiectasis
1. Epidemiology and pathogenesis
   a. Permanent dilation of the bronchi and bronchioles
      • Due to destruction of cartilage and elastic tissue by chronic necrotizing infections
   b. Causes
      (1) Cystic fibrosis
         • Most common cause in the United States
      (2) Infections
         (a) TB is the most common cause worldwide.
         (b) Adenovirus, *Staphylococcus aureus, Hemophilus influenzae*
      (3) Bronchial obstruction
         • Example—proximally located bronchogenic carcinoma occludes the lumen.
      (4) Primary ciliary dyskinesia
         (a) Absent dynein arm in cilia
         (b) Dynein arm contains ATPase (adenosine triphosphatase) for movement of the cilia.
      (5) Allergic bronchopulmonary aspergillosis
2. Gross findings
   a. Most commonly occurs in the lower lobes
   b. Dilated bronchi and bronchioles are filled with pus (Fig. 16-18).
      (1) Dilated airways extend to the lung periphery.
      (2) Dilations are tubelike and/or saccular.
3. Clinical findings
   a. Cough productive of copious sputum (often cupfuls)

Bronchiectasis: permanent dilation of bronchi and bronchioles

Primary ciliary dyskinesia: absent dynein arm in cilia

b. Hemoptysis that is sometimes massive

c. Digital clubbing, cor pulmonale

4. Chest radiograph findings
   - Crowded bronchial markings extend to the lung periphery.

5. Cystic fibrosis (CF)

   a. Epidemiology
      (1) Autosomal recessive disease
      (2) Primarily affects whites
         - Uncommon in Asians and black Americans

   b. Pathogenesis
      (1) Three nucleotide deletion on chromosome 7
         - Nucleotides normally code for phenylalanine.
      (2) Production of a defective CF transmembrane conductance regulator (CFTR) for chloride ions
      (3) CFTR Cl⁻ is degraded in the Golgi apparatus.
         - Due to defective protein folding
      (4) Loss of CFTR Cl⁻ causes decreased Na^+ and Cl^- reabsorption in sweat glands.
         - Basis of the sweat test
      (5) Effect of loss of CFTR Cl⁻ in other secretions
         (a) Increased Na^+ and water reabsorption from luminal secretions
         (b) Decreased Cl^- secretion out of epithelial cells into luminal secretions
         (c) Net effect is dehydration of body secretions due to lack of NaCl
            - Secretions are dehydrated in bronchioles, pancreatic ducts, bile ducts, meconium, and seminal fluid.

   c. Clinical findings
      (1) Nasal polyps (25% of cases)
      (2) Respiratory infections/failure
         (a) *Pseudomonas aeruginosa* is the most common respiratory pathogen.
            - Other common pathogens—*S. aureus, H. influenzae*
         (b) Cor pulmonale commonly occurs.
      (3) Malabsorption
         (a) Pancreatic exocrine deficiency
         (b) Atrophy of glands from dehydrated secretions blocking the lumens
      (4) Type 1 diabetes mellitus
         - Due to chronic pancreatitis
      (5) Infertility in males
         - Atresia of vas deferens
      (6) Meconium ileus
         - Small bowel obstruction in newborn
      (7) Secondary biliary cirrhosis
         - Due to obstruction of bile ductules by thick secretions

Cystic fibrosis: defective CFTR Cl⁻ is degraded in Golgi apparatus

Cystic fibrosis: loss NaCl in sweat, loss of NaCl in luminal secretions (dehydrated)

Respiratory infections: most common cause of death in CF

X. Lung Tumors
- Primary lung cancer is the most common cancer killer in both men and women.

A. Epidemiology
1. Incidence of lung cancer is declining in men but increasing in women.
2. Peak incidence is at 55 to 65 years of age.
3. Causes
   a. Cigarette smoking
   b. Radon gas (uranium mining)
   c. Asbestos, chromium, nickel, beryllium, arsenic, vinyl chloride

Cigarette smoking: most common cause of lung cancer

4. Primary lung cancer in decreasing incidence
   a. Adenocarcinoma
   b. Squamous cell carcinoma
   c. Small cell lung carcinoma
   d. Large cell carcinoma
   e. Bronchial carcinoid
5. Squamous and small cell lung carcinomas
   a. Greatest smoking association
   b. Tend to be centrally located (i.e., main stem bronchus) (Fig. 16-19)

Squamous cell and small cell carcinoma: centrally located

6. Adenocarcinomas
   a. Weakest smoking association
   b. Tend to be more peripherally located

Adenocarcinoma: peripherally located

B. Tumor and tumor-like disorders (Fig. 16-20 and Table 16-5)

A solitary pulmonary nodule or coin lesion is the term applied to a peripheral lung nodule smaller than 5 cm. Causes of a solitary pulmonary nodule in descending order include granulomas (e.g., TB, histoplasmosis), malignancy (usually primary cancer), and a bronchial (chondroid) hamartoma. Patients younger than 35 years old have a 1% risk of a solitary coin lesion representing a malignancy, but patients 50 years old and up have a 50% to 60% risk of malignancy, usually a primary cancer. In evaluating solitary coin lesions, comparing previous chest x-rays for changes in size of the nodule is the most important initial step.

C. Metastatic cancer
1. Epidemiology
   a. Most common lung cancer
   b. Cancers most often responsible for metastasis
      (1) Primary breast cancer most common cause
      (2) Colon cancer, renal cell carcinoma

Metastasis: most common lung cancer

2. Sites of lung metastasis
   a. Parenchyma (Fig. 16-21)
   b. Pleura and pleural space (malignant effusions)
   c. Lymphatics (causes severe dyspnea)
3. Dyspnea is the most common symptom.

D. Clinical findings in primary lung cancer
1. Cough is the most common symptom (75% of cases).

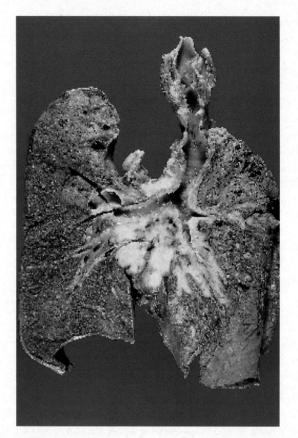

16-19: *Primary lung cancer showing the larynx, trachea, and both lungs. The white-colored cancer extends along both bifurcations of the main stem bronchus and along the tributaries and out into the lung parenchyma. Many bronchial lumens are totally occluded by tumor. The black pigment in the tumor is anthracotic pigment. The cystic spaces in both upper lobes represent centriacinar emphysema. (From Corrin B: Pathology of the Lungs. London, Churchill Livingstone, 1999, p 475, Fig. 13-1–16.)*

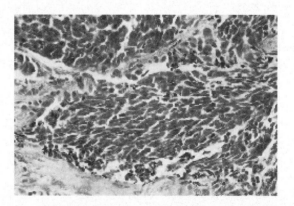

16-20: *Small cell carcinoma of the lung showing nests of basophilic staining lymphocyte-sized cells with scant cytoplasm. (From Corrin B: Pathology of the Lungs. London, Churchill Livingstone, 1999, p 476, Fig. 13-1–19.)*

Type of Tumor or Disorder	Location in Lung	Comments
Adenocarcinoma	Peripheral	More common in women Associated with cigarette smoking Tumors may develop in scars or spread along alveolar walls and mimic lobar pneumonia (bronchioloalveolar)
Squamous cell carcinoma	Central	More common in men Strong association with cigarette smoking Tend to cavitate May ectopically secrete PTH-related protein
Small cell carcinoma*	Central	More common in men Strong association with cigarette smoking Arise from neuroendocrine cells (Kulchitsky cells) Rapidly growing cancer that metastasizes early May ectopically secrete ADH or ACTH
Large cell carcinoma	Peripheral	Undifferentiated cancer that metastasizes early
Bronchial carcinoid	Central	*No* association with cigarette smoking Low-grade cancer of neuroendocrine origin Carcinoid syndrome is rare (does *not* require liver metastasis)
Carcinoma metastatic to the lung	Multifocal	More common than primary cancer Usually presents with dyspnea
Bronchial hamartoma	Peripheral (90%) Central (10%)	Non-neoplastic proliferation of cartilage and adipose tissue Appears as solitary "coin" lesion on chest radiograph

**TABLE 16-5:
Tumors and Tumor-like Disorders of the Lung**

*See Figure 16-20.
ACTH, adrenocorticotropic hormone; ADH, antidiuretic hormone; PTH, parathyroid hormone.

2. Dyspnea, hemoptysis, weight loss, chest pain
3. Pancoast tumor (superior sulcus tumor)
   a. Usually a primary squamous cancer located at the extreme apex of lung
   b. Destruction of superior cervical sympathetic ganglion produces Horner's syndrome
      (1) Ipsilateral lid lag
      (2) Miosis (pinpoint pupil)
      (3) Ipsilateral anhydrosis (lack of sweating)

Horner's syndrome: lid lag, miosis, anhydrosis

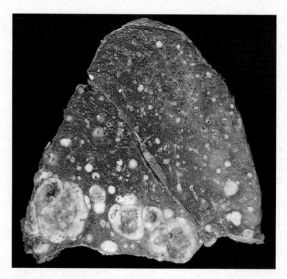

16-21: *Metastatic renal cell carcinoma showing multiple nodular lesions scattered throughout the lung parenchyma. (From Kumar V, Fausto N, Abbas A: Robbins and Cotran's Pathologic Basis of Disease, 7th ed. Philadelphia, WB Saunders, 2004, p 766, Fig. 15-47.)*

     4. Superior vena cava syndrome (see Chapter 9)
     5. Paraneoplastic syndromes
        a. Digital clubbing
           • Due to reactive periosteal changes in the underlying bone
        b. Muscle weakness (Eaton-Lambert syndrome)
        c. Ectopic hormone secretion (see above)
  E. Common sites for metastasis
     1. Hilar lymph nodes most common site
     2. Adrenal gland (50% of cases)
     3. Liver (30% of cases), brain (20% of cases), bone (usually osteolytic)
  F. Prognosis
     1. Non–small cell cancers fare better than small cell carcinoma.
     2. Overall combined 5-year survival rate is ~15%.

XI. Mediastinum Disorders
  A. Mediastinal masses
     1. Epidemiology
        a. Usually metastatic primary lung cancer in older patients
        b. Usually primary disease in younger patients
        c. Anterior compartment is the most common site.
        d. Most common primary mediastinal masses, in descending order:
           (1) Neurogenic tumors
              • Usually malignant in children and benign in adults
           (2) Thymomas (see below)
           (3) Primary cysts
              • Usually a pericardial cyst

Anterior compartment: most common site for mediastinal masses

(4) Malignant lymphomas
- Usually nodular sclerosing Hodgkin's lymphoma in a woman

(5) Teratoma

2. Thymoma
   a. Epidemiology
      (1) Located in the anterior mediastinum
      (2) Benign (70%), malignant (30%)
   b. Epithelium, *not* lymphoid tissue, is the neoplastic component.
   c. Majority express systemic symptoms of myasthenia gravis (see Chapter 23).
      (1) Less than 10% to 15% of myasthenia patients have a thymoma.
      (2) Majority (65–75%) have follicular B cell hyperplasia in the thymus.
         - Site for synthesis of antiacetylcholine receptor antibodies
   d. Other thymoma associations
      (1) Hypogammaglobulinemia, pure RBC aplasia
      (2) Increased incidence of autoimmune disease (e.g. Graves' disease)

Symptoms in thymomas: most often associated with myasthenia gravis

XII. Pleural Disorders
A. Movement of pleural fluid
- Normally moves from parietal pleura into the pleural space and into the lungs

B. Causes of pleural effusion
1. Increased hydrostatic pressure in the visceral pleura (e.g., congestive heart failure)
2. Decreased oncotic pressure (e.g., nephrotic syndrome)
3. Obstruction of lymphatic drainage from the visceral pleura (e.g., lung cancer)
4. Increased vessel permeability of visceral pleural capillaries (e.g., infarction)
5. Metastasis to the pleura (e.g., metastatic breast cancer)

C. Types of pleural effusions
1. Transudates
   a. Ultrafiltrate of plasma involving disturbances in Starling pressures
   b. Example—increased hydrostatic pressure or decreased oncotic pressure
2. Exudates
   a. Protein-rich and cell-rich fluid
      - Due to an increase in vessel permeability in acute inflammation
   b. Examples—pneumonia, infarction, metastasis
3. Laboratory findings distinguishing exudates from transudates
   a. Pleural fluid protein/serum protein ratio above 0.5
      (1) Indicates an exudate
      (2) Transudates have values below 0.5.
   b. Pleural fluid lactate dehydrogenases/serum lactate dehydrogenase ratio above 0.6
      (1) Indicates an exudate
      (2) Transudates have values below 0.6.

D. **Spontaneous pneumothorax**
   1. Causes
      a. Idiopathic (most common)
      b. Paraseptal emphysema, Marfan syndrome
   2. Pathogenesis
      a. Rupture of a subpleural or intrapleural bleb produces a hole in the pleura.
      b. Pleural cavity pressure is the *same* as the atmospheric pressure.
         (1) Loss of the negative intrathoracic pressure
         (2) Causes a portion of lung or the entire lung to collapse
   3. Clinical findings
      a. Sudden onset of dyspnea with pleuritic type of chest pain
      b. Physical examination
         (1) Tympanitic percussion note
         (2) Absent breath sounds
         (3) Trachea deviated to the side of the collapse

E. **Tension pneumothorax**
   1. Causes
      a. Penetrating trauma to the lungs (e.g., knife wound)
      b. Rupture of tension pneumatocysts (see section VI)
   2. Pathogenesis
      a. Flap-like pleural tear allows air into the pleural cavity but prevents its exit.
         • Similar in concept to filling a tire up with air
      b. Increased pleural cavity pressure
      c. Produces compression atelectasis (see section IV)
   3. Clinical findings
      a. Sudden onset of severe dyspnea
      b. Physical examination
         (1) Tympanitic percussion note and absent breath sounds
         (2) Trachea and mediastinal structures deviate to contralateral side.
            • Compromised venous return to the heart, if the pneumothorax is located on the left side
      c. Treatment
         • Insert a needle into the pleural cavity to relieve the pressure

Spontaneous pneumothorax: loss of negative intrathoracic pressure

Spontaneous pneumothorax: trachea deviates to side of pneumothorax

Tension pneumothorax: increase in pleural cavity pressure

Tension pneumothorax: trachea deviates to contralateral side

Gastrointestinal Disorders

I. **Oral Cavity and Salivary Gland Disorders**
   A. **Cleft lip**
   1. Epidemiology
      a. Most common congenital disorder of oral cavity
         • ~1:800 live births
      b. Male dominant
      c. Multifactorial inheritance
   2. Failure of fusion of facial processes
      • Cleft palate is also present in 50% of cases.

   B. **Common infections in the oral cavity (Table 17-1)**
   C. **Oral manifestation of HIV**
   1. Candidiasis (Fig. 17-1)
      • Most common oral infection
   2. Apthous ulcers (canker sores)
      • Painful ulcers covered by a shaggy gray membrane
   3. Hairy leukoplakia (Fig. 17-2)
      • Glossitis due to Epstein-Barr virus (EBV)
   4. Kaposi sarcoma
      a. Hard palate is the most common location.
      b. Due to human herpesvirus 8

   D. **Dental caries**
   1. *Streptococcus mutans* produces acid from sucrose fermentation.
      • Acid erodes enamel and exposes underlying dentine.
   2. Fluoride prevents dental caries.
      • Excess fluoride causes a chalky discoloration of the teeth.

   E. **Noninfectious ulcerations in the oral cavity**
   1. Pemphigus vulgaris and mucous membrane pemphigoid
      • Both are immunologic skin disorders (see Chapter 24).
   2. Erythema multiforme (see Chapter 24)
      a. Hypersensitivity reaction against *Mycoplasma* or drugs (e.g., sulfonamides)
      b. Called Stevens-Johnson syndrome when it involves the mouth
   3. Behçet's syndrome
      a. Autoimmune disease with recurrent aphthous ulcers
      b. Genital ulcerations, uveitis, and conjunctivitis

   F. **Pigmentation abnormalities**
   1. Peutz-Jeghers syndrome (see section IV)
      • Melanin pigmentation of the lips and oral mucosa

Cleft lip: failure of fusion of facial processes

Pre-AIDS-defining lesions: thrush, hairy leukoplakia, apthous ulcers

Dental caries: caused by *Streptococcus mutans*

TABLE 17-1:
Infections of the
Oral Cavity

Infection	Pathogen	Features
Bacterial		
Cervicofacial actinomycosis	*Actinomyces israelii*	Draining sinus tract from facial or cervical area "Sulfur granules" in pus contain gram-positive, branching filamentous bacteria Often follows extraction of abscessed tooth
Diphtheria	*Corynebacterium diphtheriae*	Toxin produces "shaggy" gray pseudomembrane in posterior pharynx and upper airways
Peritonsillar abscess	*Streptococcus pyogenes*	Uvula deviates to contralateral side Complication due to tonsillitis
Pharyngitis	*S. pyogenes*	Associated with tonsillitis Potential for acute rheumatic fever and glomerulonephritis
Scarlet fever	*S. pyogenes*	Pharyngitis, tonsillitis, glossitis Erythrogenic toxin produces rash on skin and tongue (initially white and then strawberry colored) Increased risk for glomerulonephritis
Sialadenitis	*Staphylococcus aureus*	Bacterial inflammation of major salivary gland Secondary to a calculus, which obstructs the duct in postoperative patients
Congenital syphilis	*Treponema pallidum* (spirochete)	Abnormalities involving incisors (tapered like a peg) and molar teeth (resemble mulberries)
Viral		
Exudative tonsillitis	Viruses: most cases	Culture is necessary to differentiate bacterial versus viral infection
Hairy leukoplakia	EBV	Glossitis associated with bilateral white, hairy excrescences on lateral border of tongue Pre-AIDS-defining lesion
Herpes labialis	HSV type 1	Recurrent vesicular lesions on the lips (virus remains dormant in cranial sensory ganglia) Reactivated by stress, sunlight, and menses
Mumps	Paramyxovirus	Bilateral parotitis (70%) with increased serum amylase Complications: meningoencephalitis, unilateral orchitis or oophoritis, pancreatitis
Herpangina	Coxsackievirus	Occurs in children Multiple vesicles or ulcers on soft palate and pharynx surrounded by erythema
Hand-foot-mouth disease	Coxsackievirus	Occurs in young children Vesicles located in mouth and distal extremities
Fungal		
Oral thrush	*Candida albicans* (yeast)	May occur in neonates, immunocompromised patients (common pre-AIDS-defining lesion), diabetes mellitus, and following antibiotic therapy

EBV, Epstein-Barr virus; HSV, herpes simplex virus.

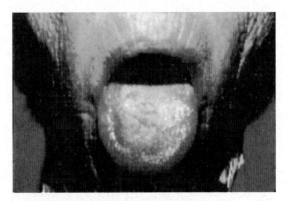

17-1: Oral thrush showing a white, creamy exudate covering the surface of the tongue. (From Goldstein BG: Practical Dermatology, 2nd ed. St. Louis, Mosby, 1997, p 108, Fig. 10-9.)

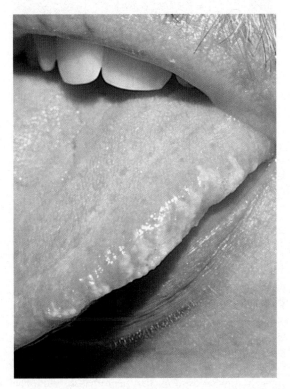

17-2: Hairy leukoplakia along the lateral border of the tongue. It is a glossitis due to Epstein-Barr virus and is a pre-AIDS-defining lesion. (From Lookingbill D, Marks J: Principles of Dermatology, 3rd ed. Philadelphia, WB Saunders, 2000, p 338, Fig. 23-7.)

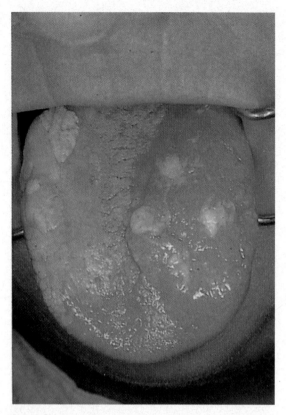

17-3: *Leukoplakia of the tongue with invasive squamous cell carcinoma. Discrete raised white patches are evident on both sides of the tongue. (From Forbes C, Jackson W: Color Atlas and Text of Clinical Medicine, 2nd ed. St. Louis, Mosby, 2003, p 362, Fig. 8-28.)*

Melanin pigmentation in oral mucosa: Addison's disease, Peutz-Jeghers syndrome

2. Addison's disease
   • Increased adrenocorticotropic hormone stimulates melanocytes.
3. Lead poisoning
   • Lead deposits along the gingival margins in adults with gingivitis

G. Tooth discoloration with tetracycline
   1. Drug discolors newly formed teeth.
   2. Drug not recommended in a child up to 12 years of age.

H. Macroglossia (enlarged tongue)
   1. Myxedema in primary hypothyroidism, Down syndrome
   2. Acromegaly, amyloidosis, mucosal neuromas in multiple endocrine neoplasia syndrome IIb

I. Glossitis (inflammation of tongue)
   1. Long-standing iron deficiency
   2. Vitamin B_{12} or folate deficiency
   3. Scurvy, scarlet fever, EBV

J. Leukoplakia and erythroplakia
   1. Leukoplakia literally means "white patch" (Fig. 17-3).

     a. Lesion does *not* wipe off.

     b. Erythroplakia is a red patch.

     c. Both lesions are due to squamous hyperplasia of the epidermis.

        • Increased risk for squamous dysplasia or invasive squamous cancer

  2. Causes

     a. Chronic irritation (e.g., dentures)

     b. All forms of tobacco use, alcohol abuse, human papillomavirus (HPV)

  3. Locations

     a. Vermilion border lower lip (most common site)

     b. Buccal mucosa, hard and soft palates, floor of the mouth

K. Dentigerous cyst

  1. Derives from epithelial elements of dental origin (odontogenic origin)

  2. Associated with the crown of an unerupted or impacted third molar tooth

  3. Association with ameloblastomas in 15% to 30% of cases

L. Benign tumors of the oral cavity (excluding salivary gland)

  1. Squamous papillomas

     a. Most common tumor in oral cavity

     b. Exophytic tumor with a fibrovascular core

     c. May occur on the tongue, gingiva, palate, or lips

  2. Ameloblastoma

     a. Arise from enamel organ epithelium or a dentigerous cyst

     b. Located in the mandible

       (1) Produces a radiolucency in bone that has a "soap bubble" appearance

       (2) Locally invasive but do *not* metastasize

> Ameloblastoma: most common odontogenic tumor

M. Malignant tumors of the oral cavity (excluding salivary gland)

  1. Epidemiology

     a. Majority are well-differentiated squamous cell carcinomas

     b. Male dominant

     c. Risk factors

       (1) Smoking is the most common risk factor.

         • Pipe, cigarettes, chewing tobacco

       (2) Alcohol abuse (synergistic with smoking)

       (3) HPV, chronic irritation from dentures

     d. Cancer sites in descending order

       (1) Lower lip (vermilion border)

       (2) Floor of mouth

       (3) Lateral border of tongue

     e. Verrucous carcinoma

       • Associated with smokeless tobacco

> Squamous cell carcinoma: most common site is lower lip

  2. Basal cell carcinoma

     a. Most common cancer of upper lip

     b. Associated with ultraviolet light B exposure

> Basal cell carcinoma: most common oral site is upper lip

N. Salivary gland disorders

  1. Sjögren's syndrome (see Chapter 23)

     a. Female dominant autoimmune disease associated with rheumatoid arthritis

     b. Autoimmune destruction of minor salivary glands and lacrimal glands

Parotid gland: most
common site for salivary
gland tumors

2. Salivary gland tumors
  a. Epidemiology
    (1) Parotid gland is the most common site.
      • Major salivary gland tumors are more likely to be benign.
    (2) Minor salivary gland tumors are more likely to be malignant.
  b. Pleomorphic adenoma (mixed tumor)
    (1) Most common benign tumor of major and minor salivary glands
      • Parotid gland is the most common site.
    (2) Female dominant
    (3) Painless, moveable mass at the angle of the jaw
    (4) Epithelial cells intermixed with myxomatous and cartilaginous stroma
      • Tumor projections through capsule increases risk of recurrence
    (5) May transform into a malignant tumor
      • Facial nerve involvement is a sign of malignancy.
  c. Warthin's tumor (papillary cystadenoma lymphomatosum)
    (1) Benign parotid gland tumor
      • Male dominant
    (2) Heterotopic salivary gland tissue trapped in a lymph node
      • Cystic glandular structures are located within benign lymphoid tissue.
  d. Mucoepidermoid carcinoma
    (1) Most common malignant salivary gland tumor
    (2) Most commonly located in the parotid gland
    (3) Mixture of neoplastic squamous and mucus-secreting cells

Pleomorphic adenoma:
most common salivary
gland tumor

Mucoepidermoid
carcinoma: most common
malignant salivary gland
tumor

II. Esophageal Disorders
A. Signs and symptoms of esophageal disease
  1. Heartburn
    • Most commonly due to gastroesophageal reflux disease
  2. Dysphagia (difficulty swallowing) for solids alone
    a. Symptom of an obstructive lesion
    b. Examples—esophageal cancer, esophageal web, stricture
  3. Dysphagia for solids and liquids
    a. Symptom of a motility disorder
    b. Oropharyngeal (upper esophageal) dysphagia
      (1) Striated muscle dysmotility
      (2) Examples—dermatomyositis, myasthenia gravis, stroke
    c. Lower esophageal dysphagia
      (1) Smooth muscle dysmotility
      (2) Examples—systemic sclerosis, CREST syndrome, achalasia
B. Tracheoesophageal (TE) fistula
  1. Characteristics
    a. Proximal esophagus ends blindly (Fig. 17-4).
    b. Distal esophagus arises from the trachea.

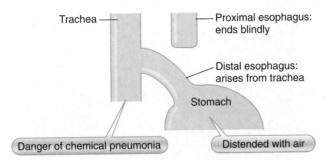

17-4: *Tracheoesophageal fistula. The proximal esophagus ends blindly, and the distal esophagus arises from the trachea. The stomach is distended with air owing to communication of the esophagus with the trachea.*

2. Clinical findings
    a. Maternal polyhydramnios (excess amniotic fluid)
        • Swallowed amniotic fluid cannot be reabsorbed in the small intestine
    b. Abdominal distention in newborn
        • Air in the stomach from tracheal fistula
    c. Difficulty with feeding
        (1) Food regurgitates out of the mouth.
        (2) Chemical pneumonia from aspiration
    d. VATER syndrome
        (1) *V*ertebral abnormalities
        (2) *A*nal atresia
        (3) *TE* fistula
        (4) *R*enal disease and absent *r*adius

> VATER syndrome: vertebral abnormalities, anal atresia, *TE* fistula, renal disease, and absent radius

C. Plummer-Vinson syndrome (see Chapter 11)
    1. Due to chronic iron deficiency
    2. Leukoplakia in oral mucosa and esophagus
    3. Intermittent dysphagia for solids
        • Due to an esophageal web or stricture
D. Esophageal diverticulum
    1. Types of diverticulum
        a. True diverticulum
            • Outpouching lined by mucosa, submucosa, muscularis propria, and adventitia
        b. False, or pulsion diverticulum
            (1) Weakness in underlying muscle wall
            (2) Outpouching of mucosa and submucosa into area of weakness
    2. Zenker's diverticulum
        a. Pulsion type located in upper esophagus
            • Area of weakness is cricopharyngeus muscle.
        b. Clinical findings
            (1) Painful swallowing (i.e., oropharyngeal dysphagia)
            (2) Halitosis (entrapped food), diverticulitis

> Zenker's diverticulum: most common esophageal diverticulum

E. Hiatal hernia
    1. Sliding hernia
        a. Most common type

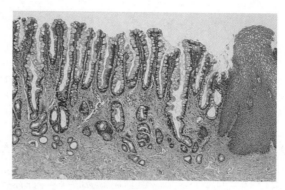

17-5: *Barrett's esophagus, showing an extensive area of glandular metaplasia with numerous goblet cells. A small section of squamous epithelium remains on the right. (From Damjanov I, Linder J: Pathology: A Color Atlas. St. Louis, Mosby, 2000, p 111, Fig. 6-26.)*

      b. Herniation of proximal stomach through a widened diaphragmatic hiatus

      c. Clinical findings

         (1) Heartburn and nocturnal epigastric distress from acid reflux

         (2) Hematemesis (vomiting blood), ulceration, stricture

   2. Paraesophageal hernia

     • Portion of stomach herniates alongside the distal esophagus.

> Pleuroperitoneal diaphragmatic hernias (Bochdalek hernia) present early in life. The visceral contents extend through the posterolateral part of the diaphragm on the left into the chest cavity causing respiratory distress at birth. Loops of bowel are present in the left pleural cavity on x-ray.

F. Gastroesophageal reflux disease (GERD)

   1. Risk factors

     • Smoking, alcohol, caffeine, fatty foods, chocolate, hiatal hernia

   2. Pathogenesis

      a. Transient relaxation of lower esophageal sphincter (LES)

        • Reflux of acid and bile into the distal esophagus

      b. Ineffective esophageal clearance of reflux material

   3. Clinical findings

      a. Noncardiac chest pain, nocturnal cough, nocturnal asthma

      b. Heartburn, acid injury to enamel

      c. Barrett's esophagus

G. Barrett's esophagus

   1. Complication of GERD

   2. Glandular metaplasia in distal esophagus due to acid injury (Fig. 17-5)

     • Gastric-type columnar cells and small intestine-type cells (goblet cells)

   3. Complications

      a. Ulceration with stricture formation (most common)

      b. Glandular dysplasia with increased risk for adenocarcinoma

GERD: relaxed LES causes acid reflux

H. Infectious esophagitis
1. Usually a complication of AIDS
2. Pathogens
   a. *Herpes simplex* virus
      - See multinucleated squamous cells with intranuclear inclusions
   b. Cytomegalovirus (CMV)
      - See basophilic intranuclear inclusions
   c. *Candida*
      - See yeasts and pseudohyphae (extended yeast forms)
3. Present with painful swallowing (i.e., odynophagia)

I. Corrosive esophagitis
1. Ingestion of strong alkali (e.g., lye) or acid (e.g., HCl)
2. Complications
   - Stricture formation, perforation, squamous cell carcinoma

J. Esophageal varices
1. Epidemiology and pathogenesis
   a. Dilated submucosal left gastric veins (Fig. 17-6)
   b. Complication of portal hypertension from cirrhosis
      - Alcohol abuse is the most common cause.
2. Clinical findings
   a. Rupture with massive hematemesis (vomiting blood)
   b. Most common cause of death in cirrhosis

K. Mallory-Weiss syndrome
1. Mucosal tear in the proximal stomach and distal esophagus
   - Due to severe retching in alcoholics or bulimia
2. Causes hematemesis

L. Boerhaave's syndrome
1. Rupture of the distal esophagus
2. Causes
   - Endoscopy (~75% of cases), retching, bulimia
3. Complications
   a. Pneumomediastinum
      (1) Air dissects into the subcutaneous tissue.
      (2) Produces a crunching sound (Hamman's crunch) on physical examination
   b. Pleural effusion contains food, acid, amylase

M. Motor disorders
1. Systemic sclerosis and CREST syndrome (see Chapter 3)
2. Achalasia
   a. Pathogenesis
      (1) Incomplete relaxation of LES
      (2) Absent ganglion cells in myenteric plexus
         (a) Decreases proximal smooth muscle contraction
         (b) Loss of vasointestinal peptide (normally relaxes LES)
      (3) Dilation of esophagus proximal to LES with absent peristalsis
      (4) Acquired cause is Chagas' disease.
         - Destruction of ganglion cells by leishmanial forms

Left gastric vein drains blood from distal esophagus and proximal stomach into the portal vein.

Esophageal varices: portal hypertension dilates left gastric veins

Mallory-Weiss syndrome: mucosal tear of distal esophagus

Boerhaave's syndrome: rupture of distal esophagus

Achalasia: most common neuromuscular disorder of the esophagus

Achalasia: absent ganglion cells in myenteric plexus

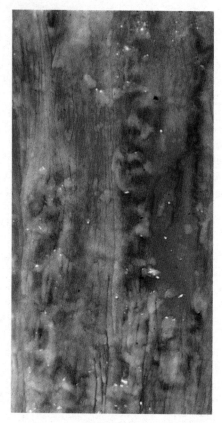

17-6: *Esophageal varices, showing many linear-oriented dilated and tortuous veins in the submucosa of the distal esophagus. (From Damjanov I, Linder J: Pathology: A Color Atlas. St. Louis, Mosby, 2000, p 110, Fig. 6-23A.)*

    b. Clinical findings
      (1) Nocturnal regurgitation of undigested food
      (2) Abnormal barium swallow
        • Dilated, aperistaltic esophagus with a beak-like tapering at distal end
      (3) Abnormal esophageal manometry
        • Detects aperistalsis and failure of LES relaxation

N. Esophageal tumors
  1. Leiomyoma
    • Most common benign tumor of esophagus
  2. Adenocarcinoma of distal esophagus
    a. Most common primary cancer of the esophagus
    b. Barrett's esophagus is most common predisposing cause.
      • Prevention of GERD decreases risk for developing adenocarcinoma.
  3. Squamous cell carcinoma
    a. Epidemiology
      (1) Most common primary cancer in developing countries

Distal adenocarcinoma of esophagus: most common esophageal cancer

      (2) More common in black Americans than whites

      (3) Male dominant

      (4) Risk factors

         (a) Smoking, alcohol abuse

         (b) Lye strictures, achalasia, Plummer-Vinson syndrome

  b. Locations

    • Midesophagus (50% of cases), lower esophagus

  c. Spreads to local nodes first and then to liver and lungs

  d. Clinical findings

    • Dysphagia for solids and weight loss

> Squamous cell carcinoma: smoking cigarettes most common cause

III. Stomach Disorders

A. Signs and symptoms of stomach disease

1. Hematemesis (vomiting blood)

  a. Most commonly due to peptic ulcer disease (PUD)

  b. Other causes—esophageal varices, hemorrhagic gastritis

2. Melena (dark, tarry stools)

  a. Hb is converted into hematin (black pigment) by acid.

  b. Signifies a bleed proximal to duodenojejunal junction

> PUD: most common cause of hematemesis and melena

> Gastric analysis includes measurement of basal acid output (BAO), maximal acid output (MAO), and the BAO:MAO ratio. BAO is the acid output of gastric juice collected via a nasogastric tube over a 1-hour period on an empty stomach. It is normally less than 5 mEq/hour. MAO is the acid output of gastric juice that is collected over 1 hour after pentagastrin stimulation. Normally, it is 5 to 20 mEq/hour. The normal BAO:MAO ratio is 0.20:1.

B. Congenital pyloric stenosis

1. Multifactorial inheritance pattern

  • 1:500 live births, male dominant

2. Progressive hypertrophy of the circular muscles in the pyloric sphincter

  • Not present at birth but occurs over the ensuing 2 to 4 weeks

3. Clinical findings

  a. Projectile vomiting of non–bile-stained fluid 2 to 4 weeks after birth

  b. Hypertrophied pylorus is palpated in the epigastrium.

4. Acquired pyloric obstruction

  • Complication of chronic duodenal ulcer disease with pyloric scarring

> Congenital pyloric stenosis: vomiting of non–bile-stained fluid

C. Gastroparesis

1. Decreased stomach motility

  • Autonomic neuropathy (e.g., diabetes mellitus), previous vagotomy

2. Clinical findings

  a. Early satiety and bloating

  b. Vomiting of undigested food a few hours after eating

D. Acute hemorrhagic (erosive) gastritis

1. Terms

  a. Erosions are a breach in the epithelium of the mucosa.

Hemorrhagic gastritis: NSAIDs most common cause

b. Ulcers are a breach in the mucosa with extension into the submucosa or deeper.
2. Causes
   a. Nonsteroidal anti-inflammatory drugs (NSAIDs)
   b. CMV (AIDS), alcohol, smoking
   c. Burns (called Curling's ulcers), CNS injury (called Cushing's ulcers)
   d. Uremia, *Anisakis* (worm associated with eating raw fish)
3. Clinical findings
   • Hematemesis, melena, iron deficiency

E. Chronic atrophic gastritis

Type A chronic atrophic gastritis: body and fundus; pernicious anemia

1. Type A chronic atrophic gastritis
   a. Involves the body and fundus
   b. Most often due to pernicious anemia (see Chapter 11)
   c. Complications
     (1) Achlorhydria with hypergastrinemia (loss of negative feedback)
     (2) Macrocytic anemia due to vitamin B_{12} deficiency
     (3) Increased risk for adenocarcinoma

Type B chronic atrophic gastritis: antrum and pylorus; *H. pylori*

2. Type B chronic atrophic gastritis
   a. Involves the antrum and pylorus
   b. Most common cause is *Helicobacter pylori*.
     (1) Gram-negative, curved rod

H. pylori: urease producer

     (2) Produces urease (converts amino groups in proteins to ammonia), proteases, cytotoxins
       • Secretion products produce chronic gastritis and PUD.
     (3) Transmitted by fecal-oral/oral-oral route
       • Common in areas of poor sanitation
     (4) Colonizes mucus layer lining (Fig. 17-7)
       • *Not* invasive
   c. Microscopic findings
     (1) Chronic inflammatory infiltrate in the lamina propria
     (2) Intestinal metaplasia (see Fig. 1-6)
       • Precursor lesion for adenocarcinoma
   d. Tests to identify *H. pylori* are highly sensitive and specific
     (1) Tests to detect urease in a gastric biopsy
     (2) Serologic tests
     (3) Radiolabeled urea breath test
     (4) Stool antigen test (excellent screen)
   e. Disease associations with *H. pylori*
     (1) Duodenal and gastric ulcers

Treatment of *H. pylori* ↓ risk of gastric cancer and lymphoma

     (2) Type B antral chronic atrophic gastritis
     (3) Gastric adenocarcinoma and low-grade B-cell malignant lymphoma
3. Menetrier's disease (hypertrophic gastropathy)
   a. Giant rugal folds
     (1) Due to hyperplasia of mucus-secreting cells
     (2) Causes hypoproteinemia (protein-losing enteropathy)
   b. Atrophy of parietal cells (achlorhydria)
     • Increased risk for adenocarcinoma

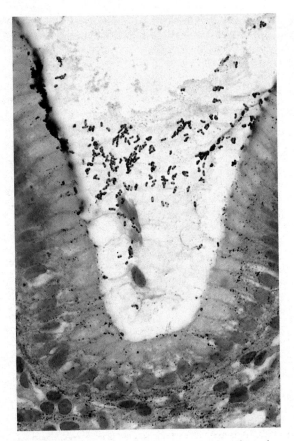

17-7: *Silver stain showing Helicobacter pylori* organisms in the mucus layer lining the gastric epithelial cells. *(From Kumar V, Fausto N, Abbas A: Robbins and Cotran's Pathologic Basis of Disease, 7th ed. Philadelphia, WB Saunders, 2004, p 815, Fig. 17-15.)*

F. Peptic ulcer disease (PUD)
1. Most often caused by *H. pylori*
2. Gross appearance of ulcers
   a. Clean, sharply demarcated, and slightly elevated around the edges
   b. Most gastric ulcers are benign.
      • Small percentage may be malignant
   c. Duodenal ulcers are *never* malignant.
   d. Four layers in sequence are noted in histologic sections of ulcers.
      (1) Necrotic debris
      (2) Inflammation with a predominance of neutrophils
      (3) Granulation tissue (repair tissue)
      (4) Fibrosis
3. Comparison of gastric and duodenal ulcers (Table 17-2)

G. Zollinger-Ellison syndrome
1. Epidemiology and pathogenesis
   a. Majority are malignant pancreatic islet cell tumors.

TABLE 17-2:
Comparison of Gastric Ulcers and Duodenal Ulcers

Feature	Gastric Ulcers	Duodenal Ulcers
Percentage of ulcer cases	25%	75%
Epidemiology	Male-female ratio 1:1 Smoking does *not* cause PUD but delays healing	Male-female ratio 2:1 Risk increased with MEN I Increased risk in cirrhosis, COPD, renal failure, hyperparathyroidism
Helicobacter pylori	~80% of cases	90–95% of cases
Pathogenesis	Defective mucosal barrier due to *H. pylori* Mucosal ischemia (reduced PGE), bile reflux, delayed gastric emptying BAO and MAO normal to decreased	Defective mucosal barrier due to *H. pylori* Increased acid production (increased parietal cell mass) BAO and MAO both increased
Location	Single ulcer on lesser curvature of antrum (same location for cancer)	Single ulcer on anterior portion of first part of duodenum followed by single ulcer on posterior portion (danger of perforation into pancreas)
Complications	Bleeding (most commonly in left gastric artery) Perforation	Bleeding (most commonly in gastroduodenal artery) Perforation (air under diaphragm, pain radiates to left shoulder) Gastric outlet obstruction, pancreatitis
Clinical findings	Burning epigastric pain soon after eating	Burning epigastric pain 1–3 hours after eating

BAO, basal acid output; COPD, chronic obstructive pulmonary disease; MAO, maximal acid output; MEN, multiple endocrine neoplasia; PGE, prostaglandin E; PUD, peptic ulcer disease.

Zollinger-Ellison syndrome: malignant islet cell tumor secreting gastrin

    b. Secrete excess gastrin producing hyperacidity
    c. Multiple endocrine neoplasia (MEN) I association (20–30% of cases)
  2. Clinical findings
    a. Epigastric pain with weight loss
    b. Peptic ulceration
      • Most are solitary duodenal ulcers rather than multiple ulcers.
    c. Acid hypersecretion with diarrhea
    d. Maldigestion of food
      • Acid interferes with pancreatic enzyme activity.
  3. Laboratory findings
    a. Increased BAO, MAO, and BAO/MAO ratio
    b. Serum gastrin level over 1000 pg/mL
H. Gastric polyps
  1. Complication of chronic gastritis and achlorhydria
  2. Hyperplastic polyp
    a. Most common type
    b. Hamartoma with no malignant potential

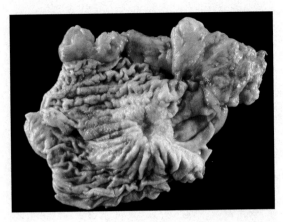

17-8: *Gastric adenocarcinoma showing an irregular ulcer crater with piling up of the mucosa around the ulcer. (From Kumar V, Fausto N, Abbas A: Robbins and Cotran's Pathologic Basis of Disease, 7th ed. Philadelphia, WB Saunders, 2004, p 825, Fig. 17-26.)*

3. Adenomatous polyp
   a. Neoplastic polyp
   b. Potential for malignant transformation

I. Gastric tumors

1. Leiomyoma
   a. Stomach is most common site.
   b. May ulcerate or bleed
2. Intestinal type of gastric adenocarcinoma
   a. Epidemiology
      (1) Decreasing incidence in United States
         • Increased incidence in Japan
      (2) Most common gastric carcinoma
   b. Risk factors
      (1) Intestinal metaplasia due to *H. pylori* (most important)
      (2) Nitrosamines, smoked foods (Japan), diets lacking fruits/vegetables
      (3) Type A chronic atrophic gastritis, Menetrier's disease
   c. Polypoid or ulcerated (Fig. 17-8)
   d. Locations
      (1) Lesser curvature of pylorus and antrum (50–60% of cases)
      (2) Cardia (25% of cases), body and fundus
3. Diffuse type of gastric adenocarcinoma
   a. Incidence has remained unchanged.
   b. *Not* associated with *H. pylori*
   c. Diffuse infiltration of malignant cells in the stomach wall
      (1) Sometimes called "linitis plastica"
      (2) Stomach does *not* peristalse.
      (3) Signet-ring cells infiltrate the stomach wall (Fig. 17-9).
      (4) Produces Krukenberg tumors of the ovaries
         • Hematogenous spread of signet-ring cells to both ovaries

Leiomyoma: most common benign tumor in gastrointestinal tract

Intestinal metaplasia: precursor lesion for gastric adenocarcinoma

Krukenberg tumor: metastatic signet-ring cells to both ovaries

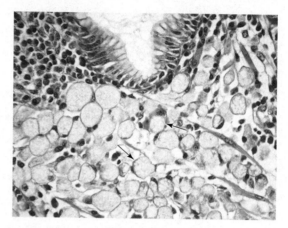

17-9: Diffuse type of gastric adenocarcinoma with signet-ring carcinoma cells (arrows). Mucin produced by the cancer cells pushes the nucleus to the periphery. (From Kumar V, Fausto N, Abbas A: Robbins and Cotran's Pathologic Basis of Disease, 7th ed. Philadelphia, WB Saunders, 2004, p 825, Fig. 17-27B.)

    d. Clinical findings of gastric adenocarcinoma
      (1) Weight loss (most common), epigastric pain with vomiting
      (2) Metastasis to left supraclavicular node (Virchow's node)
      (3) Paraneoplastic skin lesions (see Chapter 8)
        (a) Acanthosis nigricans
        (b) Multiple outcroppings of seborrheic keratoses (Leser-Trelat sign)
      (4) Metastasis to umbilicus (Sister Mary Joseph sign)
    e. Common metastatic sites
      • Liver, lung, ovaries
    f. Approximately 20% overall 5-year survival rate
  4. Primary gastric malignant lymphoma
    a. Stomach is the most common site for extranodal malignant lymphoma.
    b. Low-grade B-cell lymphoma
      (1) *H. pylori*-related
      (2) MALToma (derives from *m*ucosa-*a*ssociated *l*ymphoid *t*issue)
    c. High-grade B- or T-cell lymphomas

IV. Small Bowel and Large Bowel Disorders
  A. Signs and symptoms of small bowel disease
    1. Colicky pain
      a. Pain followed by a pain-free interval
        • Accompanied by constipation and inability to pass gas
      b. Symptom of bowel obstruction
        • Example—adhesions from previous surgery
    2. Diarrhea
      a. Sign of infection, malabsorption, osmotic diarrhea
      b. If bloody, may be a sign of infarction or dysentery

Colicky pain: symptom of bowel obstruction

3. Anemia
   - Malabsorption of iron, folate, or vitamin B_{12}
B. **Signs and symptoms of large bowel disease**
   1. Diarrhea
      a. Infection, laxative abuse, inflammatory bowel disease
      b. If bloody, may be a sign of infarction or dysentery
   2. Pain
      a. Inflammatory bowel disease
      b. Ischemic colitis
      c. Diverticulitis, appendicitis, peritonitis
   3. Iron deficiency (e.g., polyps or colorectal cancer)
   4. Hematochezia (massive loss of whole blood per rectum)
      - Sigmoid diverticulosis or angiodysplasia
C. **Diarrheal diseases (excluding malabsorption)**
   1. Diarrhea
      a. More than 250 g of stool per day
      b. Acute = less than 3 weeks, chronic = over 4 weeks
      c. Invasive, osmotic, secretory types (Table 17-3)

Hematochezia: sigmoid diverticulosis, angiodysplasia

Types of diarrhea: osmotic, secretory, invasive

TABLE 17-3: Types of Diarrhea

Type	Characteristics	Causes	Screening Tests
Invasive	Pathogens invade enterocytes Low-volume diarrhea Diarrhea with blood and leukocytes (i.e., dysentery)	*Shigella* spp., *Campylobacter jejuni*, *Entamoeba histolytica*	Fecal smear for leukocytes: positive Order stool culture and stool for ova and parasites
Secretory	Loss of isotonic fluid High-volume diarrhea Mechanisms: Laxatives Enterotoxins stimulate Cl^- channels regulated by cAMP and cGMP Serotonin increases bowel motility No inflammation in bowel mucosa	Laxatives: danger of melanosis coli (black bowel syndrome) with use of phenanthracene laxatives Production enterotoxins: *Vibrio cholerae* Enterotoxigenic *E. coli* Increased serotonin: carcinoid syndrome	Fecal smear for leukocytes: negative Increased 5-HIAA: carcinoid syndrome Stool osmotic gap < 50 mOsm/kg
Osmotic	Osmotically active substance is drawing hypotonic salt solution out of bowel High-volume diarrhea No inflammation in bowel mucosa	Disaccharidase deficiency Ingestion of poorly absorbable solutes (e.g., magnesium sulfate laxatives)	Fecal smear for leukocytes: negative Stool osmotic gap > 100 mOsm/kg

cAMP, cyclic adenosine monophosphate; cGMP, cyclic guanosine monophosphate; HIAA, hydroxyindoleacetic acid.

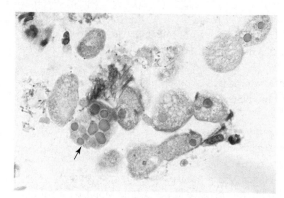

17-10: Entamoeba histolytica *trophozoites showing erythrophagocytosis* (arrow). *(From Henry JB: Clinical Diagnosis and Management by Laboratory Methods, 20th ed. Philadelphia, WB Saunders, 2001, Plate 55-7C.)*

2. Important screening tests
   a. Fecal smear for leukocytes (e.g., invasive diarrhea)
   b. Stool osmotic gap

POsm = plasma osmolality

   (1) 300 mOsm/kg (value used to represent normal POsm) − 2 × (random stool Na⁺ + random stool K⁺)
   (2) Gap of less than 50 mOsm/kg from POsm is a secretory diarrhea.
      • Indicates that diarrheal fluid approximates POsm
   (3) Gap greater than 100 mOsm/kg from POsm is an osmotic diarrhea.
      • Indicates a hypotonic loss of stool due to presence of osmotically active substances

Secretory diarrhea: loss of isotonic fluid
Osmotic diarrhea: loss of hypotonic fluid

> Lactase deficiency is a common genetic defect in Native Americans, Asian Americans, and black Americans. Colon anaerobes degrade undigested lactose into lactic acid and H₂ gas leading to abdominal distention with explosive diarrhea. Treatment is to avoid dairy products.

3. Summary table of microbial pathogens causing diarrhea (Figs. 17-10 to 17-12; Table 17-4)

D. Malabsorption
   • Increased fecal excretion of fat with concurrent deficiencies of vitamins (particularly fat soluble vitamins), minerals, carbohydrates, and proteins

Causes of malabsorption: pancreatic insufficiency, bile salt/acid deficiency, small bowel disease

1. Causes of malabsorption
   • Pancreatic insufficiency, bile salt deficiency, small bowel disease
2. Pancreatic insufficiency
   a. Most often caused by chronic pancreatitis (see Chapter 18)
      • Due to alcohol in adults and cystic fibrosis in children
   b. Maldigestion of fats due to diminished lipase activity
      • Undigested neutral fats and fat droplets are in stool.
   c. Maldigestion of proteins due to diminished trypsin
      • Undigested meat fibers are in stool.

Pancreatic insufficiency: malabsorption of fat and proteins

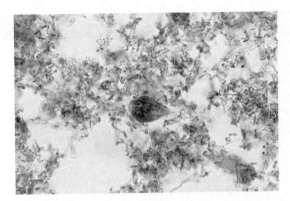

17-11: Giardia lamblia *with two nuclei and flagella. (From Henry JB: Clinical Diagnosis and Management by Laboratory Methods, 20th ed. Philadelphia, WB Saunders, 2001, Plate 55-8C.)*

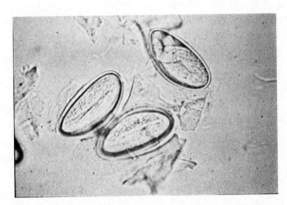

17-12: *Embryonated eggs of* Enterobius vermicularis. *(From Hart P, Shears CT: Color Atlas of Medical Microbiology. St. Louis, Mosby, 1996, p 271, Fig. 446.)*

     d. Carbohydrate digestion *not* affected
      • Amylase is present in salivary glands and brush border enzymes.
     e. Screening test
      • CT scan of pancreas shows dystrophic calcification.
   3. Bile salt deficiency; pathogenesis and causes:
     a. Inadequate production of bile salts/acids from cholesterol (e.g., cirrhosis)
     b. Intrahepatic/extrahepatic blockage of bile
      • Examples—primary biliary cirrhosis, stone in common bile duct
     c. Bacterial overgrowth in small bowel with destruction of bile salts
      • Example—small bowel diverticula
     d. Excess binding of bile salts (e.g., cholestyramine)
     e. Terminal ileal disease preventing recycling of bile salts/acids
      • Examples——Crohn's disease, resection of ileum
   4. Small bowel disease (Table 17-5; Figs. 17-13 and 17-14)
     a. Pathogenesis of malabsorption

Bile salts/acids: required to micellarize monoglycerides and fatty acids

Villi: required to reabsorb micelles

TABLE 17-4:
Microbial
Pathogens Causing
Diarrhea

Pathogen	Discussion
Viruses	
Cytomegalovirus	Common cause of diarrhea in AIDS
Norwalk virus	Most common cause of adult gastroenteritis
Rotavirus	Most common cause of childhood diarrhea Rotazyme test on stool establishes diagnosis
Bacteria	
Bacillus cereus	Gram-positive rod Food poisoning with preformed toxin Associated with fried rice or tacos
Campylobacter jejuni	Curved or S-shaped gram-negative rods Contracted by eating contaminated poultry or milk Produces dysentery with crypt abscesses and ulcers resembling ulcerative colitis
Clostridium botulinum Adult Infant	Food poisoning with preformed toxin (blocks release of acetylcholine) Causes paralysis and mydriasis Food poisoning often contracted by eating spores in honey
Clostridium difficile	Associated with pseudomembranous colitis Antibiotics (e.g., ampicillin) cause overgrowth of toxin-producing *C. difficile* in colon Pseudomembrane covers colon mucosa (see Fig. 2-7) Toxin assay of stool is best confirmatory test Rx: metronidazole; vancomycin produces resistant strains
Escherichia coli	ETEC: produces heat-stable toxin that stimulates guanylate or adenylate cyclase, causing secretory diarrhea (traveler's diarrhea) STEC (O157:H7 serotype): contracted by eating undercooked beef. Produces hemolytic uremic syndrome (see Chapter 14)
Mycobacterium avium-intracellulare complex (MAC)	Acid-fast rods Causes diarrhea with malabsorption in AIDS (CD4 count < 50 cells/µL) Foamy macrophages in lamina propria simulate Whipple's disease
Mycobacterium tuberculosis	Acid-fast organisms swallowed from primary focus in lung Invade Peyer's patches Circumferential spread in lymphatics leads to stricture formation

Salmonella species	Pathogenic *Salmonella*: *S. typhi, S. paratyphi, S. enteritidis*
	Animal reservoirs: turtles, hamsters, lizards
	Typhoid fever caused by *S. typhi*:
	  Week 1: invades Peyer's patches and produces sepsis (blood culture best for diagnosis)
	  Week 2: diarrhea (positive stool culture); classic triad of bradycardia, neutropenia, splenomegaly
	  Chronic carrier state due to gallbladder disease

Shigella species	*No* animal reservoirs Mucosal ulceration, pseudomembranous inflammation, dysentery
Staphylococcus aureus	Food poisoning with preformed toxin; culture food *not* stool Gastroenteritis occurs in 1–6 hours after eating

TABLE 17-4:
Microbial
Pathogens Causing
Diarrhea—cont'd

Pathogen	Discussion
Bacteria—cont'd	
Vibrio cholerae	Enterotoxin stimulates adenylate cyclase in small bowel
	Contracted from drinking contaminated water or eating contaminated seafood, especially crustacea
	Rx is fluid replacement; glucose and sodium required in oral supplements (cotransport system for reabsorption)
Yersinia enterocolitica	Dysentery, mesenteric lymphadenitis (granulomatous microabscesses)
Protozoa	
Balantidium coli	Produces colonic ulcers with bloody diarrhea
Cryptosporidium parvum	Most common cause of diarrhea in AIDS
	Contracted by ingesting oocysts (acid-fast positive)
Entamoeba histolytica (see Fig. 17-10)	Produces dysentery with flask-shaped ulcers in cecum
	Trophozoites phagocytose red blood cells
	Rx: metronidazole
Giardia lamblia (see Fig. 17-11)	Most common protozoal cause of diarrhea in United States
	Produces acute and chronic diarrhea with malabsorption
	Detected with antigen test of urine
	Rx: metronidazole
Isospora belli	Oocysts (acid-fast positive)
	Associated with AIDS diarrhea
Helminths	
Ascaris lumbricoides	Bowel obstruction in adult phase
Diphyllobothrium latum	Adult worms produce vitamin B_{12} deficiency
Enterobius vermicularis (see Fig. 17-12)	Eggs deposited in anus cause anal pruritus
	Urethritis in girls; appendicitis
	No eosinophilia
Necator americanus	Adults attach to villi, resulting in blood loss and iron deficiency
Strongyloides stercoralis	Abdominal pain and diarrhea
Trichuris trichiura	Abdominal pain, diarrhea
	Rectal prolapse in children

ETEC, enterotoxigenic *Escherichia coli*; Rx, treatment; STEC, Shiga toxin *E. coli*.

    (1) Inability to reabsorb micelles due to loss of villous surface
       • Examples—celiac disease, Whipple's disease
    (2) Lymphatic obstruction
       • Examples—Whipple's disease, abetalipoproteinemia (see Chapter 9)
   b. D-Xylose screening test
    (1) Xylose does *not* require pancreatic enzymes for absorption.
    (2) Lack of reabsorption of orally administered xylose indicates small bowel disease

D-Xylose: decreased reabsorption indicates small bowel disease

TABLE 17-5:
Small Bowel Disorders Causing Malabsorption

Disorder	Characteristics	Clinical Findings
Celiac disease	Autoimmune disease: antibodies against gliadin fraction in gluten Usually begins in infancy; female dominant Primarily involves duodenum and jejunum; flattened villi Hyperplastic glands with chronic inflammation (see Fig. 17-13)	Strong association with dermatitis herpetiformis (autoimmune vesicular skin disease) (see Fig. 17-14) May produce T-cell lymphoma of stomach and/or small intestine Restrict or eliminate gluten from diet Antigliadin antibodies (best screening test), antiendomysial and antireticulin antibodies
Whipple's disease	Male dominant disease Caused by *Tropheryma whippelii* bacilli (only visible by EM) Blunting of villi; foamy PAS-positive macrophages in lamina propria obstruct lymphatics and reabsorption of chylomicrons	Fever, recurrent polyarthritis, generalized lymphadenopathy, increased skin pigmentation Treat with antibiotics

EM, electron microscopy; PAS, periodic acid–Schiff.

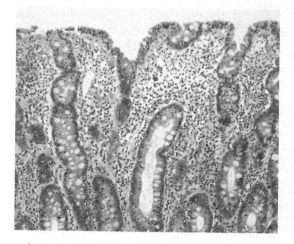

17-13: *Celiac disease showing atrophy of the villi, lengthening of the crypts, and a heavy chronic inflammatory infiltrate in the lamina propria. (From Damjanov I, Linder J: Pathology: A Color Atlas. St. Louis, Mosby, 2000, p 128, Fig. 7-25A.)*

General screening tests for malabsorption: stool for fat, serum β-carotene

5. General screening tests indicating malabsorption
   a. Increased qualitative or quantitative stool for fat
      • Best screening test
   b. Decreased serum beta carotene
      • Precursor for fat-soluble retinoic acid (vitamin A)
6. Clinical findings in malabsorption
   a. Steatorrhea
      • Excessive, large, sticky, stools that float

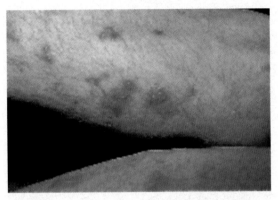

17-14: *Dermatitis herpetiformis showing groups of vesicles with erythema on the extensor surface of the forearm. Presence of this lesion has a strong association with underlying celiac disease. (From Goldstein BG: Practical Dermatology, 2nd ed. St. Louis, Mosby, 1997, p 83, Fig. 8-4.)*

    b. Fat-soluble and water-soluble vitamin deficiencies (see Chapter 7)

    c. Combined anemias (e.g., folate and iron deficiency) (see Chapter 9)

    d. Ascites and pitting edema (due to hypoproteinemia)

E. Bowel obstruction

  1. Signs of bowel obstruction

    a. Colicky pain

    b. Radiographic findings

      (1) Bowel distention

      (2) Air/fluid levels with a step-ladder appearance (Fig. 17-15)

      (3) Absence of air distal to obstruction

  2. Small bowel obstruction is the most common site for obstruction.

  3. Causes of obstruction (Table 17-6)

> Adhesions from previous surgery: most common cause of small bowel obstruction

F. Hernias

  1. Mechanisms predisposing to acquired hernias

    a. Increased intra-abdominal pressure (e.g., coughing, heavy weight lifting)

    b. Weakness in abdominal wall

  2. Types of hernias (Table 17-7)

> Indirect inguinal hernia: most common hernia

G. Vascular disorders

  1. Small bowel is more likely than large bowel to have ischemic damage.

    a. Most of the small bowel is supplied by the superior mesenteric artery (SMA).

    b. Areas supplied by SMA

      (1) Small bowel

      (2) Ascending and transverse colon

      (3) SMA and inferior mesenteric artery (IMA) overlap at the splenic flexure.

        • Splenic flexure is a watershed area (see Chapter 1).

> Occlusion of SMA: most common cause of small bowel infarction

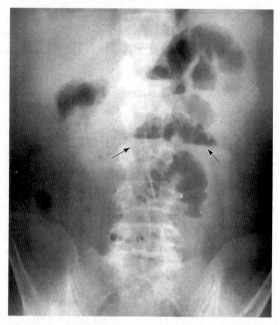

17-15: *Radiograph showing small bowel obstruction. Multiple air-fluid levels are present (arrows) in dilated small bowel. There is absence of air distal to the obstruction. (From Katz DS: Radiology Secrets. Philadelphia, Hanley & Belfus, 1998, p 117, Fig. 25-1.)*

2. Types of infarctions
    a. Transmural
        (1) Full-thickness hemorrhagic infarction
            • Usually involves all or part of the small bowel
        (2) Usually due to occlusion of SMA
    b. Mural and mucosal infarctions
        • Usually occur in hypoperfusion states (e.g., shock)
3. Causes of acute ischemia involving small bowel
    a. Acute mesenteric ischemia (50% of cases)
        (1) Embolism from the left side of the heart to the SMA
            • Atrial fibrillation is the most common predisposing arrhythmia.
        (2) Thrombosis of the mesenteric artery (usually SMA) (Fig. 17-16)
    b. Nonocclusive ischemia (25% of cases)
        (1) Hypotension secondary to heart failure (most common)
        (2) Shock, patient taking digitalis (? vasospasm)
    c. Mesenteric vein thrombosis (25% of cases)
        (1) Thrombosis states—polycythemia vera, antiphospholipid syndrome
        (2) Extension of renal cell carcinoma into vena cava
4. Clinical and radiographic findings of small bowel infarction
    a. Diffuse abdominal pain, bowel distention, and bloody diarrhea
        • Usually occurs in an elderly patient
    b. Absent bowel sounds (ileus)
    c. *No* rebound tenderness (peritonitis) early in infarction

Atrial fibrillation: most common arrhythmia associated with systemic embolization

Small bowel infarction: diffuse abdominal pain + bloody diarrhea

TABLE 17-6:
Small and Large
Bowel Obstruction

Disorder	Discussion
Adhesions	Most common cause of small bowel obstruction Adhesions from previous surgery (most common), endometriosis, radiation
Crohn's disease	Lumen in terminal ileum is narrow due to full-thickness inflammation of bowel wall Serosal adhesions from bowel-to-bowel also cause obstruction
Duodenal atresia	Atresia is distal to entry of the common bile duct Association with Down syndrome History of maternal polyhydramnios (cannot reabsorb amniotic fluid) Vomiting of bile-stained fluid at birth "Double bubble" sign: air in stomach and air in proximal duodenum
Gallstone ileus	Occurs in elderly woman with chronic cholecystitis and cholelithiasis Fistula develops between gallbladder and small bowel; stone passes into small bowel and lodges at the ileocecal valve causing obstruction Radiograph shows air in biliary tree
Hirschsprung disease	Absence of ganglion cells in Meissner's submucosal plexus and Auerbach's myenteric plexus causes localized aperistalsis; acquired Hirschsprung disease due to Chagas' disease and destruction of ganglion cells by leishmania Involves distal sigmoid and rectum; proximal bowel is dilated but has peristalsis Association with Down syndrome Alternating signs of obstruction with diarrhea; rectal examination shows *no* stool on examining finger (no stool in rectal vault) Complication: enterocolitis of dilated bowel (danger of perforation) Diagnose with rectal biopsy
Indirect inguinal hernia	Second most common cause of small bowel obstruction Common in weight lifters Bowel becomes trapped in inguinal canal
Intussusception	In children, the terminal ileum invaginates into the cecum; mounds of hyperplastic lymphoid tissue in Peyer's patches serve as the nidus for the intussusception; combination of obstruction and ischemia; colicky pain with bloody diarrhea; oblong mass palpated in midepigastrium; usually self-reduces In adults, a polyp or cancer is the nidus for intussusception
Meconium ileus	Complication of newborn with cystic fibrosis Meconium lacks NaCl and obstructs the bowel lumen
Volvulus	Bowel twists around mesenteric root producing obstruction and strangulation Sigmoid colon is most common site in elderly, while the cecum is the most common site in young adults Risk factors: chronic constipation (most common), pregnancy, laxative abuse

TABLE 17-7:
Hernias

Hernia	Discussion
Direct	Single layer of transversalis is stretched in the floor of the triangle of Hesselbach Medial border of triangle is rectus abdominis, lateral border is inferior epigastric artery, inferior border is inguinal ligament Hernia bulges through floor of triangle of Hesselbach; bulge disappears when patient reclines Small bowel cannot enter scrotal sac; therefore, there is no obstruction or incarceration
Femoral	Most common in women Bulge located below inguinal ligament Highest rate of incarceration of small bowel
Indirect	Most common hernia Pathogenesis in children: persistence of peritoneal connection between inguinal canal and tunica vaginalis Pathogenesis in adults: protrusion of new peritoneal process into inguinal canal Small bowel passes through internal inguinal ring and may enter scrotal sac; bowel directly hits the examining finger within the inguinal canal Complications: entrapped in inguinal canal (incarceration) or strangulated obstruction (hemorrhagic infarction)
Umbilical	Most common hernia in adults with ascites, pregnancy, or obesity Most common hernia in black Americans newborns Peritoneal protrusion extends into a fascial defect containing remnants of umbilical cord Majority close spontaneously by the second year Incarceration more likely in adults than children
Ventral	Hernia develops in weakened area of previous surgical excision Obesity most common cause

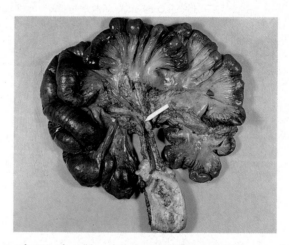

17-16: *Hemorrhagic infarction of small bowel, showing the diffuse dark discoloration of the small bowel. Arrow shows a thrombosed superior mesenteric artery attached to the aorta. (From Damjanov I, Linder J: Pathology: A Color Atlas. St. Louis, Mosby, 2000, p 124, Fig. 7-8.)*

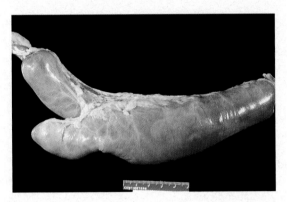

17-17: *Meckel diverticulum located on the antimesenteric side of the small intestine. (From Kumar V, Fausto N, Abbas A: Robbins and Cotran's Pathologic Basis of Disease, 7th ed. Philadelphia, WB Saunders, 2004, p 830, Fig. 17-31.)*

   d. Profound neutrophilic leukocytosis, increased amylase (bowel origin)
   e. Radiographic findings
      (1) "Thumbprint sign" due to edema in bowel wall
      (2) Bowel distention with air/fluid levels
5. Ischemic colitis
   a. Involves the splenic flexure of the large bowel
   b. Atherosclerotic narrowing of SMA or IMA causes mesenteric angina.
      (1) Severe pain occurs in splenic flexure shortly after eating.
      (2) Patient losses weight for fear of pain related to eating
   c. Clinical findings
      (1) History compatible with mesenteric angina
      (2) Pain localized to the splenic flexure
         • Accompanied by bloody diarrhea due to mucosal or mural infarction
   d. Repair of infarction site may result in fibrosis.
      • Common cause of ischemic strictures and obstruction
6. Angiodysplasia
   a. Dilation of mucosal and submucosal venules in cecum and right colon
      • Usually occurs in elderly individuals
   b. Increased wall stress in the cecum stretches the venules.
   c. Clinical findings
      (1) Hematochezia
      (2) Association with von Willebrand disease and calcific aortic stenosis
      (3) Diagnose with colonoscopy and angiography
H. Small bowel diverticula
   1. Meckel diverticulum
      a. Vitelline (omphalomesenteric) duct remnant
         (1) True diverticulum (Fig. 17-17)
         (2) Mnemonic: 2 inches long, 2 feet from ileocecal valve, 2% of population, 2% symptomatic

Ischemic colitis: splenic flexure pain + bloody diarrhea

Angiodysplasia: dilation cecal submucosal venules; hematochezia

b. Contain pancreatic rests and heterotopic gastric mucosa
  - Increase the risk for bleeding
c. Clinical findings
  (1) Newborn finding
    - Fecal material in umbilical area due to persistence of vitelline duct
  (2) Bleeding (most common finding)
    - Common cause of iron deficiency in newborns and young children
  (3) Diverticulitis
    - Clinically impossible to distinguish Meckel diverticulitis from appendicitis
d. Diagnosis
  - ^{99m}Tc nuclear scan identifies parietal cells in ectopic gastric mucosa.

2. Small bowel pulsion diverticula
  a. Duodenum is most common site.
    - Wide-mouthed diverticula suggests systemic sclerosis.
  b. Complications
    (1) Diverticulitis (danger of perforation)
    (2) Bacterial overgrowth
      - May produce bile salt deficiency and vitamin B_{12} deficiency

I. Large bowel pulsion diverticulum
  1. Pathogenesis
    a. Due to a low-fiber diet with increased constipation
    b. Sigmoid colon most common site (Fig. 17-18)
    c. Area of weakness is where vessels penetrate the muscular propria.
      - Diverticulum is juxtaposed to a blood vessel.
    d. Diverticula present in Marfan syndrome and Ehler-Danlos syndrome
  2. Complications
    a. Most common complication is diverticulitis.
      (1) Caused by stool impacted (fecalith) in diverticulum sac
        - Produces ulceration and ischemia
      (2) Diverticulitis presents as a "left-sided appendicitis."
      (3) Best diagnosed with CT scan or water-soluble barium study
      (4) Increased risk for perforation and abscess formation
    b. Most common cause of hematochezia
      (1) Refers to divertic<u>ulosis</u> *not* diverticul<u>itis</u>
      (2) Scarring of the vessel in diverticulitis prevents bleeding.
    c. Most common cause of fistulas (connection between hollow structures)

> Colovesical fistula (connection between large bowel and the bladder) is a common fistula in the gastrointestinal tract. It is associated with pneumaturia (air in urine) and recurrent urinary tract infections.

J. Inflammatory bowel disease
  1. Ulcerative colitis
    a. Most common inflammatory bowel disease

Meckel diverticulum: bleeding most common complication

Sigmoid diverticular disease: most common cause hematochezia and fistulas

Sigmoid diverticulitis: "left-sided appendicitis"

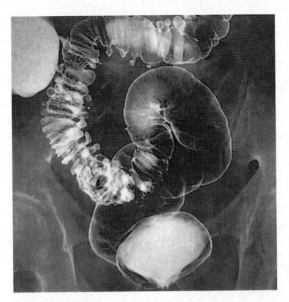

17-18: *Sigmoid diverticulosis viewed on barium enema. Multiple diverticula sacs are outlined by the double-contrast barium technique. (From Forbes C, Jackson W: Color Atlas and Text of Clinical Medicine, 2nd ed. St. Louis, Mosby, 2003, p 382, Fig. 8-110.)*

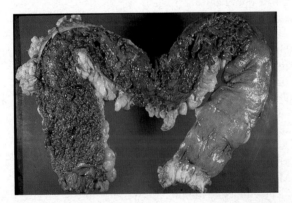

17-19: *Ulcerative colitis. The colon shows diffuse ulceration of the mucosal surface and residual islands of inflamed mucosa (pseudopolyps). (From Damjanov I: Pathology for the Health-Related Professions, 2nd ed. Philadelphia, WB Saunders, 2000, p 271, Fig. 10-10A.)*

      b. Chronic relapsing ulceroinflammatory disease
      c. Ulcerations are in continuity (Fig. 17-19).
         • Ulcerations limited to the mucosa and submucosa of rectum and colon
    2. Crohn's disease
      a. Chronic granulomatous, ulceroconstrictive disease
      b. Transmural inflammation (Fig. 17-20)
         • Discontinuous spread throughout entire gastrointestinal tract
    3. Summary of ulcerative colitis and Crohn's disease (Table 17-8)

Ulcerative colitis: mucosal/submucosal ulcerations

Crohn's disease: transmural inflammation

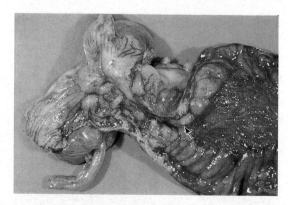

17-20: *Crohn's disease, showing a resection of the terminal ileum with attached cecum and appendix; the appendix is to the left. The thickened terminal ileal wall causes the narrowing (arrow) at the junction of the ileum and the cecum. The ileal mucosa has a cobblestone appearance due to linear ulcerations (aphthous ulcers) that cut into the underlying submucosa. (From Damjanov I: Pathology for the Health-Related Professions, 2nd ed. Philadelphia, WB Saunders, 2000, p 271, Fig. 10-10B.)*

K. **Irritable bowel syndrome**
  1. Intrinsic colonic motility disorder
     • Female dominant
  2. Alternating bouts of diarrhea and constipation
     a. Abdominal pain and bloating relieved by defecation
     b. Simulates ulcerative colitis
  3. Normal flexible sigmoidoscopy

L. **Small bowel malignancy**
  • Small bowel is the *least* common site in the gastrointestinal tract for a primary malignancy.
  1. Primary adenocarcinoma
     • Duodenum most common site
  2. Carcinoid tumor
     a. Most common small bowel malignancy
     b. Neuroendocrine tumor
        (1) Contain neurosecretory granules visible on electron microscopy
        (2) Carcinoid tumors are malignant.
        (3) Metastatic potential correlates with size and depth.
           (a) Size larger than 2 cm
           (b) Depth of invasion (>50% of bowel thickness)
        (4) Foregut (e.g., stomach) and hindgut (e.g., rectum) carcinoid tumors
           • Invade but *rarely* metastasize
        (5) Midgut carcinoid tumors (e.g., terminal ileum)
           • Invade and metastasize
     c. Locations
        (1) Tip of the vermiform appendix (most common site)
           • Usually too small to metastasize to liver

Irritable bowel syndrome: intrinsic colonic motility disorder

Carcinoid tumors: malignant neuroendocrine tumors

Vermiform appendix: most common site for carcinoid tumor

TABLE 17-8:
**Comparison of
Ulcerative Colitis
and Crohn's
Disease**

Feature	Ulcerative Colitis	Crohn's Disease
Epidemiology	More common in whites than black Americans No sex predilection Affects young adults	More common in whites than black Americans, in Jews than non-Jews More common in women Affects young adults
Extent	Mucosal and submucosal	Transmural
Location	Mainly rectum Extends continuously into left colon (may involve entire colon) Does *not* involve other areas of GI tract	Terminal ileum alone (30% of cases), ileum and colon (50% of cases), colon alone (20% of cases) Involves other areas of GI tract (mouth to anus)
Gross features	Inflammatory pseudopolyps Areas of friable, bloody residual mucosa Ulceration and hemorrhage	Thick bowel wall and narrow lumen (leads to obstruction) Aphthous ulcers (early sign) Skip lesions, strictures, fistulas Deep linear ulcers with cobblestone pattern Fat creeping around serosa
Microscopic features	Ulcers and crypt abscesses containing neutrophils Dysplasia or cancer may be present	Noncaseating granulomas (60% of cases), lymphoid aggregates Dysplasia or cancer less likely
Clinical findings	Recurrent left-sided abdominal cramping with bloody diarrhea and mucus	Recurrent right lower quadrant colicky pain (obstruction) with diarrhea Bleeding occurs only with colon or anal involvement (fistulas)
Radiography	"Lead pipe" appearance in chronic disease	"String" sign in terminal ileum from luminal narrowing by inflammation, fistulas
Complications	Toxic megacolon (hypotonic and distended bowel) Primary sclerosing cholangitis (fibrosis around common bile duct leading to jaundice) HLA-B27–positive spondyloarthropathy Adenocarcinoma: greatest risks are pancolitis, early onset, duration of disease >10 years	Fistulas, obstruction Calcium oxalate renal calculi (increased reabsorption of oxalate through inflamed mucosa) Malabsorption due to bile salt deficiency Macrocytic anemia due to vitamin B_{12} deficiency

GI, gastrointestinal.

(2) Terminal ileum
  (a) Commonly metastasize to liver
  (b) Tumor produces bioactive compounds (e.g., serotonin)
    • Compounds are delivered to the liver by the portal vein.
  (c) Serotonin is metabolized to 5-hydroxyindoleacetic acid (5-HIAA).
    • 5-HIAA is excreted in the urine.
  (d) Serotonin is completely metabolized and does *not* enter the systemic circulation.
d. Bright yellow tumor
e. Carcinoid syndrome
  (1) Liver metastasis *must* occur to produce the syndrome.
    (a) Serotonin is secreted by metastatic tumor nodules.
    (b) Serotonin entering hepatic vein tributaries gains access to the systemic circulation.
  (2) Clinical findings due to serotonin
    (a) Flushing of the skin (vasodilation) and diarrhea (increased bowel motility)
    (b) Tricuspid regurgitation and pulmonary stenosis
      • Serotonin increases collagen production in the valves.
    (c) Increase in urine 5-HIAA
3. Malignant lymphoma
a. Usually occur in Peyer's patches of terminal ileum
b. Usually B-cell origin (e.g., Burkitt's lymphoma)

M. Small and large bowel polyps
1. Non-neoplastic (hamartomatous) polyps
a. Hyperplastic polyp
  (1) Most common type in adults
  (2) Majority are in the sigmoid colon
  (3) *No* malignant potential or polyposis syndromes
  (4) Histologically have a "sawtooth" appearance
b. Juvenile (retention) polyps
  (1) Most common polyp in children
  (2) Located in the rectum
    • Sometimes prolapse out of the rectum and bleed
  (3) Solitary polyp
    • Smooth surface with enlarged cystic spaces on cut section
  (4) Juvenile polyposis
    • Autosomal dominant or nonhereditary
  (5) Cronkhite-Canada syndrome
    (a) Nonhereditary polyposis syndrome
    (b) Polyps plus ectodermal abnormalities of the nails
c. Peutz-Jeghers polyposis
  (1) Autosomal dominant
  (2) Polyps predominate in small bowel; less common in stomach and colon
  (3) Clinical findings
    (a) Mucosal pigmentation of buccal mucosa, lips
    (b) Increased risk for benign sex-cord stromal ovarian tumor

Carcinoid tumor terminal ileum: metastasis to liver causes carcinoid syndrome

Carcinoid syndrome: flushing and diarrhea

Sigmoid colon: most common site for gastrointestinal polyps

Hamartomatous polyps: no malignant potential

Hyperplastic polyp: most common polyp in adults

Juvenile polyp: most common polyp in children

Peutz-Jeghers polyposis: predominance of small intestine polyps

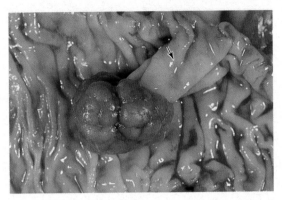

17-21: *Tubular adenoma. The head of the stalked polyp has a lobulated, mushroom-like appearance. Arrow points to the stalk. (From Damjanov I, Linder J: Pathology: A Color Atlas. St. Louis, Mosby, 2000, p 138, Fig. 7-55.)*

2. Neoplastic polyps
   - Called adenomas
   a. Premalignant dysplastic colonic polyps
      (1) Increase with age
      (2) Equal sex incidence
   b. Tubular adenoma (adenomatous polyps)
      (1) Most common polyp (60% of polyps)
      (2) Sigmoid colon is most common site.
      (3) Stalked polyp
         (a) Looks like a mushroom (Fig. 17-21)
         (b) Sections show complex branching of glands (adenomatous change) (see Fig. 8-1).
   c. Tubulovillous adenoma (20–30% of polyps)
      (1) Usually stalked polyp
      (2) Adenomatous and villous change (similar to small bowel villi)
   d. Villous adenoma (10% of polyps)
      (1) Sessile polyp (no stalk) with primarily a villous component
      (2) Rectosigmoid location
      (3) Secrete protein and potassium-rich mucus
   e. Risk factors for malignancy in adenomas
      (1) Adenoma larger than 2 cm (40% risk of malignancy)
      (2) Multiple polyps
      (3) Polyps with increased villous component
         - Villous adenomas have a 30% to 40% risk for malignancy.
   f. Familial polyposis (Fig. 17-22)
      (1) Autosomal dominant
         (a) All patients develop tubular adenomas and cancer.
         (b) Polyps begin to develop between 10 and 20 years of age.
      (2) Pathogenesis
         - Inactivation of adenomatous polyposis coli (APC) suppressor gene

Tubular adenoma: most common neoplastic polyp

Villous adenoma: greatest risk for developing colon cancer

Villous adenoma: may cause hypoproteinemia and hypokalemia

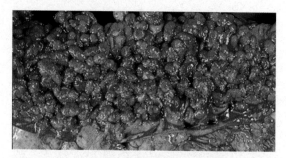

17-22: *Familial polyposis showing numerous polyps covering the large bowel mucosa. (From Damjanov I, Linder J: Anderson's Pathology, 10th ed. St. Louis, Mosby, 1996, p 1768, Fig. 56-42.)*

Familial polyposis: autosomal dominant; all patients develop colon cancer

(3) Clinical findings
  (a) Malignant transformation occurs between 35 and 40 years of age.
    • Prophylactic colectomy is recommended.
  (b) Associated with congenital hypertrophy of retinal pigment epithelium
(4) Gardner's syndrome
  (a) Autosomal dominant polyposis syndrome
  (b) Additional findings include benign osteomas and desmoid tumors.
(5) Turcot's polyposis syndrome
  (a) Autosomal recessive polyposis syndrome
  (b) Additional finding of malignant brain tumors
    • Astrocytoma and medulloblastoma

N. Colon cancer

Colon cancer: second most common cancer and cancer killer in adults

1. Risk factors for colon cancer
  a. Age older than 50 years
  b. Low-fiber/high saturated fat diet
  c. Cigarette smoking
  d. Familial polyposis syndrome, family history, ulcerative colitis
2. Carcinogenesis of colon cancer
  a. Adenoma-carcinoma sequence
    (1) Sequential mutations of different genes
      • *APC, RAS, TP53*
    (2) Accounts for 80% of sporadic colon cancers
  b. Inactivation of DNA mismatch genes (see Chapter 8)

Rectosigmoid: most common site for colon cancer

3. Locations for colon cancer
  a. Rectosigmoid (50% of cases)
  b. Ascending colon (15% of cases)
  c. Descending colon (15% of cases)
  d. Transverse colon and cecum (each 10% of cases)
4. Screening tests for colon cancer
  a. Fecal occult blood test
    • *Not* very sensitive or specific for colon cancer
  b. Colonoscopy (gold standard), barium enema

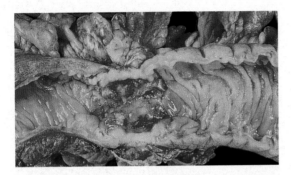

17-23: *Adenocarcinoma of the sigmoid colon. Resection of the rectosigmoid shows an annular and ulcerating growth, causing a stricture. (From Damjanov I, Linder J: Pathology: A Color Atlas. St. Louis, Mosby, 2000, p 139, Fig. 7-61.)*

5. Clinical findings in colon cancer
    a. Left-sided cancers tend to obstruct.
        (1) Bowel diameter is smaller than right colon.
        (2) Lesions have an annular, "napkin-ring" appearance (Fig. 17-23).
        (3) Change in bowel habits
            • Constipation and diarrhea with or without bleeding
    b. Right-sided cancers tend to bleed.
        (1) Bowel diameter is greater than left colon.
        (2) Tumors are more polypoid in appearance.
        (3) Blood in the stool and iron deficiency are more likely.
6. Sites of metastasis for colon cancer
     • Liver (most common), lungs, bone, and brain
7. Prognosis
    a. Approximately 35% overall 5-year survival
    b. Serum carcinoembryonic antigen (CEA) is used to detect recurrences.

O. Acute appendicitis (Fig. 17-24)
1. Pathogenesis in children
    a. Lymphoid hyperplasia (60% of cases) often secondary to a viral infection
    b. Examples—adenovirus, measles virus or immunization
2. Pathogenesis in adults
    a. Fecalith obstructs the proximal lumen
         • Increased intraluminal pressure causes mucosal injury and bacterial invasion.
    b. Other causes
         • Seeds (sunflower, persimmons), pinworm infection
    c. Primary pathogens are *Escherichia coli* (most common) and *Bacteroides fragilis.*
3. Clinical findings in sequence
    a. Initial colicky periumbilical pain
        (1) Irritation of unmyelinated afferent C fibers on visceral peritoneal surface

Left-sided colon cancer: more likely to obstruct

Right-sided colon cancer: more likely to bleed

Acute diverticulitis and appendicitis have the same pathogenesis.

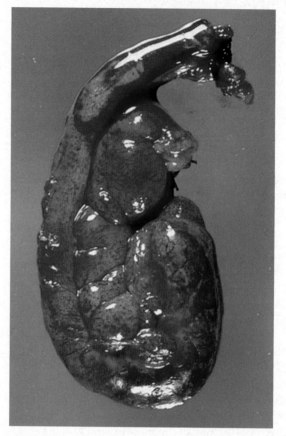

17-24: *Acute appendicitis showing erythema and vascular congestion of the serosal surface of the appendix. (From Damjanov I, Linder J: Pathology: A Color Atlas. St. Louis, Mosby, 2000, p 131, Fig. 7-30.)*

Pain in acute appendicitis: initially periumbilical and then shifts to RLQ

      (2) Refer pain to the midline

  b. Nausea, vomiting, and fever

     • Pain *precedes* nausea and vomiting

  c. Pain shifts to right lower quadrant (RLQ)

      (1) Irritation of Aδ fibers on parietal peritoneum

        • Localizes pain to the exact location

      (2) Rebound tenderness at McBurney's point (Blumberg's sign)

  d. Laboratory findings

     • Neutrophilic leukocytosis with left shift

4. Complications

  a. Periappendiceal abscess with or without perforation

      (1) Most common complication

      (2) May develop subphrenic abscess

        • Usually due to *Bacteroides fragilis*

  b. Pylephlebitis

      (1) Infection of the portal vein

(2) Danger of portal vein thrombosis

(3) Radiograph shows gas in the portal vein.

5. Diagnosis

   a. Clinical examination

   b. CT scan with oral contrast

     • Most accurate radiologic procedure for securing the diagnosis

6. Treatment is appendectomy

> There are many disorders that mimic appendicitis. These include viral gastroenteritis, ruptured follicular cyst, ruptured ectopic pregnancy, mesenteric lymphadenitis, and Meckel diverticulitis.

V. Anorectal Disorders

A. Signs and symptoms of anorectal disease

1. Bleeding

   • Internal hemorrhoids (painless), anorectal cancer, infection, fissure

2. Pain

   a. Anal fissure

   b. Thrombosed external hemorrhoids

3. Pruritus (e.g., pinworms)

4. Anal fistula (e.g., Crohn's disease)

Anorectal bleeding: internal hemorrhoids most common cause

B. Disorders

1. Internal hemorrhoids

   a. Dilated superior hemorrhoidal veins in mucosa and submucosa

   b. Causes

     (1) Straining at stool (most common)

     (2) Pregnancy, portal hypertension

   c. Clinical findings

     (1) Often prolapse out of the rectum

     (2) Commonly pass bright red blood when stooling

       • Blood coats the stool.

> In an adult, never assume that blood coating stool is always due to an internal hemorrhoid. Other causes include colorectal or anal cancer; therefore, further investigation is necessary.

     (3) Anal pruritus and soiling of underwear

2. External hemorrhoids

   a. Dilated inferior hemorrhoidal veins

   b. Painful thrombosis

3. Rectal prolapse

   a. Intussusception of the rectum through the anus

     • Due to weak rectal support mechanisms

   b. Causes in children younger than 2 years old

     (1) Whooping cough

     (2) Trichuriasis

     (3) Common sign of cystic fibrosis

    c. Common in the elderly
       • Due to straining at stool
4. Pilonidal cyst and abscess
    a. Excess hair in a deep gluteal fold becomes traumatically buried into a sinus.
    b. Painful sacrococcygeal mass with purulent drainage
5. Anal carcinoma
    a. Basaloid (epidermoid or cloacogenic) carcinoma
      (1) Most common type
      (2) Located in the transitional zone above the dentate line
      (3) Female dominant
    b. Squamous cell carcinoma
      (1) Located in the anal canal
      (2) Majority are in homosexual men (HPV association)

CHAPTER

Hepatobiliary and Pancreatic Disorders

I. Laboratory Evaluation of Liver Cell Injury
  A. Bilirubin metabolism and jaundice
  1. Bilirubin metabolism (Fig. 18-1)
     a. Unconjugated bilirubin (UCB)
        (1) Senescent red blood cells (RBCs) are phagocytosed by splenic macrophages.
        (2) UCB is the end product of heme degradation.
          • UCB is lipid-soluble (indirect bilirubin)
     b. UCB combines with albumin in the blood.
        (1) UCB is taken up by hepatocytes.
        (2) UCB is conjugated to produce conjugated bilirubin (CB).
          • CB is water-soluble (direct bilirubin)
     c. CB is secreted into the intrahepatic bile ducts.
        (1) Temporarily stored in the gallbladder
        (2) Enters the duodenum via the common bile duct
     d. Intestinal bacteria convert CB to urobilinogen (UBG).
        (1) UBG is spontaneously oxidized to urobilin.
        (2) Urobilin produces the brown color of stool.
     e. A small amount of UBG is recycled to the liver and kidneys.
        • Color of urine is due to urobilin.
  2. Jaundice
     a. Jaundice is due to an increase in UCB and/or CB.
        • Jaundice is first noticed in the sclera.
     b. Classification of causes of jaundice is based on the percentage of CB (Table 18-1).
        • Percent CB = CB/total bilirubin
     c. Schematics showing common causes of jaundice (Box 18-1)
  B. Summary of liver function tests (Table 18-2)

II. Viral Hepatitis
  A. Phases of acute viral hepatitis
  1. Prodrome
     a. Fever, painful hepatomegaly
     b. Serum transaminases increase steadily.
        • Peak just before jaundice occurs
     c. Atypical lymphocytosis

UCB: lipid soluble

UCB: end product of heme degradation in splenic macrophages

CB: water soluble

Urobilin: color of stool and urine

Viral hepatitis: most common cause of jaundice

Gilbert's disease: second most common cause of jaundice

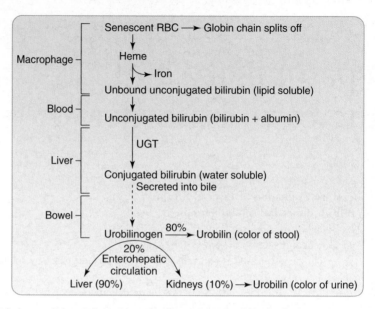

18-1: *Bilirubin metabolism. Refer to the text for discussion. RBC, red blood cell; UGT, uridine glucuronosyltransferase.*

Hepatitis A: most common viral hepatitis and cause of jaundice

2. Jaundice
   a. Variable finding depending on the type of hepatitis
   b. Increased urine bilirubin and urine UBG
3. Recovery
   • Jaundice resolves

B. Microscopic findings in acute viral hepatitis
1. Lymphocytic infiltrate with destruction of hepatocytes
   • Apoptosis of hepatocytes (Councilman bodies)
2. Persistent inflammation and fibrosis is an unfavorable sign.
   • Sign of chronic hepatitis progressing to postnecrotic cirrhosis

C. Epidemiology of viral hepatitis (Table 18-3)

D. Serologic studies in viral hepatitis
1. Hepatitis A virus (HAV)
   a. Anti-HAV-IgM indicates active infection.
   b. Anti-HAV-IgG indicates recovery from infection or vaccination.
     • Protective antibody
2. Hepatitis B virus (HBV) (Fig. 18-2 and Table 18-4)
   a. Hepatitis B surface antigen (HBsAg)
     (1) Appears within 2 to 8 weeks after exposure
       • First marker of infection
     (2) Persists up to 4 months in acute hepatitis
       • HBsAg longer than 6 months defines chronic HBV.
   b. Hepatitis B e antigen (HBeAg) and HBV-DNA
     (1) Infective particles
     (2) Appear *after* HBsAg and disappear *before* HBsAg

HBsAg > 6 months defines chronic HBV

TABLE 18-1:
Causes of Jaundice

Type of Hyperbilirubinemia	Urine Bilirubin	Urine UBG	Disorders
Unconjugated			
CB < 20%			
Increased production of UCB	Absent	↑	Extravascular hemolytic anemias: e.g., hereditary spherocytosis, Rh and ABO HDN
Decreased uptake or conjugation of UCB	Absent	Normal	Gilbert syndrome: common genetic defect in uptake/conjugation of UCB; jaundice occurs with fasting
			Crigler-Najjar syndromes: genetic disorders with decreased to absent conjugating enzymes
			Physiologic jaundice of newborn: begins on day 3 of life; caused by normal macrophage destruction of fetal RBCs
Mixed			
CB 20–50%	↑	↑	Viral hepatitis: defect in uptake, conjugation of UCB and secretion of CB
Obstructive			
CB > 50%	↑	Absent	Decreased intrahepatic bile flow Drug-induced (e.g., OCP)
			Primary biliary cirrhosis
			Dubin-Johnson syndrome: genetic defect in secretion into intrahepatic bile ducts; black pigment in hepatocytes
			Rotor's syndrome: similar to Dubin-Johnson syndrome but without black pigment in hepatocytes
			Decreased extrahepatic bile flow Gallstone in common bile duct Carcinoma of head of pancreas

CB, conjugated bilirubin; HDN, hemolytic disease of newborn; OCP, oral contraceptive pill; UBG, urobilinogen; UCB, unconjugated bilirubin.

   c. Anti-HBV core antibody IgM (anti-HBc-IgM)
     (1) Nonprotective antibody
       • Remains positive in acute infections
     (2) Persists during "window phase" or "serologic gap"
       • HBsAg, HBV DNA, and HBeAg are absent.
     (3) Converts to anti-HBc-IgG in 6 months
   d. Anti-HBV surface antibody (anti-HBs)
     (1) Protective antibody
     (2) Marker of immunization after HBV vaccination

Anti-HBc-IgM: only marker present during window phase

Anti-HBs: protective antibody; immunization or recovery from past infection

SCHEMATICS SHOWING COMMON CAUSES OF JAUNDICE

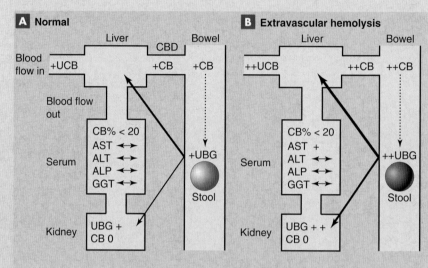

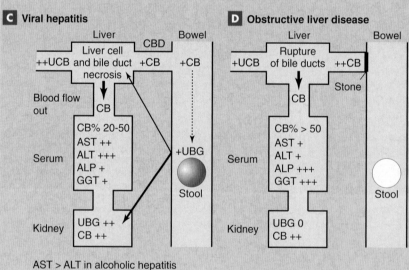

AST > ALT in alcoholic hepatitis

BOX 18-1

SCHEMATICS SHOWING COMMON CAUSES OF JAUNDICE—cont'd

In this discussion, the symbol (+) is used to indicate degrees of magnitude. **Normal bilirubin metabolism (A)** shows liver uptake of lipid-soluble unconjugated bilirubin (UCB+) and its conjugation to water-soluble conjugated bilirubin (CB+). CB is secreted into the common bile duct (CBD) and is emptied into the bowel. Intestinal bacteria convert CB to urobilinogen (UBG+), which spontaneously oxidizes to the pigment urobilin. Urobilin is responsible for the color of stool. A small percentage of UBG is reabsorbed into the blood. Most of it enters the liver *(larger arrow)* and a small percentage *(smaller arrow)* enters the urine (UBG+). Urobilin is responsible for the color of urine. All the normal bilirubin in blood is UCB (CB% < 20%) derived from macrophage destruction of senescent RBCs. UCB does not enter urine, because it is attached to albumin in the blood and is lipid, not water, soluble. CB is *never* a normal finding in urine, because it does *not* have contact with blood in its metabolism.

In **extravascular hemolysis (B)** (e.g., hereditary spherocytosis), there is increased macrophage production of UCB causing an increase in serum UCB (++; CB% < 20%). There is a corresponding increase in uptake and conjugation of UCB, conjugation to CB (++), and conversion of CB in the bowel to UBG (++). This causes darkening of the stool. There is a greater percentage of UBG recycled back to the liver *(wider arrow)* and urine *(wider arrow)*. The increase in urine UBG (++), darkens the color of urine. Because RBCs contain the enzyme aspartate aminotransferase (AST), hemolysis of RBCs causes an increase in serum AST. Alanine aminotransferase (ALT), alkaline phosphatase (ALP), and γ-glutamyltransferase (GGT) levels are normal.

In **viral hepatitis (C)**, there is generalized liver dysfunction involving uptake and conjugation of UCB, secretion of CB into bile ducts, and recycling of UBG. Serum UCB is increased (++) owing to a decrease in uptake and conjugation. Serum and urine CB are increased (++) because of liver cell necrosis and disruption of bile ductules between hepatocytes. Urine UBG is increased (++) because UBG is redirected from the liver *(smaller arrow)* to the kidneys *(larger arrow)*. Because there is an increase in serum UCB and CB, there is a mixed hyperbilirubinemia with a CB% of 20% to 50%. In viral hepatitis, ALT is higher (+++) than AST (++) and there is a slight increase in ALP and GGT (+). In alcoholic hepatitis, AST is greater than ALT, because alcohol damages mitochondria, which is where AST is normally located.

In **obstructive liver disease (D)**, an increase in serum and urine CB (++) is due to obstruction of intrahepatic or extrahepatic bile flow (stone in the CBD in this case). This causes increased pressure in the intrahepatic bile ductules leading to rupture and egress of CB into sinusoidal blood. There is absence of UBG in the stool (light-colored) and urine. CB% > 50% and there is a marked increase in serum ALP and GGT (+++) and only a slight increase in serum AST and ALT (+).

TABLE 18-2:
Liver Function Tests

Test	Significance
Liver Cell Necrosis	
Serum alanine transaminase (ALT)	Specific enzyme for liver cell necrosis Present in the cytosol ALT > AST: viral hepatitis
Serum aspartate transaminase (AST)	Present in mitochondria Alcohol damages mitochondria: AST > ALT indicates alcoholic hepatitis
Cholestasis	
Serum γ-glutamyl-transferase (GGT)	Intra- or extrahepatic obstruction to bile flow Induction of cytochrome P-450 system (e.g., alcohol): increases GGT
Serum alkaline phosphatase (ALP)	Normal GGT and increased ALP: source of ALP other than liver (e.g., osteoblastic activity in bone) Increased GGT and ALP: liver cholestasis
Bilirubin Excretion	
CB < 20%	Unconjugated hyperbilirubinemia: e.g., extravascular hemolytic anemias
CB 20–50%	Mixed hyperbilirubinemia (e.g., viral hepatitis)
CB > 50%	Conjugated hyperbilirubinemia (e.g., liver cholestasis)
Urine bilirubin	Bilirubinuria: viral hepatitis, intra- or extrahepatic obstruction of bile ducts
Urine UBG	Increased urine UBG: extravascular hemolytic anemias, viral hepatitis Absent urine UBG: liver cholestasis
Hepatocyte Function	
Serum albumin	Albumin is synthesized by the liver Hypoalbuminemia: severe liver disease (e.g., cirrhosis)
Prothrombin time (PT)	Majority of coagulation factors are synthesized in the liver Increased PT: severe liver disease
Blood urea nitrogen (BUN)	Urea cycle is present in the liver Decreased serum BUN: cirrhosis
Serum ammonia	Ammonia is metabolized in the urea cycle Increased serum ammonia: cirrhosis, Reye syndrome
Immune Function	
Serum IgM	Increased in primary biliary cirrhosis
Antimitochondrial antibody	Primary biliary cirrhosis
Anti–smooth muscle antibody	Autoimmune hepatitis
Antinuclear antibody	Autoimmune hepatitis
Tumor Marker	
α-Fetoprotein (AFP)	Hepatocellular carcinoma

CB, conjugated bilirubin; UBG, urobilinogen; UCB, unconjugated bilirubin

TABLE 18-3:
Viral Hepatitis:
Transmission and
Clinical Findings

Virus	Transmission	Clinical Findings
Hepatitis A	Fecal-oral	No carrier state Does *not* lead to chronic hepatitis Occurs in day care centers, prisons, travelers to developing countries, and male homosexuals (anal intercourse)
Hepatitis B	Parenteral, sexual, vertical (pregnancy, breast feeding)	Carrier state may occur Chronic hepatitis in 10% of immunocompetent patients Serum sickness prodrome (5–10%): vasculitis (PAN), polyarthritis, membranous GN Increased incidence of hepatocellular carcinoma
Hepatitis C	Parenteral, sexual	Carrier state may occur Mild hepatitis; jaundice uncommon Chronic hepatitis in >70% of cases Associated with posttransfusion hepatitis, type I MPGN, alcohol excess, PCT Increased incidence of hepatocellular carcinoma
Hepatitis D	Parenteral, sexual	Carrier state may occur Requires HBsAg to replicate Chronic state less likely with coinfection (HBV and HDV exposure at same time) than superinfection (HBV carrier exposed to blood containing HBV and HDV)
Hepatitis E	Fecal-oral (waterborne)	No carrier state or chronic hepatitis Fulminant hepatitis may develop in pregnant women Occurs in developing countries
Hepatitis G	Parenteral	Carrier state No chronic hepatitis

GN, glomerulopathy; MPGN, membranoproliferative glomerulonephritis; PAN, polyarteritis nodosa; PCT, porphyria cutanea tarda.

    e. Chronic HBV
      (1) Persistence of HBsAg longer than 6 months
        • Anti-HBc-IgM converts to anti-BHc-IgG.
      (2) "Healthy" chronic carrier
        (a) Presence of HBsAg and anti-HBc-IgG
        (b) Absence of DNA and e antigen
      (3) Infective chronic carrier
        (a) Presence of HBsAg, anti-HBc-IgG, and infective particles (DNA and e antigen)
        (b) Increased risk for postnecrotic cirrhosis and hepatocellular carcinoma
3. Hepatitis C virus (HCV)
    a. Screen with enzyme immunoassay
      (1) Presence of anti-HCV-IgG indicates infection or recovery.
      (2) It is *not* a protective antibody.

Extravascular hemolysis: urine UBG ++, urine bilirubin 0

Cholestasis: urine UBG 0, urine bilirubin ++

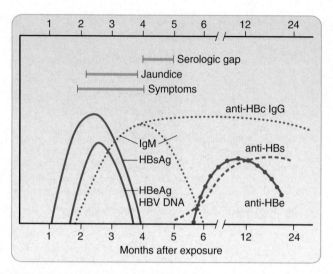

18-2: *Serologic markers in hepatitis B. Anti-HBc, anti-HBV core antigen; anti-HBe, anti-HBV e antigen; anti-HBs, anti-HBV surface antibody; HBsAg, hepatitis B surface antigen; HBeAg, hepatitis B e antigen; HBV, hepatitis B virus; IgG, immunoglobulin G; IgM, immunoglobulin M.*

TABLE 18-4:
Serologic Studies in Hepatitis B

HBsAg	HBeAg HBV DNA	Anti-HBc-IgM	Anti-HBc-IgG	Anti-HBs	Interpretation
+	–	–	–	–	Earliest phase of acute HBV
+	+	+	–	–	Acute infection
–	–	+	–	–	Window phase, or serologic gap
–	–	–	+	+	Recovered from HBV
–	–	–	–	+	Immunized
+	–	–	+	–	"Healthy" carrier if HBsAg > 6 months
+	+	–	+	–	Chronic infective carrier if > 6 months

Anti-HBc, core antibody; anti-HBs, surface antibody; HBeAg, e antigen; HBsAg, surface antigen.

    b. Confirmatory tests
      (1) Recombinant immunoblot assay (RIBA)
      (2) HCV RNA using polymerase chain reaction
      (3) Positive RIBA and HCV RNA indicate infection.
      (4) Positive RIBA and negative HCV RNA indicate recent recovery.
  4. Hepatitis D virus (HDV)
    a. Presence of anti-HDV-IgM or IgG indicates active infection.
    b. IgG is *not* a protective antibody.

5. Hepatitis E virus (HEV)
   a. Presence of anti-HEV-IgM indicates active infection.
   b. Anti-HEV-IgG indicates recovery (protective antibody).
E. **Other laboratory test findings (see Box 18-1C)**
   1. CB 20% to 50% (mixed hyperbilirubinemia)
      a. Decreased uptake/conjugation of UCB
      b. CB gains access to blood via damaged bile ductules.
   2. Increased urine UBG and urine bilirubin
      a. CB is water-soluble and is filtered in the kidneys.
      b. UBG recycled back to inflamed liver is redirected to the kidneys.
   3. Increased serum transaminases
      a. Serum ALT greater than AST
      b. Serum ALT is the last liver enzyme to return to normal.

Viral hepatitis: urine
UBG ++, urine
bilirubin ++

III. **Other Inflammatory Disorders**
   A. **Summary of important infectious diseases (Table 18-5)**
   B. **Autoimmune hepatitis**
      1. Occurs most often in young women

TABLE 18-5:
Infectious Diseases
of the Liver

Disease	Pathogen(s)	Characteristics
Amebiasis	*Entamoeba histolytica*	Usually right lobe abscess
Ascending cholangitis	*Escherichia coli*	Inflammation of bile ducts (cholangitis) from concurrent biliary infection and duct obstruction (e.g., stone) Triad of fever, jaundice, right upper quadrant pain Most common cause of multiple liver abscesses
Clonorchiasis	*Clonorchis sinensis* (Chinese liver fluke)	Contracted by ingesting encysted larvae in fish; larvae enter common bile duct and become adults May produce cholangiocarcinoma
Echinococcosis	*Echinococcus granulosus* (sheepherder's disease)	Single or multiple cysts containing larval forms Dog is definitive host; human is intermediate host Rupture of cysts can produce <u>anaphylaxis</u>
Granulomatous hepatitis	*Mycobacterium tuberculosis,* *Histoplasma capsulatum*	Sign of miliary spread
Schistosomiasis	*Schistosoma mansoni* Eggs incite a fibrotic response in the portal vein ("pipestem cirrhosis")	Complications of cirrhosis: portal hypertension, ascites, and esophageal varices
Spontaneous peritonitis	*Escherichia coli* in adults *Streptococcus pneumoniae* in children	Develops in ascites (e.g., cirrhosis, nephrotic syndrome)

—Australia, Mid east, SW US

Autoimmune hepatitis: positive serum ANA and anti–smooth muscle antibodies

2. Clinical findings
   • Fever, jaundice, hepatosplenomegaly
3. Laboratory findings
   a. Positive serum antinuclear antibody (ANA) test
   b. Anti–smooth muscle antibodies

C. Neonatal hepatitis
1. Epidemiology
   a. Idiopathic
   b. Associated with infections (e.g., cytomegalovirus)
   c. Associated with inborn errors of metabolism (e.g., α_1-antitrypsin deficiency)
2. Biopsy shows multinucleated giant cells
   • "Giant cell" hepatitis

Neonatal hepatitis: multifactorial; biopsy shows multinucleated giant cells

D. Reye syndrome
1. Usually develops in children younger than 4 years of age
   • Often follows a chickenpox or influenza infection
2. Mitochondrial damage (? virus, salicylates)
   a. Disruption of the urea cycle
      • Increase in serum ammonia
   b. Defective β-oxidation of fatty acids
3. Microvesicular type of fatty liver (? salicylate effect)
   • Small cytoplasmic globules *without* nuclear displacement
4. Clinical findings
   a. Encephalopathy
      • Cerebral edema, coma, convulsions
   b. Hepatomegaly
5. Laboratory findings
   a. Transaminasemia
   b. Normal to slight increase in total bilirubin
   c. Increased serum ammonia

Reye syndrome: encephalopathy, fatty change in liver

E. Acute fatty liver of pregnancy
1. Abnormality in β-oxidation of fatty acids
2. Fatal to mother and fetus unless the baby is delivered

F. Preeclampsia (see Chapter 21)
1. Hypertension, proteinuria, dependent pitting edema in third trimester
2. Liver cell necrosis around portal triads
   • Increased serum transaminases
3. HELLP syndrome
   a. <u>H</u>emolytic anemia with schistocytes (see Chapter 11)
   b. <u>E</u>levated serum transaminases
   c. <u>L</u>ow <u>p</u>latelets
      • Due to disseminated intravascular coagulation (see Chapter 14)

G. Fulminant hepatic failure
   • Acute liver failure with encephalopathy within 8 weeks of hepatic dysfunction
1. Causes
   a. Viral hepatitis (most common overall cause)

    b. Drugs (e.g., acetaminophen most common cause)

    c. Reye syndrome

  2. Gross and microscopic findings

    a. Wrinkled capsular surface due to loss of hepatic parenchyma

    b. Dull red to yellow necrotic parenchyma with blotches of green (bile)

  3. Clinical findings

    • Hepatic encephalopathy (see section VII), jaundice

  4. Laboratory findings

    a. Decrease in transaminases

      • Liver parenchyma is destroyed.

    b. Increase in PT and ammonia

Fulminant hepatic failure: ↓ transaminases, ↑ PT and ammonia

IV. Circulatory Disorders

  A. Prehepatic obstruction to blood flow

    • Obstruction of blood flow to the liver (i.e., hepatic artery, portal vein)

    1. Hepatic artery thrombosis with infarction

      a. Liver infarction is uncommon because of a dual blood supply.

        • Hepatic artery and portal vein tributaries normally empty blood into the sinusoids.

      b. Causes

        (1) Liver transplant rejection

        (2) Vasculitis due to polyarteritis nodosa

Hepatic artery infarction: uncommon due to dual blood supply

    2. Portal vein thrombosis

      a. Causes

        (1) Pylephlebitis (inflammation of portal vein)

          (a) Most often due to acute appendicitis

          (b) Air in biliary tree from bacterial gas

        (2) Polycythemia vera

        (3) Hepatocellular carcinoma

          • Tumor invasion of the portal vein

      b. Clinical findings

        (1) Portal hypertension, ascites, splenomegaly

        (2) *No* hepatomegaly

Portal vein thrombosis: ascites, portal hypertension, no hepatomegaly

  B. Intrahepatic obstruction to blood flow

    • Intrahepatic obstruction to sinusoidal blood flow

    1. Causes

      a. Cirrhosis (see Section VII)

      b. Centrilobular hemorrhagic necrosis

      c. Peliosis hepatis, sickle cell disease (see Chapter 11)

Intrahepatic obstruction to flood flow: cirrhosis most common cause

    2. Centrilobular hemorrhagic necrosis

      a. Most often due to left-sided heart failure (LHF) and right-sided heart failure (RHF)

        (1) LHF decreases cardiac output causing hypoperfusion of the liver.

          • Causes ischemic necrosis of hepatocytes located around central vein (see Chapter 1)

        (2) RHF causes a back-up of systemic venous blood into the central veins and sinusoids.

Centrilobular necrosis: combined LHF and RHF; "nutmeg" liver

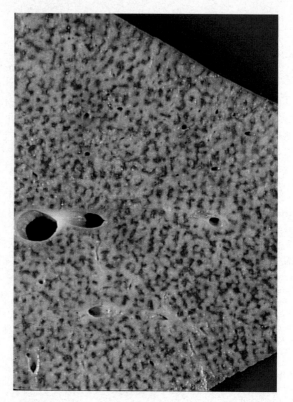

18-3: *Centrilobular hemorrhagic necrosis ("nutmeg" liver). The liver has a mottled cut surface. Dark areas represent congested central veins and sinusoids. (From Damjanov I, Linder J: Pathology: A Color Atlas. St. Louis, Mosby, 2000, p 146, Fig. 8-8.)*

    b. Enlarged liver with a mottled red appearance ("nutmeg" liver) (Fig. 18-3)
      (1) Congestion of central veins and sinusoids
      (2) Necrosis of hepatocytes around the central vein
    c. Clinical findings
      (1) Painful hepatomegaly with or without jaundice
      (2) Increased transaminases caused by ischemic necrosis
      (3) May progress to cardiac cirrhosis
         • Fibrosis around central veins
  3. Peliosis hepatis
    a. Sinusoidal dilation due to blood
    b. Causes
      (1) Anabolic steroids
      (2) *Bartonella henselae* causing bacillary angiomatosis (see Chapter 9)
         • Occurs in AIDS
    c. Potential for intraperitoneal hemorrhage
C. Posthepatic obstruction to blood flow
    • Obstruction of blood flow out of the liver (e.g., hepatic vein)

1. Causes
   a. Hepatic vein thrombosis
   b. Veno-occlusive disease
2. Hepatic vein thrombosis
   a. Causes
      (1) Polycythemia vera
      (2) Oral contraceptive pills
      (3) Hepatocellular carcinoma
         • Invades hepatic vein
   b. Clinical findings
      (1) Enlarged, painful liver
      (2) Portal hypertension, ascites, splenomegaly
      (3) High mortality rate
   c. Laboratory findings
      (1) Increased transaminases
      (2) Increased PT
3. Veno-occlusive disease
   a. Complication of bone marrow transplantation
   b. Collagen develops around the central veins.

D. Hematobilia
   • Blood in the bile in patients with trauma to the liver

Polycythemia vera: most common cause of hepatic vein thrombosis

V. Alcohol-Related and Drug- and Chemical-Induced Liver Disorders
A. Alcohol-related disorders
1. Risk factors for alcohol-related liver disease (see Chapter 6)
2. Pathways for alcohol metabolism (see Chapter 6)
3. Types of liver disease
   a. Fatty change is the most common type of disease (see Fig. 1-2).
      (1) Substrates of alcohol metabolism are used to synthesize liver triglyceride.
      (2) Clinical findings
         • Tender hepatomegaly *without* fever or neutrophilic leukocytosis
   b. Alcoholic hepatitis
      (1) Pathogenesis
         (a) Due to acetaldehyde damage to hepatocytes
         (b) Stimulation of collagen synthesis around the central vein
            • Perivenular fibrosis
      (2) Microscopic findings
         (a) Fatty change with neutrophil infiltration
         (b) Mallory bodies
            • Damaged cytokeratin intermediate filaments in hepatocytes (see Fig. 1-1)
         (c) Perivenular fibrosis
      (3) Clinical findings
         (a) Painful hepatomegaly
         (b) Fever, neutrophilic leukocytosis, ascites, hepatic encephalopathy

Alcoholic hepatitis: acetaldehyde damages hepatocytes

TABLE 18-6: Drug- and Chemical-Induced Liver Diseases

Disease	Cause
Tumors	
Angiosarcoma	Vinyl chloride, arsenic, thorium dioxide (radioactive contrast material)
Cholangiocarcinoma	Thorium dioxide
Hepatocellular carcinoma	Aflatoxin (due to *Aspergillus* mold)
Liver cell adenoma	Oral contraceptive pills
Other Liver Diseases	
Acute hepatitis	Isoniazid (caused by toxic metabolite), halothane, acetaminophen, methyldopa
Cholestasis	Oral contraceptive pills (estrogen interferes with intrahepatic bile secretion), anabolic steroids
Fatty change	Amiodarone (resembles alcoholic hepatitis; Mallory bodies and progression to cirrhosis), methotrexate
Fibrosis	Methotrexate, retinoic acid, amiodarone

        (c) May progress to alcoholic cirrhosis
     c. Cirrhosis (see section VII)
    4. Laboratory findings (see Chapter 6)
  B. Chemical- and drug-induced liver disease (Table 18-6)

VI. Obstructive (Cholestatic) Liver Disease
  A. Types of cholestatic liver disease
    1. Intrahepatic cholestasis
      a. Blockage of the intrahepatic bile ducts
      b. Causes
        (1) Drugs (e.g., oral contraceptive pills, anabolic steroids)
        (2) Neonatal hepatitis
        (3) Pregnancy-induced cholestasis (estrogen)
    2. Extrahepatic cholestasis
      a. Blockage of common bile duct (CBD)
      b. Causes
        (1) Stone usually originating from the gallbladder
        (2) Primary sclerosing pericholangitis
        (3) Extrahepatic biliary atresia
        (4) Carcinoma head of pancreas
  B. Gross and microscopic
    1. Enlarged, green-colored liver
    2. Bile ducts distended with bile, bile lakes, bile infarcts
  C. Clinical findings
    1. Jaundice with pruritus
      • Pruritus due to bile salts deposited in skin
    2. Malabsorption
      • Bile salts do *not* enter the small intestine.
    3. Cholesterol deposits in skin
      • Due to cholesterol in bile

Extrahepatic cholestasis: most commonly caused by a stone in CBD

4. Light-colored stools
- Due to a lack of urobilin

D. **Laboratory findings (see Box 18-1D)**
1. CB > 50%
2. Bilirubinuria
3. Absent urine UBG
4. Increase in serum ALP and GGT

E. **Benign intrahepatic cholestasis of pregnancy**
1. Due to estrogen inhibition of intrahepatic bile secretion
2. *Not* dangerous to the fetus or mother

F. **Extrahepatic biliary atresia**
1. Cause of jaundice in newborns
2. Inflammatory destruction of all or part of the extrahepatic bile ducts
3. Bile duct proliferation in the triads
4. Common indication for liver transplantation in a child

G. **Primary sclerosing pericholangitis**
1. Epidemiology
   a. Obliterative fibrosis of intrahepatic and extrahepatic bile ducts
   b. Male dominant
   c. Associated with ulcerative colitis
2. Clinical findings
   a. Jaundice
   b. Cirrhosis
   c. Increased incidence of cholangiocarcinoma

Primary sclerosing pericholangitis: strong association with ulcerative colitis

VII. **Cirrhosis**
- Irreversible diffuse fibrosis of the liver with formation of regenerative nodules

A. **Regenerative nodules**
1. Hepatocyte reaction to injury (Fig. 18-4)
2. Lack normal liver architecture
   - Lack of portal triads and sinusoids

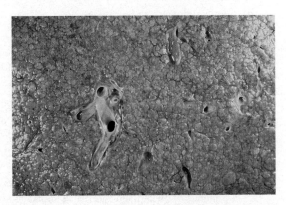

18-4: *Alcoholic cirrhosis, showing diffuse micronodular surface of the liver. The regenerative nodules are surrounded by collagen. (From Damjanov I, Linder J: Pathology: A Color Atlas. St. Louis, Mosby, 2000, p 154, Fig. 8-42.)*

3. Surrounded by bands of fibrosis
4. Compress sinusoids and central veins
   a. Intrasinusoidal hypertension
   b. Reduction in the number of functional sinusoids
   c. Increase in hydrostatic pressure in portal vein
B. **Causes**

1. Alcoholic liver disease (most common)
2. Postnecrotic cirrhosis (HBV, HCV)
3. Autoimmune disease (primary biliary cirrhosis)
4. Metabolic disease:
   a. Hemochromatosis, Wilson's disease
   b. α_1-Antitrypsin deficiency, galactosemia
C. **Complications associated with cirrhosis**
1. Hepatic failure
   • End point of progressive damage to the liver
   a. Multiple coagulation defects
      (1) Due to inability to synthesize coagulation factors
      (2) Produces a hemorrhagic diathesis
   b. Hypoalbuminemia from decreased synthesis of albumin
      • Produces dependent pitting edema and ascites
   c. Hepatic encephalopathy

      (1) Reversible metabolic disorder
      (2) Increase in aromatic amino acids (e.g., phenylalanine, tyrosine, tryptophan)
         • Converted into false neurotransmitters (e.g., gamma aminobutyric acid)
      (3) Increase in serum ammonia
         • Due to a defective urea cycle that cannot metabolize ammonia
      (4) Clinical findings
         (a) Alterations in the mental status
         (b) Somnolence and disordered sleep rhythms
         (c) Asterixis (i.e., inability to sustain posture, flapping tremor)
         (d) Coma and death in late stages

Ammonia derives from metabolism of amino acids and from the release of ammonia from amino acids by bacterial ureases in the bowel. Ammonia (NH_3) is diffusible and is reabsorbed into the portal vein for delivery to the urea cycle where it is metabolized into urea. Ammonium (NH_4^+) is *not* reabsorbed in the bowel and is excreted in stool. Methods for reducing the synthesis of ammonia in the colon include restriction of protein intake (most cost effective) and the use of oral neomycin, which destroys the colonic bacteria. Oral administration of lactulose results in the release of hydrogen ions causing NH_3 to be converted to NH_4^+, which is excreted in the feces.

2. Portal hypertension
   a. Pathogenesis
      (1) Resistance to intrahepatic blood flow due to intrasinusoidal hypertension
      (2) Anastomoses between portal vein tributaries and the arterial system
   b. Complications
      (1) Ascites (see below)
      (2) Congestive splenomegaly
          (a) Increased hydrostatic pressure in splenic vein
          (b) Hypersplenism with various cytopenias may occur (see Chapter 13)
      (3) Esophageal varices (see Chapter 17)
      (4) Hemorrhoids, periumbilical venous collaterals (caput medusae)
3. Ascites
   a. Pathogenesis
      (1) Portal hypertension
          • Increase in portal vein hydrostatic pressure
      (2) Hypoalbuminemia
          • Decreases oncotic pressure
      (3) Secondary hyperaldosteronism; causes:
          (a) Decreased cardiac output
              • Activates the renin-angiotensin-aldosterone system (retention of Na^+ and water)
          (b) Liver unable to metabolize aldosterone
   b. Clinical findings
      (1) Abdominal distention with a fluid wave
      (2) Increased risk for spontaneous bacterial peritonitis
4. Hepatorenal syndrome
   a. Renal failure *without* renal parenchymal disease
   b. Due to decreased renal blood flow
   c. Preservation of renal tubular function
5. Hyperestrinism in males
   a. Pathogenesis
      (1) Liver cannot degrade estrogen and 17-ketosteroids (e.g., androstenedione).
      (2) Androstenedione is aromatized into estrogen in the adipose cells.
   b. Clinical findings
      (1) Gynecomastia
      (2) Spider telangiectasia (see Chapter 9) (Fig. 18-5)
      (3) Female distribution of hair
D. Postnecrotic cirrhosis
   1. Most often caused by chronic hepatitis due to HBV and HCV
   2. Increased incidence of hepatocellular carcinoma
E. Primary biliary cirrhosis (PBC)
   1. Epidemiology
      a. Autoimmune disorder

> Portal vein: splenic vein + superior mesenteric vein

> Ascites: transudate due to alterations in Starling pressures + secondary aldosteronism

> Hyperestrinism in males: gynecomastia, spider telangiectasia

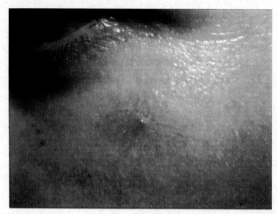

18-5: *Spider angioma (telangiectasia) on the cheek of a patient with cirrhosis. Multiple spider angiomas are common in cirrhosis and pregnancy. (From Savin J, Hunter JA, Hepburn NC: Diagnosis in Color: Skin Signs in Clinical Medicine. London, Mosby-Wolfe, 1997, p 15, Fig. 1-30.)*

PBC: autoimmune destruction of bile ducts in triads

- Granulomatous destruction of bile ducts in portal triads
  b. Occurs more often in women between 40 and 50 years of age
  c. Progresses from a chronic inflammatory reaction to cirrhosis
2. Clinical findings
  a. Pruritus
    (1) Deposition of bile salts in skin
    (2) Early finding well *before* jaundice appears
  b. Hepatomegaly
  c. Jaundice
    - Late finding *after* most of the bile ducts have been destroyed
  d. Cirrhosis with portal hypertension
  e. Increased risk for hepatocellular carcinoma

PBC: ↑ antimitochondrial antibodies and IgM

3. Laboratory findings
  a. Antimitochondrial antibodies (>90% of cases)
  b. Increase in IgM
  E. Secondary biliary cirrhosis
  1. Complication of chronic extrahepatic bile duct obstruction
    - Example—cystic fibrosis, where bile is dehydrated (see Chapter 16)
  2. *No* increase in antimitochondrial antibodies or IgM
  G. Hereditary hemochromatosis
  1. Epidemiology
    a. Autosomal recessive disorder
    b. Male dominant disorder
    c. In women, symptoms develop *after* menopause.
      - Due to menses causing loss of iron

Hemochromatosis: unrestricted reabsorption of iron

2. Pathogenesis
  a. Unrestricted reabsorption of iron in the small intestine
  b. Mutations involving hereditary hemochromatosis gene (HFE)
    - There is a 1:10 carrier rate in the population.
  c. Iron stimulates the production of hydroxyl free radicals (see Chapter 1).
    - Free radicals damage tissue and cause fibrosis.

The normal function of the HFE gene product is to facilitate the binding of plasma transferrin (binding protein of iron) with its mucosal cell transferrin receptor so that transferrin can be endocytosed by intestinal cells. The amount of endocytosed transferrin iron determines how much mucosal cell iron is released into the plasma. In hemochromatosis, when there is a mutated HFE gene, mucosal cell transfer of iron to plasma transferrin is always at a maximum resulting in iron overload.

3. Iron deposits in multiple organs
   • Liver, pancreas, heart, joints, skin, pituitary

Hemosiderosis (secondary hemochromatosis) is caused by multiple blood transfusions (e.g., sickle cell anemia, thalassemia major); alcohol abuse (alcohol increases iron reabsorption); and well water (iron pipes). Iron deposits are more prevalent in macrophages than in parenchymal tissue.

Hemosiderosis: acquired iron overload disease

4. Clinical and laboratory findings
   a. Cirrhosis
      (1) Iron deposits primarily in hepatocytes (Fig. 18-6).
      (2) Increased risk of hepatocellular carcinoma
   b. "Bronze diabetes"
      (1) Type I diabetes mellitus
         • Destruction of β-islet cells
      (2) Hyperpigmentation
         • Iron deposits in skin and increases melanin production
   c. Malabsorption
      • Destruction of exocrine pancreas

Hemochromatosis: "bronze" diabetes

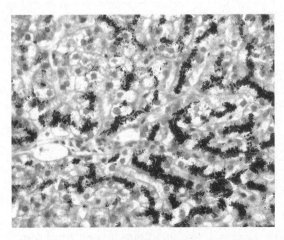

18-6: Liver biopsy stained with Prussian blue in a patient with hereditary hemochromatosis. The hepatocytes are filled with blue iron granules. This is an early stage before parenchymal damage and fibrosis develop. (From Kumar V, Fausto N, Abbas A: Robbins and Cotran's Pathologic Basis of Disease, 7th ed. Philadelphia, WB Saunders, 2004, p 910, Fig. 18-28.)

        d. Restrictive cardiomyopathy, degenerative joint disease

        e. Increased serum iron, percent saturation, and ferritin

        f. Decreased total iron-binding capacity
- Transferrin synthesis is decreased when iron stores are increased (see Chapter 11).

H. Wilson's disease (hepatolenticular degeneration)
1. Epidemiology
   - Autosomal recessive disorder
2. Pathogenesis
   a. Gene mutation
      (1) Defective hepatocyte transport of copper into bile for excretion
      (2) Decreased synthesis of ceruloplasmin (binding protein for copper in blood)
   b. Unbound copper eventually accumulates in blood
      (1) Loosely attached to albumin
      (2) Copper deposits in other tissues causing a toxic effect.

> Ceruloplasmin, the binding protein for copper, is secreted into the plasma where it represents 90% to 95% of the total serum copper concentration. The remaining 5% to 10% of copper is free copper that is loosely bound to albumin. Ceruloplasmin is eventually taken up and degraded by the liver. The copper that was bound to ceruloplasmin is excreted into the bile. The gene defect in Wilson's disease affects a copper transport system that produces a dual defect—decreased synthesis of ceruloplasmin in the liver and decreased excretion of copper into bile. Accumulation of copper in the liver increases the formation of free radicals causing damage to hepatocytes. In a few years, unbound copper is released from the liver into the circulation (increased in blood and urine) where it damages the brain, kidneys, cornea, and other tissues.

3. Clinical and laboratory findings
   a. Liver disease progresses from acute hepatitis to cirrhosis.
   b. Kayser-Fleischer ring
      - Due to free copper deposits in Descemet's membrane in the cornea (Fig. 18-7)
   c. Central nervous system disease
      (1) Copper deposits in the putamen
         - Produces a movement disorder resembling parkinsonism
      (2) Copper deposits in the subthalamic nucleus
         - Produces hemiballismus
      (3) Copper is toxic to neurons in the cerebral cortex
         - Produces dementia
   d. Decreased total serum copper
      - Due to decreased ceruloplasmin

Margin notes:

Wilson's disease:
↓ synthesis ceruloplasmin,
↓ excretion of copper in bile

Kayser-Fleischer ring: excess copper in Descemet's membrane of cornea

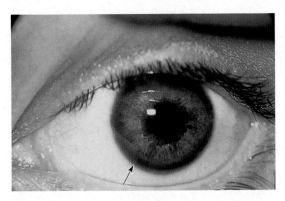

18-7: *Kayser-Fleischer ring. The arrow depicts deposition of a copper-colored pigment in Descemet's membrane in the cornea. (From Perkin GD: Mosby's Color Atlas and Text of Neurology. St. Louis, Mosby, 2002, p 151, Fig. 8-15.)*

       e. Decreased serum ceruloplasmin
- Useful in diagnosing Wilson's disease in its early stages

       f. Increased serum and urine free copper
- Useful in diagnosing Wilson's disease in the later stages

I. α₁-Antitrypsin (AAT) deficiency

1. Autosomal dominant disorder (codominant)
2. Pathogenesis
    a. Alleles are inherited codominantly (each allele expresses itself).
    b. Normal genotype is PiMM.
    c. Most common abnormal allele is Z.
    d. PiZZ variant has decreased AAT levels in serum.
      (1) Production of a mutant protein that cannot be secreted into blood
      (2) Accumulation of AAT in hepatocytes causes liver damage.
         - Periodic acid–Schiff stains show red cytoplasmic granules.
3. Clinical findings in children with PiZZ variant
    a. Neonatal hepatitis with intrahepatic cholestasis
    b. Most common cause of cirrhosis in children
    c. Increased risk for hepatocellular carcinoma
4. Young adults with panacinar emphysema
    - PiZZ variant where there is *no* synthesis of AAT in the liver

Cirrhosis in AAT deficiency: mutant AAT cannot be secreted by the liver

J. Laboratory test abnormalities in cirrhosis

1. Decreased serum blood urea nitrogen (BUN) and increased serum ammonia
    - Due to disruption of the urea cycle
2. Fasting hypoglycemia
    - Defective gluconeogenesis and decreased glycogen stores
3. Chronic respiratory alkalosis
    - Toxic products from hepatic dysfunction overstimulate respiratory center (see Chapter 4)

Cirrhosis: ↓ serum BUN, ↑ serum ammonia

4. Lactic acidosis
   - Liver dysfunction in converting lactic acid to pyruvate
5. Hyponatremia (see Chapter 4)
6. Hypokalemia
   - Secondary aldosteronism increases renal exchange of Na$^+$ for K$^+$ (see Chapter 4)
7. Increased PT
   - Decreased synthesis of coagulation factors
8. Hypoalbuminemia
   - Decreased synthesis of albumin
9. Hypocalcemia
   a. Hypoalbuminemia decreases the total serum calcium.
      - Approximately 40% of the total calcium is calcium bound to albumin.
   b. Vitamin D deficiency
      - Decreased liver 25-hydroxylation of vitamin D.
10. Mild transaminasemia
    - Enzymes are *not* markedly increased due to the loss of parenchymal cells.

Hypocalcemia in cirrhosis: ↓ serum albumin, ↓ vitamin D

VIII. Liver Tumors
   A. Benign tumors
      1. Cavernous hemangioma
         a. Most common benign tumor
         b. Rare cause of intraperitoneal hemorrhage
      2. Liver (hepatic) cell adenoma
         a. Benign tumor of hepatocytes
         b. Usually occur in women of childbearing age
            - Associated with the use of oral contraceptive pills
         c. Highly vascular tumors
            (1) Tendency to rupture during pregnancy
            (2) Produce intraperitoneal hemorrhage
   B. Malignant tumors
      1. Metastasis
         a. Most common liver cancer (see Fig. 8-7)
         b. Primary cancers of lung (most common), gastrointestinal tract, breast
         c. Multiple nodular masses
      2. Hepatocellular carcinoma
         a. Epidemiology
            (1) Most common primary liver cancer
            (2) Male dominant
               - Peaks around 60 years of age
            (3) Causes
               (a) Chronic HBV and HCV
               (b) Aflatoxins (from *Aspergillus* mold in grains and peanuts)
               (c) Hereditary hemochromatosis, alcoholic cirrhosis, PBC, AAT deficiency

Liver cell adenoma: oral contraceptive pills; intraperitoneal hemorrhage

Metastasis: most common cancer of liver; lung most common primary site

Hepatocellular carcinoma: preexisting HBV or HCV cirrhosis most common risk factor

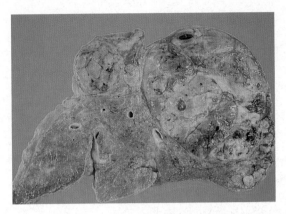

18-8: *Hepatocellular carcinoma. Multiple large, hemorrhagic tumor masses are present in the liver. There is also diffuse infiltration of tumor blending in with the remaining liver. (From Damjanov I, Linder J: Pathology: A Color Atlas. St. Louis, Mosby, 2000, p 161, Fig. 8-70.)*

     b. Pathogenesis
       (1) Most often associated with preexisting cirrhosis
       (2) Postnecrotic cirrhosis HBV/HCV most common risk factors
     c. Gross findings
       (1) Focal, multifocal, or diffusely infiltrating cancer (Fig. 18-8)
         • With or without preexisting cirrhosis (usually with preexisting cirrhosis)
       (2) Portal and hepatic vein invasion is common.
     d. Microscopic findings
       • Characteristic finding is the presence of bile in neoplastic cells. → green
     e. Clinical findings
       (1) Fever due to liver cell necrosis
       (2) Rapid enlargement of the liver
       (3) Increased ascites, blood present in ascitic fluid
     f. Laboratory findings
       (1) Increased α-fetoprotein (AFP) — non spec / think gonadal tumor
       (2) Production of ectopic hormones
         (a) Erythropoietin (secondary polycythemia)
         (b) Insulin-like factor (hypoglycemia)
     g. Lung most common metastatic site
   3. Angiosarcoma
     • Exposure to vinyl chloride (most common cause), arsenic, or thorium dioxide

Hepatocellular carcinoma: ↑ serum AFP

IX. Gallbladder and Biliary Tract Disease
  A. Cystic diseases
    1. Choledochal cyst
      a. Most common cyst in biliary tract in children younger than 10 years old

b. Clinical findings
(1) Abdominal pain with persistent or intermittent jaundice
(2) Increased incidence of cholelithiasis, cholangiocarcinoma, and cirrhosis
2. Caroli disease
a. Autosomal recessive disease
b. Segmental dilatation of intrahepatic bile ducts
c. Clinical findings
(1) Association with polycystic kidney disease
(2) Increased incidence of cholangiocarcinoma

B. Cholangiocarcinoma
1. Most common malignancy of bile ducts
2. Causes of cholangiocarcinoma
a. Primary sclerosing pericholangitis (see section VI)
• Most common cause in United States
b. *Clonorchis sinensis* (Chinese liver fluke)
c. Thorotrast (thorium dioxide)
d. Choledochal cyst and Caroli disease
3. Clinical findings
a. Obstructive jaundice
b. Palpable gallbladder (Courvoisier's sign)

C. Gallstones (cholelithiasis)
1. Types
a. Cholesterol stones (80% of cases)
• They are radiolucent.
b. Pigment stones
(1) Black and brown pigment stones
(2) Some are radiopaque.
2. Pathogenesis
a. Cholesterol stones (Fig. 18-9)
(1) Supersaturation of bile with cholesterol
(2) Decreased bile salts and lecithin
• Both normally solubilize cholesterol in bile
(3) Risk factors
(a) Female over 40 years old
(b) Obesity
• Cholesterol is increased in bile.
(c) Use of oral contraceptive pills
• Estrogen increases cholesterol in bile.
(d) Rapid weight loss, use of lipid-lowering drugs
(e) Native Americans (e.g., Pima and Navajo Indians)
b. Pigment stones
(1) Black pigment stones (Fig. 18-10)
(a) Sign of chronic extravascular hemolytic anemia (e.g., sickle cell anemia)
(b) Excess bilirubin in bile produces calcium bilirubinate

Primary sclerosing pericholangitis: most common cause cholangiocarcinoma

Cholesterol gallstones: most common stone

Cholesterol gallstones: ↑ cholesterol in bile, ↓ bile salts and lecithin

Black pigment gallstone: sign of extravascular hemolysis; calcium bilirubinate

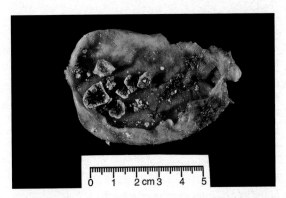

18-9: *Yellow cholesterol stones with centers containing entrapped bile pigments. The wall of the gallbladder is scarred. (From Kumar V, Fausto N, Abbas A: Robbins and Cotran's Pathologic Basis of Disease, 7th ed. Philadelphia, WB Saunders, 2004, p 930, Fig. 18-50.)*

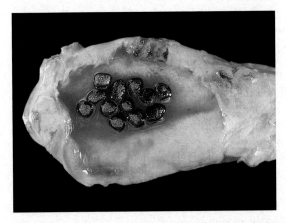

18-10: *Black pigmented stones. These are usually a sign of a chronic extravascular hemolytic anemia where there is an increase in calcium bilirubinate in bile. (From Kumar V, Fausto N, Abbas A: Robbins and Cotran's Pathologic Basis of Disease, 7th ed. Philadelphia, WB Saunders, 2004, p 931, Fig. 18-51.)*

        (2) Brown pigment stones
           • Sign of infection in the CBD
    3. Complications associated with stones
      a. Cholecystitis (most common)
      b. CBD obstruction
      c. Gallbladder cancer
      d. Acute pancreatitis
D. Acute cholecystitis
    1. Pathogenesis
      a. Obstruction of cystic duct by a stone (90% of cases)
        (1) Causes increased intraluminal pressure and ischemia to gallbladder wall
           • Mucosal ulceration predisposes to infection (usually *E. coli*).
        (2) Chemical irritation from conversion of lecithin to lysolecithin (toxic)

Brown pigment gallstones: sign of CBD infection

b. Other causes *not* associated with stones
    (1) AIDS
        • Infection with cytomegalovirus (CMV) or *Cryptosporidium*
    (2) Severe volume depletion
2. Clinical and laboratory findings
    a. Fever with nausea and vomiting
        • Usually 15 to 30 minutes after eating
    b. Initial midepigastric colicky pain
    c. Pain eventually shifts to the right upper quadrant.

Pain radiation in cholecystitis: right scapula

        (1) Pain is constant and dull
        (2) Pain may radiate to right scapula
    d. Jaundice suggests a stone in the CBD.
    e. Neutrophilic leukocytosis with left shift
    f. Tests to identify stones
        (1) Ultrasound is the gold standard
        (2) Radionuclide scan identifies stone(s) in cystic duct.

E. Chronic cholecystitis
1. Pathogenesis
    a. Cholelithiasis with repeated attacks of minor inflammation
    b. Chemical inflammation (infection is uncommon)

Chronic cholecystitis: most common symptomatic disorder of the gallbladder

2. Clinical findings
    a. Severe, persistent pain 1 to 2 hours postprandially
    b. Recurrent epigastric distress, belching, and bloating

F. Cholesterolosis
1. Excess cholesterol in bile
    a. Cholesterol deposits in macrophages
    b. Produces a yellow, speckled mucosal surface
2. *No* clinical significance

G. Gallbladder adenocarcinoma
1. Epidemiology
    a. Dominant in elderly women
    b. Poor prognosis
2. Pathogenesis
    a. Cholelithiasis (95% of cases)
    b. Porcelain gallbladder
        • Gallbladder with dystrophic calcification

X. Pancreatic Disorders
  A. Embryologic abnormalities of the pancreas
    1. Annular pancreas
        a. Dorsal and ventral buds form a ring around the duodenum.
        b. Associated with small bowel obstruction
    2. Aberrant pancreatic tissue (i.e., heterotopic rest, choristoma)
        • Locations—wall of stomach, duodenum, jejunum, or in a Meckel diverticulum
    3. Major pancreatic duct
        a. Major pancreatic duct and CBD are confluent in their terminal part

- Both empty their contents into the duodenum via the ampulla of Vater
  - b. Important in the pathogenesis of acute pancreatitis
    - (1) Stone(s) obstruct terminal part of the CBD →
    - (2) Increased back-pressure refluxes bile into the major pancreatic duct →
    - (3) Bile activates pancreatic proenzymes causing acute pancreatitis

B. Acute pancreatitis
  1. Epidemiology and pathogenesis
     a. Alcohol abuse and gallstones are the major causes
     b. Must be activation of pancreatic proenzymes (inactive enzymes)
        - Activation leads to autodigestion of the pancreas
     c. Mechanisms of activation of proenzymes
        (1) Obstruction of the main pancreatic duct or terminal CBD
            (a) Gallstones (see section IX)
            (b) Alcohol thickens ductal secretions
                - Also increases duct permeability to enzymes
        (2) Chemical injury of acinar cells
            - Examples—thiazides, alcohol, triglyceride (>1000 mg/dL)
        (3) Infectious injury of acinar cells
            - Examples—CMV, mumps, coxsackievirus
        (4) Mechanical injury of acinar cells
            - Examples—seat belt trauma, posterior penetration of duodenal ulcer
        (5) Metabolic activation of proenzymes (e.g., hypercalcemia, ischemia, shock)
     d. Trypsin is important in the activation of proenzymes.
        (1) Proteases damage acinar cell structure.
        (2) Lipases and phospholipases produce enzymatic fat necrosis.
        (3) Elastases damage vessel walls and produce hemorrhage (see Fig. 1-14).
        (4) Activated enzymes also circulate in the blood.
  3. Clinical findings
     a. Fever, nausea and vomiting
     b. Severe, boring midepigastric pain with radiation into the back
        - Radiation into back is due to its retroperitoneal location.
     c. Shock
        - Due to hemorrhage and loss of enzyme-rich fluid around the pancreas (called "third spacing")
     d. Hypoxemia
        (1) Circulating pancreatic phospholipase destroys surfactant.
            - Loss of surfactant produces atelectasis and intrapulmonary shunting.
        (2) Acute respiratory distress syndrome (ARDS) may occur.
     e. Grey-Turner's sign (flank hemorrhage), Cullen's sign (periumbilical hemorrhage)

Alcohol abuse: most common cause of acute pancreatitis

Seat belt trauma: most common cause of pancreatitis in children

    f. Tetany

       (1) Hypocalcemia is caused by enzymatic fat necrosis.

       (2) Calcium binds to fatty acids leading to a decrease in ionized calcium.

  4. Laboratory findings

    a. Increased serum amylase

       (1) Increased in 2 to 12 hours

       (2) Returns to normal in 2 to 3 days

         • Increased renal clearance

       (3) Present in urine for 1 to 14 days

> An increase in amylase is *not* specific for pancreatitis. Other causes of hyperamylasemia include mumps, small bowel infarction, and a ruptured ectopic pregnancy.

Serum lipase: more specific than amylase

    b. Increased serum lipase

       (1) More specific for pancreatitis

       (2) Serum levels return to normal in 3 to 5 days.

       (3) Is *not* excreted in urine

    c. Neutrophilic leukocytosis

    d. Hypocalcemia, hyperglycemia (destruction of β-islet cells)

    e. Computed tomographic (CT) scan is the gold standard for pancreatic imaging.

    f. Plain abdominal radiograph

       (1) Sentinel loop in subjacent duodenum or transverse colon (cut-off sign)

         • Localized ileus, where the bowel does *not* demonstrate peristalsis

       (2) Left-sided pleural effusion containing amylase (10% of cases)

Persistent increase in serum amylase: consider pancreatic pseudocyst

  5. Complications

    a. Pancreatic pseudocyst

       (1) Collection of digested pancreatic tissue around pancreas

       (2) Abdominal mass with persistence of serum amylase longer than 10 days

         • Amount of amylase in the fluid surpasses renal clearance of amylase.

    b. ARDS, pancreatic abscess, disseminated intravascular coagulation

C. Chronic pancreatitis

  1. Epidemiology

    a. Majority of cases are idiopathic.

    b. Known causes

Chronic pancreatitis: alcohol abuse is the most common known cause

       (1) Alcohol abuse is the most common known cause.

       (2) Cystic fibrosis is the most common cause in children.

       (3) Malnutrition is the most common cause in developing countries.

  2. Pathogenesis

    a. Repeated attacks of acute pancreatitis produce duct obstruction.

    b. Calcified concretions occur as well as dilation of the ducts.
- Radiographic dyes show a "chain of lakes" appearance in the major duct.

3. Clinical findings
   a. Severe pain radiating into the back
   b. Malabsorption
   c. Type 1 diabetes mellitus
   d. Pancreatic pseudocyst
4. Laboratory and radiographic findings
   a. Increased amylase and lipase
   b. Pancreatic calcifications (CT scan best study)

D. Exocrine pancreatic cancer
1. Epidemiology
   a. Adenocarcinoma
      - Varying degrees of differentiation
   b. Causes
      (1) Smoking (most common cause)
      (2) Chronic pancreatitis
      (3) Hereditary pancreatitis
2. Pathogenesis
   a. Association with *K-RAS* gene mutation
   b. Mutation of suppressor genes (*TP16* and *TP53*)
3. Location
   a. Most occur in the pancreatic head (65% of cases)
      - Often blocks CBD causing jaundice
   b. Remainder occur in the body and tail
4. Clinical and laboratory findings
   a. Epigastric pain with weight loss
   b. Signs of CBD obstruction (carcinoma of head of pancreas)
      (1) Jaundice (CB > 50%)
      (2) Light-colored stools (absent UBG)
      (3) Palpable gallbladder (Courvoisier's sign)
   c. Superficial migratory thrombophlebitis (see Chapter 8)
   d. Increased CA19–9
      - Gold standard tumor marker
5. Poor prognosis

19 CHAPTER

Kidney Disorders

I. **Renal Function Overview**
   A. **Excretes harmful waste products**
      • Examples—urea, creatinine, uric acid
   B. **Maintains acid-base homeostasis (see Chapter 4)**
      • Controls the synthesis and excretion of bicarbonate and hydrogen ions
   C. **Reabsorbs essential substances**
      • Examples—sodium, glucose, amino acids
   D. **Regulates water and sodium metabolism (see Chapter 4)**
      1. Controls water by concentrating and diluting urine
      2. Controls sodium reabsorption in the proximal and distal collecting tubules
   E. **Maintains vascular tone (see Chapter 4)**
      1. Angiotensin II (ATII)
         a. Vasoconstricts peripheral resistance arterioles and efferent arterioles
         b. Stimulates the synthesis and release of aldosterone
      2. Renal-derived prostaglandin (PGE_2)
         • Vasodilates the afferent arterioles
   F. **Produces erythropoietin (see Chapter 11)**
      • Synthesized in the endothelial cells in the peritubular capillaries
   G. **Maintains calcium homeostasis (see Chapter 22)**
      1. Second hydroxylation of vitamin D
         a. 1-α-Hydroxylase is synthesized in the proximal renal tubule cells.
         b. Converts 25-hydroxycholecalciferol to 1,25-dihydroxycholecalciferol.
      2. Functions of vitamin D
         a. Increases gastrointestinal reabsorption of calcium and phosphorus
         b. Promotes bone mineralization

> Vitamin D promotes bone mineralization by stimulating the release of alkaline phosphatase from osteoblasts. Alkaline phosphatase hydrolyzes pyrophosphate and other inhibitors of calcium-phosphate crystallization.

         c. Increases the production of osteoclasts from macrophage stem cells

II. **Important Laboratory Findings in Renal Disease**
   A. **Hematuria**
      1. Upper urinary tract (kidneys, ureter) causes of hematuria
         a. Renal stone
         b. Glomerulonephritis

Second hydroxylation vitamin D: 1-α-hydroxylase in proximal tubule

Renal stone: most common upper urinary tract cause of hematuria

- Characterized by dysmorphic RBCs (irregular membrane)
  c. Renal cell carcinoma
2. Lower urinary tract (bladder, urethra, prostate) causes of hematuria
  a. Infection
  b. Transitional cell carcinoma
    - Most common cause of gross hematuria in the absence of infection
  c. Benign prostatic hyperplasia
    - Most common cause of microscopic hematuria in adult males
3. Drugs associated with hematuria
  a. Anticoagulants (warfarin, heparin)
  b. Cyclophosphamide
    (1) Hemorrhagic cystitis
    (2) Risk factor for transitional cell carcinoma

B. Proteinuria
1. General
   a. Protein above 150 mg/24 hours or over 30 mg/dL (dipstick)
   b. Persistent proteinuria usually indicates renal disease.
   c. Qualitative tests include dipsticks and sulfosalicylic acid (SSA).
     (1) Dipsticks are specific for albumin.
     (2) SSA detects albumin and globulins.
   d. Quantitative test is a 24-hour urine collection.
2. Types of proteinuria (Table 19-1)

III. Renal Function Tests
A. Serum blood urea nitrogen (BUN)
- Normal serum BUN 7 to 18 mg/dL
1. End product of amino acid and pyrimidine metabolism
   a. Produced by the liver urea cycle
   b. Filtered in the kidneys
     - Partly reabsorbed in the proximal tubule
   c. Serum levels depend on the following:
     (1) Glomerular filtration rate (GFR)
     (2) Protein content in the diet
     (3) Proximal tubule reabsorption
     (4) Functional status of the urea cycle
2. Causes of increased and decreased serum BUN (Table 19-2)

B. Serum creatinine
- Normal serum creatinine 0.6 to 1.2 mg/dL
1. Metabolic end product of creatine in muscle
   - Creatine binds phosphate in muscle for ATP synthesis.
2. Creatinine is filtered in the kidneys and *not* reabsorbed or secreted.
   - Excellent metabolite for renal clearance testing
3. Serum concentration varies with age and muscle mass.
   - Increased with age, decreased in muscle wasting
4. Causes of increased and decreased serum creatinine
   - Similar to those for serum BUN

Infection: most common cause of lower urinary tract hematuria

Anticoagulants: most common drugs causing hematuria

Persistent proteinuria: usually indicates intrinsic renal disease

Urea: some extra-renal loss (e.g., skin) with high serum concentration

Congestive heart failure: most common cause of increased serum BUN

Creatinine: end product of creatine metabolism

Creatine supplements: ↑ serum creatinine

TABLE 19-1:
Types of
Proteinuria

Type	Definition	Causes
Functional	Protein < 2 g/24 hours *Not* associated with renal disease	Fever, exercise, congestive heart failure Orthostatic (postural): occurs with standing and is absent in the recumbent state; urine protein is absent in the first morning void; *no* progression to renal disease
Overflow	Protein loss is variable Low-molecular-weight proteinuria Amount filtered > tubular reabsorption	Multiple myeloma with BJ proteinuria Hemoglobinuria: e.g., intravascular hemolysis Myoglobinuria: crush injuries, McArdle's glycogenosis (deficient muscle phosphorylase) increase in serum creatine kinase
Glomerular	Nephritic syndrome: protein > 150 mg/24 hours but <3.5 g/24 hours Nephrotic syndrome: protein > 3.5 g/24 hours	Damage of GBM: nonselective proteinuria with loss of albumin and globulins; example is post-streptococcal glomerulonephritis Loss of negative charge on GBM: selective proteinuria with loss of albumin and *not* globulins; example is minimal change disease
Tubular	Protein < 2 g/24 hours Defect in proximal tubule reabsorption of low-molecular-weight proteins (e.g., amino acids) at normal filtered loads	Heavy metal poisoning: e.g., lead and mercury poisoning Fanconi syndrome: inability to reabsorb glucose, amino acids, uric acid, phosphate, bicarbonate, and uric acid Hartnup's disease: defect in reabsorption of neutral amino acids (e.g., tryptophan) in the gastrointestinal tract and kidneys

BJ, Bence Jones protein; GBM, glomerular basement membrane.

C. **Serum BUN:creatinine (Cr) ratio**
1. Using normal values, the normal ratio is 15 or less.
   a. Creatinine is filtered and is neither reabsorbed nor secreted.
   b. Urea is filtered and partly reabsorbed in the proximal tubule.
   c. BUN:Cr ratio depends on changes at several times:
      (1) Before the kidneys (prerenal)
      (2) Within the kidney parenchyma (renal)
      (3) After the kidneys (postrenal)
2. Prerenal, renal, and postrenal azotemia
   a. Azotemia refers to an increase in serum BUN and creatinine.
   b. Prerenal azotemia
      (1) Caused by a decrease in cardiac output
         (a) Hypoperfusion of the kidneys decreases GFR.
         (b) There is *no* intrinsic renal parenchymal disease.
      (2) Examples—blood loss, congestive heart failure
      (3) Serum BUN:Cr ratio greater than 15
         (a) Decreased GFR causes creatinine and urea to back up in blood.
         (b) After filtration, some urea is reabsorbed back into the blood.
            • All of the creatinine is excreted in the urine.

Azotemia: ↑ serum BUN and creatinine

Prerenal azotemia:
↓ cardiac output,
↓ GFR; ratio > 15

TABLE 19-2:
Causes of Increased and Decreased Serum BUN

Causes	Discussion
Increased Serum BUN	
Decreased cardiac output	CHF, shock (e.g., hemorrhage) ↓ Cardiac output → ↓ GFR → ↑ proximal tubule reabsorption of urea → ↑ serum BUN
Increased protein intake	High-protein diet, blood in gastrointestinal tract ↑ Amino acid degradation → ↑ serum BUN
Increased tissue catabolism	Third-degree burns, postoperative state ↑ Amino acid degradation → ↑ serum BUN
Acute glomerulonephritis	Poststreptococcal glomerulonephritis ↓ GFR → ↑ serum BUN
Acute or chronic renal failure	Acute tubular necrosis, diabetic glomerulopathy ↓ GFR → ↑ serum BUN
Postrenal disease	Urinary tract obstruction (e.g., urinary stone, BPH) ↓ GFR + back-diffusion of urea → ↑ serum BUN
Decreased Serum BUN	
Increased plasma volume	Normal pregnancy, SIADH ↑ Plasma volume → ↑ GFR → ↓ serum BUN
Decreased urea synthesis	Cirrhosis, Reye syndrome, fulminant liver failure Dysfunctional urea cycle → ↓ serum BUN
Decreased protein intake	Kwashiorkor, starvation ↓ Amino acid degradation → ↓ serum BUN

BPH, benign prostatic hyperplasia; BUN, blood urea nitrogen; CHF, congestive heart failure; GFR, glomerular filtration rate; SIADH, syndrome of inappropriate secretion of antidiuretic hormone; TPN, total parenteral nutrition.

      (c) Addition of urea to blood increases the ratio to over 15.
      (d) Example—serum BUN 80 mg/dL, serum creatinine 4 mg/dL
         • BUN/Cr ratio is 20.
  c. Renal azotemia (uremia)
    (1) Caused by parenchymal damage to the kidneys
    (2) Examples—acute tubular necrosis, chronic renal failure
    (3) Serum BUN:Cr ratio is 15 or below.
      (a) Decreased GFR causes creatinine and urea to back up in blood; increased extra-renal loss of urea
      (b) After filtration, both urea and creatinine are lost in the urine.
         • Proximal tubule cells are sloughed off in renal failure.
      (c) Serum BUN:Cr ratio is maintained (i.e., ≤15)
      (d) Example—serum BUN 80 mg/dL, serum creatinine 8 mg/dL
         • BUN/Cr ratio is 10.
  d. Postrenal azotemia
    (1) Caused by urinary tract obstruction below the kidneys
      • *No* intrinsic parenchymal disease
    (2) Examples—prostate hyperplasia, blockage of ureters by stones/cancer

Renal azotemia: intrinsic renal disease; extra-renal loss of urea; ratio ≤ 15

Postrenal azotemia: obstruction behind kidneys; ratio >15

(3) Serum BUN:Cr ratio greater than 15

    (a) Obstruction to urine flow decreases the GFR

    (b) Back-up of urea and creatinine in the blood

    (c) Increased tubular pressure causes back-diffusion of urea (*not* creatinine) into blood (ratio > 15).

(4) Persistent obstruction causes renal azotemia (ratio ≤ 15).

D. Creatinine clearance (CCr)

    1. Correlates with GFR

       a. Annual decrease in CCr of 1 mL/min beyond age 50

Elderly patients normally have a decrease in CCr. Therefore, it is important to calculate the dose and dose interval for drugs that are nephrotoxic (e.g., aminoglycosides) in order to avoid precipitating acute renal failure due to nephrotoxic acute tubular necrosis.

       b. Useful in detecting renal dysfunction

    2. Creatinine clearance (CCr) formula

       a. Measured CCr = UCr (mg/dL) × V (mL/min) ÷ PCr (mg/dL)

          (1) V = volume of a 24-hour urine collection in mL/min and UCr and PCr the creatinine concentration of urine and plasma, respectively.

          (2) CCr results are dependent on a correct 24-hour urine collection.

       b. Normal adult CCr is 97 to 137 mL/min.

          (1) In general, a CCr below 100 mL/min is abnormal.

          (2) CCr below 10 mL/min indicates renal failure.

    3. Causes of increased and decreased CCr (Table 19-3)

E. Urinalysis (Table 19-4)

    • Gold standard test in the initial workup of renal disease

Margin notes:

CCr: normally decreases with age

Increased CCr: normal pregnancy, early diabetic glomerulopathy

TABLE 19-3: Causes of Increased and Decreased Creatinine Clearance (CCr)

Causes	Discussion
Increased CCr	
Normal pregnancy	Normal increase in plasma volume causes an increase in the GFR leading to an increase in CCr; highest at the end of the first trimester
Early diabetic glomerulopathy	Efferent arteriole becomes constricted due to hyaline arteriolosclerosis causing an increase in the GFR and CCr Increased GFR damages the glomerulus (hyperfiltration injury)
Decreased CCr	
Elderly people	GFR normally decreases with age causing a corresponding decrease in the CCr
Acute and chronic renal disease	ARF due to acute tubular necrosis, CRF due to diabetic glomerulopathy

ARF, acute renal failure; CRF, chronic renal failure; GFR, glomerular filtration rate.

**TABLE 19-4:
Urinalysis**

Feature Tested	Result	Cause
General Examination		
Color	Dark yellow	Concentrated urine (e.g., volume depletion), bilirubinuria, increased UBG
	Red or pink	Hematuria, hemoglobinuria, myoglobinuria
Specific gravity	Fixed (e.g., 1.010)	Lack of concentration and dilution (e.g., chronic renal failure)
	Inability to concentrate urine	First sign of intrinsic renal disease
Chemical Dipsticks		
pH	Acid or alkaline pH	Determined by diet and acid-base status
		Alkaline urine in *Proteus* infections: urease converts urea to ammonia
Protein	Proteinuria	Detects albumin (*not* globulins)
		SSA: detects albumin and globulins (e.g., BJ protein)
		Albuminuria: dipstick and SSA have the same results
		BJ protein: SSA greater than dipstick result
Glucose	Increased serum glucose + glucosuria	Diabetes mellitus
	Normal serum glucose + glucosuria	Normal pregnancy, benign glucosuria: both conditions have decreased renal threshold for glucose
Ketones	Ketonuria	Diabetic ketoacidosis, starvation, ketogenic diets, pregnancy
		Test only detects acetone and AcAc (*not* β-OHB)
Bilirubin	Bilirubinuria	Viral hepatitis, obstructive jaundice
Urobilinogen (trace amount normal)	Absent	Obstructive jaundice
	Increased	Viral hepatitis, extravascular hemolytic anemia (e.g., spherocytosis)
Blood	Hemoglobinuria	Intravascular hemolytic anemia
	Hematuria	Renal calculus, infection, cancer (renal cell carcinoma, transitional cell carcinoma)
	Myoglobinuria	Crush injuries
Nitrites	Increased	Produced by nitrate-reducing uropathogens (e.g., *Escherichia coli*)

continued

TABLE 19-4:
Urinalysis—cont'd

Feature Tested	Result	Cause
Chemical Dipsticks—cont'd		
Leukocyte esterase	Presence of esterase in neutrophils (pyuria)	Infections (e.g., urethritis, cystitis, pyelonephritis)
	Sterile pyuria (neutrophils present but *negative* standard urine culture)	*Chlamydia trachomatis* urethritis, renal tuberculosis
Sediment		
Cells	Bacteria	Usually sign of UTI
	Red blood cells (hematuria)	Renal stone, cancer (bladder, renal), glomerulonephritis (RBCs are dysmorphic), infection, BPH
	Neutrophils (pyuria)	Infection, sterile pyuria
	Oval fat bodies	Renal tubular cells with lipid (nephrotic syndrome)
Casts	Hyaline	*No* significance in absence of proteinuria
	Red blood cell	Nephritic type of glomerulonephritis (e.g., poststreptococcal glomerulonephritis)
	White blood cell	Acute pyelonephritis, acute tubulointerstitial nephritis (drugs)
	Renal tubular cell	Acute tubular necrosis
	Fatty	Nephrotic syndrome (e.g., minimal change disease)
	Waxy (refractile, acellular)	Sign of chronic renal failure Often have a large diameter due to tubular atrophy (broad casts)
	Broad	Sign of chronic renal failure Waxy cast with an increased diameter
Crystals	Calcium oxalate	Pure vegan diet, ethylene glycol poisoning, calcium oxalate calculi
	Uric acid	Hyperuricemia associated with gout or massive destruction of cells after chemotherapy
	Cystine	Cystinuria, hexagonal cystine crystals

AcAc, acetoacetic acid; BJ, Bence Jones; BPH, benign prostatic hyperplasia; β-OHB, hydroxybutyric acids; SSA, sulfosalicylic acid; UBG, urobilinogen; UTI, urinary tract infection.

IV. **Clinical Anatomy of the Kidney**
   A. **Blood supply of the kidney**
      1. Renal cortex receives ~90% of the blood supply.
      2. Renal medulla is relatively ischemic due to reduced blood supply.
      3. Renal vessels are end arteries.
         a. *No* collateral circulation
         b. Occlusion of any branch of a renal artery produces infarction.

Renal medulla: relatively ischemic

4. Afferent arterioles
   a. Contain the juxtaglomerular apparatus
      • Produces the enzyme renin
   b. Blood flow is controlled by renal-derived PGE_2 (vasodilator).
   c. Direct blood into the glomerular capillaries
5. Efferent arterioles
   a. Drain the glomerular capillaries
   b. Blood flow controlled by ATII (vasoconstrictor)
   c. Eventually become the peritubular capillaries

   > Nonsteroidal anti-inflammatory drugs (NSAIDs) inhibit production of PGE_2; therefore, intrarenal blood flow is controlled by the efferent arterioles, whose blood flow is maintained by ATII, a vasoconstrictor. This increases the risk of ischemic damage to the medulla.

B. **Structure of the glomerulus (Fig. 19-1)**
   1. Glomerular capillaries contain fenestrated epithelium.
      • Holes in the endothelial surface are important in the filtration process.
   2. Glomerular basement membrane (GBM)
      a. Composed of type IV collagen
      b. Size and charge are the primary determinants of protein filtration.
         (1) Heparan sulfate produces the negative charge of the GBM.
         (2) Cationic proteins of low molecular weight (LMW) are permeable.
         (3) Albumin has a strong negative charge and is *not* permeable.
            • Loss of the negative charge causes loss of albumin in the urine.
         (4) GBM is permeable to water and LMW (<70,000) proteins (e.g., amino acids).
      c. Causes of GBM thickening
         (1) Deposition of immunocomplexes
            • Example—membranous glomerulopathy
         (2) Increased synthesis of type IV collagen
            • Example—diabetes mellitus

   GBM: size and charge determine protein filtration

   3. Visceral epithelial cells (VEC)
      a. Primarily responsible for production of the GBM
      b. Contain podocytes (foot-like processes) and slit pores between the podocytes
         • Serve as a distal barrier for preventing protein loss in the urine
      c. Fusion of the podocytes is present in any cause of the nephrotic syndrome.

   Fusion of the podocytes: sign of nephrotic syndrome

   4. Mesangial cells
      a. Support the glomerular capillaries
      b. Can release inflammatory mediators and proliferate
         • Example—IgA glomerulonephritis
   5. Parietal epithelial cells
      a. Lining cells of Bowman's capsule
      b. Proliferation causes "crescents" that destroy the glomerulus.

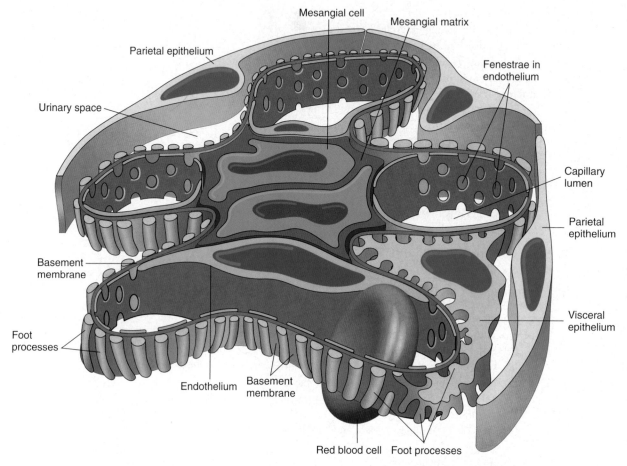

19-1: *Schematic of a normal glomerulus. See text for discussion. (From Kumar V, Fausto N, Abbas A: Robbins and Cotran's Pathologic Basis of Disease, 7th ed. Philadelphia, WB Saunders, 2004, p 511, Fig. 14-1.)*

Renal dysplasia: most common cystic disease in children

V. Congenital Disorders and Cystic Diseases of the Kidneys

A. Horseshoe kidney

1. Most common congenital kidney disorder
2. Majority (90%) are fused at the lower pole
   - Kidney is trapped behind the root of the inferior mesenteric artery.
3. Clinical findings
   a. Increased incidence with Turner's syndrome
   b. Danger of infection and stone formation

B. Cystic diseases of the kidney (Table 19-5 and Fig. 19-2)

VI. Glomerular Disorders

A. Terminology of glomerular disease (Table 19-6)
   - Normal glomerulus (Fig. 19-3)

TABLE 19-5:
Cystic Diseases of the Kidneys

Cystic Disease	Discussion
Renal dysplasia	Most common cystic disease in children No inheritance pattern Abnormal development of one or both kidneys; abnormal structures persist in the kidneys (e.g., cartilage, immature collecting ductules) Present as an enlarged, irregular, cystic, unilateral (bilateral) flank mass Bilateral dysplastic kidneys may lead to renal failure; account for ~20% of cases of CRF in children
Juvenile polycystic kidney disease	Autosomal recessive inheritance Bilateral cystic disease; cysts in the cortex and medulla Cysts also occur in the liver; association with congenital hepatic fibrosis leading to portal hypertension Enlarged kidneys at birth; most serious types are incompatible with life Maternal oligohydramnios (decreased amniotic fluid); newborns have Potter's facies, a deformation due to oligohydramnios; findings include low-set ears, parrot beak nose, and lung hypoplasia
Adult polycystic kidney disease (Fig. 19-2)	Autosomal dominant inheritance Bilateral cystic disease develops by 20–25 years of age; bilaterally palpable kidneys; cysts involve all parts of nephron in cortex and medulla Cysts are present in the liver (40% of cases) and pancreas Hypertension (>80% of cases); associated with stroke due to rupture of intracranial berry aneurysms (aneurysms in 10–30% of cases) or intracerebral hemorrhage CRF begins at age 40–60 years; due to destruction of kidneys by slowly expanding cysts; accounts for ~10% of cases of CRF; most common cause of death from cystic disease Other findings: sigmoid diverticulosis, hematuria, mitral valve prolapse, risk for developing renal cell carcinoma
Medullary sponge kidney	No inheritance pattern Most commonly discovered with an IVP; striations are present in the papillary ducts of the medulla ("Swiss-cheese" appearance); multiple cysts of the collecting ducts are present in the medulla Recurrent UTIs, hematuria, and renal stones
Acquired polycystic kidney disease	Most common cause is renal dialysis; occurs in ~50% of patients on long-term dialysis Tubules are obstructed by interstitial fibrosis or oxalate crystals Small risk for developing renal cell carcinoma
Simple retention cysts	Most common adult renal cyst Derived from tubular obstruction May produce hematuria Requires needle aspiration to distinguish it from renal cell carcinoma

CRF, chronic renal failure; IVP, intravenous pyelogram; UTIs, urinary tract infections.

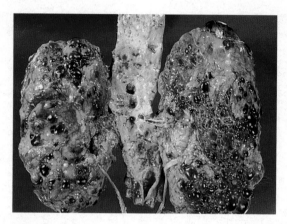

19-2: *Adult polycystic kidney disease. There is complete effacement of normal kidney architecture by cysts within the cortex and medulla of both kidneys. (From Damjanov I, Linder J: Pathology: A Color Atlas. St. Louis, Mosby, 2000, p 212, Fig. 11-7.)*

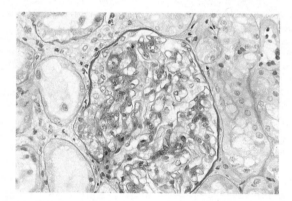

19-3: *Normal glomerulus. (From Damjanov I: Pathology for the Health-Related Professions, 2nd ed. Philadelphia, WB Saunders, 2000, p 329, Fig. 13-5A.)*

**TABLE 19-6:
Nomenclature and Description of Glomerular Disorders**

Term	Description
Focal glomerulonephritis	Only a few glomeruli are abnormal
Diffuse glomerulonephritis	All glomeruli are abnormal
Proliferative glomerulonephritis	>100 nuclei in affected glomeruli
Membranous glomerulopathy	Thick GBM, no proliferative change
Membranoproliferative glomerulonephritis	Thick GBM, hypercellular glomeruli
Focal segmental glomerulosclerosis	Fibrosis involving only a segment of the involved glomerulus
Crescentic glomerulonephritis	Proliferation of parietal epithelial cells around glomerulus
Primary glomerular disease	Involves only glomeruli and *no* other target organs (e.g., minimal change disease)
Secondary glomerular disease	Involves glomeruli and other target organs (e.g., SLE)

GBM, glomerular basement membrane; SLE, systemic lupus erythematosus.

B. Routine studies on biopsy specimens
    1. H&E (hematoxylin and eosin) and other special stains
        • Used to help classify the type of glomerular disease
    2. Immunofluorescence (IF) stain
        a. Identifies patterns and type of protein deposition
        b. Linear pattern (Fig. 19-4)
            (1) It is a characteristic finding in anti-GBM disease.
                • Example—Goodpasture syndrome
            (2) Antibodies line up against evenly distributed antigens in the GBM
        c. Granular ("lumpy-bumpy") pattern (Fig. 19-5)
            • Usually indicates immunocomplex (IC) deposition in the glomerulus

Linear IF: anti-GBM disease (e.g., Goodpasture syndrome)

Granular pattern: immunocomplex type of glomerulonephritis

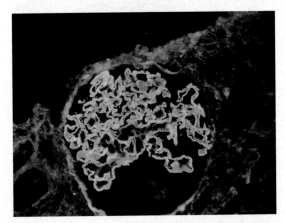

19-4: *Linear immunofluorescence. The uninterrupted smooth immunofluorescence along the glomerular basement membrane is caused by deposition of IgG antibodies directed against the membrane (e.g., Goodpasture syndrome). (From Kumar V, Fausto N, Abbas A: Robbins and Cotran's Pathologic Basis of Disease, 7th ed. Philadelphia, WB Saunders, 2004, p 969, Fig. 20-10E.)*

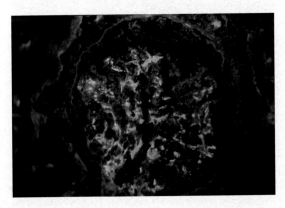

19-5: *Granular immunofluorescence. Granular irregular deposits in the capillaries are caused by immunocomplex deposition (e.g., poststreptococcal glomerulonephritis). (From Damjanov I, Linder J: Pathology: A Color Atlas. St. Louis, Mosby, 2000, p 224, Fig. 11-46.)*

3. Electron microscopy
   a. Detects submicroscopic defects in the glomerulus; examples:
      (1) Fusion of podocytes in the nephrotic syndrome (Fig. 19-6)
      (2) Damage to visceral epithelial cells
   b. Detects the site(s) of IC deposition
      (1) Deposits are electron-dense
      (2) Sites are designated
         (a) Subendothelial (Fig. 19-7)

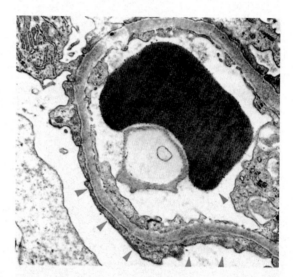

19-6: *Fusion of the podocytes. Arrowheads show fusion of the podocytes, which should be separated by slit pores. This finding occurs in all glomerular diseases that present with the nephrotic syndrome (e.g., minimal change disease).*

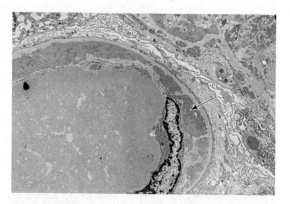

19-7: *Subendothelial immunocomplex deposits viewed with electron microscopy. The band of electron-dense material extends around the glomerular basement membrane and hugs the interface of the membrane with the capillary lumen. Arrow points to immune deposits directly beneath the nucleus of the endothelial cell. A thin rim of normal basement membrane (light gray) separates the deposits from the epithelial side of the membrane. The patient had diffuse proliferative glomerulonephritis due to systemic lupus erythematosus. (From Damjanov I, Linder J: Pathology: A Color Atlas. St. Louis, Mosby, 2000, p 224, Fig. 11-54.)*

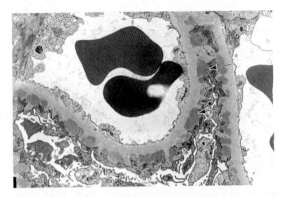

19-8: *Subepithelial immunocomplex deposits viewed with electron microscopy. Arrows point to electron-dense deposits directly beneath the visceral epithelial cells in a patient with poststreptococcal glomerulonephritis. The normal basement membrane has a light gray appearance. (From Damjanov I: Pathology for the Health-Related Professions, 2nd ed. Philadelphia, WB Saunders, 2000, p 341, Fig. 13-8C.)*

  (b) Subepithelial (Fig. 19-8)
  (c) Intramembranous, mesangial
C. **Mechanisms producing glomerular disease**
 1. Immunocomplexes (type III hypersensitivity)
  a. Circulate and deposit in glomeruli or they develop in situ
   • Example: DNA–anti-DNA complexes in SLE
  b. ICs activate the complement system.
   (1) C5a is produced, which is chemotactic to neutrophils
   (2) Neutrophils damage the glomeruli.
 2. Antibodies directed against GBM antigens
  • Example—Goodpasture syndrome
 3. T-cell production of cytokines
  a. Cytokines cause the GBM to lose its negative charge.
  b. Example—minimal change disease
D. **Clinical manifestations of glomerular diseases**
 1. Nephritic syndrome
 2. Nephrotic syndrome
 3. Chronic glomerulonephritis
E. **Nephritic syndrome**
 1. Clinical and laboratory findings
  a. Hypertension
   • Due to salt retention
  b. Periorbital puffiness
   • Due to salt retention in the loose skin in that area
  c. Oliguria (<400 mL urine/day)
   • Due to decreased GFR from inflamed glomeruli
  d. Hematuria
   • Dysmorphic RBCs with irregular membranes

Immunocomplexes: most common mechanism causing glomerulonephritis

Nephritic syndrome: moderate proteinuria; RBC casts

Nephrotic syndrome: proteinuria > 3.5 g/24 hours; fatty casts

Nephrotic syndrome: less glomerular inflammation than nephritic syndrome

   e. Neutrophils in the sediment
      • Particularly in IC types
   f. RBC casts are a key finding (Fig. 19-9).
      • Occasionally, white blood cell (WBC) casts are also present.
   g. Proteinuria greater than 150 mg/day but less than 3.5 g/day
   h. Azotemia with a BUN:Cr ratio greater than 15
      • Tubular function is intact in acute glomerulonephritis.
   2. Primarily nephritic types of glomerular disease (Table 19-7; Figs. 19-10 and 19-11)
F. **Nephrotic syndrome**
   1. Clinical and laboratory findings
      a. Key finding is proteinuria greater than 3.5 g/24 hours.
      b. Generalized pitting edema and ascites
         (1) Due to hypoalbuminemia
         (2) Increased risk for developing spontaneous peritonitis (see Chapter 18)
            • Due to *Streptococcus pneumoniae*

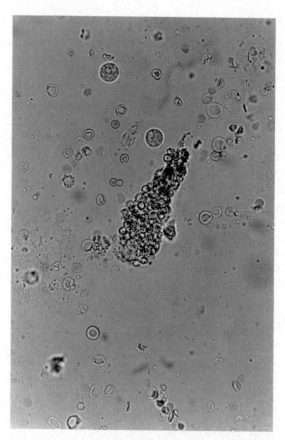

19-9: *Red blood cell cast in the urine. Note the cylindrical cast composed of red-staining cells. (From Forbes C, Jackson W: Color Atlas and Text of Clinical Medicine, 2nd ed. St. Louis, Mosby, 2003, p 276, Fig. 6-11.)*

TABLE 19-7: Primarily Nephritic Types of Glomerular Disease

Glomerular Disease	Clinicopathologic Findings
IgA glomerulopathy (Berger's disease)	Most common GN; almost equal incidence of nephritic or nephrotic presentation Affects children and adults Increased mucosal synthesis and decreased clearance of IgA; increased serum IgA (50% of cases) Mesangial IgA IC deposits with granular IF; ICs activate alternative complement pathway Overlapping features with HSP may occur Episodic bouts of hematuria (microscopic or gross) usually following an upper respiratory infection Slow progression to CRF (40–50% of cases)
Poststreptococcal glomerulonephritis (Fig. 19-10)	Most common type of postinfectious GN Usually follows group A streptococcal infection of skin (e.g., scarlet fever) or pharynx Subepithelial IC deposits with granular IF; ICs activate alternative complement pathway Diffuse proliferative pattern with neutrophil infiltration Hematuria 1–3 weeks following group A streptococcal infection Increased anti-DNAase B titers; ASO is degraded in skin and is not increased Usually resolves; CRF is uncommon
Diffuse proliferative glomerulonephritis (SLE)	Diffuse proliferative GN is most common subtype of glomerular disease in SLE Subendothelial IC deposits with granular IF; DNA–anti-DNA ICs activate classical complement pathway "Wire looping" of capillaries (subendothelial ICs); neutrophil infiltration with hyaline thrombi in capillary lumens Kidneys are major target organ in SLE (~90% of cases) Serum ANA test usually has a rim pattern, which corresponds with the presence of anti-ds DNA antibodies Evolves into CRF in most cases; common cause of death in SLE

Rapidly progressive glomerulonephritis (Fig. 19–11)	Clinical syndrome that may be primary or secondary types of glomerular disease
	Rapid loss of renal function progresses to ARF over days to weeks; very poor prognosis
	May or may not be associated with crescent formation (crescentic GN)
	Clinical associations: Goodpasture syndrome, microscopic polyarteritis (p-ANCA), Wegener's granulomatosis (c-ANCA)
	Goodpasture syndrome:
	  Male dominant disease
	  Anti–basement membrane antibodies against collagen in glomerular and pulmonary capillaries
	  Linear IF; EM has *no* electron dense deposits; crescentic GN begins with hemoptysis and ends with renal failure

ANA, antinuclear antibody; ANCA, antineutrophil cytoplasmic antibody; ARF, acute renal failure; ASO, antistreptolysin O; CRF, chronic renal failure; ds, double-stranded; EM, electron microscopy; GN, glomerulonephritis; HSP, Henoch-Schönlein purpura; IC, immunocomplex; IF, immunofluorescence; SLE, systemic lupus erythematosus.

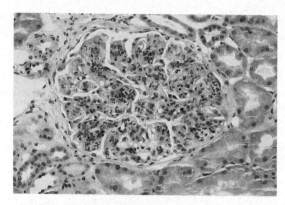

19-10: *Poststreptococcal diffuse proliferative glomerulonephritis. The glomerulus is hypercellular due to an increase in neutrophils and mesangial cells. (From Damjanov I: Pathology for the Health-Related Professions, 2nd ed. Philadelphia, WB Saunders, 2000, p 329, Fig. 13-5B.)*

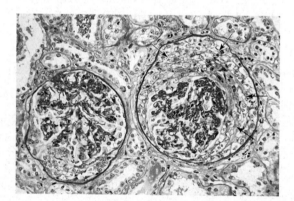

19-11: *Crescentic glomerulonephritis. Arrows point to a proliferation of parietal epithelial cells in Bowman's capsule, occupying approximately 50% of the entire urinary space. The cells encase and compress the glomerular tuft. (From Kumar V, Fausto N, Abbas A: Robbins and Cotran's Pathologic Basis of Disease, 7th ed. Philadelphia, WB Saunders, 2004, p 977, Fig. 20-17.)*

    c. Hypertension in some types
      • Due to salt retention
    d. Hypercoagulable state due to loss of antithrombin III
      • Potential for renal vein thrombosis
    e. Hypercholesterolemia
      • Hypoalbuminemia increases synthesis of cholesterol (unknown mechanism).
    f. Hypogammaglobulinemia
      • Due to the loss of γ-globulins in the urine
    g. Fatty casts with Maltese crosses and oval fat bodies (Fig. 19-12)
      • Key finding of the nephrotic syndrome

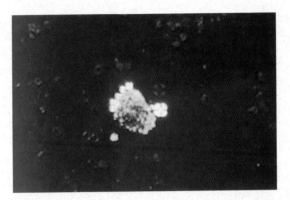

19-12: *Fatty cast under polarization showing classic Maltese crosses. The Maltese crosses are due to cholesterol, which is always increased in the nephrotic syndrome. (From Henry JB: Clinical Diagnosis and Management by Laboratory Methods, 20th ed. Philadelphia, WB Saunders, 2001, Plate 18–12.)*

2. Primarily nephrotic types of glomerular disease (Table 19-8 and Fig. 19-13)

G. **Systemic diseases with nephrotic syndrome**
  1. Diabetic glomerulopathy
     • Nodular glomerulosclerosis, Kimmelstiel-Wilson disease
     a. Glomerulopathy occurs in type 1 and 2 diabetes.
        (1) Occurs in type 1 more than type 2 diabetes
        (2) Most common cause of chronic renal failure in United States
     b. Risk factors
        (1) Poor glycemic control
        (2) Hypertension
        (3) Diabetic retinopathy
           • High correlation with coexisting glomerulopathy
     c. Pathogenesis
        (1) Nonenzymatic glycosylation (NEG) of the GBM
           • Also affects tubule basement membranes
           (a) Glycosylation refers to glucose attaching to amino acids.
           (b) Increases vessel and tubular cell permeability to proteins
        (2) NEG of the afferent and efferent arterioles
           (a) Produces hyaline arteriolosclerosis (see Chapter 9)
           (b) Involves efferent arterioles *before* afferent arterioles
        (3) Osmotic damage to glomerular capillary endothelial cells
           (a) Glucose is converted by aldose reductase into sorbitol.
           (b) Sorbitol is osmotically active.
           (c) Water enters the cells causing damage.
        (4) Hyperfiltration damage to the mesangium
           (a) Selective hyaline arteriolosclerosis of efferent arterioles
           (b) Increases the GFR, which damages mesangial cells
        (5) Diabetic microangiopathy; increased deposition of type IV collagen
           • GBM, tubular cell basement membranes, mesangium

Diabetic glomerulopathy: poor glycemic control is the most common cause

Hyaline arteriolosclerosis of efferent arteriole: ↑ GFR producing hyperfiltration injury

TABLE 19-8:
Primarily Nephrotic Types of Glomerular Disease

Glomerular Disease	Clinicopathologic Findings
Minimal change disease (lipoid nephrosis)	Most common cause of nephrotic syndrome in children; more common in girls than boys; occurs in ~15% of adults with nephrotic syndrome T-cell cytokines cause the GBM to lose its negative charge; selective proteinuria (albumin *not* globulins) Secondary causes: NSAIDs, Hodgkin's lymphoma Structurally normal glomeruli; positive fat stains in glomerulus and tubules Negative IF; EM shows fusion of podocytes and *no* deposits Often preceded by respiratory infection or routine immunization Normotensive, unlike other types of nephrotic syndrome Children respond well to steroid therapy; CRF is rare
Focal segmental glomerulosclerosis	Primary or secondary disease; secondary causes—HIV (most common glomerular disease) and intravenous heroin abuse Negative IF; EM focal damage of VECs Nonselective proteinuria, microscopic hematuria Poor prognosis; commonly progresses to CRF
Diffuse membranous glomerulopathy (Fig. 19-13A and B)	Most common cause of nephrotic syndrome in adults Primary and secondary types; secondary causes— Drugs: e.g., captopril Infections: HBV, *Plasmodium malariae*, syphilis Malignancy: carcinomas, non-Hodgkin's lymphoma Autoimmune disease: SLE (nephrotic presentation) Diffuse thickening of membranes; silver stains show "spike and dome" pattern beneath VECs (subepithelial deposits) Subepithelial ICs with granular IF
Type I MPGN	Most common type of MPGN; some cases have a nephritic presentation Associated with HBV, HCV, or cryoglobulinemia Subendothelial ICs with granular IF; ICs activate classical and alternative complement pathways; EM shows tram tracks caused by splitting of the GBM by an ingrowth of mesangium Majority progress to CRF
Type II MPGN	Associated with the C3 nephritic factor (C3NeF), an autoantibody that binds to C3 convertase (C3bBb); prevents degradation of C3 convertase causing sustained activation of C3 resulting in very low C3 levels Diffuse intramembranous deposits ("dense deposit disease"); EM shows tram tracks Majority progress to CRF

CRF, chronic renal failure; EM, electron microscopy; GBM, glomerular basement membrane; HBV, hepatitis B; HCV, hepatitis C; ICs, immunocomplexes; IF, immunofluorescence; MPGN, membranoproliferative glomerulonephritis; NSAIDs, nonsteroidal anti-inflammatory drugs; SLE, systemic lupus erythematosus; VECs, visceral epithelial cells.

  d. Nonspecific immunofluorescence
  e. Electron microscope shows fusion of podocytes.
  f. Microscopic findings (Fig. 19-14)
    (1) Afferent and efferent hyaline arteriolosclerosis

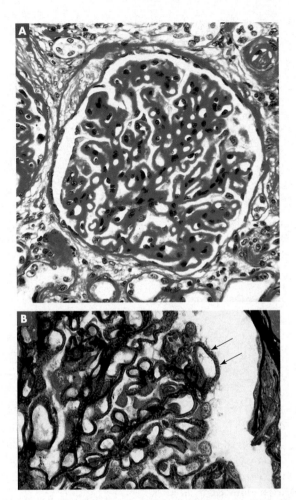

19-13: *Diffuse membranous glomerulonephritis. The H&E (hematoxylin & eosin)-stained biopsy (**A**) shows glomerular basement membranes that are uniformly thickened. There is no proliferative component. The silver stain of the biopsy (**B**) shows numerous silver-positive spikes (arrows) on the epithelial side of the glomerular basement membrane (subepithelial immunocomplex deposits). (From Kern WF, Silva FG, Kern W (eds): Atlas of Renal Pathology. Philadelphia, WB Saunders, 1999, p 53, Figs. 5-30 and 5-33.)*

- When the afferent arteriole becomes hyalinized, the GFR decreases.
  (2) Nodular masses develop in the mesangial matrix.
  - Due to increased type IV collagen synthesis and trapped proteins
  g. Clinical and laboratory findings
  (1) Microalbuminuria
  (a) Initial laboratory manifestation of diabetic glomerulopathy
  - Usually begins after ~10 years of poor glycemic control
  (b) Microalbuminuria dipsticks detect albumin levels in the range of 1.5 to 8 mg/dL.

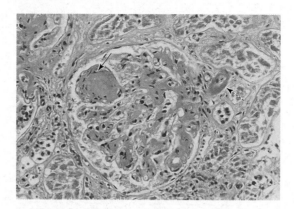

19-14: *Diabetic glomerulosclerosis. Broken arrow points to an afferent or efferent arteriole that has hyaline arteriolosclerosis, with an increase in proteinaceous material in the wall of the vessel. Solid arrow shows a mesangial nodule containing type IV collagen and trapped protein. (From Damjanov I, Linder J: Pathology: A Color Atlas. St. Louis, Mosby, 2000, p 229, Fig. 11-64.)*

An angiotensin-converting enzyme inhibitor is prescribed when microalbuminuria is first detected. It slows the progression of diabetic glomerulopathy by decreasing pressure in the glomerular capillaries by decreasing ATII vasoconstriction of the hyalinized efferent arterioles.

(2) Other renal diseases associated with diabetes mellitus
  • Renal papillary necrosis, acute and chronic pyelonephritis
2. Renal amyloidosis (see Chapter 3)
  • Associated with primary and secondary amyloidosis

H. Hereditary glomerular diseases
  1. Alport's syndrome
    a. X-linked dominant disease (85% of cases)
      • Defect in the synthesis of α_5-subtype of type IV collagen in GBM
    b. *No* specific immunofluorescence or electron microscopic findings
    c. Microscopic findings
      • Lipid accumulation in VECs producing foam cells
    d. Sensorineural hearing loss and ocular abnormalities
  2. Thin basement membrane disease
    • "Benign familial hematuria"
    a. Autosomal dominant disorder
    b. Extremely thin GBMs
      • Normal renal function
    c. Mild proteinuria, persistent microscopic hematuria

I. Chronic glomerulonephritis
  1. Causes in descending order of incidence
    a. Rapidly progressive glomerulonephritis (RPGN)
    b. Focal segmental glomerulosclerosis

Alport's syndrome: hereditary nephritis, sensorineural hearing loss, ocular defects

RPGN: most common cause of chronic glomerulonephritis

   c. Type I membranoproliferative glomerulonephritis
   d. IgA glomerulonephritis
 2. Gross and microscopic findings
   a. Shrunken kidneys
   b. Glomerular sclerosis and tubular atrophy

VII. Disorders Affecting Tubules and Interstitium
A. Acute tubular necrosis (ATN)
 1. Epidemiology
   a. Acute renal failure (ARF)
    (1) Acute suppression of renal function developing in 24 hours
    (2) Accompanied by anuria or oliguria (<400 mL/24 hours)
    (3) Acute tubular necrosis (ATN) is the most common cause of ARF.
     • Subdivided into ischemic and nephrotoxic types
   b. Other causes of ARF
    (1) Postrenal obstruction
     • Examples—prostate hyperplasia, invasive cervical cancer
    (2) Vascular disease
     • Example—malignant hypertension
    (3) RPGN, drugs, DIC, urate nephropathy
 2. Ischemic ATN
   a. Most often caused by prerenal azotemia due to hypovolemia
   b. Ischemia damages endothelial cells.
    (1) Causes decrease in vasodilators
     • Examples—nitric oxide, PGI_2
    (2) Increase in vasoconstrictors
     • Example—endothelin
    (3) Net effect is vasoconstriction of afferent arterioles, which decreases GFR.
   c. Ischemia damages tubule cells
    (1) Causes detachment of tubular cells into the lumen causing obstruction
     • Produces pigmented renal tubular cell casts
    (2) Casts obstruct the lumen causing an increase in intratubular pressure
     (a) Decreases GFR
     (b) Pushes fluid into the interstitium
     (c) Net effect is oliguria
   d. Sites of tubular damage
    (1) Straight segment of proximal tubule
     • Part of the nephron most susceptible to hypoxia
    (2) Medullary segment of the thick ascending limb (TAL)
    (3) Tubular basement membranes are disrupted at these sites.
     • Prevents renal tubular cell regeneration
 3. Nephrotoxic type
   a. Causes
    (1) Aminoglycosides are the most common cause (e.g., gentamicin)

ATN: most common cause of ARF

Ischemic ATN: most common type of ATN

Prerenal azotemia: most common cause of ischemic ATN

Renal tubular cell cast: key cast of ATN

Aminoglycosides: most common cause of nephrotoxic ATN

(2) Radiocontrast agents

(3) Heavy metals (e.g., lead and mercury)

 b. Microscopic findings

  (1) Primarily damages the proximal tubule cells

  (2) Tubular basement membrane is intact.

4. Clinical and laboratory findings in ATN

 a. Oliguria, in most cases

  • Some cases have polyuria (>800 mL/24 hours)

 b. Pigmented renal tubular cell casts

 c. Hyperkalemia, increased anion gap metabolic acidosis (see Chapter 4)

 d. Increased serum BUN and creatinine (ratio ≤ 15)

 e. Hypokalemia (diuresis phase) and infection are common problems

5. Differential diagnosis of oliguria (Box 19-1)

B. Tubulointerstitial nephritis (TIN)

 • Acute or chronic inflammation of tubules and interstitium

1. Causes of TIN

 a. Acute pyelonephritis (most common)

 b. Drugs

 c. Infections

  • Examples—Legionnaires' disease, leptospirosis

 d. SLE, lead poisoning, urate nephropathy, multiple myeloma

2. Acute pyelonephritis (APN)

 a. Epidemiology

  (1) More common in women than men

   • Women have a short urethra.

  (2) Risk factors

   (a) Urinary tract obstruction

   (b) Medullary sponge kidney

   (c) Diabetes mellitus, pregnancy, sickle cell trait/disease

Acute pyelonephritis: most common cause of TIN

BOX 19-1

DIFFERENTIAL DIAGNOSIS OF OLIGURIA

Oliguria is defined as a urine output < 400 mL/day or < 20 mL/hour. The major causes of oliguria include prerenal azotemia (most common cause), acute glomerulonephritis (nephritic type), acute tubular necrosis (renal azotemia), and postrenal azotemia.

 Laboratory tests that are commonly used in differentiating the types of oliguria include urine osmolality (UOsm), fractional excretion of sodium (FENa⁺), random urine sodium (UNa⁺), and the serum BUN:Cr (blood urea nitrogen/creatinine) ratio (see section III). These tests evaluate tubular function.

A UOsm > 500 mOsm/kg indicates good concentrating ability and intact tubular function, but a UOsm < 350 mOsm/kg indicates poor concentrating ability and tubular dysfunction. The FENa$^+$ represents the amount of sodium excreted in the urine divided by the amount of sodium that is filtered by the kidneys. The calculation is as follows:

$$FENa^+ = [(UNa^+ \times PCr) \div (PNa^+ \times UCr)] \times 100$$

where UNa$^+$ is a random urine sodium, PNa$^+$ is serum sodium, UCr is random urine creatinine, and PCr is plasma creatinine. Creatinine is used in the formula, because the amount of sodium filtered is dependent on the glomerular filtration rate (GFR), which closely approximates the creatinine clearance (CCr). An FENa$^+$ < 1% indicates good tubular function and *excludes* acute tubular necrosis (ATN) as a cause of oliguria. An FENa$^+$ > 2% indicates tubular dysfunction and is highly predictive of ATN as the cause of oliguria. A random UNa$^+$ < 20 mEq/L indicates intact tubular function, and a random UNa$^+$ > 40 mEq/L indicates tubular dysfunction. A serum BUN:Cr ratio > 15 indicates intact tubular function, and a serum BUN:Cr ratio ≤ 15 indicates tubular dysfunction. Prerenal azotemia and acute glomerulonephritis (nephritic type) have preservation of tubular function. In order to distinguish the two, the urine sediment examination is most useful. In prerenal azotemia, the urine sediment has *no* abnormal findings or may have a few hyaline casts. The sediment in acute glomerulonephritis (nephritic type) has hematuria and RBC casts. ATN and postrenal azotemia (long-standing obstruction) both have tubular dysfunction. Postrenal azotemia of short duration has normal tubular function and has laboratory findings similar to prerenal azotemia. In order to distinguish ATN from postrenal azotemia as a cause of tubular dysfunction and oliguria, the urine sediment is most useful. In ATN, the sediment has pigmented renal tubular cell casts, but in postrenal azotemia, the sediment is usually normal. In addition, the patient will likely have a history of a renal stone, benign prostatic hyperplasia, or cervical cancer, which commonly obstructs the ureters where they enter the urinary bladder.

Disorder	FENa$^+$%	BUN:Cr	UNa$^+$	UOsm	Urinalysis
Prerenal azotemia	<1	>15	<20	>500	Normal sediment or few hyaline casts
Acute glomerulonephritis	<1	>15	<20	>500	RBC casts, hematuria
Acute tubular necrosis	>2	≤15	>40	<350	Renal tubular cell casts
Postrenal azotemia (prolonged obstruction)	>2	≤15	>40	<350	Normal sediment

b. Pathogenesis
  (1) Vesicoureteral reflux (VUR) with ascending infection (most common)
    (a) Intravesical portion of the ureter is normally compressed with micturition.
      • Prevents reflux of urine into the ureter(s)
    (b) In VUR, the intravesical portion of the ureter is *not* compressed during micturition.
      • Urine refluxes into the ureter(s).
  (2) Ascending infection
    (a) Most common mechanism for lower and upper UTIs in females
    (b) Distal urethra and vaginal introitus are normally colonized by *Escherichia coli.*
    (c) Organisms ascend into the urethra and bladder.
      • Causes urethritis and cystitis
    (d) If VUR is present, infected urine ascends to the renal pelvis and renal parenchyma.
      • Causes APN
c. Gross and microscopic findings
  (1) Grayish white areas of abscess formation are in the cortex and medulla.
  (2) Microabscess formation occurs in the tubular lumens and interstitium (Fig. 19-15).
d. Clinical findings
  (1) Spiking fever, flank pain
  (2) Increased frequency of urination
  (3) Painful urination (dysuria)
e. Laboratory findings
  (1) WBC casts (key finding)

VUR: urine refluxes into the ureters during micturition

Ascending infection: most common mechanism for upper and lower UTIs in females

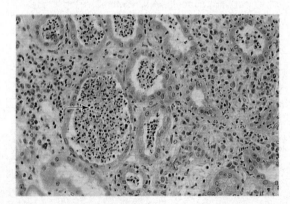

19-15: *Acute pyelonephritis showing a neutrophil-dominant infiltrate in the tubular lumens (arrow) and interstitium. The neutrophils in the lumens are molded into white blood cell (WBC) casts, which are passed in the urine along with free neutrophils and bacteria (pyuria). (From Kern WF, Silva FG, Kern W (eds): Atlas of Renal Pathology. Philadelphia, WB Saunders, 1999, p 149, Fig. 13-15B.)*

(2) Pyuria, bacteriuria (usually *E. coli*), hematuria

  f. Complications

    (1) Chronic pyelonephritis

    (2) Perinephric abscess

    (3) Renal papillary necrosis, septicemia with endotoxic shock

3. Chronic pyelonephritis (CPN)

  a. Pathogenesis

    (1) VUR starting in young girls

    (2) Lower urinary tract obstruction

      (a) Produces hydronephrosis

      (b) Examples—prostatic hyperplasia, renal stones

  b. Gross and microscopic findings

    (1) Reflux type of CPN

      (a) U-shaped cortical scars overlying a blunt calyx

      (b) Visible with an intravenous pyelogram (IVP)

    (2) Obstructive type CPN

      (a) Uniform dilation of the calyces

      (b) Diffuse thinning of cortical tissue

    (3) Microscopic findings

      (a) Chronic inflammation

        • Secondary scarring of the glomeruli

      (b) Tubular atrophy

        • Tubules contain eosinophilic material resembling thyroid tissue ("thyroidization").

  c. Clinical and laboratory findings

    (1) Usually a history of recurrent APN

    (2) May cause hypertension

      • Reflux nephropathy is a cause of hypertension in children.

    (3) May cause CRF

4. Acute drug-induced TIN

  a. Common drug associations

    (1) Penicillin, particularly methicillin

    (2) Rifampin, sulfonamides

    (3) NSAIDs, diuretics

  b. Pathogenesis

    (1) Combination of type I and type IV hypersensitivity

    (2) Occurs ~2 weeks after beginning a drug

  c. Clinical and laboratory findings

    (1) Abrupt onset of fever, oliguria, and rash

      • Withdrawal of the drug causes reversal of the disease.

    (2) Laboratory findings

      (a) BUN : Cr ratio ≤ 15

      (b) Eosinophilia and eosinophiluria (highly predictive)

5. Analgesic nephropathy

  a. Epidemiology

    (1) Common cause of chronic drug-induced TIN

    (2) More common in women than men

Findings in APN and not lower UTIs: fever, flank pain, WBC casts in urine

CPN: VUR in young girls, chronic hydronephrosis

Acute drug-induce TIN: abrupt onset fever, oliguria, rash

(3) Usually occurs in patients with chronic pain

b. Pathogenesis

(1) Chronic use of acetaminophen plus aspirin for 3 or more years

(2) Acetaminophen free radicals damage renal tubules in medulla (see Chapter 1)

(3) Aspirin inhibits renal synthesis of PGE_2 leaving ATII unopposed.
- Decreased blood flow to the renal medulla

Analgesic nephropathy: combination of acetaminophen + aspirin; renal papillary necrosis

c. Complications

(1) Renal papillary necrosis (Fig. 19-16)

(a) Sloughing of renal papillae
- Produces gross hematuria, proteinuria, and colicky flank pain

(b) An IVP shows a "ring defect" where one or more papillae used to reside.

(c) Other causes of renal papillary necrosis
- Diabetes, sickle cell trait/disease, APN

(2) Hypertension, CRF

(3) Renal pelvic and bladder transitional cell carcinomas

6. Urate nephropathy

a. Deposition of urate crystals in the tubules and interstitium

b. Causes

(1) Massive release of purines (precursor of uric acid)
- Usually following aggressive treatment of disseminated cancer (e.g., leukemia)

(2) Lead poisoning, gout

Prevention of urate nephropathy: allopurinol *before* aggressive cancer therapy

c. May produce ARF

> Patients with disseminated cancers should receive allopurinol, an xanthine oxidase inhibitor, *before* being treated with chemotherapy. This prevents urate nephropathy (tumor lysis syndrome) and acute renal failure.

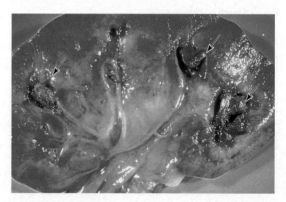

19-16: *Analgesic nephropathy showing multiple brownish necrotic papillae (arrows). (From Kumar V, Fausto N, Abbas A: Robbins and Cotran's Pathologic Basis of Disease, 7th ed. Philadelphia, WB Saunders, 2004, p 1003, Fig. 20-45.)*

7. Chronic lead poisoning
   a. Pathogenesis
      (1) Decreases secretion of uric acid (urate nephropathy)
      (2) Direct toxic effect produces TIN
   b. Proximal tubule cells contain characteristic nuclear acid-fast inclusions.
8. Multiple myeloma: mechanisms for renal disease
   a. Bence Jones (BJ) proteinuria (see Chapter 13)
      (1) BJ protein produces tubular casts
         • Light chains are toxic to renal tubular epithelium.
      (2) Casts obstruct the lumen and incite a foreign body giant cell reaction.
         • Reaction involves tubules and interstitium leading to renal failure.
   b. Nephrocalcinosis (see Chapter 1)
      (1) Due to hypercalcemia
         • Metastatic calcification of the basement membrane of collecting tubules
      (2) Causes polyuria and renal failure
   c. Primary amyloidosis producing nephrotic syndrome (see Chapter 3)
      • Light chains are converted to amyloid.

> BJ proteinuria: casts with foreign body giant cell reaction

VIII. Chronic Renal Failure (CRF)

A. Epidemiology and pathogenesis
1. Progressive irreversible azotemia that develops over months to years
2. Culminates in end-stage renal disease
   a. Kidneys no longer function well enough to sustain life.
   b. GFR is below 10 mL/min.
3. Primary causes, in descending order
   a. Diabetic mellitus
   b. Hypertension
   c. Glomerulonephritis
      • Particularly RPGN and focal segmental glomerulosclerosis
   d. Cystic renal disease
      • Renal dysplasia in children, adult polycystic kidney disease

B. Gross appearance
• Bilateral, small shrunken kidneys

C. Hematologic findings
1. Normocytic anemia (see Chapter 11)
   • Primarily due to decreased erythropoietin
2. Qualitative platelet defects (see Chapter 14)

D. Renal osteodystrophy
1. Osteitis fibrosa cystica
   a. Due to hypovitaminosis D (see Chapter 7)
      (1) Causes hypocalcemia, which stimulates production of parathyroid hormone
      (2) Called secondary hyperparathyroidism (HPTH) (Chapter 22)
   b. Secondary HPTH increases bone resorption.

(1) Causes cystic lesions in bone (e.g., jaw)

(2) Hemorrhage into cysts causes a brown discoloration.

2. Osteomalacia

a. Decreased mineralization of the organic bone matrix (osteoid)

b. In CRF, it is due to hypovitaminosis D.

• Causes hypocalcemia, leading to decreased bone mineralization

c. Produces fractures and bone pain

3. Osteoporosis (see Chapter 23)

a. Loss of organic bone matrix and minerals

• Causes an overall reduction in bone mass

b. In CRF, it is due to chronic metabolic acidosis.

• Excess H^+ ions are buffered by bone.

c. Produces fractures and bone pain

E. **Cardiovascular findings**

1. Hypertension from salt retention

2. Hemorrhagic fibrinous pericarditis

3. Congestive heart failure, accelerated atherosclerosis

F. **Miscellaneous findings**

1. Hemorrhagic gastritis

2. Uremic frost (urea crystals deposit on skin)

G. **Laboratory findings**

1. Acid-base and electrolyte abnormalities

a. Hyperkalemia and increased anion gap metabolic acidosis (see Chapter 4)

b. Sodium is usually normal except in salt losing types of CRF.

2. Hypocalcemia; causes:

a. Hypovitaminosis D

(1) Due to decreased synthesis of 1-α-hydroxylase

(2) Decreased reabsorption of calcium from the small intestine

b. Hyperphosphatemia

(1) Due to decreased renal excretion

(2) Drives calcium into bone and soft tissue

• Metastatic calcification (see Chapter 1)

3. Urinalysis findings

a. Fixed specific gravity

• Tubular dysfunction causes lack of concentration and dilution.

b. Waxy and broad casts (Fig. 19-17)

IX. **Vascular Disorders**

A. **Benign nephrosclerosis (BNS)**

1. Most common renal disease in essential hypertension

2. Pathogenesis

a. Hyaline arteriolosclerosis of arterioles in the renal cortex.

b. Causes tubular atrophy, interstitial fibrosis, glomerular sclerosis

3. Small kidneys with a finely granular cortical surface (Fig. 19-18)

4. Laboratory findings

a. Mild proteinuria

Renal osteodystrophy: due to secondary HPTH, osteomalacia, osteoporosis

Waxy casts: sign of CRF

BNS: kidney of essential hypertension; due to hyaline arteriolosclerosis

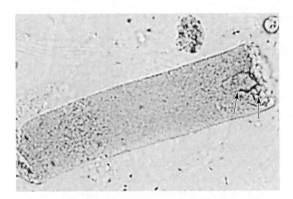

19-17: Waxy cast in the urine sediment. The diameter of the cast is increased due to tubular atrophy. It has a refractile quality, with distinct margins. Arrows show degenerating renal tubular cells. (From Henry JB: Clinical Diagnosis and Management by Laboratory Methods, 20th ed. Philadelphia, WB Saunders, 2001, Plate 18-14.)

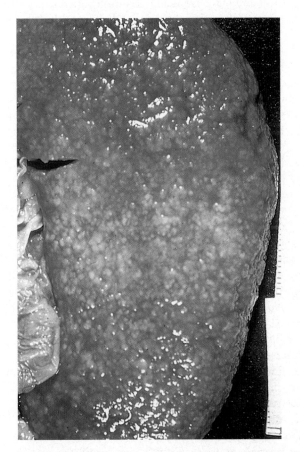

19-18: Benign nephrosclerosis showing a finely granular cortical surface due to atrophy of tubules, glomerular sclerosis, and interstitial fibrosis in the renal cortex. (From Kumar V, Fausto N, Abbas A: Robbins and Cotran's Pathologic Basis of Disease, 7th ed. Philadelphia, WB Saunders, 2004, p 1007, Fig. 20-48.)

      b. Hematuria (no RBC casts)

      c. Renal azotemia

B. Malignant hypertension

  1. Epidemiology

    a. Sudden onset of accelerated hypertension

      (1) May occur in normotensive individuals

      (2) May occur in those with BNS (most common)

      (3) May occur as a complication of various disorders

    b. Risk factors

      (1) Preexisting BNS (most common)

      (2) Hemolytic-uremic syndrome

      (3) Thrombotic thrombocytopenic purpura

      (4) Systemic sclerosis

  2. Pathogenesis

    a. Vascular damage to arterioles and small arteries

    b. Gross and microscopic changes

      (1) Fibrinoid necrosis and necrotizing arteriolitis and glomerulitis

        • Pinpoint hemorrhages on the cortical surface ("flea-bitten" kidneys)

      (2) Hyperplastic arteriolosclerosis ("onion skin" lesion; see Chapter 9)

        • Smooth muscle hyperplasia and reduplication of basement membrane

  3. Clinical findings

    a. Rapid increase in blood pressure to or over 210/120 mm Hg

    b. Hypertensive encephalopathy

      (1) Cerebral edema

      (2) Papilledema

        • Loss of the normal optic nerve disc margin

      (3) Retinopathy

        • Flame hemorrhages, exudates

      (4) Potential for an intracerebral bleed

    c. Oliguric acute renal failure

  4. Laboratory findings

    a. Azotemia with BUN:Cr ratio ≤ 15

    b. Hematuria with RBC casts

    c. Proteinuria

  5. Initial treatment is intravenous sodium nitroprusside.

C. Renal infarction

  1. Causes

    a. Embolization from thrombi in the left side of the heart (most common)

    b. Atheroembolic renal disease

    c. Vasculitis, particularly polyarteritis nodosa

  2. Gross and microscopic appearance

    a. Irregular, wedge-shaped pale infarctions in the cortex

    b. Old infarcts have a V-shaped appearance due to scar tissue

  3. Sudden onset of flank pain and hematuria

Malignant hypertension: ≥210/≥120 mm Hg, encephalopathy, renal failure

Renal infarction: hematuria and flank pain

D. **Sickle cell nephropathy**
1. Occurs with sickle cell trait or disease
2. Clinical presentations
   a. Asymptomatic hematuria (most common) (see Chapter 11)
   • Due to infarctions in the medulla
   b. Loss of concentrating ability
   c. Renal papillary necrosis
   d. Pyelonephritis
E. **Diffuse cortical necrosis**
1. Complication of an obstetric emergency
   • Examples—preeclampsia, abruptio placentae
2. Due to DIC limited to the renal cortex
   a. Fibrin clots in arterioles and glomerular capillaries
   b. Bilateral, diffuse, pale infarct of the renal cortex
3. Anuria (no urine) in a pregnant woman followed by ARF

X. **Obstructive Disorders**
A. **Hydronephrosis**
1. Causes
   a. Renal stone (most common)
   b. Retroperitoneal fibrosis
   c. Cervical cancer, benign prostatic hyperplasia
2. Gross findings
   a. Dilated ureter and renal pelvis (see Fig. 1-3)
   b. Compression atrophy of the renal medulla and cortex
3. May produce postrenal azotemia

B. **Renal stones (urolithiasis)**
1. Risk factors
   a. Hypercalciuria in the absence of hypercalcemia
      (1) Most common metabolic abnormality
      (2) Due to increased gastrointestinal reabsorption of calcium
   b. Decreased urine volume concentrates the urine
   c. Reduced urine citrate
      • Citrate normally chelates calcium
   d. Primary hyperparathyroidism
   e. Diets high in dairy products (contain phosphate) or oxalates
   f. Urinary infections due to urease producers (e.g., *Proteus*)
2. Types of renal stones
   a. Calcium stones
      (1) Calcium oxalate stones is the most common type in adults.
         • Increased incidence in pure vegans and Crohn's disease
      (2) Calcium phosphate stones are the most common type in children.
         • Associated with dairy products and distal renal tubular acidosis
   b. Magnesium ammonium phosphate
      (1) "Staghorn calculus" or struvite stone

Hydronephrosis: most common complication of upper urinary tract obstruction

Renal stone: most common cause of upper urinary tract obstruction

Hypercalciuria: most common metabolic abnormality causing calcium stones

(2) Associated with urease producers (e.g., *Proteus*)

(3) Urine is alkaline and smells like ammonia.

c. Uric acid, cystine

3. Clinical and laboratory findings

   a. Ipsilateral colicky pain in the flank with radiation to the groin

   b. Gross and microscopic hematuria

4. Majority of stones contain calcium (~80% of cases).

   a. Often visualized on a routine radiograph

   b. Renal ultrasound and IVP detect stones that do *not* visualize.

XI. **Tumors of the Kidney and Renal Pelvis**

  A. **Angiomyolipoma**

    1. Hamartoma composed of blood vessels, smooth muscle, and adipose cells

    2. Associated with tuberous sclerosis (see Chapter 25)

      a. Mental retardation

      b. Multisystem hamartomas

  B. **Renal cell carcinoma**

    • Alias Grawitz tumor, clear cell carcinoma, hypernephroma

    1. Epidemiology

      a. Sporadic (most common) and hereditary types

      b. Male dominant

        • Occur in the sixth to seventh decades

      c. Cytogenetic abnormalities occur in sporadic and hereditary cancers

        • Involve translocations with loss of the von Hippel–Lindau suppressor gene

      d. Cancer derives from proximal tubule cells

      e. Risk factors

        (1) Smoking (most common)

        (2) Von Hippel–Lindau disease (VHL)

          (a) Autosomal dominant

          (b) Hemangioblastomas of cerebellum and retina

          (c) Bilateral renal cell carcinoma (50–60% of cases)

        (3) Adult polycystic kidney disease

    2. Gross and microscopic findings

      a. Clear cell carcinoma

        (1) Most common type (70–80% of cases)

        (2) Most are sporadic

          • Remainder are associated with VHL.

        (3) Upper pole mass with cysts and hemorrhage (Fig. 19-19)

          • Tumor is a bright yellow mass larger than 3 cm in 75% to 80% of cases.

        (4) Composed of clear cells that contain lipid and glycogen

        (5) Tendency for renal vein invasion

          • Yellow tumor may invade the inferior vena cava and extend to the right side of the heart.

        (6) Metastasis

          (a) Lungs are the most common site

Thiazides: increase reabsorption of calcium out of urine

Renal cell carcinoma: yellow tumor with renal vein invasion

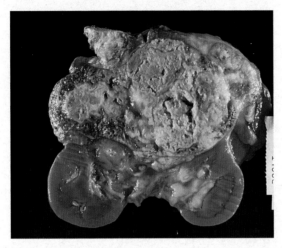

19-19: *Renal cell carcinoma. The large, yellow upper pole mass with multifocal areas of hemorrhage extends into the renal pelvis. (From Damjanov I, Linder J: Pathology: A Color Atlas. St. Louis, Mosby, 2000, p 234, Fig. 11-79.)*

- Often hemorrhagic, "cannonball" appearance on radiographs
  (b) Bone (lytic lesions)
  (c) Hemorrhagic nodules in the skin
    - Due to increased vascularity in the tumor
3. Clinical findings
   a. Triad of hematuria, flank mass, and costovertebral angle pain
      - Fever may also occur.
   b. May produce a left-sided varicocele if left renal vein is invaded (see Chapter 20)
   c. Ectopic secretion of hormones
      (1) Erythropoietin
         - Produces secondary polycythemia
      (2) Parathyroid hormone-related protein
         - Produces hypercalcemia
4. Prognosis
   a. Characteristically has late metastases
      - May recur 10 to 20 years after the tumor has been removed.
   b. Average 5-year survival rate is 45% with metastasis.
      - Up to 70% of cases do not have metastasis.
   c. Extension into the renal vein or through the renal capsule has a poor prognosis
      - 10% to 15% 5-year survival rate
C. **Cancers of the renal pelvis**
   1. Transitional cell carcinoma
      a. Most common type
         - Approximately 50% have similar tumors elsewhere in the urinary tract.

      b. Risk factors

         (1) Smoking (most common)

         (2) Phenacetin abuse

         (3) Aromatic amines (aniline dyes)

         (4) Cyclophosphamide

  2. Squamous cell carcinoma

     • Risk factors include renal stones and chronic infection.

D. Wilms' tumor

  1. Epidemiology

      a. Most common primary renal tumor in children

      b. Occurs between 2 and 5 years of age

      c. Sporadic type (most common)

      d. Genetic type

         (1) Autosomal dominant inheritance (chromosome 11)

         (2) WAGR syndrome

            • <u>W</u>ilms' tumor, <u>a</u>niridia (absent iris), <u>g</u>enital abnormalities, <u>r</u>etardation

         (3) Beckwith-Wiedemann syndrome

            • Wilms' tumor, enlarged body organs, hemihypertrophy of extremities

  2. Large, necrotic, gray-tan tumor

      a. Derived from mesonephric mesoderm

      b. Contains abortive glomeruli and tubules, primitive blastemal cells, and rhabdomyoblasts

  3. Clinical findings

      a. Unilateral palpable mass in a child with hypertension

         • Hypertension due to renin secretion

      b. Lungs are the most common site of metastasis.

      c. With combined therapies 2-year survival rate is above 90%.

Wilms' tumor: child with unilateral flank mass and hypertension

20 CHAPTER

Lower Urinary Tract and Male Reproductive Disorders

I. Common Ureteral Disorders

A. Congenital anomalies
1. Double ureters
   - Due to a double or split ureteral bud
2. Congenital megaloureter
   - May be associated with Hirschsprung's disease

B. Ureteritis cystica
1. Manifestation of chronic inflammation
2. Smooth cysts project from the mucosa into the lumen.
   - Similar findings may be present in the bladder.
3. May undergo glandular metaplasia and predispose to adenocarcinoma

C. Ureteral stones
   - Ureters are the most common site for stones to cause obstruction.

D. Retroperitoneal fibrosis
1. Causes
   a. Majority are idiopathic.
   b. Ergot derivatives used in the treatment of migraines
   c. Association with other sclerosing periconditions
      (1) Primary sclerosing pericholangitis
      (2) Sclerosing mediastinitis, Ridel's fibrosing thyroiditis
   d. Retroperitoneal malignant lymphoma
2. Complications
   a. Hydronephrosis is the most common complication.
   b. May cause right scrotal varicocele (see section V)
      - Blocks the drainage of the right spermatic vein into the vena cava

Hydronephrosis: most common complication of retroperitoneal fibrosis

E. Ureteral cancers
   - Transitional cell carcinoma is the most common cancer.

II. Urinary Bladder Disorders

A. Congenital disorders
1. Exstrophy of the bladder
   a. Developmental failure of the anterior abdominal wall and bladder
      (1) Bladder mucosa is exposed to the body surface.
      (2) Often associated with epispadias (see section IV)

b. Complications
   (1) Inflammation predisposes to glandular metaplasia.
   (2) Predisposition for adenocarcinoma of the bladder
2. Urachal cyst remnants
   a. Drainage of urine from the umbilicus in a newborn
   b. Predispose to adenocarcinoma of the bladder
      • Most common cause of bladder adenocarcinoma

B. Acute and chronic cystitis
1. Risk factors for lower urinary tract (LUT) infection
   a. Female sex
      (1) Short urethra
      (2) Ascending infection (see Chapter 19)
   b. Indwelling urinary catheter
      • Most common cause of sepsis in hospitalized patients

   c. Sexual intercourse
      • "Honeymoon cystitis" from trauma to the urethra
   d. Diabetes mellitus
   e. Cyclophosphamide
      • Produces hemorrhagic cystitis
   f. *Schistosoma hematobium*
2. Causes of acute cystitis
   a. *E. coli*
      (1) Most common uropathogen (80–90% of cases)
      (2) Most common cause of sepsis in a hospitalized patient

   b. Adenovirus
      • Causes hemorrhagic cystitis
   c. *Staphylococcus saprophyticus*
      (1) Causes acute cystitis in young sexually active women
         • Accounts for ~10% to 20% of LUT infections
      (2) Coagulase negative
   d. Acute urethral syndrome in women
      • Female counterpart to nonspecific urethritis (NSU) in men
      (1) *Chlamydia trachomatis*

         (a) Most common cause of acute urethral syndrome
         (b) Identification of *Chlamydia*
            • Polymerase chain reaction (PCR) testing of voided urine
      (2) Other pathogens
         • *Mycoplasma hominis, Ureaplasma urealyticum, Neisseria gonorrhoeae*
   e. Clinical findings in LUT infections
      (1) Dysuria (painful urination)
      (2) Increased frequency, urgency, nocturia
      (3) Suprapubic discomfort
      (4) Gross hematuria
   f. Laboratory findings in LUT infections
      (1) Pyuria at or above 10 white blood cells (WBCs) per high-power field (HPF) in a centrifuged specimen

- More than 2 WBCs/HPF in an uncentrifuged specimen
      (2) Bacteriuria, hematuria
      (3) Positive dipstick for leukocyte esterase and nitrite (see Chapter 19)
      (4) At or above 10^5 colony-forming units (CFUs)/mL
        - Gold standard criterion of infection

$\geq 10^5$ CFUs/mL: gold standard for LUT infection

   g. Asymptomatic bacteriuria in women
      (1) Two successive cultures with 10^5 or more CFUs/mL in an asymptomatic patient
      (2) Causes
        (a) Pregnancy
          - Acute pyelonephritis may occur in 1% to 2% of cases.
        (b) Elderly women in nursing homes
        (c) Diabetes mellitus
  3. Sterile pyuria
   a. Neutrophils in the urine and negative standard culture after 24 hours
      - Positive leukocyte esterase, negative nitrite

Sterile pyuria: neutrophils in the urine, negative standard culture

   b. Causes
      (1) *Chlamydia trachomatis*
      (2) Renal tuberculosis
      (3) Acute tubulointerstitial nephritis (see Chapter 19)
  4. Malacoplakia
   a. Associated with a chronic *E. coli* infection of the bladder
   b. Microscopic findings
      (1) Yellow, raised mucosal plaques
      (2) Foamy macrophages filled with laminated mineralized concretions

Malacoplakia: Michaelis-Gutmann bodies

        (a) Called Michaelis-Gutmann bodies
        (b) Defective phagosomes that cannot degrade bacterial products

C. Miscellaneous disorders

  1. Acquired diverticula
   a. Most are due to benign prostatic hyperplasia (BPH)
   b. Causes obstruction of urine outflow and increased intravesical pressure

Acquired bladder diverticula: most common cause is BPH

   c. Diverticulitis and stone formation are common complications
  2. Cystocele
   a. Common in middle-aged to elderly women
   b. Mechanism
      (1) Relaxation of pelvic support causes descent of the uterus
      (2) Bladder wall protrudes into the vagina
        - Creates a pouch that collects residual urine
  3. Cystitis cystica and glandularis
   a. Bladder rendition of ureteritis cystica
   b. Increased risk for developing bladder adenocarcinoma

D. Bladder tumors

  1. Bladder papilloma
     - Very uncommon benign tumor

2. Transitional cell carcinoma (TCC)
   a. Most common bladder cancer (>95% of cases)
   b. Male dominant
   c. Multifocality and recurrence are the rule.
      (1) Common malignant stem cell abnormality
      (2) Reimplantation of the tumor from another site
   d. Causes

Smoking cigarettes: most common cause of TCC of bladder

      (1) Smoking cigarettes
      (2) Aniline dyes
      (3) Cyclophosphamide
      (4) *Schistosoma hematobium*
         • 70% produce squamous cell carcinoma, 30% TCC
   e. Gross and microscopic findings
      (1) Low-grade cancers
         • Usually papillary and are *not* usually invasive
      (2) High-grade cancers
         • Papillary or flat and are usually invasive
      (3) Most common sites
         • Lateral or posterior walls at the base of the bladder
      (4) Significance of blood group antigens (A, B, or H)
         • Better prognosis if the tumor has the antigens
   f. Clinical findings
      (1) Painless gross/microscopic hematuria
         • Most common sign (70–90% of cases)
      (2) Dysuria, increased frequency of urination
3. Squamous cell carcinoma of the bladder
   a. Epidemiology
      (1) Association with *Schistosoma hematobium*
         • Eggs are located in the urinary bladder venous plexus.
      (2) Common cancer in Egypt
      (3) 70% of cancers are squamous cell carcinoma, 30% are TCC
   b. Pathogenesis of squamous cell carcinoma

Squamous cell carcinoma of bladder: *S. hematobium* infection

      (1) Eggs are surrounded by eosinophils.
      (2) IgE antibodies are attached to the eggs.
      (3) Eosinophils have Fc receptors for IgE.
      (4) Eosinophils attach to receptors and release major basic protein, which destroys the egg.
         • Type II hypersensitivity reaction
      (5) Chronic bladder irritation/infection produces squamous metaplasia
         • Metaplasia can progress to dysplasia and squamous cell carcinoma.
4. Adenocarcinoma of the bladder; causes:
   a. Urachal remnants (most common cause)
   b. Cystitis glandularis
   c. Exstrophy of the bladder
5. Embryonal rhabdomyosarcoma (sarcoma botryoides)

a. Most common sarcoma in children
b. Most common site for boys is urinary system.
  • Presents as grape-like masses protruding from the urethral orifice
c. Most common site in girls is the vagina.
6. Cancers invading the bladder
  a. Invasive cervical cancer and prostate cancer
  b. Produce obstruction of the urethra and the ureters
  c. Produces hydronephrosis, postrenal azotemia, and death by renal failure

III. Urethral Disorders
A. Infections
  1. *Chlamydial* and gonococcal infections in men and women
    • Most common site for these sexually transmitted diseases
  2. Nonvenereal diseases causing urethritis
    a. Most commonly due to *E. coli*
    b. Complications
      (1) Cystitis in women
      (2) Prostatitis in men
  3. *Chlamydial* urethritis is a common component of Reiter's syndrome in men.
    a. Urethritis
    b. Sterile conjunctivitis
    c. HLA-B27-associated arthritis (see Chapter 23)
B. Urethral caruncle
  1. Female dominant disease
  2. Friable, red painful mass is present at the urethral orifice.
  3. Chronically inflamed granulation tissue causes bleeding.
C. Squamous cell carcinoma
  • Most common cancer of the urethra

IV. Penis Disorders
A. Malformations of the urethral groove
  1. Types of malformations
    a. Hypospadias
      • Most common malformation
    b. Epispadias
  2. Pathogenesis
    a. Hypospadias
      (1) Abnormal opening on the ventral surface of the penis
      (2) Due to faulty closure of the urethral folds
    b. Epispadias
      (1) Abnormal opening on the dorsal surface of the penis
      (2) Due to a defect in the genital tubercle
B. Phimosis
  1. Orifice of the prepuce is too small to retract over the head of the penis
  2. Commonly associated with infections

Hypospadias: faulty closure of urethral folds

Epispadias: defect genital tubercle

C. Balanoposthitis
1. Infection of the glans and prepuce
    a. Usually occurs in uncircumcised males with poor hygiene
    b. Accumulation of smegma leads to infection.
        • *Candida,* pyogenic bacteria, and anaerobes
2. Inflammatory scarring may produce an acquired phimosis.

D. Miscellaneous disorders
1. Peyronie's disease
    a. Type of fibromatosis (see Chapter 23)
    b. Painful contractures of the penis
        • Causes lateral curvature of the penis
    c. May cause infertility
2. Priapism
    a. Persistent and painful erection
    b. Causes include sickle cell disease, penile trauma

E. Carcinoma in situ (CIS)
1. Bowen's disease
    a. Leukoplakia involving the shaft of the penis and scrotum
        (1) Patients usually over 35 years old
        (2) Association with human papillomavirus (HPV) type 16
    b. Precursor for invasive squamous cell carcinoma (~10% of cases)
    c. Association with other types of visceral cancer
2. Erythroplasia of Queyrat
    a. Erythroplakia located on the mucosal surface of the glans and prepuce
    b. HPV type 16 association
    c. Precursor for invasive squamous cell carcinoma
3. Bowenoid papulosis
    a. Multiple pigmented reddish brown papules on the external genitalia
    b. Association with HPV type 16
    c. Does *not* develop into invasive squamous cell carcinoma
        • Only CIS with no predisposition for invasion

F. Squamous cell carcinoma
1. Most common cancer of the penis
    a. Usually affects men 40 to 70 years old
    b. Most common sites
        • Glans or mucosal surface of prepuce
2. HPV type 16, 18 association in two thirds of cases
    • Smoking may act as a cocarcinogen with HPV.
3. Risk factors
    a. Lack of circumcision
        • Greatest risk factor
    b. Bowen's disease, erythroplasia of Queyrat
4. Metastasizes to inguinal and iliac nodes

Margin notes:

Risk factors invasive squamous cell carcinoma: Bowen's disease, erythroplasia of Queyrat

Circumcision: protects against developing cancer of the penis

V. Testis, Scrotal Sac, Epididymis Disorders
  A. Cryptorchidism
    1. Normal descent of testes
      a. Transabdominal phase
        (1) Testes descend to lower abdomen or pelvic brim
        (2) Müllerian inhibitory factor is responsible for this phase
      b. Inguinoscrotal phase
        (1) Descent through the inguinal canal into the scrotum
        (2) Androgen-dependent
    2. Cryptorchidism
      a. Complete or incomplete descent of the testis into the scrotal sac
      b. Locations
        (1) Inguinal canal most common site
          (a) Palpable mass
          (b) Majority are unilateral
        (2) Intra-abdominal (5–10% of cases)
      c. Complications if uncorrected
        (1) Potential for infertility
          (a) Arrest in germ cell maturation
          (b) Testicular atrophy
          (c) Similar changes occur in the normally descended
              contralateral testis.
        (2) Increased risk for developing a seminoma
          (a) Five- to tenfold increased risk for cancer in cryptorchid testis
          (b) Risk also applies to the normally descended testicle

> Cryptorchid testis: risk for seminoma of cryptorchid testis and normally descended testis

  B. Orchitis
    1. Mumps
      a. Infertility is uncommon.
      b. Most cases are unilateral.
      c. Orchitis is more likely in an older child or adult.
    2. Congenital or acquired syphilis
    3. Human immunodeficiency virus
    4. Extension of acute epididymitis
  C. Epididymitis
    1. Causes
      a. Pathogens in patients youngers than 35 years old
        (1) *Neisseria gonorrhoeae*
        (2) *Chlamydia trachomatis*
      b. Pathogens in patients over 35 years of age
        (1) *E. coli*
        (2) *Pseudomonas aeruginosa*
      c. Tuberculosis
        (1) Begins in the epididymis
          • Spreads to the seminal vesicles, prostate, and testicles
        (2) Caseating granulomatous inflammation
    2. Signs and symptoms of acute epididymitis
      a. Scrotal pain with radiation into spermatic cord or flank

> Epididymitis: scrotal pain with radiation into spermatic cord

b. Scrotal swelling, epididymal tenderness
c. Urethral discharge
  • If it is sexually transmitted
d. Prehn's sign
  • Elevation of the scrotum decreases pain.

D. Varicocele

1. Most common cause of left-sided scrotal enlargement in an adult
   a. "Bag of worms" appearance
   b. Left spermatic vein drains into the left renal vein
      (1) Increased resistance to blood flow
      (2) Blockage of left renal vein can also produce a varicocele.
         • Example—renal cell carcinoma invading renal vein
   c. Right spermatic vein drains into the vena cava
      (1) Blockage of right spermatic vein produces right-sided varicocele.
      (2) Example—retroperitoneal fibrosis
2. Very common cause of infertility
   • Heat decreases spermatogenesis.

Varicocele: most often left-sided; spermatic vein empties into left renal vein

E. Torsion of the testicle

1. Predisposing factors
   a. Violent movement or physical trauma
      • Most common causes
   b. Cryptorchid testis
   c. Atrophy of testis
2. Twisting of the spermatic cord cuts off the venous/arterial blood supply
   • Danger for hemorrhagic infarction of the testicle
3. Clinical findings
   a. Sudden onset of testicular pain
   b. Absent cremasteric reflex
      • Stroking the inner thigh with a tongue blade normally causes the scrotum to retract.
   c. Testicle is drawn up into the inguinal canal.
4. Surgery is imperative.

Torsion of testicle: absent cremasteric reflex, testis high in inguinal canal

F. Hydrocele

1. Most common cause of scrotal enlargement
   • Due to a persistent tunica vaginalis
2. Diagnosis
   • Ultrasound distinguishes fluid versus a testicular mass causing scrotal enlargement.
3. Other fluid accumulations
   a. Hematocele contains blood.
   b. Spermatocele contains sperm.

Hydrocele: persistent tunica vaginalis

G. Testicular tumors

1. Epidemiology
   a. Most common malignancy between ages 15 and 35
   b. Occurs more often in whites than black Americans
2. Types of testicular tumors

Unilateral, painless testicular mass: testicular cancer

      a. Malignant testicular tumors are most often germ cell in origin (95% of cases).

      b. Benign testicular tumors are usually sex-cord stromal tumors (5% of cases).

      c. Classification of germ cell tumors

        (1) 40% are of one cell type

          • Seminoma is the most common type.

        (2) 60% are mixtures of two or more patterns

          • Most common mixture is embryonal carcinoma, teratoma, choriocarcinoma, yolk sac tumor.

        (3) Best classified as seminomas or nonseminomatous

  3. Risk factors

      a. Cryptorchid testicle

        (1) Overall most common risk factor

        (2) Greatest risk is an intra-abdominal cryptorchid testis.

      b. Testicular feminization (see Chapter 5)

      c. Klinefelter's syndrome (XXY) (see Chapter 5)

  4. Clinical finding

      • Unilateral, painless enlargement of the testis

  5. Tumor markers

      a. α-Fetoprotein (AFP)

        • Yolk sac (endodermal sinus) tumor origin

      b. Human chorionic gonadotropin (hCG)

        • Choriocarcinoma

      c. Lactate dehydrogenase

        (1) Nonspecific cancer enzyme

        (2) Degree of elevation correlates with tumor mass

  6. Summary of testicular tumors (Table 20-1)

> Testicular cancer markers: AFP, hCG

VI. Prostate Disorders

A. Clinical anatomy

  1. Dihydrotestosterone (DHT) is responsible for developing the prostate.

  2. Zones of the prostate

      a. Peripheral zone

        (1) Palpated during a digital rectal examination (DRE)

        (2) Primary site for prostate cancer

      b. Transitional zone

        • Primary site for the glandular component of BPH

      c. Periurethral zone

        • Primary site for the fibromuscular (stromal) component of BPH

B. Acute/chronic prostatitis

  1. Causes

      a. Acute prostatitis

        (1) Intraprostate reflux of urine from the posterior urethra or urinary bladder

        (2) Pathogens

          • *E. coli, P. aeruginosa, K. pneumoniae*

TABLE 20-1:
Testicular Tumors

Tumor	Age (Years)	Morphologic/ Clinical Findings	Tumor Marker(s)	Prognosis
Seminoma	30–35; >65	Most common germ cell tumor Gray tumor *without* hemorrhage or necrosis; composed of large cells with centrally located nucleus containing prominent nucleoli; lymphocytic infiltrate. Metastasis: lymphatic (para-aortic lymph nodes) *before* hematogenous (lungs) Spermatocytic variant occurs in older individuals and rarely metastasizes	hCG increased in 10% of cases	Excellent Extremely radiosensitive
Embryonal carcinoma	20–25	Bulky tumor with hemorrhage and necrosis; other tumor types often present Metastasis: hematogenous *before* lymphatic spread	AFP and hCG increased in 90% of cases	Intermediate Less radiosensitive than seminomas
Yolk sac (endodermal sinus) tumor	Most common testicular tumor in children < 4	Characteristic Schiller-Duval bodies resemble primitive glomeruli	AFP increased in all cases	Good
Choriocarcinoma	20–30	Most commonly mixed with other tumor types Contains trophoblastic tissue (syncytiotrophoblast and cytotrophoblast) May produce gynecomastia (hCG is an LH analogue)	hCG increased in all cases	Poor Most aggressive tumor; hematogenous spread to lungs
Teratoma	Affects males of all ages	Contains derivatives from ectoderm, endoderm, mesoderm Mixed with embryonal carcinoma (teratocarcinoma)	AFP and/or hCG increased in 50% of cases	Good Usually benign in children and malignant in adults (usually squamous cell carcinoma)
Malignant lymphoma	Most common testicular cancer in men > 60	Secondary involvement of both testes by diffuse large cell lymphoma	None	Poor

AFP, α-fetoprotein; hCG, human chorionic gonadotropin; LH, luteinizing hormone.

b. Chronic prostatitis
  (1) Majority are abacterial
  (2) Chronic bacterial infection
    • Due to recurrent acute prostatitis
2. Clinical findings
  a. Fever occurs in acute prostatitis.

   b. Lower back, perineal, or suprapubic pain
   c. Painful/swollen gland on rectal examination
   d. Dysuria, hematuria
3. Fractionated urine culture and examination for WBCs
   a. Specimen collections
      (1) First 10 mL is the urethral component.
      (2) Second midstream sample is the bladder component.
      (3) Third specimen at the end of micturition is the prostate component.
      (4) Fourth specimen is secretions milked out after prostate massage.
   b. Diagnosis of prostatitis
      (1) More than 20 WBCs/HPF in the third and fourth sample suggests acute prostatitis.
      (2) Increased bacterial count in third and fourth specimens is confirmatory.

C. **Benign prostatic hyperplasia (BPH)**
1. Epidemiology
   a. Age-dependent change
      • All men develop BPH as they age.
   b. More common in black Americans than whites
   c. Develops in the transitional and periurethral zones
   d. DRE has a sensitivity of 50% in detecting BPH.
2. Pathogenesis
   a. DHT is the primary mediator.
      • Causes hyperplasia of glandular and stromal cells
   b. Stromal cells are the site of DHT synthesis.
   c. Estrogen is a co-mediator.
      • Increases the synthesis of androgen receptors
3. Gross and microscopic findings
   a. Hyperplasia of glandular cells and stromal cells
      (1) Leads to nodule formation (Fig. 20-1)
      (2) Nodules are yellow-pink and are soft.
   b. Glandular hyperplasia develops nodules in the transitional zone.
   c. Stromal hyperplasia develops nodules in the periurethral zone.
      • Most responsible for obstruction of the urethra
4. Clinical and laboratory findings
   a. Signs of obstruction
      (1) Trouble initiating and stopping the urinary stream
      (2) Dribbling, incomplete emptying
      (3) Nocturia, dysuria
   b. Hematuria
   c. Prostate-specific antigen (PSA)
      (1) Proteolytic enzyme
         (a) Increases sperm motility
         (b) Maintains seminal secretions in the liquid state
      (2) PSA is neither sensitive nor specific for BPH.

BPH: most common cause of enlarged prostate in men over 50 years old

DHT: primary mediator for developing BPH

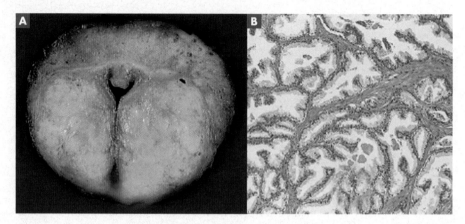

20-1: *Benign prostatic hyperplasia. The gross section of prostate* **(A)** *shows yellow periurethral nodular masses, causing narrowing of the lumen of the urethra. The microscopic section* **(B)** *shows hyperplastic glands with infolding of the epithelium into the gland lumens. (From Damjanov I, Linder J: Pathology: A Color Atlas. St. Louis, Mosby, 2000, p 249, Figs. 12-31 and 12-32.)*

(3) Usually normal (0–4 ng/mL) or between 4 and 10 ng/mL
  • Rarely over 10 ng/mL

Obstructive uropathy: most common complication of BPH

d. Complications
  (1) Obstructive uropathy
    (a) Most common complication
    (b) Postrenal azotemia
      • Potential for progressing to acute renal failure if left untreated
    (c) Bilateral hydronephrosis
    (d) Bladder diverticula from increased pressure
    (e) Bladder wall smooth muscle hypertrophy
  (2) Bladder infections due to residual urine
  (3) Prostatic infarcts
    (a) Pain on DRE
    (b) Enlarged, indurated gland

BPH is *not* a risk factor for prostate cancer.

    (c) Increased PSA values due to infarction
  (4) *No* risk for progression into carcinoma

D. Prostate cancer
  1. Epidemiology
    a. Most common cancer in adult males
      • Second most common cause of death due to cancer in adult males
    b. Universal in all men if they live long enough
    c. More common in black Americans than whites
      • Rare in Asians
    d. Usually asymptomatic until advanced
    e. Risk factors

Advancing age: greatest risk factor for prostate cancer

      (1) Advancing age
        • Most important risk factor

      (2) First-degree relatives (father and brothers)

      (3) Black Americans

      (4) Smoking cigarettes, high saturated fat diet

2. Pathogenesis
   - DHT-dependent

3. Gross and microscopic findings
   a. Develops in the peripheral zone
      (1) Palpable by DRE
      (2) Obstructive uropathy is *not* an early finding.
   b. Prostate intraepithelial neoplasia (PIN)
      (1) Foci of atypia/dysplasia
      (2) May be a precursor lesion for prostate cancer
   c. Invasive cancer has a firm, gritty yellow appearance (Fig. 20-2).
   d. Hallmarks of malignancy
      (1) Invasion of the capsule around the prostate
      (2) Blood vessel/lymphatic invasion
      (3) Perineural invasion
      (4) Extension into the seminal vesicles or base of the bladder

4. Clinical findings in symptomatic prostate cancer
   a. Obstructive uropathy implies extension into the bladder base
   b. Low back/pelvic pain
      (1) Portends bony metastases to vertebra and pelvic bones
         - Due to spread via the Batson venous plexus (see Chapter 8)
      (2) Alkaline phosphatase is increased.
         - Due to osteoblastic metastases
   c. Compression of the spinal cord

5. Diagnosis of prostate cancer
   a. Screening
      (1) DRE/PSA annually beginning at 50 years of age

PSA: more sensitive than specific in prostate cancer

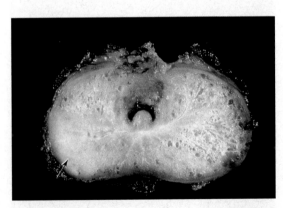

20-2: *Prostate cancer. Arrow points to a triangular area of prostate cancer located at the periphery of the gland. The remainder of the gland has a normal, spongy appearance. (From Kumar V, Fausto N, Abbas A: Robbins and Cotran's Pathologic Basis of Disease, 7th ed. Philadelphia, WB Saunders, 2004, p 1052, Fig. 21-34.)*

(2) PSA is sensitive but *not* specific for cancer.
   - BPH and prostatic infarcts can increase PSA; hence, lowering its specificity by increasing false positives.

(3) PSA over 10 ng/mL is highly predictive of cancer.
   - 70% positive predictive value

(4) PSA between 4 and 10 ng/mL is a gray zone.
   - Overlap between early cancer and BPH

(5) Other more sensitive methods of reporting PSA
   - (a) Rate of change of PSA values with time (PSA velocity)
   - (b) Ratio between serum PSA and volume of the prostate gland (prostate density)
   - (c) Measurement of free versus bound forms of circulating PSA

b. Confirmatory test
   - Needle biopsies of suspicious sites if screening tests are abnormal

6. Spread of prostate cancer
   a. Perineural invasion
   b. Lymphatic spread to regional lymph nodes
   c. Hematogenous spread
      (1) Bone is the most common extranodal site (Fig. 20-3)
         - In descending order—lumbar spine, proximal femur, and pelvis
      (2) Lungs and liver

7. Prognosis
   - With treatment, over 90% live for more than 15 years.

VII. Male Hypogonadism
   A. Normal male reproductive physiology
      1. Follicle-stimulating hormone (FSH)
         a. Stimulates spermatogenesis in the seminiferous tubules

Prostate cancer: osteoblastic metastases; lumbar spine, pelvis

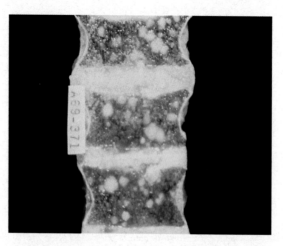

20-3: *Prostate cancer metastatic to the vertebral column. Multiple white foci of metastatic prostate cancer produce an osteoblastic response in the bone. (From Kumar V, Fausto N, Abbas A: Robbins and Cotran's Pathologic Basis of Disease, 7th ed. Philadelphia, WB Saunders, 2004, p 1052, Fig. 21-35.)*

b. Negative feedback relationship with inhibin
  (1) Inhibin is synthesized in Sertoli cells in seminiferous tubules.
  (2) Decreased inhibin causes an increase in FSH.
2. Luteinizing hormone (LH)
  a. Testosterone synthesis occurs in the Leydig cells.
  b. Testosterone has a negative feedback with LH.
    • Decreased testosterone causes an increase in LH.
3. Prolactin
  a. Prolactin enhances testosterone function and spermatogenesis.
  b. Increased prolactin inhibits gonadotropin-releasing hormone (GnRH)
    • Decreases LH and FSH
4. Testosterone
  a. Maintains male secondary sex characteristics
  b. Enhances spermatogenesis in the seminiferous tubules
  c. Increases libido (sexual desire)
  d. Decreased testosterone causes male hypogonadism and infertility.
5. Sex hormone-binding globulin (SHBG or androgen-binding globulin)
  a. Binding protein for testosterone and estrogen
    (1) In both men and women, SHBG is mainly synthesized in the liver.
    (2) In men, the Sertoli cells also synthesizes SHBG.
    (3) Estrogen increases synthesis of SHBG in the liver.
    (4) Androgens, insulin, obesity, and hypothyroidism all cause decreased synthesis of SHBG.
  b. SHBG has a higher binding affinity for testosterone than estrogen.
    • "Estrogen amplifier"
    (1) Increased SHBG decreases free testosterone levels.
    (2) Decreased SHBG increases free testosterone levels.

↑SHBG causes ↓ free testosterone
↓SHBG causes ↑ free testosterone

B. **Pathogenesis of male hypogonadism**
1. Decreased production of testosterone
  • Examples—hypopituitarism, Leydig cell dysfunction
2. Resistance to testosterone
  • Example—androgen receptor deficiency in testicular feminization

C. **Clinical presentations**
1. Impotence
  a. Most common manifestation
  b. Failure to sustain an erection during attempted intercourse or during intercourse

Impotence: most common manifestation of male hypogonadism

Testosterone, per se, does *not* have any role in producing an erection (parasympathetic response) or ejaculation (sympathetic response). However, decreased testosterone decreases libido, which decreases psychic desire.

2. Loss of male secondary sex characteristics
  a. Estrogen activity is unopposed.
  b. Findings include female hair distribution, gynecomastia

3. Osteoporosis
- Testosterone normally inhibits osteoclastic activity and increases osteoblastic activity.
4. Infertility
- Decreased spermatogenesis

D. **Classification of male hypogonadism**
1. Primary hypogonadism
- Due to Leydig cell dysfunction
a. Luteinizing hormone (LH) is increased.
- Loss of negative feedback imposed by testosterone
b. Hypergonadotropic (increased LH) hypogonadism
2. Secondary hypogonadism
- Due to hypothalamic/pituitary dysfunction
a. Decreased LH
b. Hypogonadotropic (decreased LH) hypogonadism

E. **Primary hypogonadism: Leydig cell dysfunction**
1. Causes
a. Chronic alcoholic liver disease
- Inhibits binding of LH to Leydig cells (? mechanism)
b. Chronic renal failure
- Toxins have a direct toxic effect on Leydig cell
c. Irradiation, orchitis, trauma
2. Laboratory findings in Leydig cell dysfunction
a. Decreased testosterone
- Due to destruction of Leydig cells
b. Increased LH
- Due to decreased testosterone
c. Decreased sperm count
- Due to testosterone deficiency
d. Normal FSH
- Inhibin is present in Sertoli cells.

F. **Primary hypogonadism: Leydig cell and seminiferous tubule dysfunction**
1. Causes
- Same causes as Leydig cell dysfunction
2. Laboratory findings
a. Decreased testosterone
- Due to destruction of Leydig cells
b. Increased LH
- Due to decreased testosterone
c. Decreased sperm count
- Due to testosterone deficiency and seminiferous tubule dysfunction
d. Increased FSH
- Due to decrease in inhibin

G. **Causes of secondary hypogonadism**
1. Constitutional delay in puberty
- A testicular volume greater than 4 mL indicates puberty has begun.

Dysfunction	Testosterone	Sperm Count	LH	FSH
Primary				
Leydig dysfunction	↓	↓	↑	N
Leydig cell and seminiferous tubule dysfunction	↓	↓	↑	↑
Secondary				
Hypopituitarism	↓	↓	↓	↓

TABLE 20-2: Summary of Causes of Male Hypogonadism

FSH, follicle-stimulating hormone; LH, luteinizing hormone; N, normal.

2. Kallmann's syndrome
   a. Autosomal dominant disorder
   b. Maldevelopment of the olfactory bulbs and GnRH-producing cells
   c. Clinical findings
      (1) Delayed puberty
      (2) Anosmia, color blindness
   d. Laboratory findings
      • Decreased FSH, LH, testosterone, and sperm count
3. Hypopituitarism (see Chapter 22)
   a. Causes
      (1) Craniopharyngioma in children
      (2) Nonfunctioning pituitary adenoma in adults
   b. Laboratory findings
      • Decreased FSH, LH, testosterone, and sperm count
H. **Summary of causes of male hypogonadism (Table 20-2)**

VIII. **Male Infertility**
   A. **Epidemiology and pathogenesis**
      1. Decreased sperm count
         a. Primary testicular dysfunction
            (1) Leydig cell dysfunction (see Male Hypogonadism, section VII)
            (2) Seminiferous tubule dysfunction
               (a) Causes
                  • Varicocele (see section V), Klinefelter's syndrome (see Chapter 5), orchitis
               (b) Normal testosterone and LH
                  • Leydig cells are intact
               (c) Decreased sperm count
                  • Loss of seminiferous tubules and decreased testosterone
               (d) Increased FSH
                  • Inhibin is decreased
         b. Secondary hypogonadism
            • Pituitary and hypothalamic dysfunction (see Male Hypogonadism, section VII)

Seminiferous tubule dysfunction: accounts for 90% of cases of male infertility

2. End-organ dysfunction
   a. Causes
      (1) Obstruction of vas deferens
      (2) Disorders involving accessory sex organs or ejaculation
   b. Normal testosterone, FSH, LH, prolactin
   c. Sperm count variable

B. Laboratory tests for male infertility
1. Semen analysis
   a. Gold standard test for infertility
   b. Components of semen
      (1) Spermatozoa derive from the seminiferous tubules.
      (2) Coagulant derives from the seminal vesicles
      (3) Enzymes to liquefy semen derive from the prostate gland.
   c. Components evaluated in a standard semen analysis
      (1) Volume
         • Volume does *not* correlate with the number of sperm.
      (2) Sperm count
         • Normal is 20 to 150 million sperm/mL.
      (3) Sperm morphology
         • Morphology is very abnormal in reconnections of a vasectomy.
      (4) Sperm motility
2. Serum gonadotropins, testosterone, prolactin

IX. Erectile Dysfunction
   A. Causes of impotence
   1. Psychogenic
      a. Most common cause of impotence in young men
      b. Stress at work, marital conflicts, performance anxiety
      c. Nocturnal penile tumescence (NPT)
         (1) Average male has ~5 erections while sleeping at night.
         (2) NPT is preserved in impotence that is due to psychogenic causes.
         (3) All other causes of impotence have a loss of NPT.
   2. Decreased testosterone
      • Decreased libido (see Male Hypogonadism, section VII)
   3. Vascular insufficiency
      a. Most common cause of impotence in men over 50 years old
      b. Example—Leriche syndrome
         (1) Impotence due to vascular insufficiency
         (2) Aortoiliac atherosclerosis involving hypogastric arteries
         (3) Calf claudication with atrophy
         (4) Diminished femoral pulse
   4. Neurologic disease
      a. Parasympathetic system (S2–S4) is necessary for erection.
      b. Sympathetic system (T12–L1) is necessary for ejaculation.
      c. Neurogenic causes of impotence

Impotence + preserved NPT: psychogenic cause of impotence

Vascular insufficiency: most common cause impotence men over 50 years old

(1) Multiple sclerosis

(2) Autonomic neuropathy due to diabetes mellitus

(3) Radical prostatectomy

5. Drug effects; examples:

a. Leuprolide (GnRH agonist)

b. Methyldopa, psychotropics

6. Endocrine disease

a. Diabetes mellitus

• Autonomic neuropathy + vascular insufficiency

b. Primary hypothyroidism

• Increased prolactin inhibits GnRH release

c. Prolactinoma

7. Penis disorders

a. Peyronie's disease (fibromatosis)

b. Priapism

B. **Drugs used in erectile dysfunction**

1. Sildenafil (Viagra)

a. Most common drug used for the treatment of erectile dysfunction

b. Mechanism

(1) Inhibits the breakdown of cyclic guanosine monophosphate (cGMP) by type 5 phosphodiesterase

(2) Increases levels of cGMP causes vasodilation in the corpus cavernosum and the penis.

2. Yohimbe

• Herb that produces vasodilatation of vessels

Sildenafil: increases cGMP, which causes vasodilation in corpus cavernosum

Female Reproductive Disorders and Breast Disorders

Chlamydia trachomatis: most common STD in adult men and women

I. **Sexually Transmitted Diseases (STDs) and Other Genital Infections**
   - Summary of infections (Table 21-1 and Fig. 21-1)

II. **Vulva Disorders**
   A. **Bartholin gland abscess**
      - Most often caused by *Neisseria gonorrhoeae*
   B. **Non-neoplastic dermatoses**
      1. Lichen sclerosis
         a. Usually occurs in postmenopausal women
         b. Thinning of the epidermis
            - Parchment-like appearance of skin
         c. Small risk for developing squamous cell carcinoma
      2. Lichen simplex chronicus
         a. White plaque-like lesion (leukoplakia)
            - Due to squamous cell hyperplasia
         b. Small risk for developing squamous cell carcinoma
   C. **Benign and malignant tumors**
      1. Papillary hidradenoma
         a. Benign tumor of the apocrine sweat gland
         b. Painful nodule on the labia majora
      2. Vulvar intraepithelial neoplasia (VIN)
         a. Dysplasia ranges from mild to carcinoma in situ
         b. Strong human papillomavirus (HPV) type 16 association
         c. Precursor for developing squamous cell carcinoma
      3. Squamous cell carcinoma
         a. Most common cancer
         b. Risk factors
            (1) HPV type 16
            (2) Smoking cigarettes
            (3) Immunodeficiency (e.g., AIDS)
         c. Metastasize first to the inguinal nodes
      4. Extramammary Paget's disease
         a. Red, crusted vulvar lesion

VIN: HPV association

Extramammary Paget's disease: intraepithelial adenocarcinoma

Pathogen	Description and Treatment
Calymmatobacterium granulomatis	STD; gram-negative coccobacillus that causes granuloma inguinale Organism phagocytized by macrophages (Donovan bodies) Creeping, raised, sore that heals by scarring; *no* lymphadenopathy Rx: doxycycline or trimethoprim-sulfamethoxazole
Candida albicans (Fig. 21-1A)	Yeasts and pseudohyphae (elongated yeasts) Risk factors: diabetes, antibiotics, pregnancy, OCP Pruritic vaginitis with a white discharge and fiery red mucosa Rx: fluconazole (single dose)
Chlamydia trachomatis (Fig. 21-1B)	Most common STD; often coexists with *Neisseria gonorrhoeae* Incubation period 2–3 weeks after exposure; red inclusions (reticulate bodies) in infected metaplastic squamous cells Infections in males: NSU, epididymitis, proctitis Infections in females: urethritis, cervicitis, PID, perihepatitis (FHC syndrome—scar tissue between peritoneum and surface of liver from pus from PID), proctitis Infections in newborns: conjunctivitis (ophthalmia neonatorum), pneumonia PCR test for quick diagnosis Rx: azithromycin 1 g (single dose), doxycycline
C. trachomatis subspecies	Lymphogranuloma venereum Papules with *no* ulceration; inguinal lymphadenitis with granulomatous microabscesses and draining sinuses Lymphedema of scrotum or vulva; women may also develop rectal strictures Rx: doxycycline
Gardnerella vaginalis (Fig. 21-1C)	Gram-negative rod that causes bacterial vaginosis Malodorous vaginal discharge; vaginal pH > 5.5 Organisms adhere to squamous cells producing "clue cells" Rx: metronidazole
Hemophilus ducreyi	STD; gram-negative rod that causes chancroid Painful genital and perianal ulcers with suppurative inguinal nodes Rx: ceftriaxone or azithromycin 1 g (single dose)
HSV-2 (Fig. 21-1D, E)	STD; virus remains latent in sensory ganglia Recurrent vesicles that ulcerate; locations—penis, vulva, cervix, perianal area Tzanck preparation: scrapings removed from the base of an ulcer; see multinucleated cells with eosinophilic intranuclear inclusions Pregnancy: if virus is shedding, baby is delivered by cesarean section Rx: acyclovir (decreases recurrences)
HPV (Fig. 21-1F)	STD; types 6 and 11 associated with condylomata acuminata (venereal warts); fernlike or flat lesions in genital area (e.g., penis, vulva, cervix, perianal) Types 16 and 18 associated with dysplasia and squamous cancer

continued

TABLE 21-1:
Sexually Transmitted Diseases and Other Genital Infections—cont'd

Pathogen	Description and Treatment
	Virus produces koilocytic change in squamous epithelium; cells have wrinkled pyknotic nuclei surrounded by a clear halo Rx: topical podophyllin
Neisseria gonorrhoeae (Fig. 21-1G)	STD; gram-negative diplococcus that infects glandular or transitional epithelium; symptoms appear 2–5 days after sexual exposure Infection sites similar to *C. trachomatis* Complications: ectopic pregnancy, male sterility, disseminated gonococcemia (C6–C9 deficiency), septic arthritis, FHC syndrome PCR test for quick diagnosis Rx: ceftriaxone
Treponema pallidum (Fig. 21-H, I)	STD; spirochete that causes syphilis Primary syphilis: solitary painless, indurated chancre; locations—penis, labia, mouth Secondary syphilis: maculopapular rash on trunk, palms, soles; generalized lymphadenopathy; condylomata lata, which are flat lesions in same area as condylomata acuminata Tertiary syphilis: neurosyphilis, aortitis, gummas Congenital syphilis (see Chapter 5) Nonspecific screening tests: RPR or VDRL; titers decrease after Rx Confirmatory treponemal test: FTA-ABS; positive with or without Rx Jarisch-Herxheimer reaction: intensification of rash in primary or secondary syphilis may occur due to proteins released from dead organisms after Rx with penicillin Rx: penicillin
Trichomonas vaginalis (Fig. 21-1J)	STD; flagellated protozoan with jerky motility Produces vaginitis, cervicitis, and urethritis; strawberry-colored cervix and fiery red vaginal mucosa; greenish, frothy discharge Rx: metronidazole (both partners)

FHC, Fitz-Hughes-Curtis; FTA-ABS, fluorescent treponeme antibody-absorption test; HPV, human papillomavirus; HSV, herpes simplex virus; NSU, nonspecific urethritis; OCP, oral contraceptive pill; PCR, polymerase chain reaction; PID, pelvic inflammatory disease; RPR, rapid plasma reagin; Rx, treatment; STD, sexually transmitted disease; VDRL, Venereal Disease Research Laboratory.

    b. Intraepithelial adenocarcinoma
      (1) Tumor derives from primitive epithelial progenitor cells
      (2) Malignant Paget's cells contain mucin (Fig. 21-2)
        • Mucin is PAS (periodic acid–Schiff) positive.
      (3) Spreads along the epithelium
        • Rarely invades the dermis
  5. Malignant melanoma
    a. Melanoma cells are histologically similar to Paget's cells
    b. Unlike Paget's cells, melanoma cells are PAS negative.

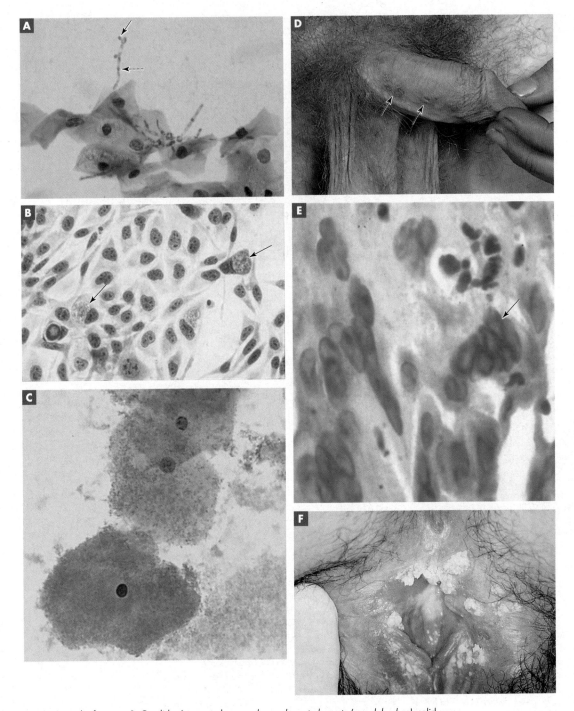

21-1: *Genital infections.* ***A,*** *Candida. Interrupted arrow shows elongated yeasts (pseudohyphae), solid arrow shows yeasts.* ***B,*** *Chlamydia trachomatis. Arrows show metaplastic squamous cells containing vacuoles with an reticulate bodies.* ***C,*** *Gardnerella vaginalis. Superficial squamous cells are covered by granular material representing bacterial organisms attached to the surface.* ***D,*** *Herpes type 2. Arrows show ulcerated, red lesions on the shaft of the penis.* ***E,*** *Herpes type 2. Tzanck preparation showing a multinucleated squamous cell with smudged, "ground glass" nuclei with intranuclear inclusions (arrow).* ***F,*** *Human papillomavirus. Numerous keratotic papillary processes are present on the surface of the labia. These are called venereal warts or condylomata acuminata.*

continued

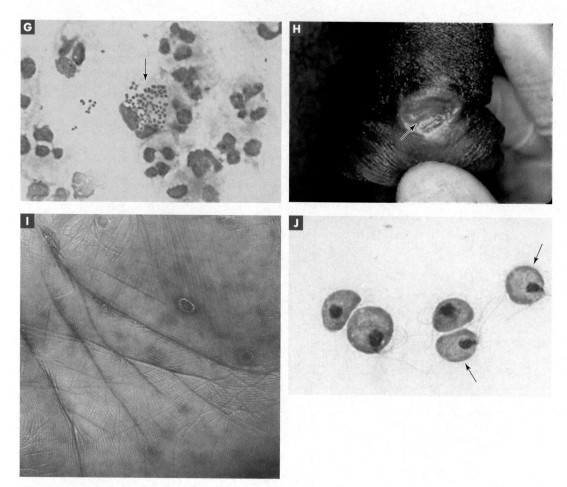

21-1, cont'd: G, Neisseria gonorrhoeae. *Neutrophils (arrow) show numerous, phagocytosed gram-negative diplococci.* ***H,*** Treponema pallidum. *Note the well-demarcated primary chancre with a clean base just distal to the glans penis.* ***I,*** Treponema pallidum. *Note the characteristic palmar papules and plaques of secondary syphilis.* ***J,*** Trichomonas vaginalis. *Note the numerous pear-shaped, flagellated organisms (arrows). (Parts A, B, and E from Atkinson BF: Atlas of Diagnostic Cytopathology. Philadelphia, WB Saunders, 1992, pp 76, 78 and 80, Figs. 2-49B, 2-55, and 2-63, respectively; parts C and F from Damjanov I, Linder J: Pathology: A Color Atlas. St. Louis, Mosby, 2000, pp 261 and 260, Figs. 13-10B and 13-8, respectively; part D from Bouloux P-M: Self-Assessment Picture Tests: Medicine, vol 1. St. Louis, Mosby, 1996, p 17, Fig. 33; part G from Greer I, Cameron IT, Kitchener HC, Prentice A: Mosby's Color Atlas and Text of Obstetrics and Gynecology. St. Louis, Mosby, 2000, p 274, Fig. 10-50; part H from Goldstein BG: Practical Dermatology, 2nd ed. St. Louis, Mosby, 1997, p 197, Fig. 15-5; part I from Lookingbill D, Marks J: Principles of Dermatology, 3rd ed. Philadelphia, WB Saunders, 2000, p 124, Fig. 10-17; part J from Kumar V, Fausto N, Abbas A: Robbins and Cotran's Pathologic Basis of Disease, 7th ed. Philadelphia, WB Saunders, 2004, p 1064, Fig. 22-4.)*

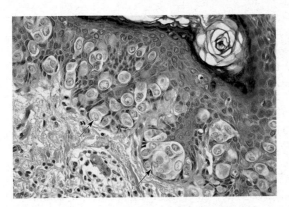

21-2: *Extramammary Paget's disease. Large, pink-staining, malignant Paget's cells (arrows) are disposed singly and in clusters within the epidermis. (From Rosai J, Ackerman LV: Surgical Pathology, 9th ed. St. Louis, Mosby, 2004, p 1492, Fig. 19-17B.)*

III. Vagina Disorders
A. Rokitansky-Kuster-Hauser syndrome
1. Absence of the upper vagina and uterus
2. Anatomic cause of primary amenorrhea

B. Gartner's duct cyst
1. Remnant of the wolffian (mesonephric) duct
2. Presents as a cyst on the lateral wall of the vagina

C. Benign and malignant tumors
1. Rhabdomyoma
   a. Benign tumor of skeletal muscle
   b. Other locations are the tongue and heart.
2. Embryonal rhabdomyosarcoma
   a. Occurs in girls younger than 5 years old
   b. Necrotic, grape-like mass protrudes from the vagina
3. Clear cell adenocarcinoma of the vagina
   a. Epidemiology
      (1) Occurs in women with intrauterine exposure to diethylstilbestrol (DES)
         • DES was used to prevent a threatened abortion.
      (2) DES inhibits müllerian differentiation.
         • Mullerian structures: tubes, uterus, cervix, upper one third of vagina
      (3) Vaginal adenosis
         (a) Remnants of müllerian glands
            • Produces a ridge in the upper portion of the vagina
         (b) Precursor lesion for clear cell adenocarcinoma
      (4) Small risk for developing the cancer (1:1000)
      (5) Cancer may involve upper vagina or cervix.
   b. Other DES abnormalities
      (1) Abnormally shaped uterus that thwarts implantation

DES: inhibits müllerian differentiation

Clear cell adenocarcinoma of vagina: associated with DES exposure

(2) Cervical incompetence
- Common cause of recurrent abortions

4. Vaginal squamous cell carcinoma
   a. Primary squamous cell carcinoma has an HPV type 16 association.
   b. Most cancers are an extension of a cervical squamous cancer into the vagina.

IV. **Cervix Disorders**
   A. **Clinical anatomy and histology**
      1. Cervix includes the endocervix + exocervix
         - The exocervix begins at the cervical os.
      2. Exocervix is normally lined by squamous epithelium.
      3. Endocervical glands are normally lined by mucus-secreting columnar cells.
      4. Endocervical epithelium normally migrates down to the exocervix.
         a. Exposure to the acid pH of the vagina produces squamous metaplasia.
         b. The area undergoing metaplasia is called the transformation zone.
            (1) This zone is where squamous dysplasia and cancer develop.
            (2) It must be sampled when performing a cervical Papanicolaou (Pap) smear.
         c. Metaplastic squamous cells block endocervical gland orifices.
            (1) Obstruction of outflow of mucus produces nabothian cysts.
            (2) Nabothian cysts are a normal finding in adult women.

   B. **Acute and chronic cervicitis**
      1. Acute cervicitis
         a. Acute inflammation is normally present in the transformation zone.
         b. Pathologic acute cervicitis
            - Causative agents: *Chlamydia trachomatis, N. gonorrhoeae, Trichomonas vaginalis, Candida,* and herpes simplex virus (HSV-2)
         c. Follicular cervicitis
            (1) Caused by *C. trachomatis*
            (2) Pronounced lymphoid infiltrate with germinal centers
            (3) *Chlamydia* infects metaplastic squamous cells.
               (a) Cells contain vacuoles with red inclusions (reticulate bodies).
               (b) Elementary bodies are infective particles.
            (4) Cervicitis is the primary source for conjunctivitis and pneumonia in newborns.
      2. Chronic cervicitis occurs when acute cervicitis persists.

   C. **Cervical Pap smear**
      1. Purpose
         a. Screening test to rule out squamous dysplasia and cancer
         b. To evaluate the hormone status of the patient
      2. Sample sites
         - Vagina, exocervix, transformation zone

Transformation zone: site where squamous dysplasia and cancer develop

Reticulate bodies: produce elementary bodies, the infective particle of *Chlamydia*

Because the transformation zone is the site for squamous dysplasia and squamous cancer, it must be adequately sampled. The presence of metaplastic squamous cells or mucus-secreting columnar cells indicates proper sampling. Absence of these cells means that the Pap smear must be repeated.

Cervical Pap smear: screen for dysplasia/cancer, evaluates hormonal status

3. Interpretation of the Pap smear
   a. Superficial squamous cells indicate adequate estrogen.
   b. Intermediate squamous cells indicate adequate progesterone.
   c. Parabasal cells indicate a lack of estrogen and progesterone.
   d. Normal nonpregnant adult woman
      • 70% superficial squamous cells, 30% intermediate squamous cells
   e. Pregnant woman
      • 100% intermediate squamous cells from progesterone effect
   f. Elderly woman with lack of estrogen and progesterone
      • Atrophic smear with parabasal cells and inflammation
   g. Woman with continuous exposure to estrogen without progesterone
      • 100% superficial squamous cells

D. Cervical polyp
1. Non-neoplastic polyp
2. Protrudes from the cervical os
   • Produces postcoital bleeding
3. *Not* precancerous

E. Cervical intraepithelial neoplasia (CIN)
1. Epidemiology
   a. Majority of cases are associated with HPV.
      (1) Low risk—types 6, 11
      (2) High risk—types 16, 18
      (3) HPV produces koilocytosis in squamous cells (Fig. 21-3).
         • Clear halo containing a wrinkled, pyknotic nucleus

CIN: most cases associated with HPV

Koilocytosis: HPV effect in squamous cells

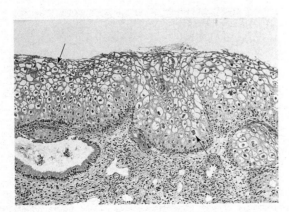

21-3: Koilocytosis caused by human papillomavirus. The squamous cells have wrinkled pyknotic nuclei surrounded by a clear halo (arrows). (From Damjanov I, Linder J: Pathology: A Color Atlas. St. Louis, Mosby, 2000, p 267, Fig. 13-32.)

     b. Risk factors
       (1) Early age of onset of sexual intercourse
       (2) Multiple, high-risk partners
       (3) High-risk types of HPV in the biopsy
       (4) Smoking, oral contraceptive pills (OCPs), immunodeficiency

  2. Classification of CIN
     a. CIN I
       • Mild dysplasia involving the lower third of the epithelium
     b. CIN II
       • Moderate dysplasia involving the lower two thirds of the epithelium
     c. CIN III (see Fig. 1-7)
       • Severe dysplasia to CIS involving the full thickness of the epithelium

  3. Progression from CIN I to CIN III is *not* inevitable.
     a. Reversal to normal is more likely in CIN I.
     b. Requires ~10 years to progress from CIN I to CIN III
     c. Requires ~10 years to progress from CIN III to invasive cancer
       • Average age for cervical cancer is ~45 years old.

F. Cervical cancer
  1. Epidemiology
     a. Least common gynecologic cancer
       • Due to early detection of CIN with Pap smears
     b. Majority are squamous cell carcinoma (75–80% of cases)
       • Small cell cancer and adenocarcinoma are less common types.
     c. Cause and risk factors
       • Same as those listed for CIN

  2. Clinical findings (Fig. 21-4)
     a. Malodorous discharge
     b. Postcoital bleeding

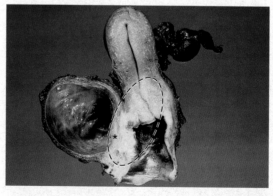

21-4: *Squamous cell carcinoma of cervix with extension down into the vagina and into the wall of the urinary bladder. The white area encompassed within interrupted lines represents the extent of tumor invasion. Asterisk marks a tumor invading the wall of the urinary bladder. (From Rosai J, Ackerman LV: Surgical Pathology, 9th ed. St. Louis, Mosby, 2004, p 1538, Fig. 19-85C.)*

3. Cancer characteristics
   a. Extends down into the vagina
   b. Extends out into the lateral wall of the cervix and vagina
   c. Infiltrates the bladder wall and obstructs the ureters
     • Postrenal azotemia leading to renal failure is the most common cause of death.
   d. Distant metastases (e.g., lungs)

> Cervical cancer: renal failure is the most common cause of death.

V. Reproductive Physiology and Selected Hormone Disorders
A. Sequence to menarche
1. Breast budding (thelarche)
2. Growth spurt
3. Pubic hair
4. Axillary hair
5. Menarche
   a. Mean age of 12.8 years
   b. Anovulatory cycles for 1 to 1.5 years
B. Summary of the normal menstrual cycle
• Synthesis of sex hormones in the ovary (Fig. 21-5)

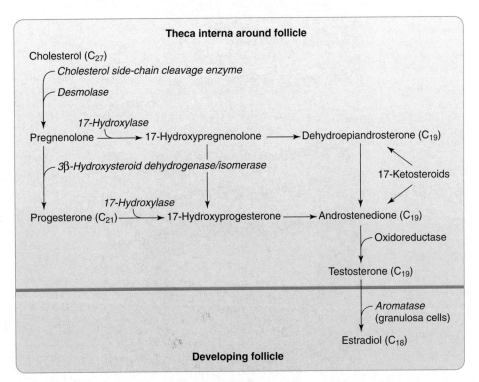

21-5: *Synthesis of sex hormones in the ovaries. Luteinizing hormone is responsible for stimulation of hormone synthesis in the theca interna surrounding the developing follicle. Follicle-stimulating hormone increases the synthesis of aromatase in granulosa cells. Aromatase converts testosterone to estradiol. (From Goljan EF: Star Series: Pathology. Philadelphia, WB Saunders, 1998, Fig. 18-1.)*

Proliferative phase:
estrogen-mediated

1. Proliferative phase
   a. Estrogen-mediated proliferation of glands
      • *Most* variable phase of the cycle
   b. Estrogen surge occurs 24 to 36 hours prior to ovulation.
      (1) Stimulates luteinizing hormone (LH)
         • Positive feedback
      (2) Inhibits follicle-stimulating hormone (FSH)
         (a) Negative feedback
         (b) Serum LH greater than FSH
      (3) LH surge initiates ovulation.
2. Ovulation
   a. Occurs between days 14 and 16
   b. Ovulation indicators
      (1) Increase in body temperature
         • Effect of progesterone
      (2) Subnuclear vacuoles in endometrial cells (Fig. 21-6)

Subnuclear vacuoles:
sign of ovulation

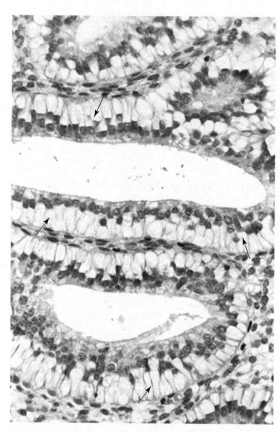

21-6: *Subnuclear vacuoles* (arrows) *containing mucin push the nuclei of the endometrial cells toward the apex of the cell. Eventually the mucin passes the nucleus and enters the lumen marking the beginning of the secretory phase. (From Kumar V, Fausto N, Abbas A: Robbins and Cotran's Pathologic Basis of Disease, 7th ed. Philadelphia, WB Saunders, 2004, p 1081, Fig. 21-5B.)*

      (3) Mittelschmerz
          • Peritoneal irritation from blood from the ruptured follicle
  3. Secretory phase
    a. Progesterone-mediated
      • *Least* variable phase of the cycle
    b. Increased gland tortuosity and secretion
    c. Edema of stromal cells

> Secretory phase: progesterone-mediated

> In fertility workups, endometrial biopsies are commonly performed on day 21 to see if ovulation has occurred. Presence of secretory endometrium on day 21 confirms that ovulation has occurred.

    d. Changes occurring after fertilization
      (1) Fertilization usually occurs in the ampullary portion of the fallopian tube.
      (2) Fertilized egg spends 3 days in the fallopian tube.
      (3) Fertilized egg spends 2 days in the uterine cavity.
          • Implants in the endometrial mucosa on day 21
      (4) An exaggerated secretory phase occurs in pregnancy.
          • Called the Arias-Stella phenomenon
  4. Menses
    a. Initiated by dropoff in serum levels of estrogen and progesterone
      • Cells undergo apoptosis.
    b. Plasmin prevents menstrual blood from clotting.
      • Excess clotting is a sign of menorrhagia.
  5. Functions of FSH
    a. Prepares the follicle of the month
    b. Increases aromatase synthesis in the granulosa cells
    c. Increases the synthesis of LH receptors
  6. Functions of LH
    a. LH in the proliferative phase
      (1) Increases the synthesis of 17-ketosteroids (KS) in the theca interna (see Fig. 21-5)
          • 17-KS are dehydroepiandrosterone (DHEA) and androstenedione.
      (2) DHEA is converted to androstenedione.
      (3) An oxidoreductase converts androstenedione to testosterone.
      (4) Testosterone enters granulosa cells and is aromatized to estradiol.
    b. LH surge is induced by a sudden increase in estrogen.
      • Ovulation occurs when LH is higher than FSH.
    c. LH in the secretory phase (see Fig. 21-5)
      • Theca interna primarily synthesizes 17-hydroxyprogesterone.
  7. Hormone changes in pregnancy
    a. Human chorionic gonadotropin (hCG)
      (1) Synthesized in the syncytiotrophoblast lining the chorionic villus
      (2) Acts as an LH analogue by maintaining the corpus luteum of pregnancy.
      (3) Corpus luteum synthesizes progesterone for ~8 to 10 weeks.

> hCG: maintains corpus luteum of pregnancy

b. Corpus luteum involutes after ~8 to 10 weeks.
   (1) Placenta synthesizes progesterone for the remainder of the pregnancy.
   (2) Spontaneous abortion may occur if placental production of progesterone is inadequate.

C. **Oral contraceptive pills (OCPs)**
   1. Mixture of estrogen + progestins (progesterone)
      a. Baseline levels of estrogen prevent the midcycle estrogen surge.
         • Prevents the LH surge and ovulation
      b. Progestins arrest the proliferative phase and cause gland atrophy.
      c. Progestins inhibit LH, which also prevents the LH surge.
   2. OCPs render the cervical mucus hostile to sperm.
   3. OCPs alter fallopian tube motility.

D. **Sources and types of estrogen**
   1. Estradiol
      a. Primary estrogen in nonpregnant women
      b. Derived from aromatization of testosterone in granulosa cells
   2. Estrone
      a. Weak estrogen produced during menopause
      b. Derived from adipose cell aromatization of androstenedione
         • Androstenedione is synthesized in the adrenal cortex.
   3. Estriol
      a. End product of estradiol metabolism
      b. Primary estrogen of pregnancy
         • Derives from fetal adrenal, placenta, and maternal liver (see section IX)

E. **Sources and types of androgens**
   1. Androstenedione
      • Equal derivation from ovaries and adrenal cortex
   2. DHEA
      a. Mainly synthesized in the adrenal cortex (80%)
      b. Remainder is synthesized in the ovaries.
   3. DHEA-sulfate
      • Almost exclusively synthesized in the adrenal cortex
   4. Testosterone
      a. Derived from conversion of androstenedione to testosterone
      b. Majority of testosterone is synthesized in the ovaries.
         • Smaller amount is synthesized in the adrenal cortex

F. **Sex hormone-binding globulin (SHBG)**
   1. Binding protein for testosterone and estrogen (see Chapter 20)
      a. In both men and women, SHBG is primarily synthesized in the liver.
      b. Estrogen increases synthesis of SHBG in the liver.
      c. Androgens, obesity, hypothyroidism all decrease the synthesis of SHBG.
   2. SHBG has a greater binding affinity for testosterone than estrogen.
      a. Increased SHBG decreases free testosterone levels.
      b. Decreased SHBG increases free testosterone levels.
         • Common cause of hirsutism in women (see below)

OCP: prevents LH surge and ovulation

Estrogens: estradiol (reproductive life), estriol (pregnancy), estrone (menopause)

DHEA-sulfate: almost exclusively synthesized in the adrenal cortex

G. Normal changes in pregnancy
1. Plasma volume and red blood cell (RBC) mass
   a. Both are increased
      - Increase in plasma volume is greater than the increase in RBC mass.
   b. Causes a 1 g/dL drop in hemoglobin (Hb) (dilutional effect)
   c. Increases glomerular filtration rate
      (1) Creatinine clearance is increased.
      (2) Increased clearance of urea and creatinine.
         - Serum levels are at the lower limit of normal.
2. Respiratory alkalosis
   a. Effect of estrogen and progesterone stimulating respiratory center
   b. Decrease in $Paco_2$ causes a corresponding increase in Pao_2.
3. Increased serum thyroxine and cortisol
   a. Estrogen stimulates synthesis of thyroid-binding globulin and transcortin.
   b. Increased binding proteins increases total thyroxine and cortisol.
   c. Metabolically active free hormone levels are normal (see Chapter 22).
      - *No* clinical signs of overactivity

Pregnancy: ↑ serum T_4/cortisol; due to increase in binding proteins

H. Menopause
1. Mean age 52 years old
2. Increase in FSH and LH
   a. Due to drop in estrogen and progesterone, respectively
   b. Serum FSH is the best screen.
3. Clinical findings
   a. Secondary amenorrhea
   b. Hot flushes, night sweats

Menopause: ↑ FSH best marker; absence of menses for 12 months

I. Hirsutism and virilization
1. Epidemiology and pathogenesis
   a. Hirsutism is excess hair in normal hair-bearing areas.
      - Virilization is hirsutism + male secondary sex characteristics.
   b. Male secondary sex characteristics
      (1) Increased muscle mass
      (2) Acne
      (3) Enlarged clitoris (clitoromegaly)
         - Most important finding
   c. Both conditions are due to increased androgens of ovarian or adrenal origin
      (1) Ovarian origin—testosterone is primarily increased
      (2) Adrenal origin—DHEA-sulfate is primarily increased

Hirsutism and virilization: hyperandrogenicity of ovarian or adrenal origin

2. Selected ovarian disorders
   a. Polycystic ovarian syndrome (POS)
      (1) Increased pituitary synthesis of LH and decreased synthesis of FSH
      (2) Increased LH increases androgen synthesis.
         - Hirsutism occurs more often than virilization.
      (3) Androgens are aromatized to estrogen in the adipose cells.

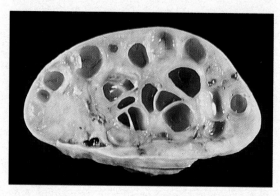

21-7: *Polycystic ovarian syndrome showing an enlarged ovary with multiple subcortical cysts. (From Damjanov I, Linder J: Pathology: A Color Atlas. St. Louis, Mosby, 2000, p 262, Fig. 13-17A.)*

          (a) Causes an increase in estrogen
          (b) Increases the risk for developing endometrial hyperplasia and cancer
      (4) Increased estrogen has a positive feedback on LH and negative feedback on FSH.

POS: ↑ LH, ↓ FSH;
LH:FSH ratio > 2

          (a) Suppression of FSH causes follicle degeneration.
          (b) Fluid accumulation produces subcortical cysts that enlarge the ovaries (Fig. 21-7).
      (5) Clinical findings
          (a) Menstrual irregularities
             • Oligomenorrhea is the most common complaint.
          (b) Hirsutism, infertility, obesity (50% of cases)
      (6) Laboratory findings
          (a) LH:FSH ratio above 2
          (b) Increased testosterone and androstenedione
          (c) Increased estrogen
    b. Obesity, hypothyroidism
      • Decreased SHBG causes an increase in free testosterone.
    c. Ovarian tumors with increased androgen production
  3. Adrenal disorders
    • Adrenogenital syndrome and Cushing syndrome (see Chapter 22)

J. Menstrual dysfunction
  1. Menorrhagia
    • Loss of blood greater than 80 mL per period
  2. Dysmenorrhea
    a. Painful menses
    b. Primary type
      (1) Due to increased prostaglandin $F_{2\alpha}$ ($PGF_{2\alpha}$)
      (2) Increases uterine contractions
    c. Secondary type
      • Most often due to endometriosis

3. Dysfunctional uterine bleeding (DUB)
   a. Definition
      (1) Bleeding *unrelated* to an anatomic cause
      (2) Caused by a hormonal imbalance
   b. Anovulatory DUB
      (1) Occurs at the extremes of reproductive life
         (a) Menarche to age 20 years
         (b) Perimenopausal period
      (2) Excessive estrogen stimulation relative to progesterone
         (a) Absent secretory phase of the cycle
         (b) Produces endometrial hyperplasia and bleeding
   c. Inadequate luteal phase
      (1) Ovulatory type of DUB
      (2) Inadequate maturation of the corpus luteum
         (a) Inadequate synthesis of progesterone
            • Delay in development of the secretory phase
         (b) Decreased serum 17-hydroxyprogesterone on day 21
   d. Irregular shedding of the endometrium
      (1) Ovulatory type of DUB
      (2) Persistent luteal phase with continued secretion of progesterone
      (3) Mixture of proliferative and secretory glands in the menstrual effluent
4. Causes of abnormal bleeding by age (Table 21-2)

K. Amenorrhea
1. Epidemiology
   a. Primary amenorrhea
      (1) Absence of menses by 16 years of age
      (2) Most cases are due to constitutional delay.
         • Family history of delayed onset of menses
   b. Secondary amenorrhea

Anovulatory DUB: most common type of DUB

Primary amenorrhea: most cases due to constitutional delay

Age Bracket	Causes of Bleeding
Prepubertal	Vulvovaginitis: poor hygiene, infection (e.g., gonorrhea), sexual abuse, foreign bodies Embryonal rhabdomyosarcoma
Menarche to 20 years old	Anovulatory DUB (most common cause) Von Willebrand's disease (see Chapter 14)
20 to 40 years old	Pregnancy and its complications (most common cause) Ovulatory types of DUB PID, hypothyroidism, submucosal leiomyomas, adenomyosis, endometrial polyp, endometriosis
40 years or older	Anovulatory DUB (most common cause in perimenopausal period) Endometrial hyperplasia/cancer (most common cause in menopause)

TABLE 21-2:
Causes of Abnormal Bleeding by Age

DUB, dysfunctional uterine bleeding; PID, pelvic inflammatory disease.

Secondary amenorrhea: most cases due to pregnancy

(1) Absence of menses for 3 months
(2) Most cases are due to pregnancy.

2. Pathogenesis

   a. Hypothalamic or pituitary disorder
     (1) Decreased synthesis of FSH and LH
       (a) Decreased synthesis of estrogen and progesterone
       (b) Hypogonadotropic (↓ FSH and LH) hypogonadism
     (2) *No* withdrawal bleeding after receiving progesterone
       • Endometrial mucosa is *not* estrogen-stimulated.
     (3) Examples
       (a) Hypopituitarism, prolactinoma (see Chapter 22)
       (b) Anorexia nervosa (see Chapter 7)

   b. Ovarian disorder
     (1) Decreased synthesis of estrogen and progesterone
       (a) Increase in serum FSH and LH, respectively
       (b) Hypergonadotropic (↑ FSH and LH) hypogonadism
     (2) *No* withdrawal bleeding after receiving progesterone
       • Endometrial mucosa is *not* estrogen-stimulated.
     (3) Examples
       (a) Turner's syndrome (see Chapter 5)
       (b) Surgical removal of ovaries

Primary amenorrhea + poor female secondary sex characteristics: probable Turner's syndrome

   c. End-organ defect
     (1) Prevents the normal egress of blood
       • More likely cause of primary amenorrhea
     (2) Normal levels of FSH, LH, estrogen, and progesterone
     (3) *No* withdrawal bleeding after receiving progesterone
     (4) Examples
       (a) Imperforate hymen, Rokitansky-Kuster-Hauser syndrome
       (b) Asherman syndrome
         • Removal of stratum basalis owing to repeated curettage

   d. Summary of amenorrhea (Table 21-3)

TABLE 21-3: Differential Diagnosis of Amenorrhea

Disorder	FSH/LH	Estrogen	Examples
Hypothalamic/pituitary disorder	↓	↓	Hypopituitarism Anorexia nervosa, prolactinoma
Ovarian disorder	↑	↓	Turner's syndrome
End-organ defect	N	N	Imperforate hymen, Asherman syndrome
Constitutional delay	N	N	Family history of delayed onset of menses

VI. Uterine Disorders
  A. Endometritis
   1. Acute endometritis
     a. Most often due to bacterial infection following delivery or miscarriage
     b. Group B streptococcus (*Streptococcus agalactiae*) is a common pathogen.

Acute endometritis: group B streptococcus

   2. Chronic endometritis
     a. Causes
       (1) Retained placenta
       (2) Gonorrhea, intrauterine device (*Actinomyces israeli*)
     b. Key histologic finding is the presence of plasma cells
  B. Adenomyosis
   1. Invagination of the stratum basalis into the myometrium
     a. Glands and stroma thicken myometrial tissue
     b. Produces uterine enlargement

Adenomyosis: glands and stroma in myometrium

   2. Clinical findings
     • Menorrhagia, dysmenorrhea, pelvic pain
  C. Endometriosis
   1. Functioning glands and stroma are located *outside* the uterus.
   2. Pathogenesis
     a. Reverse menses through fallopian tubes (most common)
     b. Coelomic metaplasia, vascular or lymphatic spread
   3. Cyclic bleeding of gland and stromal implants
   4. Common sites
     • Ovaries (most common), rectal pouch, fallopian tubes, intestine

Endometriosis: functioning glands and stroma outside the confines of the uterus

> The rectal pouch of Douglas is anterior to the rectum and posterior to the uterus. It is the most dependent portion of the female pelvis. It can be palpated by digital rectal examination. It is a common site to collect blood (e.g., ruptured tubal pregnancy), malignant cells (e.g., seeding by ovarian cancer), endometrial implants, and pus (e.g., pelvic inflammatory disease).

   5. Clinical findings
     a. Dysmenorrhea
     b. Painful stooling during menses
       • Implants located in rectal pouch
     c. Intestinal obstruction and bleeding during menses
     d. Increased risk for ectopic pregnancy
     e. Enlargement of ovaries
       • Blood-filled cysts
   6. Laparoscopy useful for diagnosis and treatment
     • Implants have a "powder burn" appearance
  D. Endometrial hyperplasia
   1. Epidemiology and pathogenesis
     a. Prolonged estrogen stimulation
     b. Risk factors
       (1) Early menarche or late menopause

Endometrial hyperplasia: prolonged estrogen stimulation

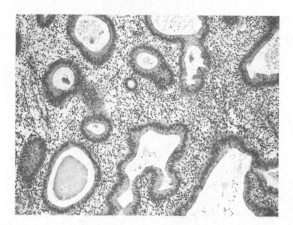

21-8: *Simple hyperplasia of endometrial glands showing cystic dilation and focal areas of glandular outpouching. There is no gland crowding or stratification of the epithelial lining. (From Kumar V, Fausto N, Abbas A: Robbins and Cotran's Pathologic Basis of Disease, 7th ed. Philadelphia, WB Saunders, 2004, p 1086, Fig. 22-31A.)*

    (2) Nulliparity
    (3) Obesity
      • Increased aromatization of androgens to estrogen
    (4) POS, taking estrogen without progesterone
   c. Classification
    (1) Simple hyperplasia (Fig. 21-8)
     (a) Increased number of cystically dilated glands
     (b) *No* glandular crowding
    (2) Complex hyperplasia
     (a) Increased number of dilated glands with branching
     (b) Glandular crowding
    (3) Atypical hyperplasia
     (a) Glandular crowding and dysplastic epithelium
     (b) Increased risk for endometrial cancer
  2. Clinical findings
   a. Menorrhagia or irregular uterine bleeding
   b. Increased risk for progression to endometrial carcinoma
 E. Endometrial polyp
  1. Benign polyp that enlarges with estrogen stimulation
  2. Does *not* progress to endometrial carcinoma
  3. Common cause of menorrhagia in 20- to 40-year-old age bracket
 F. Endometrial carcinoma
  1. Epidemiology and pathogenesis
   a. Most common gynecologic tumor
   b. Prolonged estrogen stimulation
    • Same risk factors as endometrial hyperplasia
   c. OCPs decrease risk
   d. Increased risk for breast cancer

Endometrial carcinoma: most common gynecologic cancer; best prognosis

      e. Types of endometrial cancer
        (1) Well-differentiated adenocarcinoma
          (a) Most common type
          (b) Adenoacanthoma
            • Contains foci of benign squamous tissue (no prognostic significance)
          (c) Adenosquamous carcinoma
            • Contain foci of malignant squamous cancer (worse prognosis)
        (2) Papillary adenocarcinoma
          • Highly aggressive cancer
  2. Cancer characteristics
    a. Spreads down into the endocervix
    b. Spreads out into the uterine wall (Fig. 21-9)
    c. Lungs are the most common site of metastasis
  3. Clinical findings
    • Postmenopausal bleeding
G. Leiomyoma ("fibroids")
  1. Epidemiology
    a. Benign smooth muscle tumor (Fig. 21-10)
    b. More common in black Americans than whites
    c. Estrogen sensitive tumors
      • May become larger during pregnancy
  2. Tumor characteristics
    a. Commonly undergo
      (1) Degeneration
      (2) Dystrophic calcification
      (3) Hyalinization
        • Reason for the term "fibroids"
    b. They do *not* transform into leiomyosarcomas.
  3. Clinical findings
    a. Menorrhagia (when located in submucosa)
    b. Obstructive delivery

> Leiomyoma: most common benign connective tissue tumor in women

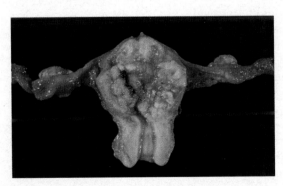

21-9: *Endometrial carcinoma showing necrotic tumor filling the uterine cavity and extending completely through the uterine wall. (From Damjanov I, Linder J: Pathology: A Color Atlas. St. Louis, Mosby, 2000, p 268, Fig. 13-37.)*

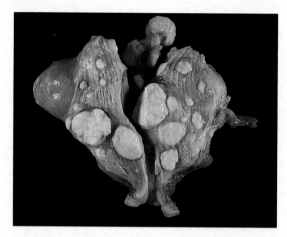

21-10: *Leiomyomas. In sagittal section, multiple well-circumscribed, gray-white nodules (leiomyomas) are dispersed throughout the myometrium. (From Damjanov I, Linder J: Pathology: A Color Atlas. St. Louis, Mosby, 2000, p 271, Fig. 13-49.)*

    H. Leiomyosarcoma
        1. Most common sarcoma of the uterus
        2. Tumor characteristics
          • Numerous atypical mitoses and foci of necrosis
    I. Malignant mixed müllerian tumors (carcinosarcomas)
        1. Endometrial adenocarcinoma + malignant mesenchymal (stromal) tumor
          a. Primarily occur in postmenopausal women
          b. Bulky, necrotic tumors that often protrude through the cervical os
        2. Mesenchymal component may include muscle, cartilage, and bone
        3. Strong association with previous irradiation
        4. Poor prognosis

VII. Fallopian Tube Disorders
    A. Hydatids of Morgagni
        1. Cystic müllerian remnants
        2. Most often located around the fimbriated end of the tube
    B. Pelvic inflammatory disease (PID)
        1. Causes of PID
          a. Most often due to *N. gonorrhoeae* or *C. trachomatis*
          b. Other pathogens
            • *Bacteroides fragilis,* streptococci, *Clostridium perfringens*
        2. Most common cause of hydrosalpinx
          • Pus resorbs leaving a clear fluid distending the tube
    C. Salpingitis isthmica nodosa (SIN)
        1. Invagination of the mucosa into the muscle
          a. Produces nodules
          b. Analogous to adenomyosis

PID: most common cause is *N. gonorrhoeae*

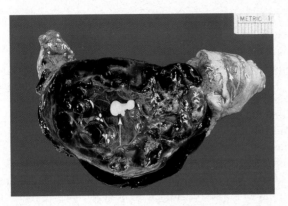

21-11: *Ruptured ectopic tubal pregnancy showing marked hemorrhage (hematosalpinx) and an embryo (arrow) in the center of the clot material. (From Rosai J, Ackerman LV: Surgical Pathology, 9th ed. St. Louis, Mosby, 2004, p 1639, Fig. 19-198.)*

2. Complications
   - Infertility, ectopic pregnancy

D. Ectopic pregnancy
   1. Epidemiology and pathogenesis
      a. Implantation of a fetus outside the normal uterine location
      b. Sites of implantation
         (1) Majority occur within the tubes (Fig. 21-11)
            - Most are in the broad ampullary portion below the fimbriae.
         (2) Ovaries, abdominal cavity
      c. Causes
         (1) Most common cause is scarring from previous PID.
         (2) Endometriosis, altered tubal motility, SIN
   2. Clinical findings
      a. Sudden onset of lower abdominal pain
         - Usually ~6 weeks after a previous normal menstrual period
      b. Abnormal uterine bleeding, adnexal mass, hypovolemic shock
   3. Complications
      a. Rupture with intra-abdominal bleed
         - Most common cause of death in early pregnancy
      b. Most common cause of hematosalpinx
         - Blood in the tube
   4. Diagnosis
      a. β-hCG is the best screening test.
         (1) Urine screen is usually sensitive enough.
         (2) Serum test is used if the urine screen is negative.
         (3) Positive test does *not* prove that an ectopic pregnancy is present.
      b. Vaginal ultrasound is the confirmatory test.
         - Check for an amniotic sac
      c. Laparoscopy is used in equivocal cases.

Ectopic tubal pregnancy: most common cause is previous PID

Follicular cyst: most common ovarian mass

OCPs decrease risk for endometrial and ovarian cancers.

Surface-derived tumors: most common group of ovarian tumors

Serous cystadenocarcinoma: most common ovarian cancer; bilaterality; psammoma bodies

VIII. Ovarian Disorders

A. Follicular cyst
1. Most common ovarian mass
2. Non-neoplastic cyst
   - Accumulation of fluid in a follicle or previously ruptured follicle
3. Rupture produces sterile peritonitis with pain.
4. Ultrasound is the best screening test.

B. Corpus luteum cyst
1. Most common ovarian mass in pregnancy
2. Non-neoplastic cyst
   a. Accumulation of fluid in the corpus luteum during pregnancy
   b. May be confused with an amniotic sac

C. Oophoritis
- May be a complication of mumps or pelvic inflammatory disease

D. Stromal hyperthecosis
1. Occurs primarily in postmenopausal women
   - Causes ovarian enlargement
2. Hypercellular ovarian stroma
   a. Vacuolated stromal hilar cells are present that synthesize androgens
   b. May cause hirsutism or virilization
3. Association with acanthosis nigricans and insulin resistance

E. Ovarian tumors
1. Epidemiology and pathogenesis
   a. Tumors are more likely benign in women younger than 45 years of age.
   b. Risk factors
      (1) Nulliparity
         (a) Increased number of ovulatory cycles increases risk.
         (b) Increased risk for surface-derived ovarian tumors
      (2) Genetic factors
         (a) Mutations of *BRCA1* and *BRCA2* suppressor genes
         (b) Lynch syndrome (see Chapter 8)
         (c) Turner's syndrome (see Chapter 5)
            - Increased risk for dysgerminoma
         (d) Peutz-Jeghers syndrome (see Chapter 17)
            - Increased incidence of sex cord tumors with annular tubules
      (3) Smoking cigarettes
      (4) OCPs decrease risk
         - Decreased number of ovulatory cycles
2. Classification of ovarian tumors (Table 21-4)
   a. Surface-derived tumors
      (1) Account for 65% to 70% of ovarian tumors
      (2) Derive from coelomic epithelium
      (3) Account for the greatest number of malignant ovarian tumors
      (4) Malignant tumors commonly seed the omentum (see Chapter 8)

TABLE 21-4:
Classification of Ovarian Tumors

Tumor	Characteristics
Surface-Derived Tumors	
Serous tumors	Most common group of primary benign and malignant tumors Most common group of tumors that can be bilateral Cysts are lined by ciliated cells (similar to fallopian tube) Serous cystadenoma (benign); serous cystadenocarcinoma has psammoma bodies (dystrophically calcified tumor cells); most common tumor that is bilateral
Mucinous tumors	Cysts lined by mucus-secreting cells (similar to endocervix) Large, multiloculated tumors Seeding produces pseudomyxoma peritonei Mucinous cystadenoma (benign); may be associated with Brenner's tumors; mucinous cystadenocarcinoma
Endometrioid	Malignant tumors associated with endometrial carcinoma (15–30% of cases); tumor resembles endometrial carcinoma Commonly bilateral
Brenner tumor	Usually benign Contain Walthard's rests (transitional-like epithelium)
Germ Cell Tumors	
Cystic teratoma	Usually benign; less then 1% become malignant (usually squamous cancer) Ectodermal differentiation (hair, sebaceous glands, teeth) most prominent Most of these derivatives are found in a nipple-like structure in the cyst wall called Rokitansky tubercle Immature malignant types contain mature and immature components (e.g., muscle, neuroepithelium) Struma ovarii type has functioning thyroid tissue
Dysgerminoma	Most common malignant germ cell tumor; characteristic increase in serum LDH; same histologic picture as seminoma of testis Associated with streak gonads of Turner's syndrome
Yolk sac tumor	Malignant tumor; most common ovarian cancer in girls < 4 years old Contain Schiller-Duval bodies (resemble yolk sac) Increased α-fetoprotein
Sex-Cord Stromal Tumors	
Thecoma-fibroma	Benign tumor associated with Meigs' syndrome (ascites, right-sided pleural effusion); regression of effusions follows removal of tumor Commonly calcify
Granulosa-thecal cell tumor	Low-grade malignant tumor Feminizing tumor (produces estrogen) that contains Call-Exner bodies
Sertoli-Leydig cell	Benign masculinizing tumor (produces androgens) Pure Leydig cell tumors contain cells with crystals of Reinke
Gonadoblastoma	Malignant tumor with mixture of germ cell tumor (dysgerminoma) and sex-cord stromal tumor; associated with abnormal sexual development in 80% of cases Commonly calcify
Tumors Metastatic to Ovary	
Krukenberg tumor	May affect both ovaries; contains signet-ring cells from hematogenous spread of a gastric cancer

LDH, lactate dehydrogenase.

        b. Germ cell tumors
           (1) Account for 15% to 20% of ovarian tumors
           (2) Cancers are similar to those seen in the testicle (see Chapter 20).
           (3) A relatively small number of tumors are malignant.
        c. Sex cord-stromal tumors
           (1) Account for 3% to 5% of ovarian tumors
           (2) Derive from stromal cells
           (3) May be hormone-producing
           (4) Majority of tumors are benign
        d. Metastasis
           (1) Accounts for 5% of ovarian tumors
           (2) Common primary cancers metastasizing to ovaries
              • Breast, stomach (e.g., Krukenberg tumors)
    3. Clinical findings
        a. Signs of seeding from malignant surface-derived cancers
           (1) Malignant ascites and increased abdominal girth
           (2) Induration in the rectal pouch on digital rectal examination
           (3) Intestinal obstruction with colicky pain

> Malignant surface-derived cancers: commonly seed the abdominal cavity

        b. Palpable ovarian mass in a postmenopausal woman
           • Ovaries should *not* be palpable in menopausal women.
        c. Malignant pleural effusion
           • Common site for ovarian cancer metastasis
        d. Cystic teratomas undergo torsion leading to infarction.
           • Radiographs show calcification from bone or teeth (see Fig. 8-3).
        e. Signs of hyperestrinism from estrogen-secreting tumors.
           (1) Bleeding from endometrial hyperplasia/cancer
           (2) 100% superficial squamous cells in a cervical Pap smear
        f. Hirsutism or virilization from androgen-secreting tumors
    4. Tumor markers
        a. Increased serum cancer antigen 125 (CA 125)
        b. Only increased in surface-derived malignant tumors

IX. Gestational Disorders
    A. Placental anatomy
        1. Maternal surface
           • Contains cotyledons covered by a layer of decidua basalis
        2. Fetal surface
         a. Entirely covered by the chorionic plate
         b. Chorionic villi vessels converge with the umbilical cord.
         c. Chorion is covered by the amnion.
        3. Chorionic villus/umbilical cord
         a. Chorionic villi project in the intervillous space.
           (1) Space contains maternal blood from which oxygen is extracted.
           (2) Spiral arteries from the uterus empty into the space.
         b. Chorionic villi are lined by trophoblastic tissue.
           (1) Outside layer is composed of syncytiotrophoblast.
               (a) Synthesizes hCG (see above)

      (b) Synthesizes human placental lactogen (HPL)
- Directly correlates with placental mass and has anti-insulin activity

    (2) Inside layer is composed of cytotrophoblast.

  c. Chorionic villus vessels coalesce to form the umbilical vein.

  d. Umbilical cord

    (1) Contains one umbilical vein and two umbilical arteries
- Umbilical vein contains oxygenated blood.

    (2) Single umbilical artery
- Increased incidence of congenital anomalies

B. Infections

  1. Epidemiology

    a. Most are due to ascending bacterial infections

      (1) Complication of premature rupture of membranes

      (2) Group B streptococcus is the most common pathogen.

    b. Congenital infections (e.g., cytomegalovirus, syphilis)

  2. Funisitis and placentitis
- Infection of the umbilical cord and placenta, respectively

  3. Chorioamnionitis

    a. Infection of the fetal membranes

    b. Danger of neonatal sepsis and meningitis

C. Selected placental abnormalities

  1. Placenta previa

    a. Implantation over cervical os

    b. Painless vaginal bleeding

  2. Abruptio placentae

    a. Premature separation of placenta due to formation of a retroplacental clot
- Separates the placenta from the implantation site

    b. Risk factors

      (1) Hypertension

      (2) Smoking cigarettes

      (3) Cocaine addiction, advanced maternal age

    c. Painful vaginal bleeding

  3. Placenta accreta

    a. Direct implantation into muscle *without* intervening decidua

    b. Requires a hysterectomy after delivery of the baby

  4. Succenturiate lobes

    a. Accessory lobes of the placenta located along the margin

    b. Risk for hemorrhage if the accessory lobes are detached

  5. Enlarged placenta

    a. Diabetes mellitus

    b. Rh hemolytic disease of newborn

    c. Congenital syphilis

  6. Twin placentas (Fig. 21-12)

    a. Monochorionic types are associated with identical twins.

      (1) Identical twins derive from a single fertilized egg.

HPL: directly correlates with placental mass, anti-insulin activity

Abruptio placentae: retroplacental clot; painful vaginal bleeding

Monochorionic twin placentas: identical twins, single fertilized egg

Type		Identical	Fraternal
A. Monochorionic monoamniotic		X	
B. Monochorionic diamniotic		X	
C. Dichorionic diamniotic (fused)		X	X
D. Dichorionic diamniotic (separate)		X	X

21-12: *Twin placentas. See text for description. (Redrawn from Goljan EF: Star Series: Pathology. Philadelphia, WB Saunders, 1998, Fig. 18-2.)*

(2) Monoamniotic with a single amniotic sac (see Fig. 21-12A)
  • Type for Siamese twins or tangling of umbilical cords
(3) Diamniotic with separate amniotic sacs (see Fig. 21-12B)
(4) Fetal-to-fetal transfusion can occur in either type.
  b. Dichorionic placentas
(1) Can be identical or fraternal twins
  • Fraternal twins occur when separate eggs are fertilized.
(2) Placentas can be diamniotic (see Fig. 21-12C) or separated (see Fig. 21-12D).

D. **Preeclampsia/eclampsia**
  • Toxemia of pregnancy
  1. Epidemiology
    a. Usually occurs in the third trimester (24th to 25th week)
    b. Preeclampsia in the first trimester
      • Associated with a molar pregnancy (see below)
    c. More common in women older than 35 years of age
  2. Pathogenesis
    a. Abnormal placentation
      • Causes mechanical or functional obstruction of the spiral arteries
    b. Normal vasodilators are decreased.
      • Examples—PGE_2, nitric oxide
    c. Vasoconstrictors are increased.
      • Examples—thromboxane A_2, angiotensin II
    d. Net effect is placental hypoperfusion.
  3. Pathologic findings
    a. Premature aging of the placenta

Dichorionic twin placentas: identical or fraternal (separate fertilized eggs)

Preeclampsia: placental hypoperfusion

b. Multiple placental infarctions

c. Spiral arteries show intimal atherosclerosis

4. Clinical findings

  a. Diastolic hypertension (increased vasoconstrictors)

  b. Proteinuria often in nephrotic range

  c. Dependent pitting edema

    • Due to loss of albumin in the urine

  d. Generalized seizures

    (1) Preeclampsia + seizures is called eclampsia.

    (2) Magnesium sulfate is used for treatment.

  e. Renal disease

    • Swollen endothelial cells in the glomerular capillaries

  f. Liver disease

    • Periportal necrosis with increased transaminases

  g. HELLP syndrome (see Chapter 18)

    • Hemolytic anemia and disseminated intravascular coagulation

E. Gestational trophoblastic neoplasms

1. Hydatidiform moles

  a. Benign tumors of the chorionic villus

    • Complete and partial moles

  b. Complete mole is the most common type.

    (1) The entire placenta is neoplastic.

    (2) Dilated, swollen villi without fetal blood vessels (Fig. 21-13)

    (3) *No* embryo is present.

    (4) 46XX (90% of cases)

      (a) Both chromosomes are of male origin.

      (b) Egg is fertilized by two haploid spermatozoa with X chromosomes.

    (5) Increased risk for developing choriocarcinoma

    (6) Clinical findings

> Preeclampsia: hypertension, proteinuria, pitting edema

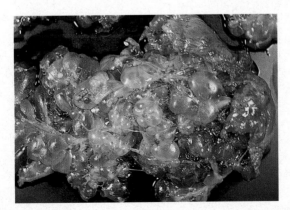

21-13: *Complete hydatidiform mole. The enlarged and edematous villi are interconnected by thin cord-like structures. (From Damjanov I, Linder J: Pathology: A Color Atlas. St. Louis, Mosby, 2000, p 290, Fig. 13-111A.)*

Preeclampsia first trimester: complete mole

(a) Preeclampsia develops in the first trimester
(b) Uterus is too large for gestational age
(c) Increased hCG for the gestational age
(d) "Snowstorm appearance" with ultrasound

  c. Partial mole
    (1) Not all villi are neoplastic or dilated.
    (2) Embryo is present.
      (a) Triploid (69XXY)
      (b) Egg with 23X is fertilized by a 23X and a 23Y sperm.
    (3) *No* increased risk for developing a choriocarcinoma

2. Choriocarcinoma
  a. Malignant tumor composed of syncytiotrophoblast and cytotrophoblast
    • Chorionic villi are *not* present.

Choriocarcinoma: malignancy of trophoblastic tissue

  b. Risk factors
    (1) Complete mole (50% of cases)
    (2) Spontaneous abortion (25% of cases)
    (3) Normal pregnancy (25% of cases)
  c. Common sites of metastasis
    (1) Lungs and vagina
    (2) Lesions are hemorrhagic
  d. Excellent response to chemotherapy
    • Good response does *not* apply to non–gestationally derived cancer.

F. Amniotic fluid
1. Composition
  a. Fetal urine
  b. High salt content causes ferning when dried on a slide
    • Excellent sign of premature rupture of the amniotic sac
  c. Swallowed and recycled by the fetus
  d. Polyhydramnios
    (1) Excessive amniotic fluid
    (2) Causes
      • Tracheoesophageal fistula, duodenal atresia (see Chapter 17)
  e. Oligohydramnios
    (1) Decreased amount of amniotic fluid
    (2) Juvenile polycystic kidney disease (see Chapter 19)

Increased AFP in pregnancy: open neural tube defect

2. α-Fetoprotein (AFP) in pregnancy
  a. Increased maternal AFP
    (1) Open neural tube defect
    (2) Related to folate deficiency
    (3) Folate stores should be adequate *before* pregnancy.
      • Neural tube is already developed by the end of the first month of gestation.
  b. Decreased maternal AFP
    • Down syndrome
3. Lecithin/sphingomyelin (L:S) ratio
  a. Lecithin

(1) Synthesized by type II pneumocytes

(2) Decreases alveolar surface tension to prevent atelectasis

b. L:S ratio greater than 2 in amniotic fluid indicates adequate surfactant.

c. Cortisol and thyroxine increase surfactant synthesis.

   • Maternal administration of glucocorticoids increases surfactant synthesis if babies must be delivered before term.

d. Insulin inhibits surfactant synthesis.

G. Urine estriol in pregnancy

1. Derived from the fetal adrenal gland, placenta, and maternal liver

   a. Fetal zone of the adrenal cortex

      (1) Converts pregnenolone synthesized in the placenta to DHEA-sulfate

      (2) Fetal zone is absent in anencephaly (absent brain).

   b. Fetal liver

      • DHEA-sulfate is 16-hydroxylated to 16-OH-DHEA-sulfate.

   c. Maternal placenta

      (1) Placental sulfatase cleaves off the sulfate from 16-OH-DHEA-sulfate.

      (2) 16-OH-DHEA is converted by aromatase to free unbound estriol.

   d. Maternal liver

      (1) Free estriol is conjugated to estriol sulfate and estriol glucosiduronate.

      (2) Both compounds are excreted in maternal urine and bile.

2. Decreased levels of estriol

   • Sign of fetal-maternal-placental dysfunction

3. Down syndrome triad

   a. Decreased urine estriol

   b. Decreased AFP

   c. Increased β-hCG

X. Breast Disorders

A. Clinical anatomy

1. High-density locations of breast tissue

   a. Upper outer quadrant

      • Underscores why cancer is most commonly located in this quadrant

   b. Beneath the nipple

2. Hormone effects during menstrual cycle

   a. Estrogen

      • Stimulates ductal and alveolar growth

   b. Progesterone

      • Stimulates alveolar differentiation

3. Hormone effects in lactation

   a. Prolactin

      • Stimulates and maintains lactogenesis

L:S ratio > 2: adequate surfactant

Estriol: derived from fetal adrenal gland, placenta, maternal liver

      b. Oxytocin
        (1) Released by suckling reflex
        (2) Expulsion of milk into ducts
    4. Lymph nodes
      a. Outer quadrant cancers
        • Drain to the axillary lymph nodes
      b. Inner quadrant cancers
        • Drain to the internal mammary nodes

B. Locations for breast lesions (Fig. 21-14)

C. Nipple discharges
    1. Galactorrhea; causes other than lactation:
      a. Mechanical stimulation of the nipple
        • Most common physiologic cause of galactorrhea
      b. Prolactinoma (see Chapter 22)
        • Most common pathologic cause of galactorrhea
      c. Primary hypothyroidism (see Chapter 22)
        (1) Most common nonpituitary endocrine disease causing galactorrhea
        (2) Decreased serum thyroxine increases thyrotropin-releasing factor (TRF).
          • TRF stimulates prolactin.
      d. Drugs (e.g., OCPs)
    2. Bloody nipple discharge
      • Intraductal papilloma, ductal cancer
    3. Purulent nipple discharge
      a. Acute mastitis due to *Staphylococcus aureus*
      b. Usually occurs during lactation or breast-feeding
    4. Greenish brown nipple discharge
      • Mammary duct ectasia (plasma cell mastitis)

D. Breast pain
    1. Most common cause is fibrocystic change
    2. Mondor's disease
      a. Superficial thrombophlebitis of veins overlying the breast
      b. Presents as a palpable, painful cord

Nipple/areola complex	Lactiferous sinus	Major duct	Terminal duct	Lobule	Stroma
Paget's disease Breast abscess	Intraductal papilloma Breast abscess Plasma cell mastitis	Fibrocystic change Ductal cancer	Tubular carcinoma	Lobular carcinoma Sclerosing adenosis	Fibroadenoma Phyllodes tumor

21-14: *Locations for breast lesions. See text for discussion. (Redrawn from Goljan EF: Star Series: Pathology. Philadelphia, WB Saunders, 1998, Fig. 18-3.)*

E. Fibrocystic change
1. Epidemiology and pathogenesis
   a. Most common breast mass in women younger than 50 years old
   b. Limited to the reproductive period of life
   c. Distortion of normal cyclic breast changes
2. Small and large cysts
   a. Some cysts have hemorrhage into the cyst fluid.
      • Called "blue domed" cysts
   b. Vary in size with the menstrual cycle
   c. *No* malignant potential
3. Fibrosis
   • *No* malignant potential
4. Sclerosing adenosis
   a. Proliferation of small ductules/acini in the lobule
      • Pattern is often confused with infiltrating ductal cancer.
   b. Often contain microcalcifications
5. Ductal hyperplasia
   a. Ducts are estrogen-sensitive.
   b. Pathologic findings
      (1) Papillary proliferation is called papillomatosis.
      (2) Apocrine metaplasia refers to the presence of large, pink-staining cells.
      (3) Atypical ductal hyperplasia
         • Increased risk for developing cancer

F. Inflammation
1. Acute mastitis (see above)
2. Mammary duct ectasia (plasma cell mastitis)
   a. Nonbacterial infection
   b. Main ducts fill up with debris.
      • Causes dilation, rupture, and inflammation
   c. May produce skin and nipple retraction simulating cancer
3. Traumatic fat necrosis
   a. Trauma to breast tissue
   b. Microscopic findings
      (1) Lipid-laden macrophages with foreign body giant cells
      (2) Fibrosis, dystrophic calcification
   c. Painless, indurated mass
      • Painful in acute stage
   d. May produce skin retraction simulating cancer
4. Silicone breast implant
   a. Polymer of silica, oxygen, and hydrogen
   b. Silicone gel can leak or the implant can rupture
      (1) Produces foreign body giant cells and chronic inflammation
      (2) Association with autoimmune disease is *not* proved.

G. Benign breast tumors
1. Fibroadenoma
   a. Most common breast tumor in women younger than 35 years old

Fibrocystic change: most common breast mass in women < 50 years old

Cysts and fibrosis: "lumpy bumpy" feeling on breast examination

Fibroadenoma: most common breast tumor women < 35 years old

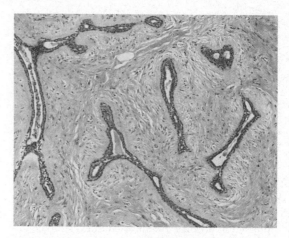

21-15: Fibroadenoma showing compressed, elongated ducts surrounded by neoplastic stromal tissue. (From Damjanov I: Pathology for the Health-Related Professions, 2nd ed. Philadelphia, WB Saunders, 2000, p 405, Fig. 16-5B.)

   - Stroma proliferates and compresses the ducts (Fig. 21-15).
   c. Discrete movable, painless or painful mass
      - Multiple lesions may be present.
   d. Increases in size during pregnancy
      - Estrogen-sensitive
   e. Rarely becomes malignant
2. Phyllodes tumor
   a. Bulky tumor derived from stromal cells
   b. Most often benign but can be malignant in some cases
      - Hypercellular stroma with mitoses are signs of malignancy.
   c. Lobulated tumor with cystic spaces containing leaf-like extensions
      - Often reach massive size
3. Intraductal papilloma
   a. Most common cause of bloody nipple discharge in women younger than 50 years old
   b. Develop in the lactiferous ducts or sinuses
   c. No increased risk for cancer

H. **Breast cancer**
1. Epidemiology
   a. Most common cancer in adult women (1 : 8 lifetime risk)
      - Mean age is 64 years old.
   b. Second most common cancer producing death in women
   c. Most common breast mass in women over 50 years old
2. Risk factors
   a. Family history and genetics
      (1) Increased risk if breast cancer involves first-generation relatives
         - Mother, sister
      (2) Genetic basis is involved in fewer than 10% of cases (see Chapter 8).

Intraductal papilloma: most common cause of bloody nipple discharge in women < 50 years old

Breast cancer risk: prolonged estrogen stimulation, genetically susceptible background

       (a) Autosomal dominant *BRCA1* and *BRCA2* association

       (b) Li-Fraumeni multicancer syndrome

         • Inactivation of *TP53* suppressor gene

     (3) Other gene relationships

       • *RAS* oncogene, *ERBB2, RB* suppressor gene

  b. Prolonged estrogen stimulation

     (1) Early menarche/late menopause

     (2) Nulliparity

     (3) Postmenopausal obesity

       • Aromatization of androstenedione to estrone

     (4) Hormone replacement therapy

  c. Atypical ductal hyperplasia

  d. Endometrial cancer, ionizing radiation, smoking cigarettes

  e. Common denominators for increased risk of cancer

     (1) Prolonged estrogen stimulation

     (2) Genetically susceptible background

3. Clinical findings

  a. Painless mass in the breast

    • Usually in the upper outer quadrant

  b. Skin or nipple retraction

  c. Painless axillary lymphadenopathy

> Initial management of breast mass: fine needle aspiration

4. Mammography

  a. Primarily a screening test

    • Detects nonpalpable breast masses

  b. Does *not* distinguish benign from malignant lesions

  c. Screening usually starts annually at age 40.

  d. Identifies microcalcifications

    • Most often occur in ductal carcinoma in situ and sclerosing adenosis

5. Types of breast cancer (Table 21-5; Figs. 21-16 to 21-19)

6. Natural history, treatment, and prognosis

  a. Spread first by lymphatics and then hematogenously

     (1) Outer quadrant cancer spreads to axillary nodes.

     (2) Inner quadrant cancers spread to internal mammary nodes.

  b. Extranodal metastasis

     (1) Common sites of metastasis

       • Lungs, bone, liver, brain, ovaries

     (2) May metastasize 10 to 15 years after treatment

     (3) Pain in bone metastasis is relieved with radiation.

> Breast cancer: most common cancer metastatic to lungs and bone

  c. Staging

     (1) Extranodal metastasis has greater significance than nodal metastasis

     (2) Sentinel node biopsy

      (a) Sampling of the initial node that drains the tumor

      (b) If negative for metastasis, the other nodes in that group are usually negative.

TABLE 21-5:
Types of Breast
Cancer

Type	Comments
Noninvasive	
Ductal carcinoma in situ (DCIS) (Fig. 21-16)	Nonpalpable Patterns: cribriform (sieve-like), comedo (necrotic center) Commonly contain microcalcifications One third eventually invade
Lobular carcinoma in-situ (Fig. 21-17)	Nonpalpable; virtually always an incidental finding in a breast biopsy for other reasons Lobules distended with bland neoplastic cells; one third eventually invade Increased incidence of cancer in the opposite breast
Invasive	
Infiltrating ductal carcinoma (Fig. 21-18)	One third overexpress $ERBB_2$ oncogene Stellate-shaped, indurated, gray-white tumor Gritty on cut section Induration caused by reactive fibroplasia (desmoplasia)
Paget's disease of nipple (Fig. 21-19)	Extension of DCIS into lactiferous ducts and skin of nipple producing a rash with or without nipple retraction Paget's cells
Medullary carcinoma	Associated with *BRCA1* mutations Bulky, soft tumor with large cells and lymphoid infiltrate
Inflammatory carcinoma	Erythematous breast with dimpling like an orange (peau d'orange) Plugs of tumor blocking lumen of dermal lymphatics cause localized lymphedema Very poor prognosis
Invasive lobular carcinoma	Neoplastic cells arranged in linear fashion or form concentric circles (bull's-eye appearance)
Tubular carcinoma	Develops in terminal ductules Increased incidence of cancer in opposite breast
Colloid (mucinous) carcinoma	Usually occurs in elderly women Neoplastic cells are surrounded by extracellular mucin

        (c) If positive for metastasis, there is a one-third chance that other nodes in that group have metastases.

    d. Estrogen and progesterone receptor assays

       (1) Most often positive in postmenopausal women

       (2) Clinical significance

          (a) Confers an overall better prognosis

          (b) Candidate for antiestrogen therapy with tamoxifen

    e. Other tests performed on tissue

       (1) S phase fraction

         • Above 5% is poor prognosis.

       (2) DNA ploidy

         • Diploid tumor is better than an aneuploid tumor.

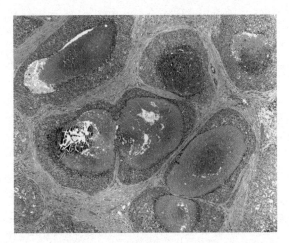

21-16: *Ductal carcinoma in situ (DCIS) showing dilated ducts lined by layers of neoplastic cells. Central areas of necrosis (comedo pattern) are present, some of which contain microcalcifications (arrow). (From Kumar V, Fausto N, Abbas A: Robbins and Cotran's Pathologic Basis of Disease, 7th ed. Philadelphia, WB Saunders, 2004, p 1139, Fig. 23-16B.)*

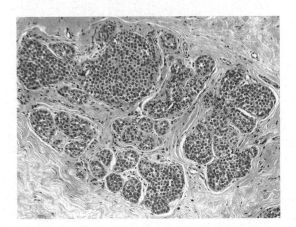

21-17: *Lobular carcinoma in situ showing complete replacement and expansion of a lobule by a monomorphic population of cells. (From Kumar V, Fausto N, Abbas A: Robbins and Cotran's Pathologic Basis of Disease, 7th ed. Philadelphia, WB Saunders, 2004, p 1142, Fig. 23-20.)*

        (3) *ERBB2* oncogene status
           • Poor prognosis if amplification is present.
    f. Surgical procedures
       (1) Modified radical mastectomy
           • Removal of nipple-areolar complex, breast tissue, pectoralis minor, axillary nodes

> A winged scapula may occur due to damage of the long thoracic nerve. There is also a danger for developing lymphedema.

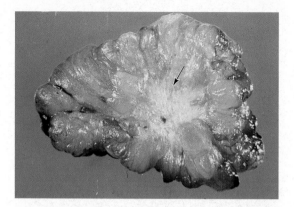

21-18: *Infiltrating ductal carcinoma showing a stellate-shaped scar (arrow) in the fat tissue of the breast. (From Damjanov I, Linder J: Pathology: A Color Atlas. St. Louis, Mosby, 2000, p 304, Fig. 14-14A.)*

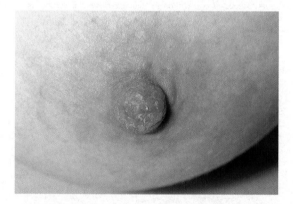

21-19: *Paget's disease of the breast showing erythema around a nipple that has a scaly-appearing rash on the surface. (From Rosai J, Ackerman LV: Surgical Pathology, 9th ed. St. Louis, Mosby, 2004, p 1813, Fig. 20-87.)*

        (2) Breast conservation therapy
           (a) Lumpectomy with microscopically free margins
           (b) Removal of level I and II axillary nodes
           (c) Breast radiation
     g. Overall, 25% of women with breast cancer die from their disease.

I. Gynecomastia
    1. Benign glandular proliferation in the male breast due to estrogen
      a. Subareolar mass (see Fig. 5-8)
      b. More often unilateral than bilateral
      c. Due to estrogen stimulation
    2. Physiologic gynecomastia
      a. Normal in newborn, puberty, elderly
      b. In general, surgery is *not* indicated.

3. Pathologic gynecomastia
   a. Cirrhosis
      - Inability to metabolize estrogen
   b. Klinefelter's syndrome
   c. Drugs
      - Example—spironolactone, which blocks androgen receptors

J. Breast cancer in men
   1. Risk factors
      a. *BRCA2* suppressor gene
      b. Klinefelter's syndrome
   2. Usually have a poor prognosis

Endocrine Disorders

I. **Overview of Endocrine Disease**
   A. **Negative feedback loops**
      1. Control an increase or decrease in hormone production
      2. Example—increased calcium decreases parathyroid hormone (PTH).
   B. **Stimulation tests**
      1. Evaluate hypofunctioning disorders
         • Example—adrenocorticotropic hormone (ACTH) stimulation test is used in the workup of hypocortisolism.
      2. Causes of hypofunction
         a. Autoimmune destruction
            • Examples—Addison's disease, Hashimoto's thyroiditis
         b. Infarction
            • Example—Sheehan's postpartum necrosis, Waterhouse-Friderichsen syndrome
         c. Decreased hormone stimulation
            • Example—decreased thyroid stimulating hormone in hypopituitarism
         d. Enzyme deficiency, infection, neoplasia, congenital disorder
   C. **Suppression tests**
      1. Evaluate hyperfunctioning disorders
         • Example—dexamethasone suppression test evaluates hypercortisolism.
      2. Most hyperfunctioning disorders *cannot* be suppressed.
         • Notable *exceptions* are prolactinoma and pituitary Cushing syndrome.
      3. Causes of hyperfunction
         • Adenoma, acute inflammation, hyperplasia, cancer

II. **Hypothalamus Disorders**
   A. **Tumors altering hypothalamic function**
      1. Pituitary adenoma (see section IV)
         • Most common tumor affecting the hypothalamus
      2. Craniopharyngioma (see section IV)
      3. Midline hamartoma
         • *Not* a neoplasm
      4. Langerhans histiocytosis (see Chapter 13)
   B. **Inflammatory disorders altering hypothalamic function**
      1. Sarcoidosis (see Chapter 16)
         • Produces granulomatous inflammation
      2. Meningitis (see Chapter 25)
   C. **Clinical findings of hypothalamic dysfunction**

Endocrine gland hypofunction: most common cause is autoimmune disease

Endocrine gland hyperfunction: most common cause is a benign adenoma

1. Secondary hypopituitarism
   - *No* releasing hormones to stimulate the anterior pituitary
2. Central diabetes inspidus
   - Antidiuretic hormone (ADH) is synthesized in the hypothalamus.
3. Hyperprolactinemia
   - Loss of dopamine inhibition causes galactorrhea.
4. Precocious puberty
   - Most common cause in boys is a midline hamartoma.

   > "True" precocious puberty implies a central nervous system (CNS) origin for the disorder, but pseudo-precocious puberty implies a peripheral cause (e.g., adrenogenital syndrome). True precocious puberty in boys is the onset of puberty before 9 years of age. The most common cause is a midline hamartoma in the hypothalamus. True precocious puberty in girls is the onset of puberty before 8 years of age. In most cases, it is idiopathic and less likely to be caused by a midline hamartoma.

5. Visual field disturbances
   - Usually bitemporal hemianopsia
6. Mass effects
   - Produces obstructive hydrocephalus (see Chapter 25)
7. Growth disorders
   - Dwarfism in children
8. Kallmann's syndrome (see Chapter 20)

III. Pineal Gland Disorders
A. Clinical anatomy
1. Midline location above the quadrigeminal plate
2. Site for melatonin production
   a. Superior cervical sympathetic ganglia stimulates receptors on pinealocytes.
      - Causes release of melatonin into spinal fluid and blood
   b. Melatonin functions
      (1) Important in sleep/moods and circadian rhythms
         - Released at night
      (2) Used in the treatment of sleep and mood disorders

Melatonin: chemical messenger of darkness

B. Disorders
1. Dystrophic calcification of the pineal gland begins in childhood.
   - Useful in showing shifts due to mass lesions in the brain
2. Pineal tumors
   a. Majority are germ cell tumors resembling seminomas.
   b. Minority of tumors are teratomas.
C. Clinical findings
1. Visual disturbances
   - Paralysis of upward conjugate gaze (Parinaud's syndrome)
2. Obstructive hydrocephalus
   - Due to compression of the aqueduct of Sylvius in the third ventricle

IV. **Pituitary Gland Disorders**
A. **Anterior pituitary hypofunction**
1. Causes
a. Pituitary disease (most common)
• Approximately 75% of the gland must be destroyed.
b. Hypothalamic disorder (see section II)
2. Causes of hypopituitarism
a. Nonfunctioning (null) pituitary adenoma
(1) Association with multiple endocrine neoplasia (MEN) I syndrome
• Pituitary adenoma, hyperparathyroidism, pancreatic tumor (Zollinger-Ellison syndrome or insulinoma)
(2) Clinical findings
(a) Loss of trophic hormones and hypofunction of target organs
(b) Enlarged sella turcica with erosions of the clinoid processes
(c) Bitemporal hemianopia, headache
b. Sheehan's postpartum necrosis
(1) Hypovolemic shock (e.g., blood loss) causes infarction.
(2) Sudden cessation of lactation due to loss of prolactin
• Eventual development of hypopituitarism

> The pituitary gland doubles in size during pregnancy due to synthesis of prolactin. Prolactin release is inhibited by estrogen and progesterone during pregnancy.

c. Craniopharyngioma
(1) Most common cause of hypopituitarism in children
(2) Benign pituitary tumor derived from Rathke's pouch remnants

> Rathke's pouch is an ectodermal derivative derived from the oral cavity. It develops into the anterior lobe of the pituitary gland.

(3) Located *above* the sella turcica
• Extends into sella turcica and destroys the gland
(4) Cystic tumor with hemorrhage and calcification
(5) Commonly causes bitemporal hemianopsia
(6) May produce central diabetes insipidus
d. Pituitary apoplexy
• Hemorrhage/infarction of a pituitary adenoma
e. Lymphocytic hypophysitis
(1) Female dominant autoimmune destruction of the pituitary gland
(2) Occurs during or after pregnancy
3. Clinical findings of pituitary hypofunction (Table 22-1)
B. **Posterior pituitary hypofunction**
1. Central diabetes insipidus (CDI)
a. Lack of ADH
b. Causes of CDI
(1) Hypothalamic disease (see section II)

Hypopituitarism in adults: most common cause is nonfunctioning adenoma

Hypopituitarism in children: most common cause is craniopharyngioma

TABLE 22-1:
Clinical Findings in
Hypopituitarism

Trophic Hormone Deficiency	Discussion

Gonadotropins (FSH, LH)	Children have delayed puberty
	Adult females have secondary amenorrhea
	Males have impotence (see Chapter 20)
	GnRH stimulation test:
	   No significant increase of FSH/LH in hypopituitarism
	   Eventual increase of FSH/LH in hypothalamic disease

Growth hormone (GH)	Decreased GH decreases synthesis and release of IGF-1 Children have growth delay: delayed fusion of epiphyses; bone growth does *not* match the age of the child Adults have hypoglycemia: decreased gluconeogenesis Arginine and sleep stimulation tests: *no* increase in GH or IGF-1; normally, GH and IGF-1 are released at 5 AM
Thyroid-stimulating hormone (TSH)	Secondary hypothyroidism: decreased serum T_4 and TSH Cold intolerance, constipation, weakness *No* increase in TSH after TRF stimulation
Adrenocorticotropic hormone (ACTH)	Secondary hypocortisolism: decreased ACTH and cortisol Hypoglycemia: decreased gluconeogenesis Hyponatremia: mild SIADH (loss of inhibitory effect of cortisol on ADH) Metyrapone test: stimulation test of pituitary ACTH reserve; metyrapone inhibits adrenal 11-hydroxylase, which causes a decrease in cortisol and a corresponding increase in plasma ACTH (pituitary) and 11-deoxycortisol (adrenal), which is proximal to the enzyme block; in hypopituitarism, neither ACTH or 11-deoxycortisol are increased Short ACTH stimulation test: *no* increase in serum cortisol over decreased baseline levels Prolonged ACTH stimulation test: eventual increase in cortisol over the decreased baseline value once the adrenal gland is restimulated

FSH, follicle-stimulating hormone; GnRH, gonadotropin-releasing hormone; IGF, insulin growth factor; LH, luteinizing hormone; SIADH, syndrome of inappropriate antidiuretic hormone; T_4, thyroxine; TRF, thyrotropin-releasing factor.

      (2) Transection of the pituitary stalk (e.g., trauma)

      (3) Posterior pituitary disease (e.g., metastasis)

   2. Nephrogenic diabetes insipidus (NDI)

     a. Collecting tubule is refractory to ADH stimulation.

     b. Causes of NDI

      (1) Drugs

        • Lithium, demeclocycline

      (2) Hypokalemia

        • Vacuolar nephropathy of collecting tubules (see Chapter 4)

      (3) Nephrocalcinosis (see Chapters 1 and 19)

        • Metastatic calcification of the collecting tubule basement membranes

   3. Clinical findings

     • Excessive thirst, polyuria

Diabetes insipidus: polyuria and thirst

Water deprivation test: defines the type of diabetes insipidus

4. Laboratory findings
  a. Hypernatremia and a hypotonic urine
    • Cannot concentrate urine and lose free water (see Chapter 4)
  b. Water deprivation test
    (1) Normal findings
      (a) Increased plasma osmolality (POsm)
        • Stimulates release of ADH
      (b) Increased urine osmolality (UOsm)
        • Urine is concentrated by ADH reabsorption of free water.
    (2) Findings in CDI and NDI
      (a) Increased POsm (hypernatremia)
      (b) Decreased UOsm
    (3) Findings in CDI and NDI after injection of ADH
      (a) In CDI, UOsm increases more than 50% from the baseline.
      (b) In NDI, UOsm increases less than 50% from the baseline.
5. Differential diagnosis of polyuria
  a. Excessive drinking of water
  b. Osmotic diuresis
    • Glucosuria in diabetes mellitus, use of diuretics
6. Treatment of CDI
  a. Treat the underlying disease
  b. Desmopressin
7. Treatment of NDI
  • Thiazides—volume depletion increases proximal tubule reabsorption of water.

C. **Pituitary hyperfunction disorders**
  1. Prolactinoma
    a. Benign adenoma
      • Overall most common pituitary tumor
    b. Clinical and laboratory findings
      (1) Women
        (a) Secondary amenorrhea
          • Prolactin inhibits gonadotropin-releasing hormone (GnRH).
        (b) Galactorrhea
      (2) Men
        (a) Impotence
          • Loss of libido due to decrease in testosterone
        (b) *Not* enough breast tissue to produce galactorrhea
      (3) Serum prolactin level is usually above 200 ng/mL.
      (4) Decreased follicle-stimulating hormone (FSH) and luteinizing hormone (LH)
        • Due to decreased GnRH
    c. Other causes of galactorrhea (see Chapter 21)
    d. Treatment
      • Dopamine analogues (e.g., cabergoline) or surgery

Secondary amenorrhea + galactorrhea: prolactinoma

2. Growth hormone (GH) adenoma
   a. Functions of GH
      (1) Stimulates liver synthesis/release of insulin growth factor (IGF)-1
      (2) Stimulates gluconeogenesis and amino acid uptake in muscle
      (3) Negative feedback relationship with glucose and IGF-1
   b. Functions of IGF-1
      • Stimulates growth of bone (linear and lateral), cartilage, soft tissue
   c. Clinical and laboratory findings
      (1) Children develop gigantism
         • Due to increased linear bone growth
      (2) Adults develop acromegaly (Fig. 22-1)
         (a) Increased lateral bone growth (e.g., hands, feet, jaw)
            • *No* linear growth because epiphyses are fused.
         (b) Prominent jaw
            • Spacing between the teeth
         (c) Frontal bossing
            • Enlarged frontal sinus increases the hat size.
         (d) Macroglossia, cardiomyopathy (cause of death)
      (3) Increased GH and IGF-1
         • Hormones are *not* suppressed by glucose administration.
      (4) Hyperglycemia
         • Due to increase in gluconeogenesis
3. Syndrome of inappropriate ADH (SIADH)
   a. Causes
      (1) Small cell carcinoma of lung
         • Most common cause
      (2) Central nervous system injury
      (3) Drugs
         • Example—chlorpropamide, an oral sulfonylurea
      (4) Lung infections (e.g., tuberculosis)

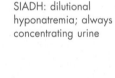

Acromegaly: increased lateral bone growth, organomegaly, hyperglycemia

SIADH: dilutional hyponatremia; always concentrating urine

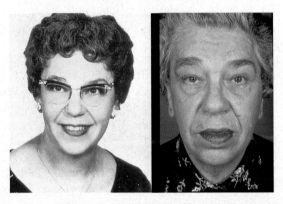

22-1: *Acromegaly showing the patient before development of the tumor (left) and after development of the tumor (right). Note the coarse facial features and enlargement of the jaw and lips. (From Damjanov I: Pathology for the Health-Related Professions, 2nd ed. Philadelphia, WB Saunders, 2000, p 407.)*

b. Clinical and laboratory findings
   (1) Mental status dysfunction
       • Due to cerebral edema
   (2) Hyponatremia (see Chapter 4)
       • Serum Na^+ is usually below 120 mEq/L.
c. Treatment is to restrict water.

> Demeclocycline is a nephrotoxic drug that produces NDI. It is frequently used in treating ectopic ADH from small cell carcinoma of the lung because the patient does not have to be deprived of water.

V. Thyroid Gland Disorders

A. Steps in thyroid hormone synthesis

1. Trapping of iodide is TSH-mediated.
2. Oxidation of iodides to iodine is peroxidase-mediated.
3. Organification

   Thyroid hormone: iodide attached to tyrosine

   a. Iodine is incorporated into tyrosine to form MIT (monoiodotyrosine) and DIT (diiodotyrosine).
   b. It is TSH-mediated.
4. Coupling of MIT with DIT produces triiodothyronine (T_3).
5. Coupling of DIT with DIT produces thyroxine (T_4).
6. Hormones are stored as colloid.
7. Proteolysis of colloid by lysosomal proteases is TSH-mediated.
8. T_4 and T_3 bind to thyroid-binding globulin (TBG).
   • One third of TBG binding sites are normally occupied.
9. Free T_4 (FT_4) is peripherally converted to free T_3 (FT_3) by an outer ring deiodinase.

   FT_4/FT_3: negative feedback with TSH

   a. FT_3 is a metabolically active hormone.
   b. FT_4 is considered a prohormone.
   c. FT_4 and FT_3 have a negative feedback relationship with TSH.
      (1) An increase in FT_4/FT_3 should produce a decrease in TSH.
      (2) A decrease in FT_4/FT_3 should produce an increase in TSH.

B. Thyroid function tests

1. Total serum T_4 (Fig. 22-2A)
   a. Represents T_4 bound to TBG and free (unbound) T_4 (FT_4)
      (1) Figure 22-2A shows one third of TBG binding sites on two TBGs occupied by T_4.
          • Total of 6 T_4 bound to TBG
      (2) There are 4 FT_4.
      (3) The total serum T_4 is 10.
      (4) TSH is normal, because FT_4 is normal.

   Total serum T_4: T_4 bound to TBG + FT_4

   b. Increase in TBG synthesis increases total serum T_4 (see Fig. 22-2B).
      (1) Estrogen increases the synthesis of TBG.
          • Pregnancy, oral contraceptive pill, hormone replacement
      (2) Extra TBG automatically has one third of its binding sites occupied by T_4.

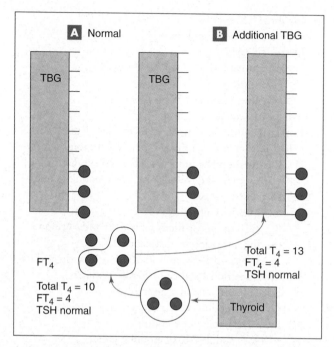

22-2: *Schematic of total serum thyroxine (T₄) in a normal individual (A) and an individual with an increase in thyroid-binding globulin (TBG) (B). The actual numbers do not represent the true concentration of T₄ and free T₄ (FT₄). The bars represent TBG and the circles are T₄ bound to TBG and T₄ that is free (FT₄). FT₄ normally has a negative feedback with thyroid-stimulating hormone (TSH). Refer to the text for a complete discussion. (From Goljan EF: Star Series: Pathology. Philadelphia, WB Saunders, 1998, Fig. 19-1.)*

- Total of 9 T_4 bound to TBG
  - (3) The 3 T_4 used to bind to the extra TBG is replaced by 3 T_4 released from the thyroid gland.
  - (4) FT_4 remains normal (4).
  - (5) Total serum T_4 is increased (9 + 4 = 13).
  - (6) TSH is normal, because FT_4 is normal.
  - (7) *No* signs of thyrotoxicosis are present.
  - c. Decrease in TBG synthesis decreases total serum T_4.
    - (1) Causes of a decreased TBG
      - Anabolic steroids, nephrotic syndrome (urinary loss)
    - (2) Total serum T_4 is decreased.
    - (3) FT_4 and TSH remain normal.
    - (4) *No* signs of hypothyroidism
  - d. Normal TBG with increase or decrease in total serum T_4
    - (1) Increase or decrease in FT_4 must be present.
    - (2) Increased FT_4—Graves' disease, thyroiditis
    - (3) Decreased FT_4—hypothyroidism
  2. Serum TSH
    - a. Best overall screening test for thyroid function

Alterations in TBG: alter total serum T_4; no effect on FT_4 and TSH

b. Increased TSH
- Primary hypothyroidism

c. Decreased TSH
  (1) Thyrotoxicosis (e.g., Graves' disease)
  (2) Hypopituitarism
    - Causes secondary hypothyroidism

3. ^{131}I radioactive uptake

  a. Evaluates synthetic activity of the thyroid gland
    - Iodide is used to synthesize thyroid hormone.
    (1) Increased uptake indicates increased synthesis of T_4.
      - Examples—Graves' disease, toxic nodular goiter
    (2) Decreased uptake
      (a) Inactivity of the gland
        - Example—patient taking thyroid hormone
      (b) Inflammation of the gland
        - Example—acute/subacute/chronic thyroiditis

  b. Evaluates functional status of thyroid nodules
    (1) Decreased uptake in a nodule
      - "Cold" nodule—cyst, cancer
    (2) Increased uptake in a nodule
      - "Hot" nodule—toxic nodular goiter

4. Thyroglobulin
- Marker for thyroid cancer

C. Lingual thyroid

1. Failed descent of thyroid anlage from the base of the tongue
- Usually represents all of the thyroid tissue

2. Clinical findings
  a. Dysphagia for solids
  b. Mass lesion

3. ^{131}I scan locates the lesion
- Also identifies any other thyroid tissue that is present

D. Thyroglossal duct cyst
- Cystic midline mass that is close to or within the hyoid bone

E. Thyroiditis

1. Acute thyroiditis
  a. Bacterial infection (e.g., *Staphylococcus aureus*)
  b. Clinical findings
    (1) Fever
    (2) Tender gland with painful cervical adenopathy
    (3) Initial thyrotoxicosis from gland destruction
      - Increased serum T_4, decreased serum TSH
    (4) Permanent hypothyroidism is uncommon.
  c. Decreased ^{131}I uptake

2. Subacute granulomatous thyroiditis
  a. Viral infection (e.g., coxsackievirus)
  b. Occurs most often in women 40 to 50 years old
  c. Granulomatous inflammation with multinucleated giant cells

Mass at base of the tongue: lingual thyroid

Branchial cleft cyst: located in the anterolateral neck

Subacute granulomatous thyroiditis: most common cause of painful thyroid

   d. Clinical findings
      (1) Most common cause of a painful thyroid gland
      (2) Often preceded by an upper respiratory infection
      (3) Cervical adenopathy is *not* prominent.
      (4) Initial thyrotoxicosis from gland destruction
         • Increased serum T_4, decreased serum TSH
      (5) Permanent hypothyroidism is uncommon.
   e. Decreased ^{131}I uptake
3. Hashimoto's thyroiditis
   a. Autoimmune thyroiditis
      (1) HLA-Dr3 and Dr5 association
      (2) Cytotoxic T cells destroy parenchyma.
         • Initial thyrotoxicosis, eventual hypothyroidism
      (3) Blocking IgG autoantibodies against the TSH receptor
         • Decrease hormone synthesis
      (4) Antimicrosomal and thyroglobulin antibodies
         • Develop as a *result* of gland injury
   b. Enlarged, gray gland
      • Lymphocytic infiltrate with prominent germinal follicles
   c. Clinical findings
      (1) Most common cause of primary hypothyroidism
      (2) Initial thyrotoxicosis from gland destruction
         • Called Hashitoxicosis
      (3) Signs of hypothyroidism (see below)
      (4) Risk factor for primary B-cell malignant lymphoma of the thyroid
4. Reidel's thyroiditis
   a. Fibrous tissue replacement of the gland
   b. Extension of fibrosis into surrounding tissue
      • Can produce tracheal obstruction
   c. Associated with other sclerosing conditions
      • Example—sclerosing mediastinitis
   d. Hypothyroidism may occur.
5. Subacute painless lymphocytic thyroiditis
   a. Autoimmune disease that develops postpartum
   b. Gland lacks germinal follicles.
   c. Clinical findings
      (1) Abrupt onset of thyrotoxicosis due to gland destruction
      (2) Gland is slightly enlarged and painless.
      (3) Progresses to primary hypothyroidism in 40% to 50% of cases
      (4) Lacks immunologic markers seen in Hashimoto's thyroiditis

F. Hypothyroidism
   1. Reduced secretion of thyroid hormone
      a. Patients are hypometabolic.
      b. Decrease in the basal metabolic rate
   2. Causes
      a. Hashimoto's thyroiditis

Hashimoto's thyroiditis: most common cause of hypothyroidism

Reidel's thyroiditis: fibrous tissue replacement of gland and surrounding tissue

Subacute painless lymphocytic thyroiditis: develops postpartum

b. Subacute painless lymphocytic thyroiditis

c. Hypopituitarism, iodine deficiency, enzyme deficiency

3. Cretinism

a. Hypothyroidism in infancy or early childhood

b. Brain requires thyroxine for its maturation.

c. Causes

(1) Maternal hypothyroidism
  - *Before* the fetal thyroid is developed

(2) Enzyme or iodine deficiency

d. Clinical findings

(1) Severe mental retardation

(2) Increased weight and short stature
  - Pituitary dwarfism—decreased weight and short stature

4. Clinical findings in adult hypothyroidism

a. Proximal muscle myopathy

(1) Very common finding

(2) Increased serum creatine kinase

b. Weight gain
  - Due to hypometabolic state with retention of water and salt

c. Dry and brittle hair, coarse yellow skin
  - Yellow skin due to less conversion of β-carotenes into retinoic acid

d. Periorbital puffiness, hoarse voice, myxedema (Fig. 22-3)

e. Fatigue, cold intolerance, constipation

f. Diastolic hypertension
  - Due to retention of sodium and water

g. Congestive (dilated) cardiomyopathy with biventricular heart failure

h. Atherosclerotic coronary artery disease

i. Delayed recovery of Achilles reflex, mental slowness, dementia

5. Laboratory findings

a. Decreased serum T_4, increased serum TSH

b. Antimicrosomal and antithyroglobulin antibodies
  - Present in Hashimoto's thyroiditis

c. Hypercholesterolemia
  - Due to decreased synthesis of low-density lipoprotein (LDL) receptors

6. Treatment

a. Levothyroxine

b. Bring serum TSH into the normal range

G. Thyroid hormone excess

1. Classification

a. Thyrotoxicosis
  - Describes hormone excess regardless of cause

b. Hyperthyroidism

(1) Describes hormone excess due to increased synthesis

(2) Examples—Graves' disease, toxic nodular goiter

2. Patients are hypermetabolic.
  - Increase in the basal metabolic rate

Cretinism: most often caused by maternal hypothyroidism

Primary hypothyroidism: ↓ serum T_4, ↑ serum TSH

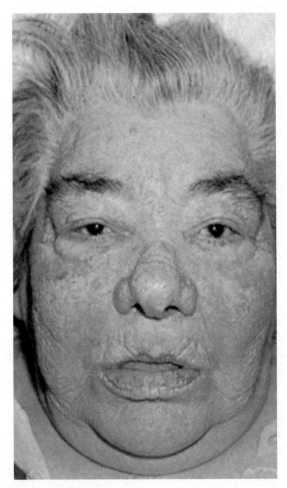

22-3: *Primary hypothyroidism in a patient with Hashimoto's thyroiditis. The patient has a puffy face, particularly around the eyes, and coarse hair. (From Forbes C, Jackson W: Color Atlas and Text of Clinical Medicine, 2nd ed. St. Louis, Mosby, 2003, p 325, Fig. 7-72.)*

3. Graves' disease
    a. Most common cause of hyperthyroidism and thyrotoxicosis
    b. Female dominant autoimmune disease
        (1) HLA-Dr3 association
        (2) Thyroid-stimulating (IgG) antibodies against TSH receptor
            (a) Causes hyperthyroidism
            (b) Type II hypersensitivity reaction
        (3) Antimicrosomal and thyroglobulin antibodies are present.
        (4) Inciting events that may initiate onset of the disease
            • Infection, withdrawal of steroids, iodide excess, postpartum
    c. Symmetrical, nontender thyromegaly
        (1) Scant colloid
        (2) Papillary infolding of the glands

Graves' disease: anti-TSH receptor antibody, type II hypersensitivity

498 PATHOLOGY

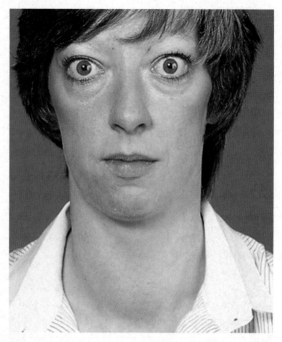

22-4: *Graves' disease. The patient has exophthalmos and a diffuse enlargement of the thyroid gland (goiter). (From Forbes C, Jackson W: Color Atlas and Text of Clinical Medicine, 2nd ed. St. Louis, Mosby, 2003, p 323, Fig. 7-61.)*

Exophthalmos: proptosis of eye; unique to Graves' disease

Atrial fibrillation: always order a TSH test to rule out hyperthyroidism

  d. Clinical features unique to Graves' disease
    (1) Infiltrative ophthalmopathy (exophthalmos)
      (a) Proptosis and muscle weakness of the eye (Fig. 22-4)
      (b) Due to adipose and glycosaminoglycans deposited in orbital tissue
    (2) Pretibial myxedema
      • Due to excess glycosaminoglycans in the dermis
4. Graves' disease in the elderly (apathetic hyperthyroidism)
    a. Cardiac abnormalities
      • Atrial fibrillation, congestive heart failure
    b. Muscle weakness, apathy
    c. Thyromegaly
5. Toxic multinodular goiter (Plummer's disease)
    a. One or more nodules in a multinodular goiter become TSH-independent.
    b. Distinctions from Graves' disease
      • *Lack* exophthalmos and pretibial myxedema
6. Clinical findings in all causes of thyrotoxicosis
    a. Constitutional signs
      (1) Weight loss (good appetite)
      (2) Fine tremor of the hands

(3) Heat intolerance, diarrhea, anxiety
(4) Lid stare
  • Due to increased sympathetic stimulation of eyelid muscles
  b. Cardiac findings
  (1) Sinus tachycardia
  (2) Increased risk for atrial fibrillation
  (3) Systolic hypertension, high-output heart failure
    (a) Thyroid hormone increases β-receptor synthesis in the heart.
    (b) Excess hormone increases inotropic and chronotropic effect on the heart.
  c. Brisk reflexes, osteoporosis (increased bone turnover)
7. Laboratory findings
  a. Increased serum T_4, decreased serum TSH
  b. Increased ^{131}I uptake
    • Graves' disease and toxic multinodular goiter
  c. Decreased ^{131}I uptake
    • Thyroiditis, patient taking excess thyroid hormone
  d. Hyperglycemia
    • Increased glycogenolysis
  e. Hypocholesterolemia
    • Increased LDL receptor synthesis
  f. Hypercalcemia
    • Increased bone turnover
  g. Absolute lymphocytosis
8. Treatment of Graves' disease
  a. β-Blockers decrease adrenergic effects.
  b. Thionamides decrease hormone synthesis.

H. Summary of laboratory findings in thyroid disorders (Table 22-2)
I. Nontoxic goiter
1. Thyroid enlargement from excess colloid
2. Types of goiter
  a. Endemic type
    • Due to iodide deficiency (most common)
  b. Sporadic type
    • Due to goitrogens (e.g., cabbage), enzyme deficiency, puberty, pregnancy
3. Pathogenesis
  a. Absolute or relative deficiency of thyroid hormone
  b. Hyperplasia/hypertrophy
    • Attempt to increase hormone synthesis
  c. Hyperplasia/hypertrophy is followed by gland involution.
    • Failure of gland to sustain synthesis
  d. Initial diffuse thyromegaly is followed by multinodular goiter
4. Complications
  a. Hemorrhage into cyst
    • Produces sudden, painful, gland enlargement
  b. Primary hypothyroidism

Graves' hyperthyroidism: ↑ serum T_4, ↑ ^{131}I uptake, ↓ serum TSH

Treatment for Graves' disease: β-blockers, thionamides

Nontoxic goiter: absolute or relative deficiency of thyroid hormone

**TABLE 22-2:
Laboratory
Findings in Thyroid
Disease**

Disorder	Serum T$_4$	Free T$_4$	Serum TSH	^{131}I Uptake
Graves' disease	↑	↑	↓	↑
Patient taking excess hormone	↑	↑	↓	↓
Initial phase of thyroiditis	↑	↑	↓	↓
Primary hypothyroidism	↓	↓	↑	↔
Secondary hypothyroidism (hypopituitarism)	↓	↓	↓	↔
Increased TBG (e.g., excess estrogen)	↑	Normal	Normal	↔
Decreased TBG (e.g., anabolic steroids)	↓	Normal	Normal	↔

T$_4$, thyroxine; TBG, thyroid-binding globulin; TSH, thyroid-stimulating hormone; ↔, not indicated.

   c. Toxic nodular goiter
      • One or more nodules become TSH-independent.
   d. Hoarseness (compresses laryngeal nerve)
   e. Dyspnea (compresses trachea)
5. Treatment
      • Levothyroxine reduces gland size and achieves the euthyroid state.

J. Solitary thyroid nodule
   1. Majority are cold nodules.
   2. Causes in adult women
      a. Majority are cysts in a goiter or a follicular adenoma.
      b. Approximately 15% are malignant.
   3. Causes in adult men and children
      • Similar to women, but there is a greater chance of malignancy
   4. Prior history of radiation to head and neck
      • Nodule is more likely to be malignant.

K. Benign and malignant tumors
   1. Follicular adenoma
      a. Most common benign tumor
         • Surrounded by a complete capsule
      b. "Cold" nodule
      c. Approximately 10% progress into a follicular carcinoma.
   2. Papillary adenocarcinoma
      a. Epidemiology
         (1) Most common primary cancer in adults and children
         (2) Female dominant
         (3) Associated with radiation exposure
      b. Gross and microscopic findings
         (1) Usually multifocal
         (2) Papillary fronds intermixed with follicles
         (3) Psammoma bodies
            • Dystrophically calcified cancer cells (Fig. 22-5)

First step in management
of thyroid nodule: fine
needle aspiration

Papillary carcinoma:
most common cancer;
psammoma bodies

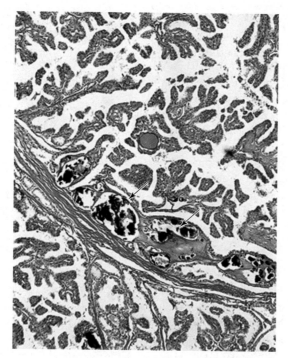

22-5: *Papillary carcinoma of thyroid showing branching papillae and blue concretions* (arrows) *representing psammoma bodies. (From Damjanov I, Linder J: Pathology: A Color Atlas. St. Louis, Mosby, 2000, p 191, Fig. 10-27.)*

        (4) Empty-appearing nuclei
           • Called Orphan Annie nuclei
        (5) Lymphatic invasion
    c. Metastasize to cervical nodes, lung
    d. Good prognosis
  3. Follicular carcinoma
    a. Epidemiology
        (1) Most common thyroid cancer presenting as a solitary cold nodule
        (2) Female dominant cancer
    b. Gross and microscopic findings
        (1) Encapsulated or invasive
        (2) Neoplastic follicles invade blood vessels.
        (3) Lymph node metastasis is uncommon.
    c. Metastasize to lung and bone
    d. Intermediate prognosis
  4. Medullary carcinoma
    a. Types
        (1) Sporadic (80% of cases)
        (2) Familial (20% of cases)
    b. Familial type
        (1) Associated with autosomal dominant MEN IIa/IIb

> Follicular carcinoma: hematogenous rather than lymphatic spread

(2) MEN IIa syndrome
- Medullary carcinoma, hyperparathyroidism, pheochromocytoma
(3) MEN IIb (III) syndrome
- Medullary carcinoma, mucosal neuromas (lips/tongue), pheochromocytoma

c. Tumors derive from parafollicular C cells.

Medullary carcinoma: derives from C cells; calcitonin is tumor marker

    (1) C cells synthesize calcitonin.
        (a) Tumor marker
        (b) May produce hypocalcemia
        (c) Converted into amyloid
    (2) C-cell hyperplasia is a precursor lesion.
      - Calcitonin levels increase with infusion of pentagastrin.
    (3) Genetic testing for familial cases
      - Detection of mutation of *RET* proto-oncogene

Medullary carcinoma: calcitonin is converted into amyloid

    (4) Familial type has a better prognosis than sporadic type.
    (5) Ectopic hormones
      - ACTH, which can produce Cushing syndrome

5. Primary B-cell malignant lymphoma
- Most often develop from Hashimoto's thyroiditis
6. Anaplastic thyroid cancer
  a. Most often occurs in elderly women
  b. Risk factors
    - Multinodular goiter, history of follicular cancer
  c. Rapidly aggressive and uniformly fatal

VI. Parathyroid Gland Disorders
  A. Clinical anatomy and physiology
    1. Superior and inferior parathyroid glands
      - Derive from fourth pharyngeal pouch and third pharyngeal pouch, respectively
    2. Parathyroid hormone (PTH)
      a. Increases calcium reabsorption in the early distal tubule
      b. Decreases bicarbonate reclamation in the proximal tubule
      c. Decreases phosphorus reabsorption in the proximal tubule
      d. Maintains ionized calcium level in blood
        - Increases bone resorption and renal reabsorption of calcium
      e. Stimulated by hypocalcemia and hyperphosphatemia
      f. Suppressed by hypercalcemia and hypophosphatemia

Total serum calcium: calcium bound + calcium free (ionized)

    3. Total serum calcium
      a. Components of the total serum calcium (Fig. 22-6A)
        (1) Calcium bound to albumin (40%) and phosphorus and citrate (13%)

Hypoalbuminemia: ↓ total serum calcium, normal ionized calcium

        (2) Free, ionized calcium (47%)
          - Metabolically active fraction has a negative feedback with PTH.

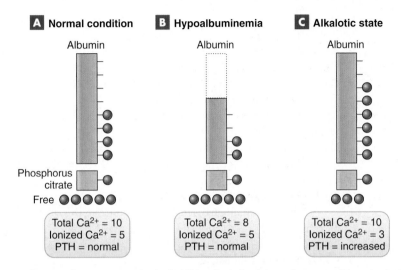

22-6: *Total serum calcium in a normal individual (**A**), individual with hypoalbuminemia (**B**), and individual with alkalosis (**C**). Refer to the text for discussion. PTH, parathyroid hormone.*

b. Hypoalbuminemia (Fig. 22-6B)
   (1) Decreased total serum calcium
       • Due to a decrease in calcium bound to albumin
   (2) Normal free ionized level, normal PTH
   (3) *No* evidence of tetany
c. Effect of respiratory or metabolic alkalosis (see Fig. 22-6C)
   (1) Increases negative charges on albumin
       (a) Due to fewer hydrogen ions on the COOH groups of acidic amino acids
           • Change of COOH groups to COO⁻
       (b) Extra negative charges bind some of the ionized calcium (arrows in schematic).
   (2) Total serum calcium remains normal.
   (3) Decreased ionized calcium, increased PTH
   (4) Patient develops tetany.
d. Tetany is due to a decreased ionized calcium level.
   (1) Causes partial depolarization of nerves and muscle
       (a) Lowers the threshold potential (E_t)
           • Comes closer to the resting membrane potential (E_m)
       (b) A smaller stimulus is required to initiate an action potential.
   (2) Clinical findings of tetany
       (a) Carpopedal spasm
           • Thumb flexes into the palm.
       (b) Chvostek's sign
           • Facial twitch after tapping the facial nerve

B. Hypoparathyroidism
   • Hypofunction of the parathyroid glands leads to hypocalcemia.

Alkalosis: normal total serum calcium, decreased ionized calcium

1. Causes
   a. Previous thyroid surgery (most common cause)
   b. Autoimmune hypoparathyroidism
   c. DiGeorge syndrome
      (1) Failure of descent of third and fourth pharyngeal pouches
         • Absence of parathyroid glands
      (2) Absent thymus (pure T-cell deficiency)
   d. Hypomagnesemia
      (1) Magnesium is a cofactor for adenylate cyclase.
         • Cyclic adenosine monophosphate (cAMP) is required for PTH activation.
      (2) Causes of hypomagnesemia
         • Diarrhea, aminoglycosides, diuretics, alcoholism
2. Clinical findings
   a. Tetany
   b. Calcification of basal ganglia
      (1) Due to metastatic calcification
      (2) Increased phosphorus drives calcium into the brain tissue.
   c. Cataracts, *Candida* infections (? cause)
3. Laboratory findings
   • Hypocalcemia, hyperphosphatemia, decreased PTH
4. Other causes of hypocalcemia (Table 22-3)

C. Primary hyperparathyroidism (HPTH)
   1. Most common nonmalignant cause of hypercalcemia
   2. Female dominant (>50 years old)
   3. Association with MEN I and MEN IIa

Hypomagnesemia: most common pathologic cause of hypocalcemia in the hospital

Chronic renal failure: most common cause of hypocalcemia; causes hypovitaminosis D

TABLE 22-3: Other Causes of Hypocalcemia

Disorder	Comments
Acute pancreatitis	Calcium is bound to fatty acids in enzymatic fat necrosis Poor prognostic sign
Hypovitaminosis D	Lack of sunlight: decreased photoconversion of cholesterol to vitamin D in the skin Malabsorption (e.g., celiac disease): decreased reabsorption of fat soluble vitamin D Cirrhosis: decreased synthesis of 25-hydroxyvitamin D (decreased 25-hydroxylation) Drugs enhancing cytochrome system (e.g., alcohol, phenytoin): increased metabolism of precursor vitamin D Chronic renal failure: decreased synthesis of 1,25-hydroxyvitamin D (decreased 1-α-hydroxylation)
Pseudohypoparathyroidism	autosomal dominant disease End-organ resistance to PTH Mental retardation, basal ganglia calcification, short fourth and fifth metacarpals ("knuckle-knuckle-dimple-dimple" sign) Hypocalcemia, normal to increased PTH

PTH, parathyroid hormone.

4. Causes
   a. Adenoma (85% of cases)
      (1) Sheets of chief cells with *no* intervening adipose
      (2) Remainder of the gland plus all other glands show atrophy.
         • Hypercalcemia suppresses PTH produced from normal tissue.
      (3) Right inferior parathyroid gland is most often involved.
   b. Primary hyperplasia
      (1) All four glands are involved.
      (2) Usually a chief cell hyperplasia
      (3) Clear cell hyperplasia (wasserhelle cell hyperplasia)
         • Associated with markedly increased serum calcium levels
   c. Carcinoma (uncommon)
5. Clinical findings
   a. Renal
      (1) Calcium stones
         • Most common presentation.
      (2) Nephrocalcinosis (see Chapters 1 and 19)
         • Causes polyuria and renal failure
   b. Gastrointestinal
      (1) Peptic ulcer disease
         • Calcium stimulates gastrin, which increases gastric acid.
      (2) Acute pancreatitis
         • Calcium activates phospholipase.
      (3) Constipation
   c. Bone
      (1) Osteitis fibrosa cystica
         (a) Cystic and hemorrhagic bone lesion
            • Caused by increased osteoclastic activity
         (b) Commonly involves the jaw
      (2) Radiographic findings
         (a) Subperiosteal bone resorption of phalanges and tooth sockets
         (b) "Salt and pepper" appearance of the skull
   d. Diastolic hypertension
      • Due to hypercalcemia
   e. Eyes
      (1) Band keratopathy in the limbus of the eye
      (2) Due to metastatic calcification
6. Laboratory findings
   a. Increased serum PTH, increased calcium, decreased phosphorus
   b. Normal anion gap metabolic acidosis
      (1) Due to decreased proximal tubule reclamation of bicarbonate
      (2) Type II renal tubular acidosis (see Chapter 4)
   c. Chloride:phosphorus ratio above 33
      • Ratio below 29:1 *excludes* primary HPTH.
7. Diagnosis
   • Technetium-99m-sestamibi radionuclide scan

> Most common cause of primary HPTH: benign adenoma

> Malignancy: most common cause of hypercalcemia in the hospital

8. Treatment
  - Surgical removal of the adenoma
9. Other causes of hypercalcemia (Table 22-4)

D. Secondary hyperparathyroidism
1. Hyperplasia of all four parathyroid glands
    a. Compensation for hypocalcemia
    b. Example—hypovitaminosis D due to renal failure and malabsorption
2. Decreased calcium, increased PTH
3. May develop tertiary hyperparathyroidism
    a. Glands become resistant to the hypocalcemic stimulus.
    b. May bring serum calcium into a normal or increased range

E. Phosphorus disorders
1. Causes of hypophosphatemia (Table 22-5)
2. Clinical findings in hypophosphatemia
    a. Muscle weakness
      (1) Decreased synthesis of ATP causes muscle weakness.
      (2) Muscle paralysis and rhabdomyolysis may occur.

Secondary HPTH: compensation for hypocalcemia

TABLE 22-4:
Other Causes of Hypercalcemia

Disorder	Comments
Hypervitaminosis D	Increased calcium reabsorption in the jejunum and kidneys
Malignancy-induced	Mechanisms: bone metastasis with activation of osteoclasts (most common), ectopic secretion of a PTH-related protein (squamous cell carcinoma of lung, renal cell carcinoma) Multiple myeloma: increased secretion of osteoclast-activating factor (IL-1) by malignant plasma cells Laboratory findings: hypercalcemia with decreased serum PTH
Sarcoidosis	Mechanism: macrophages in granulomas synthesize 1-α-hydroxylase, causing hypervitaminosis D
Thiazides	Mechanism: volume depletion increases renal tubule reabsorption of calcium

IL, interleukin; PTH, parathyroid hormone.

TABLE 22-5:
Causes of Hypophosphatemia

Disorder	Comments
Hypovitaminosis D (extrarenal causes)	Decreased reabsorption of phosphorus from the small intestine and kidneys
Insulin Rx in DKA	Increased uptake of glucose into cells requires phosphorus for phosphorylation
Primary HPTH	Increased PTH decreases phosphorus reabsorption in the proximal tubules
Respiratory/metabolic alkalosis	Alkalosis activates phosphofructokinase, the rate-limiting reaction of glycolysis, causing increased phosphorylation of glucose
Vitamin D–resistant rickets	X-linked dominant disorder Defect in renal and gastrointestinal reabsorption of phosphorus

DKA, diabetic ketoacidosis; HPTH, hyperparathyroidism; PTH, parathyroid hormone; Rx, treatment.

Disorder/Condition	Comments
Chronic renal failure	Decreased excretion of phosphorus as titratable acid
Normal child	Children require increased serum phosphorus to drive calcium into bone for mineralization
Primary hypoparathyroidism	Decreased excretion of phosphorus as titratable acid

TABLE 22-6:
Causes of Hyperphosphatemia

Disorder	Serum Calcium	Serum Phosphorus	Serum PTH
Primary hypoparathyroidism	↓	↑	↓
Vitamin D deficiency: e.g., renal failure	↓	↑	↑
Vitamin D deficiency: e.g., malabsorption	↓	↓	↑
Primary HPTH	↑	↓	↑
Malignancy-induced hypercalcemia	↑	↑	↓

TABLE 22-7:
Summary of Calcium and Phosphorus Disorders

HPTH, hyperparathyroidism; PTH, parathyroid hormone.

   b. Red blood cell (RBC) hemolysis
      • RBCs require ATP to maintain pumps and membrane integrity.
3. Causes of hyperphosphatemia (Table 22-6)
4. Clinical finding in hyperphosphatemia
   a. Metastatic calcification
      • Excess phosphorus drives calcium into normal tissue
   b. Hypovitaminosis D
      • Hyperphosphatemia inhibits the synthesis of 1-α-hydroxylase.
F. **Summary of laboratory findings in calcium and phosphorus disorders (Table 22-7)**

VII. **Adrenal Gland Disorders**
   A. **Adrenal cortex hormones (Fig. 22-7)**
      1. Zona glomerulosa produces mineralocorticoids (e.g., aldosterone).
      2. Zona fasciculata produces glucocorticoids.
         • 11-Deoxycortisol and cortisol are 17-hydroxycorticoids (17-OH).
      3. Zona reticularis produces sex hormones.
         a. 17-Ketosteroids (17-KS)
            • Dehydroepiandrosterone (DHEA) and androstenedione
         b. Testosterone
            • Converted to dihydrotestosterone (DHT) by 5α-reductase
   B. **Adrenal medulla**
      1. Neural crest origin
      2. Produces catecholamines
         • Epinephrine (EPI) and norepinephrine (NOR)

Insulin therapy: danger of developing hypophosphatemia

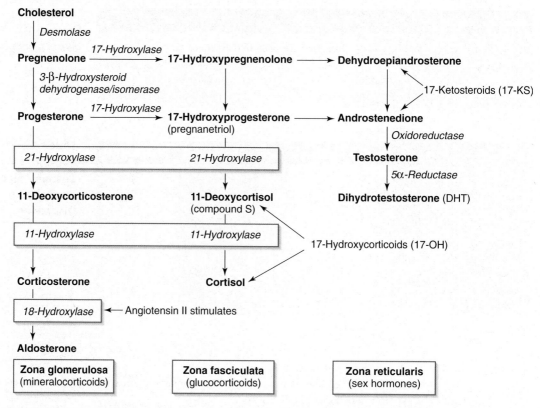

22-7: *Adrenocortical hormone synthesis. The zona glomerulosa produces mineralocorticoids (e.g., aldosterone), the zona fasciculata produces glucocorticoids (e.g., cortisol), and the zona reticularis produces sex hormones (e.g., testosterone). The 17-hydroxycorticoids (17-OH) are 11-deoxycortisol and cortisol. The 17-ketosteroids (17-KS, weak androgens) are dehydroepiandrosterone and androstenedione. Testosterone is converted to dihydrotestosterone (DHT) by 5α-reductase.*

3. Metabolic products of EPI and NOR
   - Metanephrine and vanillylmandelic acid (VMA)
4. Metabolic product of dopamine is homovanillic acid (HVA).

C. Adrenocortical hypofunction (primary hypocortisolism)

1. Acute adrenocortical insufficiency
   a. Causes
      (1) Abrupt withdrawal of corticosteroids
      (2) Waterhouse-Friderichsen syndrome (see below)
      (3) Anticoagulation therapy
   b. Waterhouse-Friderichsen syndrome
      (1) Usually associated with septicemia from *Neisseria meningitidis*
      (2) Patients develop endotoxic shock.
         - Release of tissue thromboplastin causes disseminated intravascular coagulation (DIC).
      (3) Bilateral adrenal hemorrhage
         - Fibrin clots in vessels cause hemorrhagic infarction.

Abrupt withdrawal of corticosteroids: most common cause of acute adrenocortical insufficiency

2. Chronic adrenal insufficiency (Addison's disease)
   a. Causes
      (1) Autoimmune destruction
         • Most common cause
      (2) Miliary tuberculosis/histoplasmosis
      (3) Adrenogenital syndrome (see below)
      (4) Metastasis
         • Most often from a primary lung cancer
   b. Clinical findings
      (1) Weakness and hypotension
         • Due to sodium loss from mineralocorticoid and glucocorticoid deficiency
      (2) Diffuse hyperpigmentation
         • Increased plasma ACTH stimulates melanocytes.
   c. Laboratory findings
      (1) Short and prolonged ACTH stimulation test
         • *No* increase in cortisol or 17-OH
      (2) Metyrapone test (see section IV)
         • Increased ACTH but *no* increase in 11-deoxycortisol
      (3) Increased plasma ACTH
      (4) Electrolyte findings (see Chapter 4)
         • Hyponatremia, hyperkalemia, and metabolic acidosis

   > Aldosterone enhances the exchange of sodium for potassium in the kidneys. Hence, its deficiency leads to a hypertonic loss of sodium in the urine (hyponatremia) and retention of potassium (hyperkalemia). Aldosterone also enhances the proton pump. Deficiency leads to retention of protons and metabolic acidosis (normal anion gap type).

      (5) Fasting hypoglycemia
         • Due to decrease in cortisol (cortisol is gluconeogenic)
      (6) Eosinophilia, lymphocytosis, and neutropenia
         • Due to decrease in cortisol (see Chapter 12)
3. Adrenogenital syndrome (see Fig. 22-7)
   a. Autosomal recessive disorders
   b. Enzyme deficiency causes hypocortisolism and corresponding increase in ACTH.
      (1) Increase in ACTH
         • Causes adrenocortical hyperplasia and diffuse skin pigmentation
      (2) Increase in 17-KS, testosterone, and DHT; causes:
         (a) Ambiguous genitalia in females
            • Primarily due to DHT
         (b) Precocious puberty in males
      (3) Increase in mineralocorticoids
         • Causes sodium retention leading to hypertension
      (4) Decrease in mineralocorticoids; causes:

Miliary TB: most common cause of Addison's disease in developing countries

Most common cause of Addison's disease in children: adrenogenital syndrome

21-Hydroxylase deficiency: most common adrenogenital syndrome

(a) Sodium loss (hyponatremia), hyperkalemia

(b) Hypotension

  c. Substrates proximal to the enzyme block increase.

  d. Substrates distal to the enzyme block decrease.

  e. 21-Hydroxylase deficiency

    (1) Most common enzyme deficiency (95% of cases)

    (2) Ambiguous genitalia in females

     • Increase in 17-KS, testosterone, and DHT

    (3) Precocious puberty in males

     • Increase in 17-KS, testosterone, and DHT

    (4) Hypotension

     • Sodium loss due to decrease in mineralocorticoids

    (5) Decrease in 17-OH

    (6) Increase in 17-hydroxyprogesterone

  f. 11-Hydroxylase deficiency

    (1) Ambiguous genitalia in females

     • Increase in 17-KS, testosterone, and DHT

    (2) Precocious puberty in males

     • Increase in 17-KS, testosterone, and DHT

    (3) Hypertension

     • Increase in mineralocorticoids (11-deoxycorticosterone)

    (4) Increase in 17-OH (11-deoxycortisol)

    (5) Increase in 17-hydroxyprogesterone

  g. 17-Hydroxylase deficiency

    (1) Hypogonadism in females

     (a) Decrease in 17-KS, testosterone, and DHT

     (b) Recall that estrogen comes from aromatization of androgens.

    (2) Male pseudohermaphroditism

     • Male external genitalia development requires DHT (see Chapter 5).

    (3) Hypertension

     • Due to sodium retention from increase in mineralocorticoids

    (4) Decrease in 17-OH and 17-hydroxyprogesterone

  h. Summary of adrenogenital syndrome (Table 22-8)

D. Adrenocortical hyperfunction

  1. Cushing syndrome

    a. Causes

     (1) Prolonged corticosteroid therapy

TABLE 22-8: Summary of Adrenogenital Syndromes

Laboratory	21-OHase Deficiency	11-OHase Deficiency	17-OHase Deficiency
17-Ketosteroids	↑	↑	↓
17-Hydroxyprogesterone	↑	↑	↓
17-Hydroxycorticoids	↓	↑	↓
Mineralocorticoids	↓	↑	↑

*OHase, hydroxylase.

- Most common cause
  - (2) Pituitary Cushing syndrome (Cushing disease)
    - (a) 60% of cases
    - (b) Due to a pituitary adenoma
    - (c) Increased ACTH and cortisol
  - (3) Adrenal Cushing syndrome
    - (a) 25% of cases
    - (b) Most often due to an adenoma
    - (c) Decreased ACTH and increased cortisol
  - (4) Ectopic Cushing syndrome
    - (a) 15% of cases
    - (b) Usually small cell carcinoma of lung
      - Ectopic ACTH production
    - (c) Markedly increased ACTH and cortisol
- b. Clinical findings
  - (1) Weight gain
    - (a) Due to hyperinsulinism from hyperglycemia
      - Insulin increases storage of fat (triglyceride) in adipose.
    - (b) Fat deposition in face ("moon facies"), upper back ("buffalo hump"), and trunk (truncal obesity) (Fig. 22-8)
  - (2) Muscle weakness
    - (a) Cortisol breaks down muscles in the extremities (thin extremities).
    - (b) Muscles supply amino acids (e.g., alanine) for gluconeogenesis.
  - (3) Diastolic hypertension
    - (a) Due to increase in weak mineralocorticoids and glucocorticoids
    - (b) Aldosterone is *not* increased (requires angiotensin II)
  - (4) Hirsutism
    - Due to increased androgens
  - (5) Purple abdominal stria
    - Cortisol weakens collagen, causing rupture of blood vessels in stretch marks.
  - (6) Osteoporosis
    - Hypercortisolism causes increased breakdown of bone.
- c. Laboratory findings
  - (1) Increased urine for free cortisol
    - Very high positive and negative predictive value
  - (2) Low-dose dexamethasone (cortisol analogue) suppression test
    - *Cannot* suppress cortisol in all types
  - (3) High-dose dexamethasone suppression test
    - Can suppress cortisol in pituitary Cushing syndrome but *not* the other types
  - (4) Hyperglycemia
    - Cortisol enhances gluconeogenesis.

Cushing syndrome: truncal obesity, thin extremities, purple stria

Pituitary Cushing syndrome: suppression of cortisol by high-dose dexamethasone

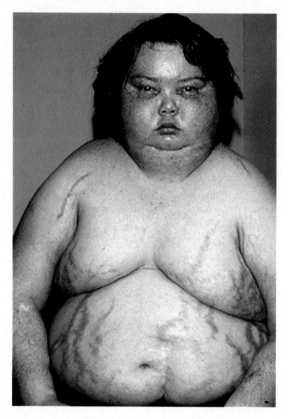

22-8: *Patient with Cushing syndrome, showing "moon facies," truncal obesity, and purple abdominal striae. (From Damjanov I: Pathology for the Health-Related Professions, 2nd ed. Philadelphia, WB Saunders, 2000, p 426.)*

        (5) Hypokalemic metabolic alkalosis
          • Due to increased weak mineralocorticoids
    d. Nelson's syndrome
        (1) Bilateral adrenalectomy causes enlargement of a preexisting pituitary adenoma.
          • Sudden drop in cortisol causes an increase in synthesis of ACTH.
        (2) Clinical findings of headache and diffuse hyperpigmentation
    e. Summary of Cushing syndrome (Table 22-9)
  2. Hyperaldosteronism
    a. Primary aldosteronism (Conn's syndrome)
        (1) Most often due to a benign adenoma in the zona glomerulosa
        (2) Clinical findings
          (a) Diastolic hypertension
          (b) Muscle weakness, tetany (from metabolic alkalosis)
        (3) Laboratory findings (see Chapter 4)
          (a) Hypernatremia, hypokalemia, metabolic alkalosis
          (b) Decreased plasma renin activity

Primary hyperaldosteronism: hypertension, hypernatremia, hypokalemia, metabolic alkalosis

TABLE 22-9:
Summary of
Pituitary, Adrenal,
and Ectopic
Cushing Syndrome
(CS)

Laboratory Test	Pituitary CS	Adrenal CS	Ectopic CS
Serum cortisol	↑	↑	↑
Urine free cortisol	↑	↑	↑
Low-dose dexamethasone	Cortisol *not* suppressed	Cortisol *not* suppressed	Cortisol *not* suppressed
High-dose dexamethasone	Cortisol suppressed	Cortisol *not* suppressed	Cortisol *not* suppressed
Plasma adrenocorticotropic hormone (ACTH)	"Normal*" to ↑	↓	Markedly ↑

*"Normal": a plasma ACTH in the normal range is *not* normal in the presence of an increase in serum cortisol.

> In primary hyperaldosteronism, there is increased exchange of sodium (hypernatremia) for potassium (hypokalemia). Sodium exchanges with hydrogen ions when potassium is depleted, causing a loss of hydrogen ions in the urine and a corresponding increase in bicarbonate reabsorption (metabolic alkalosis). Hypernatremia increases plasma volume, which increases renal blood flow and inhibits plasma renin activity. Chronic retention of sodium produces hypertension. Hypokalemia produces muscle weakness.

   b. Secondary aldosteronism
     (1) Compensatory reaction related to a decrease in cardiac output
     (2) Decreased renal blood flow activates the renin-angiotensin-aldosterone system.
     (3) Plasma renin activity is increased.

E. Adrenal medulla hyperfunction
   • Increased production of catecholamines causes hypertension.
   1. Pheochromocytoma
     a. Unilateral (~90% of cases)
     b. Benign adenoma (~90% of cases)
     c. Arises in the adrenal medulla (~90% of cases)
      • Other sites—bladder, organ of Zuckerkandl near the bifurcation of the aorta, posterior mediastinum
     d. *N*-methyltransferase converts NOR to EPI.
      (1) Adrenal medulla and the organ of Zuckerkandl contain the enzyme.
       • Pheochromocytoma produces NOR and EPI.
      (2) Other sites lack the enzyme.
       • Pheochromocytoma produces only NOR.
     e. Associations
      (1) Neurofibromatosis
      (2) MEN IIa and IIb
      (3) Von Hippel–Lindau disease (often bilateral tumors)

f. Tumor characteristics
- Brown, hemorrhagic, and often necrotic

g. Clinical findings
  (1) Diastolic hypertension
     - Sustained with occasional paroxysmal bursts
  (2) Palpitations
     - *Not* present in essential hypertension
  (3) Anxiety
     - *Not* present in essential hypertension
  (4) Drenching sweats
     - *Not* present in essential hypertension
  (5) Headache, chest pain from subendocardial ischemia

h. Laboratory findings
  (1) Increased 24-hour urine for VMA and metanephrine
  (2) Hyperglycemia
     - Increased glycogenolysis and gluconeogenesis
  (3) Neutrophilic leukocytosis
     - Inhibition of neutrophil adhesion molecules

2. Neuroblastoma
  a. Malignant tumor
    (1) Most often occurs in children under 5 years old
    (2) Primarily located in the adrenal medulla
       - Occasionally located in the posterior mediastinum
    (3) Amplification of *N-MYC* oncogene (nuclear transcriber)
  b. "Small cell" tumor
    (1) Composed of malignant neuroblasts
    (2) Presence of Homer-Wright rosettes
       - Neuroblasts located around a central space
    (3) Electron microscopy shows neurosecretory granules.
  c. Clinical findings
    (1) Palpable abdominal mass
    (2) Diastolic hypertension
  d. Commonly metastasize to skin and bones
  e. Prognosis depends on age
     - Children under 1 year old have a good prognosis.
  f. Laboratory findings
     - Increased urine VMA, metanephrines, and HVA

VIII. Islet Cell Tumors (Table 22-10)
IX. Diabetes Mellitus
  A. Classification
    1. Type 1 and type 2 diabetes mellitus (Table 22-11)
    2. Secondary causes
      a. Pancreatic disease
        - Examples—cystic fibrosis, chronic pancreatitis
      b. Drugs
        - Examples—glucocorticoids, pentamidine, thiazides, α-interferon

---

Margin notes:

Unique findings in pheochromocytoma: palpitations, anxiety, drenching sweats

Neuroblastoma: abdominal mass + hypertension

TABLE 22-10:
Summary of Islet Cell Tumors

Tumor	Description
Glucagonoma	Malignant tumor of α-islet cells Clinical: hyperglycemia, rash (necrolytic migratory erythema)
Insulinoma	Benign tumor of β-islet cells; most common islet cell tumor; approximately 80% have MEN I syndrome Clinical: fasting hypoglycemia causing mental status abnormalities Laboratory: fasting hypoglycemia; increase in serum insulin and C peptide, which is an endogenous marker of insulin produced in β-islet cells Surreptitious injection of insulin: fasting hypoglycemia, increased insulin, *decreased* C peptide
Somatostatinoma	Malignant tumor of δ-islet cells; somatostatin is an inhibitory hormone Inhibition of gastrin causes achlorhydria Inhibition of cholecystokinin causes cholelithiasis and steatorrhea Inhibition of gastric inhibitory peptide causes diabetes mellitus Inhibition of secretin causes steatorrhea
VIPoma (pancreatic cholera)	Malignant tumor with excessive secretion of vasoactive intestinal peptide (VIP) Clinical: secretory diarrhea, achlorhydria Laboratory: hypokalemia, normal anion gap metabolic acidosis (loss of bicarbonate in stool)
Zollinger-Ellison (see Chapter 17)	Malignant islet cell tumor that secretes gastrin producing hyperacidity; MEN I association (20–30% of cases) Clinical: peptic ulceration, diarrhea, maldigestion of food Laboratory: serum gastrin > 1000 pg/mL

MEN, multiple endocrine neoplasia.

   c. Endocrine disease
- Examples—pheochromocytoma, glucagonoma, Cushing syndrome

   d. Genetic disease
- Examples—hemochromatosis, syndrome X, maturity onset diabetes of the young

   e. Insulin-receptor deficiency
- Acanthosis nigricans is a phenotypic marker.

   f. Infections
- Examples—mumps, cytomegalovirus (AIDS patients)

3. Impaired glucose tolerance (IGT)
4. Gestational diabetes mellitus (GDM)

B. Maturity onset diabetes of the young (MODY)

1. Autosomal dominant inheritance
2. Patients are under 25 years old and are *not* obese.
3. Mild hyperglycemia
- Impaired glucose-induced secretion of insulin release
4. Resistance to ketosis
5. May progress into type 2 diabetes mellitus

TABLE 22-11:
Comparison Between Types 1 and 2 Diabetes Mellitus

Characteristic	Type 1	Type 2
Prevalence	5–10%	90–95%
Age of onset	<20 years	>30 years
Speed of onset	Rapid	Insidious
Body habitus	Usually thin	Usually obese (80% of cases)
Genetics	Family history uncommon HLA-DR3 and HLA-DR4	Family history common No HLA association Increased in Native Americans and American blacks
Pathogenesis	Lack of insulin Pancreas devoid of β-islet cells Insulitis: T-cell cytokine destruction and autoantibodies against β-islet cells and insulin; triggers for destruction include viruses	Insulin resistance Decreased insulin receptors: downregulation by increased adipose tissue Postreceptor defects: most important factor; examples—tyrosine kinase defects, GLUT-4 abnormalities Fibrotic β-islet cells contain amyloid
Clinical findings	Polyuria, polydipsia, polyphagia, weight loss Ketoacidosis (hyperglycemia, coma; production of ketone bodies)	Insidious onset of symptoms Recurrent blurry vision: alteration in lens refraction from sorbitol Recurrent infections: bacterial, *Candida* Target organ disease: nephropathy, retinopathy, neuropathy, coronary artery disease Reactive hypoglycemia: too much insulin is released for a glucose load (early finding) HNKC: enough insulin to prevent ketoacidosis but not enough to prevent hyperglycemia; lactic acidosis may occur due to shock
Treatment	Insulin	Weight loss: upregulates insulin receptor synthesis Oral hypoglycemic agents; may require insulin

GLUT, glucose transport unit; HLA, human leukocyte antigen; HNKC, hyperosmolar nonketotic coma.

Syndrome X: insulin resistance exacerbated by obesity

C. Syndrome X (metabolic syndrome)
  1. Insulin resistance syndrome
     - Genetic defect causes insulin resistance that is exacerbated by obesity.
  2. Clinical findings
     a. Hyperinsulinemia:
        (1) Increased synthesis of VLDL (hypertriglyceridemia)
        (2) Hypertension
           - Increased insulin increases sodium retention by the renal tubules.

TABLE 22-12:
Complications of
Diabetes Mellitus

Complication	Discussion
Atherosclerotic disease	Increased incidence of strokes, CAD, and peripheral vascular disease Acute MI is the most common cause of death Gangrene of the lower extremities; diabetes is the most common cause of nontraumatic amputation of the lower extremity
Renal disorders	Renal failure due to nodular glomerulosclerosis Renal papillary necrosis
Ocular disorders	Increased risk for cataracts and glaucoma Retinopathy: microaneurysm formation; increased risk for retinal detachment and blindness; annual ophthalmologic examination is mandatory
Peripheral nerve disorders	Diabetes mellitus is the most common cause of peripheral neuropathy in the United States Sensory (paresthesias) and motor dysfunction (muscle weakness) Neuropathy is the most important risk factor for pressure ulcers on the bottom of the feet (cannot feel pain)
Autonomic nervous system disorders	Autonomic neuropathy: gastroparesis (delayed emptying of stomach), impotence, cardiac arrhythmias
Cranial nerve disorders	Diabetes is the most common cause of multiple cranial nerve palsies Cranial nerves most often involved: CNIII, IV, and VI
Infectious disorders	Urinary tract infections *Candida* infections: e.g., vulvovaginitis Malignant external otitis due to *Pseudomonas aeruginosa* Rhinocerebral mucormycosis: *Mucor* extends from the frontal sinuses to the frontal lobes producing infarction (vessel invader) and abscesses Cutaneous infections: usually *Staphylococcus aureus* abscesses
Skin disorders	Necrobiosis lipoidica diabeticorum: well-demarcated yellow plaques over the anterior surface of the legs/dorsum of ankles Lipoatrophy: atrophy at insulin injection sites due to impure insulin Lipohypertrophy: increased fat synthesis at insulin injection sites

CAD, coronary artery disease; MI, myocardial infarction.

(3) Coronary artery disease
  • Increased insulin damages endothelial cells.
  b. Obesity exacerbates insulin resistance.
  • Increased adipose downregulates insulin receptor synthesis.
D. Pathologic processes in diabetes mellitus (Table 22-12)
  1. Poor glycemic control
    a. Hyperglycemia is the key factor that produces organ damage.
    b. Glucose control reduces onset and severity of complications.
    • Complications are related to retinopathy, neuropathy, and nephropathy in descending order.
  2. Nonenzymatic glycosylation (NEG)
    a. Glucose combines with amino groups in proteins.

Good glycemic control prevents complications of diabetes.

b. Produces advanced glycosylation products
  (1) Increased vessel permeability to protein
  (2) Increased atherogenesis
c. Role in diabetes
  (1) Production of glycosylated HbA1c
  (2) Hyaline arteriolosclerosis (see Chapter 9)
  (3) Diabetic glomerulopathy (see Chapter 19)
  (4) Ischemic heart disease, strokes, peripheral vascular disease
3. Osmotic damage
  a. Aldose reductase
    (1) Converts glucose to sorbitol
    (2) Sorbitol draws water into tissue causing damage.
  b. Role in diabetes mellitus
    (1) Formation of cataracts
    (2) Peripheral neuropathy
      • Osmotic damage of Schwann cells produces demyelination.
    (3) Retinopathy
      • Osmotic damage to pericytes produces microaneurysms of retinal vessels.
4. Diabetic microangiopathy
  a. Increased synthesis of type IV collagen in basement membranes and mesangium
  b. Important in diabetic glomerulopathy (see Chapter 19)
E. Clinical findings
1. Insulin-induced hypoglycemia
  a. Most common complication
  b. Produces irreversible brain damage by destroying neurons
  c. Clinical findings
    (1) Sympathetic nervous system signs
      • Sweating, tachycardia, palpitations, and tremulousness
    (2) Parasympathetic nervous system signs
      • Nausea and hunger
    (3) Focal neurologic deficits, mental confusion, coma
2. Diabetic ketoacidosis (Fig. 22-9)
  a. Complication of type 1 diabetes
  b. Precipitated by medical illness or omission of insulin
  c. Produces severe volume depletion and coma
    • Volume depletion due to loss of sodium and water with osmotic diuresis
  d. Mechanisms for hyperglycemia
    (1) Increased gluconeogenesis
      (a) Due to increase in glucagon and epinephrine
      (b) Most important mechanism of hyperglycemia
    (2) Increased glycogenolysis in the liver
  e. Mechanism for ketone bodies
    (1) Increased lipolysis with release of fatty acids
      • *No* inhibition of hormone-sensitive lipase

Aldose reductase: converts glucose to sorbitol; osmotic damage

Insulin-induced hypoglycemia: most common complication of diabetes

Gluconeogenesis: most important mechanism of hyperglycemia in diabetic ketoacidosis

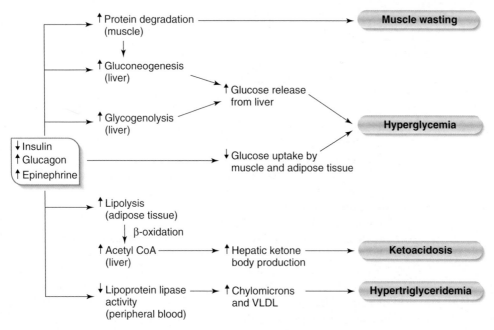

22-9: *Metabolic changes in diabetic ketoacidosis (DKA). Refer to the text for discussion. VLDL, very low-density lipoprotein. (From Pelley J, Goljan EF: Rapid Review: Biochemistry. St. Louis, Mosby, 2004, p 176, Fig. 9-5.)*

(2) Increased β-oxidation of fatty acids increases production of acetyl CoA.
  • *No* malonyl Co-A to inhibit carnitine acyltransferase, the rate-limiting enzyme of β-oxidation
(3) Acetyl CoA is converted by the liver to ketone bodies.
  • Acetone (fruity odor), acetoacetic and β-hydroxybutyric acid
f. Mechanism for hypertriglyceridemia
  (1) Lack of insulin decreases capillary lipoprotein lipase activity in peripheral blood.
  (2) Accumulation of chylomicrons and VLDL in the blood
    • Type V hyperlipoproteinemia (see Chapter 9)
  (3) May precipitate acute pancreatitis and eruptive xanthomas in the skin
    • Called the hyperchylomicronemia syndrome
g. Laboratory findings
  (1) Hyperglycemia
    • Glucose ranges from 250 to 1000 mg/dL.
  (2) Dilutional hyponatremia (see Chapter 4)
    (a) Glucose overrides sodium in controlling the osmotic gradient.
    (b) Water shifts out of the intracellular fluid compartment into the extracellular fluid compartment.

Ketoacids: synthesized from acetyl CoA derived from β-oxidation of fatty acids

       (3) Hyperkalemia (see Chapter 4)
- Transcellular shift as excess H^+ ions enter cells in exchange of potassium

       (4) Increased anion gap metabolic acidosis (see Chapter 4)
- Due to ketoacidosis and lactic acidosis

       (5) Prerenal azotemia (see Chapter 19)
- Due to volume depletion

  3. Hyperosmolar nonketotic coma (see Table 22-11)

    a. Complication of type 2 diabetes

    b. Increased mortality rate (20–50%)
- Patients are older and usually have underlying cardiac and renal problems.

F. Laboratory diagnosis

  1. Criteria

    a. Random plasma glucose at or above 200 mg/dL plus classic symptoms

    b. Fasting plasma glucose at or above 126 mg/dL
- Set for high sensitivity

    c. Two-hour glucose level after 75-g glucose challenge is at or above 200 mg/dL.

    d. One of the preceding three criteria must be present on a subsequent day to confirm the diagnosis of diabetes.

> HbA1c: marker long-term glycemic control

  2. Glycosylated hemoglobin (HbA1c)

    a. Evaluates long-term glycemic control

    b. Represents the mean glucose value for the preceding 8 to 12 weeks

    c. Test is *not* used to diagnose diabetes.

  3. Fructosamine
- Reflects glycemic control for the preceding 2 weeks

G. Impaired glucose tolerance

  1. Patient has hyperglycemia that is nondiagnostic of diabetes.

  2. Increased risk for macrovascular disease and neuropathy

  3. Approximately 30% develop diabetes within 10 years.

H. Gestational diabetes

  1. Glucose intolerance develops during pregnancy.
- Due to increased placental size and anti-insulin effect of human placental lactogen

  2. Screening

    a. All pregnant women are screened between 24 and 28 weeks' gestation.

    b. 50-g glucose challenge followed by 1-hour glucose level
- Above 140 mg/dL is a positive screen.

    c. Positive screen is confirmed with a 3-hour oral glucose tolerance test.

  3. Newborn risks

    a. Macrosomia

      (1) Hyperglycemia in the fetus causes release of insulin.

      (2) Insulin increases fat stored in adipose tissue.

      (3) Insulin increases muscle mass by increasing amino acid uptake in muscle.

    b. Respiratory distress syndrome
- Insulin inhibits fetal surfactant production.

    c. Increased risk for open neural tube defects

    d. Neonatal hypoglycemia
- High insulin levels at birth drives glucose into the hypoglycemic range (give newborn glucose after birth).

  4. Maternal risk
- Diabetes may develop at a later date.

X. Hypoglycemia

A. Reactive type of hypoglycemia

  1. Fed state hypoglycemia

  2. Causes

    a. Insulin treatment in type 1 diabetes

      (1) Most common cause

      (2) Sulfonylurea-related hypoglycemia is less common.

    b. IGT or type 2 diabetes
- Excessive amount of insulin is released for the glucose absorbed.

    c. Idiopathic postprandial syndrome

      (1) Lack of energy, mental dullness, chronic anxiety

      (2) Symptoms are *rarely* accompanied by hypoglycemia.

      (3) Treatment is frequent high-protein meals.

  3. Develop adrenergic symptoms ~1 to 5 hours after eating
- Sweating, trembling, anxiety

B. Fasting type of hypoglycemia

  1. Fasting state hypoglycemia

  2. Causes

    a. Alcohol

      (1) Increased NADH converts pyruvate to lactate.
- Less pyruvate for gluconeogenesis

      (2) Decreased glycogen stores in severe liver disease

    b. Renal failure
- Kidney is a site of gluconeogenesis.

    c. Malnutrition

    d. Chronic liver disease
- Decreased gluconeogenesis, glycogen depletion

    e. Insulinoma, hypopituitarism

    f. Ketotic hypoglycemia in childhood

      (1) Most common cause of hypoglycemia from 18 months to mid-childhood

      (2) Multiple etiologies
- Maple syrup urine disease, galactosemia, hereditary fructose intolerance, von Gierke's glycogen storage disease (see Chapter 5)

  3. Neuroglycopenic symptoms

    a. Dizziness, confusion, headache, inability to concentrate

    b. Motor disturbances, seizures, visual disturbances, coma

Musculoskeletal Disorders

I. Bone Disorders

A. Osteogenesis imperfecta ("brittle bone" disease)

1. Autosomal dominant
2. Defective synthesis of type I collagen
3. Clinical findings
   a. Pathologic fractures at birth
   b. Blue sclera, deafness

Blue sclera: reflection of underlying choroidal veins

B. Achondroplasia

1. Autosomal dominant
2. Impaired proliferation of cartilage at the growth plate
3. Clinical findings
   a. Normal-sized head and vertebral column
   b. Shortened arms and legs
   c. Normal growth hormone and insulin growth factor-1 levels

C. Osteopetrosis ("marble bone" disease)

1. Autosomal recessive (severe)
   • Autosomal dominant (less severe)
2. Defect in osteoclasts
   • Overgrowth and sclerosis of cortical bone ("too much bone")
3. Clinical findings
   a. Pathologic fractures
   b. Anemia
      • Replacement of marrow cavity
   c. Cranial nerve compression
      • Visual and hearing loss

Osteopetrosis: defect in osteoclasts; "too much bone"

D. Osteomyelitis

1. Osteomyelitis in children and adults
   a. Metaphysis is the most common site.
      • Hematogenous spread
   b. Most often due to *Staphylococcus aureus* (90% of cases)
      • Other pathogens: *Streptococcus pyogenes, Hemophilus influenzae*
   c. Neutrophils enzymatically destroy bone.
      • Devitalized bone is called sequestra.
   d. Chronic disease produces reactive bone formation in periosteum.
      • Called involucrum
   e. Draining sinus tracts to the skin surface
      • Danger of squamous cell carcinoma developing at orifice of sinus tract
   f. Clinical findings
      • Fever, bone pain

Staphylococcus aureus: most common pathogen causing osteomyelitis

2. Osteomyelitis in sickle cell disease
   - Due to *Salmonella paratyphi*
3. Tuberculous osteomyelitis
   a. Hematogenous spread from a primary lung focus
   b. Targets vertebral column (Pott's disease)
4. *Pseudomonas aeruginosa* osteomyelitis
   - Most often due to puncture of foot through rubber footwear

E. Osteoporosis
1. Most common metabolic abnormality of bone
   a. Loss of organic bone matrix and minerals
      (1) Decreased bone mass and density
      (2) Decreased thickness of cortical and trabecular bone
   b. Types of osteoporosis
      (1) Primary
         - Idiopathic, senile, postmenopausal
      (2) Secondary
         (a) Underlying disease (e.g., hypercortisolism)
         (b) Drugs (e.g., heparin)
         (c) Space travel
            - Lack of gravity reduces bone stress
2. Postmenopausal osteoporosis
   a. Due to estrogen deficiency
      (1) Increased resorption of bone by osteoclasts
      (2) Decreased formation of bone by osteoblasts
   b. Clinical findings
      (1) Compression fractures of vertebral bodies (Fig. 23-1)
      (2) Colles' fracture of distal radius
   c. Dual-photon absorptiometry
      - Noninvasive test that evaluates bone density
   d. Prevention
      (1) Role of estrogen replacement is being reevaluated.
      (2) Calcium and vitamin D supplements

P. aeruginosa osteomyelitis: puncture of foot through rubber footwear

Estrogen: inhibits production of osteoclasts; enhances osteoblasts

Postmenopausal osteoporosis: compression vertebral fractures most common

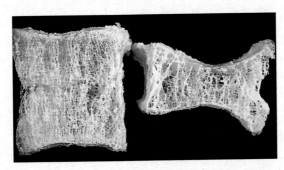

23-1: *Osteoporosis of vertebral column. The vertebral body on the right shows decreased bone mass caused by compression fractures when compared with a normal vertebral body on the left. (From Kumar V, Fausto N, Abbas A: Robbins and Cotran's Pathologic Basis of Disease, 7th ed. Philadelphia, WB Saunders, 2004, p 1284, Fig. 26-12.)*

(3) Weight-bearing exercise
  • Excludes swimming, which decreases bone stress
  e. Treatment
    (1) Bisphosphonates inhibit bone resorption.
    (2) Calcitonin inhibits osteoclasts.
3. Senile osteoporosis
  • Decreased ability of osteoblasts to divide and produce osteoid

F. Avascular (aseptic) necrosis of bone
1. Disruption of microcirculation causes bone infarctions.
  a. Femoral head
    (1) Fracture in elderly persons
    (2) Sickle cell disease
    (3) Long-term use of corticosteroids
  b. Scaphoid bone
  c. Digits
  • Dactylitis in sickle cell anemia
2. Bone shows increased density on radiographs.
  • MRI is the most sensitive test.
3. Osteochondrosis
  a. Aseptic necrosis of ossification centers in children
  b. Legg-Calvé-Perthes disease
    (1) Aseptic necrosis involving the femoral head ossification center
    (2) Occurs most often in boys 3 to 10 years of age
    (3) Presents with pain in the knee or a limp
    (4) Secondary osteoarthritis is common.

> Legg-Calvé-Perthes disease: aseptic necrosis of femoral head in children

G. Osgood-Schlatter disease
1. Affects physically active boys 11 to 15 years of age
2. Inflammation of proximal tibial apophysis at insertion of patellar tendon
3. Produces permanent knobby-appearing knees
4. *No* effect on bone growth

H. Paget's disease of bone (osteitis deformans)
1. Epidemiology
  a. Primarily occurs in elderly men
  b. Cause unknown (? virus)
  c. Targets the pelvis, skull (enlarged), and femur
2. Pathogenesis
  a. Early phase of osteoclastic resorption of bone
  • Causes shaggy-appearing lytic lesions
  b. Late phase of increased osteoblastic bone formation
    (1) Markedly increased serum alkaline phosphatase
    (2) Production of thick, weak bone (mosaic bone)

> Paget's disease: osteoblastic phase has increased alkaline phosphatase

3. Clinical findings
  a. Pathologic fractures
  b. Risk for developing osteogenic sarcomas
  c. Risk for developing high-output heart failure
  • Due to arteriovenous connections in vascular bone

I. Fibrous dysplasia
1. Benign, non-neoplastic process of single or multiple bones
2. Targets ribs, femur, or cranial bones of children and young adults
3. Replacement of marrow by fibrous tissue
   - Risk for a pathologic fracture
4. Multiple bone involvement is associated with Albright's syndrome.
   a. Café-au-lait spots on skin
   b. Precocious sexual development

J. Neoplastic disorders of bone
1. Metastasis is the most common malignancy of bone.
   - Breast cancer is the most common primary site.
2. Primary malignant tumors of bone, in descending order of frequency
   - Osteogenic sarcoma, chondrosarcoma, Ewing's sarcoma
3. Summary of bone tumors (Table 23-1)

Metastasis: most common bone malignancy

Osteochondroma: most common benign bone tumor

II. Joint Disorders
A. Synovial fluid (SF) analysis
1. Routine studies
   - White blood cell (WBC) count and differential, crystal analysis, culture, Gram stain
2. Crystal identification
   a. Monosodium urate (MSU)
      (1) Needle-shaped (monoclinic) crystal
      (2) Special polarization shows negative birefringence.
         - Crystal is yellow when parallel to the slow ray (Fig. 23-2).
   b. Calcium pyrophosphate
      (1) Monoclinic-like or triclinic (rhomboid) crystals
      (2) Special polarization shows positive birefringence.
         - Crystal is blue when parallel to the slow ray.

MSU crystals: negatively birefringent

Calcium pyrophosphate: positively birefringent

B. Osteoarthritis
1. Epidemiology
   a. Noninflammatory joint disease
   b. More common in women
   c. Universal after 65 years of age
   d. Secondary causes
      - Obesity, trauma, ochronosis

Most common disabling joint disease: osteoarthritis

> Ochronosis (alkaptonuria) is an autosomal recessive disease caused by deficiency of homogentisic acid oxidase and accumulation of homogentisic acid (urine turns black when oxidized). Homogentisic acid deposits in the intervertebral disks, causing osteoarthritis and other systemic findings.

2. Progressive degeneration of articular cartilage
   a. Primarily targets weight-bearing joints
   b. Joint findings
      (1) Erosion and clefts in articular cartilage

TABLE 23-1:
Tumors of Bone

Tumor Type	Epidemiology	Primary Location	Characteristics
Benign			
Osteochondroma	Males, 10–30 years old Solitary or multiple	Metaphysis of distal femur	Outgrowth of bone (exostosis) capped by benign cartilage Most common benign tumor
Enchondroma	Equal distribution 20–50 years old Solitary or multiple	Medullary location Small tubular bones in hands and feet	Multiple enchondromas Risk for chondrosarcoma
Osteoma	Males, any age	Facial bones	Associated with Gardner's polyposis syndrome
Osteoid osteoma	Males, 10–20 years old	Cortex of proximal femur	Radiographic finding: radiolucent focus surrounded by sclerotic bone Nocturnal pain relieved by aspirin
Osteoblastoma	Males, 10–20 years old	Vertebra	Similar to osteoid osteoma
Giant cell tumor	Females, 20–40 years old	Epiphysis of distal femur or proximal tibia	Reactive multinucleated giant cells resemble osteoclasts Neoplastic mononuclear cells
Malignant			
Chondrosarcoma	Males, 30–60 years old	Pelvic bones, proximal femur	Grade determines biologic behavior Metastasizes to lungs
Osteogenic sarcoma (Fig. 8-6)	Males, 10–25 years old Risk factors: Paget's disease, familial retinoblastoma, irradiation Most common primary bone cancer	Metaphysis of distal femur, proximal tibia	Malignant osteoid Radiographic findings: "sunburst" appearance (spiculated pattern from calcified malignant osteoid), Codman's triangle (tumor lifting periosteum) Metastasizes to lungs
Ewing's sarcoma	Males, 10–20 years old	Pelvic girdle, diaphysis and metaphysis of proximal femur or rib	Small, round cell tumor Radiographic finding: "onion skin" appearance around bone (periosteal reaction) Possible fever and anemia

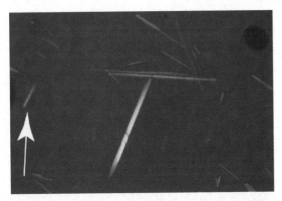

23-2: *Synovial fluid with special polarization. Special red filter causes the background to be red. Crystals are aligned parallel to the slow ray (axis) of the compensator (arrow). If the crystal is yellow when parallel to the slow ray, as in this figure, the crystal demonstrates negative birefringence. If the crystal is blue when parallel to the slow ray, the crystal demonstrates positive birefringence. (From Henry JB: Clinical Diagnosis and Management by Laboratory Methods, 20th ed. Philadelphia, WB Saunders, 2001, Plate 19-7.)*

    (2) Reactive bone formation at joint margins (osteophytes)
- Causes a slight increase in serum alkaline phosphatase

    (3) Subchondral cysts

    (4) Bone eventually rubs on bone.
- Produces dense, sclerotic bone

    (5) *No* ankylosis (fusion) of the joint

3. Clinical findings
   a. Hand involvement (Fig. 23-3)

    (1) Enlargement of distal interphalangeal joints (DIP)
- Called Heberden's nodes (osteophytes)

    (2) Enlargement of proximal interphalangeal joints (PIP) joint
- Called Bouchard's nodes (osteophytes)

   b. Pain with passive motion of the joint
- Due to secondary synovitis

   c. Vertebral findings
- Degenerative disk disease and compressive neuropathies

C. Neuropathic arthropathy (Charcot's joint)
1. Noninflammatory joint disease
2. Secondary to a neurologic disease
- Joint destruction is due to insensitivity to pain (neuropathy).
3. Causes
   a. Diabetes mellitus
- Primarily affects the tarsometatarsal joint
   b. Syringomyelia
- Primarily affects the shoulder, elbow, wrist joints
   c. Tabes dorsalis
- Primarily affects the hip, knee, ankle joints

> Osteoarthritis: wearing down of articular cartilage

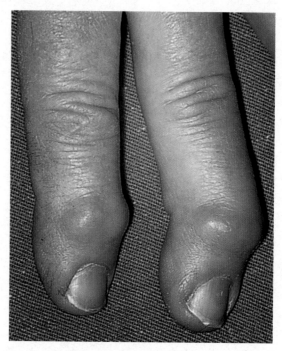

23-3: Osteoarthritis. Bony protuberances (Heberden's nodes) from the base of the terminal phalanx (distal interphalangeal joints) represent osteophytes at the margin of the joint. (From Forbes C, Jackson W: Color Atlas and Text of Clinical Medicine, 2nd ed. St. Louis, Mosby, 2003, p 137, Fig. 3-66.)

D. Rheumatoid arthritis

1. Epidemiology
   a. Occurs more often in women 30 to 50 years of age
   b. HLA-DR4 association
   c. Initial inciting agent may be the Epstein-Barr virus.
2. Pathogenesis of joint disease involves a series of inflammatory responses.
   a. B cells in the joint produce rheumatoid factor (RF) complexes.
      (1) RF complexes are IgM autoantibodies against the Fc receptor of IgG.
      (2) RF complexes are also present in serum in 70% to 90% of cases.
      (3) Type III hypersensitivity reaction
   b. RF complexes activate complement, which attracts neutrophils.
      (1) Neutrophils produce acute inflammation of synovial tissue.
      (2) Neutrophil phagocytosis of RF complexes produces ragocytes.
   c. Chronically inflamed synovial tissue proliferates (forms a pannus).
      (1) Pannus releases cytokines that destroy articular cartilage.
      (2) End result is reactive fibrosis and joint fusion (ankylosis).
3. Clinical and laboratory findings
   a. Symmetric involvement of second/third metacarpophalangeal (MCP) and PIP joints
      (1) Produces ulnar deviation, morning stiffness (Fig. 23-4)

Rheumatoid factor: IgM autoantibody directed against Fc receptor of IgG

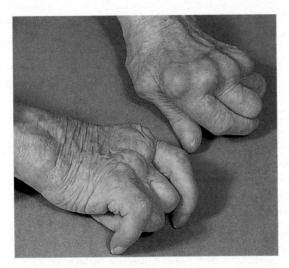

23-4: *Rheumatoid arthritis showing bilateral ulnar deviation of the hands and prominent swelling of the second and third metacarpophalangeal joints. (From Forbes C, Jackson W: Color Atlas and Text of Clinical Medicine, 2nd ed. St. Louis, Mosby, 2003, p 121, Fig. 3-3.)*

      (2) Other joints commonly involved
         • Knees, ankles, hips, cervical spine
   b. Lung disease
     • Chronic pleuritis with effusions, interstitial fibrosis
   c. Hematologic disease
     (1) Anemia of chronic disease
     (2) Felty's syndrome
        • Autoimmune neutropenia and splenomegaly
   d. Carpal tunnel syndrome (see section V)
     • Entrapment of median nerve under transverse carpal ligament
   e. Rheumatoid nodules
     • Extensor surface of the forearm, lungs
   f. Vasculitis (around ankles), pericarditis, and aortitis
   g. Popliteal (Baker's) cyst
     • Outpouching of joint space due to increased intra-articular pressure
   h. Positive serum antinuclear antibody test (30% of cases)
4. Sjögren's syndrome (SS)
   a. Female dominant autoimmune disease
   b. Pathogenesis
     • Autoimmune destruction of minor salivary glands and lacrimal
      glands
   c. Clinical findings
     (1) Rheumatoid arthritis
     (2) Keratoconjunctivitis sicca
       (a) Dry eyes described as "sand in my eyes."
       (b) Due to autoimmune destruction of lacrimal glands

> Caplan syndrome: rheumatoid nodules in the lung plus pneumoconiosis

(3) Xerostomia or dry mouth
    (a) Autoimmune destruction of minor salivary glands
        • "Doctor, I can't swallow dry crackers."
    (b) Dental caries
  d. Laboratory findings
    (1) Anti-SS-A antibodies (Ro; 70–95% of cases)
    (2) Anti-SS-B antibodies (La; 60–90% of cases)
  e. Confirm with lip biopsy
    • Must demonstrate lymphoid destruction of minor salivary glands

E. Juvenile rheumatoid arthritis (JRA)
  1. Epidemiology
    a. Occurs in children younger than 16 years of age
    b. More common in girls
    c. RF is usually absent.
  2. Still's disease (20% of cases)
    a. Commonly presents as an "infectious disease"
    b. Fever, rash, polyarthritis
    c. Generalized lymphadenopathy
    d. Neutrophilic leukocytosis
  3. Polyarticular JRA (40% of cases)
    • Disabling arthritis predominates.
  4. Pauciarticular JRA (40% of cases)
    a. Arthritis limited to a few joints.
    b. Uveitis with the potential for blindness

F. Gouty arthritis
  1. Epidemiology
    a. Multifactorial inheritance pattern
    b. Occurs more often in men older than 30 years of age
    c. Most often due to underexcretion of uric acid in the kidneys
      • Overproduction of uric acid is less common.
  2. Secondary causes
    a. Increased nucleated cell turnover
      • Example—leukemia
    b. Decreased renal excretion
      • Examples—lead poisoning, alcoholism
  3. Recurrent acute arthritis
    a. Commonly involves the first metatarsophalangeal joint
      • Called podagra
    b. Fever, pain, and neutrophilic leukocytosis
    c. MSU phagocytosed by neutrophils in synovial fluid.
  4. Chronic gout
    a. Tophi are produced.
      (1) Deposits of MSU in soft tissue around joints (Fig. 23-5)
      (2) Granulomatous reaction with multinucleated giant cells
    b. Tophi destroy subjacent bone causing erosive arthritis.
  5. Clinical conditions associated with gout
    a. Urate nephropathy, renal stones (see Chapter 19)

JRA: RF is usually negative

Gout: most cases due to underexcretion of uric acid

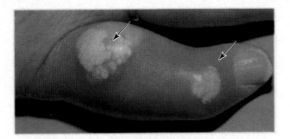

23-5: *Tophi (arrows) involving the soft tissue around joints in the hand. (From Forbes C, Jackson W: Color Atlas and Text of Clinical Medicine, 2nd ed. St. Louis, Mosby, 2003, Fig. 3-72.)*

    b. Hypertension, coronary artery disease
    c. Lead poisoning
        • Produces interstitial nephritis, which interferes with uric acid excretion

Tophus: MSU in soft tissue around joints

  6. Laboratory findings
    a. Hyperuricemia
    b. Joint aspiration is confirmatory.
G. Chondrocalcinosis (pseudogout)
  1. Degenerative joint disease
    a. Usually involves the knee
    b. Crystals produce linear deposits in articular cartilage.
  2. Crystals phagocytosed by neutrophils show positive birefringence.
H. Seronegative spondyloarthropathies
  1. Characteristics
    a. RF negative (meaning of seronegative)
    b. Individuals HLA-B27 positive
    c. Male dominant
    d. Sacroiliitis with or without peripheral arthritis
  2. Types of spondyloarthropathy
    a. Ankylosing spondylitis
    b. Reiter's syndrome
    c. Arthritis
        • Associated with ulcerative colitis, shigellosis, psoriasis
  3. Ankylosing spondylitis
    a. Initially targets sacroiliac joint in young men
        • Bilateral sacroiliitis with morning stiffness
    b. Eventually involves the vertebral column (Fig. 23-6)
        • Fusion of vertebrae ("bamboo spine") causes forward curvature.
    c. Aortitis with aortic regurgitation
    d. Uveitis (blurry vision)

Ankylosing spondylitis: HLA-B27+, vertebral fusion

  4. Reiter's syndrome
    a. Urethritis due to *Chlamydia trachomatis*
    b. Arthritis and Achilles tendon periostitis
        • Achilles tendon periostitis is a confirmatory radiologic sign.
    c. Conjunctivitis (noninfectious)

Reiter's syndrome: *C. trachomatis* urethritis, arthritis, conjunctivitis

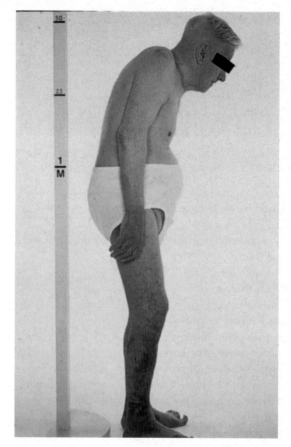

23-6: *Man with ankylosing spondylitis. The patient cannot bend forward owing to fusion of the vertebra. (From Forbes C, Jackson W: Color Atlas and Text of Clinical Medicine, 2nd ed. St. Louis, Mosby, 2003, Fig. 3-48.)*

     5. Psoriatic arthritis
        a. Sausage-shaped DIP joints (finger or toe)
        b. Radiographs show erosive joint disease.
          • "Pencil-in-cup" deformity
        c. Extensive nail pitting
I. Septic arthritis
     1. *Staphylococcus aureus*
        • Most common nongonococcal cause of septic arthritis
     2. *Neisseria gonorrhoeae*
        a. Most common cause of septic arthritis in urban populations
        b. May produce disseminated gonococcemia
          (1) More common in young women
             • Deficiency of C6–C9 predisposes to dissemination
          (2) Septic arthritis (knee)

        (3) Tenosynovitis (wrists and ankles)

        (4) Dermatitis (pustules on wrists or ankles)

3. Lyme disease

  a. Epidemiology

        (1) Caused by *Borrelia burgdorferi* (spirochete)

        (2) Transmitted by bite of the *Ixodes* tick

        (3) White-tailed deer is a reservoir for the organism.

  b. Early disease

        (1) Erythema chronicum migrans develops at tick bite site (Fig. 23-7).

        (2) Red, expanding lesion with concentric circles ("bull's-eye" lesion)

        (3) Pathognomonic lesion of Lyme disease

  c. Late disease

        (1) Disabling arthritis (usually involves the knee)

        (2) Bilateral Bell's palsy

          • Highly predictive of Lyme disease

        (3) Myocarditis and pericarditis

  d. Babesiosis

        (1) Intraerythrocytic protozoal disease due to *Babesia microti*

        (2) Secondary infection transmitted by *Ixodes*

          • Often presents concurrently with Lyme disease

        (3) Fever, headache, hemolytic anemia

  e. Diagnosis of Lyme disease

        (1) Serologic tests

        (2) Culture biopsy specimens

        (3) Silver stains of synovial biopsy to identify spirochetes

4. Septic arthritis and tendinitis due to cat bite

    • Causal agent is *Pasteurella multocida.*

Cause of Lyme disease: Borrelia burgdorferi, a gram-negative spirochete

Erythema chronicum migrans: pathognomonic of Lyme disease

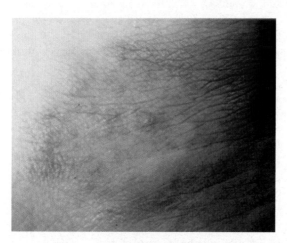

23-7: *Erythema chronicum migrans in a patient with Lyme disease. Raised central area is the site of the tick bite. Concentric area of erythema surrounds the bite site. (From Lookingbill D, Marks J: Principles of Dermatology, 3rd ed. Philadelphia, WB Saunders, 2000, p 269, Fig. 17-5A.)*

III. Muscle Disorders

A. Muscle fibers

1. Type I fibers
   a. Slow-twitch (red) fibers
   b. Rich in mitochondria and oxidative enzymes
2. Type II fibers
   a. Fast-twitch (white) fibers
   b. Poor in mitochondria

B. Muscle disorders

1. Pathogenesis of muscle weakness
   a. Abnormality in the motor neuron pathways
      • Example—poliomyelitis
   b. Abnormality in the neuromuscular synapse
      • Example—myasthenia gravis
   c. Abnormality in muscle
      • Example—muscular dystrophy
2. Neurogenic atrophy
   a. Motor neuron or its axon degenerates.
   b. Produces atrophy of type I and type II fibers
3. Duchenne's muscular dystrophy
   a. X-linked recessive
   b. Pathogenesis
      (1) Deficiency of dystrophin
         (a) Dystrophin normally anchors actin to membrane glycoprotein
         (b) Becker's type has defective dystrophin.
      (2) Progressive degeneration of type I and type II fibers
      (3) Fibrosis and infiltration of muscle tissue by fatty tissue
         • Produces pseudohypertrophy of calf muscles
   c. Clinical findings
      (1) Symptoms occur between 2 and 5 years of age.
      (2) Weakness and wasting of pelvic muscles
         (a) Child places hands on the knees for help in standing.
         (b) Waddling gait (duck-like)
      (3) Death usually occurs by 20 years of age.
   d. Laboratory findings
      (1) Serum creatine kinase (CK) increased at birth.
         • Progressively declines as muscle degenerates
      (2) Female carriers have increased levels of serum CK.
4. Myotonic dystrophy
   a. Epidemiology and pathogenesis
      (1) Autosomal dominant
      (2) Most common adult muscular dystrophy
      (3) Trinucleotide repeat disorder (see Chapter 5)
      (4) Selective atrophy of type I fibers
   b. Clinical findings
      (1) Facial weakness

Duchenne's muscular dystrophy: waddling gait due to weakness of pelvic muscles

Myotonic dystrophy: most common muscular dystrophy in adults

(2) Myotonia
- Inability to relax muscles (sustained grip)

(3) Frontal balding, cataracts

(4) Testicular atrophy, cardiac involvement

c. Increased serum CK

5. Myasthenia gravis

   a. Epidemiology

     (1) Afflicts men in sixth and seventh decades of life

     (2) Afflicts women in second and third decades of life

   b. Pathogenesis

     (1) Autoantibody against acetylcholine receptors

       (a) Type II hypersensitivity reaction

       (b) Antibodies inhibit and/or destroy the receptors.

     (2) Antibody is synthesized in the thymus.

      - Thymic hyperplasia with germinal follicles (85% of cases)

   c. Clinical findings

     (1) Ptosis is the most common initial finding (Fig. 23-8).

      - Diplopia due to eye muscle weakness

     (2) Muscle weakness improves with rest

> Myasthenia gravis: autoantibodies against ACh receptors

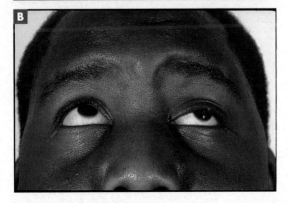

23-8: *Patient with myasthenia gravis showing ptosis of the left eye* (**A**) *followed by opening of the eye* (**B**) *after intravenous injection of Tensilon. (From Perkin GD: Mosby's Color Atlas and Text of Neurology. St. Louis, Mosby, 2002, p 263, Fig. 14-5A and B.)*

      (3) Dysphagia for solids and liquids
          • Occurs in the upper esophagus (striated muscle)
      (4) Increased risk for developing a thymoma
          • Occurs in 15% of cases
    d. Tensilon (edrophonium) test facilitates diagnosis
      (1) Inhibits acetylcholinesterase
      (2) Increase in acetylcholine reverses muscle weakness

IV. Soft Tissue Disorders
A. Fibromatosis
   1. Non-neoplastic, proliferative connective tissue disorder
   2. Fibrous tissue infiltrates tissue (usually muscle).
   3. Dupuytren's contracture
     a. Fibromatosis involving palmar fascia
     b. Causes contraction of single or multiple fingers
     c. Associated with alcoholism
   4. Desmoid tumor

TABLE 23-2:
Soft Tissue Tumors

Tumor Type	Location	Comment
Lipoma (Fig. 8-2)	Trunk, neck, proximal extremities	Most common benign soft tissue tumor Arises in subcutaneous tissue *No clinical significance*
Liposarcoma	Thigh, retroperitoneum	Most common adult sarcoma Lipoblasts identified with fat stains
Fibrosarcoma	Thigh, upper limb	May arise after irradiation
Dermatofibroma	Lower extremities	Benign, nonencapsulated proliferation of spindle cells confined to the dermis Red nodule that umbilicates (has a central dimple) when squeezed
Malignant fibrous histiocytoma	Retroperitoneum, thigh	Associated with radiation therapy and scarring
Rhabdomyoma	Heart, also tongue and vagina	Benign heart tumor associated with tuberous sclerosis
Embryonal rhabdomyosarcoma	Penis and vagina	Most common sarcoma in children Grape-like, necrotic mass protrudes from penis or vagina
Leiomyoma	Uterus, stomach	Most commonly located in uterus Most common benign tumor in gastrointestinal tract
Leiomyosarcoma	Gastrointestinal tract, uterus	Most common sarcoma of gastrointestinal tract and uterus
Neurofibrosarcoma	Major nerve trunks	Associated with neurofibromatosis
Synovial sarcoma	Around joints	Does not arise from synovial cells in joints but from mesenchymal cells around joints Biphasic pattern: epithelial cells forming glands + intervening spindle cells

TABLE 23-3:
Selected Orthopedic Disorders

Disorder	Description and Comments
Rotator cuff tear	Components: tendon insertions of supraspinatus, infraspinatus, teres minor, subscapularis muscles Pain/weakness with active shoulder abduction
Tennis elbow	Causes: raquet sports, repetitive use of a hammer or screwdriver Pain where extensor muscle tendons insert near the lateral epicondyle
Golfer's elbow	Pain where the flexor muscle tendons insert near the medial epicondyle
DeQuervain's tenosynovitis	Chronic stenosing tenosynovitis of the first dorsal compartment of the wrist Overuse of the hands and wrist; first dorsal compartment has abductor pollicis longus and extensor pollicis brevis; excessive friction thickens tendon sheath causing stenosis of the osseofibrous tunnel Pain on the radial aspect of the wrist aggravated by moving the thumb
Ganglion (synovial) cyst	Bulge on the dorsum of the wrist when the wrist is flexed Cyst communicates with synovial sheaths on the dorsum of the wrist
Compartment syndrome	Increase of pressure in a confined space; pressure reduces perfusion, which may cause ischemic contractures of the muscle(s) Pain, paresthesias, pallor, paralysis, pulselessness Risk factors: fractures, injuries to arteries or soft tissue Volkmann's ischemic contracture: supracondylar fracture of humerus causing compression of brachial artery and median nerve; forearm muscles may undergo contracture
Carpal tunnel syndrome	Entrapment syndrome of the median nerve in the transverse carpal ligament of the wrist Causes: rheumatoid arthritis and pregnancy most common causes Pain, numbness, or paresthesias in the thumb, index finger, second finger, third finger, and the radial side of fourth finger; thenar atrophy produces "ape" hand appearance
Ulnar nerve injury	Fracture of medial epicondyle of the humerus Injury produces a "claw hand" (loss of interosseous muscles)
Radial nerve injury	Midshaft fractures of humerus; draping the arm over a park bench (called "Saturday night palsy") Injury produces wrist drop
Erb-Duchenne palsy	Brachial plexus lesion involving C5 and C6 "Waiter's tip deformity"
Axillary nerve injury	Fracture of surgical neck of humerus; anterior dislocation of the shoulder joint (may also injury the axillary artery) Cannot abduct the arm to horizontal position or hold the horizontal position when a downward force is applied to the arm (paralysis of deltoid muscle)
Intervertebral disk disease	Degeneration of fibrocartilage/nucleus pulposus; ruptured disk material may herniate posteriorly and compress the nerve root and/or spinal cord Radicular pain; leg pain aggravated by straight leg raising Herniation of L3–L4 disk: loss of knee jerk (femoral nerve L2–L4) Herniation of L4–L5 disk: *no* loss of reflexes (ankle and knee reflexes intact) Herniation L5–S1 disk: loss of ankle reflex (tibial nerve L4–S3)
Knee joint injuries	Valgus injury: angulation *away* from the midline; laterally originating force is applied to the knee (e.g., clipping injury in football) Varus injury: angulation *toward* the midline; medially originating force is applied to the knee McMurray test: meniscus injuries Anterior and posterior draw test: cruciate injuries Unhappy triad: most common internal derangement of knee joint; valgus injury; damage to medial meniscus, medial collateral ligament, anterior cruciate ligament

Unhappy triad: damage to medial meniscus, medial collateral ligament, anterior cruciate ligament

a. Fibromatosis of the anterior abdominal wall in women
b. Associated with previous trauma
c. Associated with Gardner's polyposis syndrome

B. Selected soft tissue tumors (Table 23-2)

V. Selected Orthopedic Disorders (Table 23-3)

24 CHAPTER

Skin Disorders

I. Skin Histology and Terminology
A. Normal skin histology
1. Epidermis
   a. Stratum basalis
      (1) Actively dividing stem cells along the basement membrane
      (2) Mitoses should be limited to this area.
   b. Stratum spinosum
      - Contains prominent desmosome attachments
   c. Stratum granulosum
      - Granular layer with keratohyaline granules
   d. Stratum corneum
      (1) Anucleate cells with keratin
      (2) Site for superficial dermatophyte infections

Stratum corneum: site for superficial dermatophyte infections

2. Dermis
   a. Papillary
      - Loose connective tissue beneath the epidermis
   b. Reticular
      - Dense dermal collagen
3. Melanocytes
   a. Derived from neural crest cells
   b. Located in stratum basalis
      - Dendritic processes extend between keratinocytes.
   c. Melanin is synthesized in membrane-bound melanosomes.
      (1) Tyrosinase converts tyrosine to 3,4-dihydroxyphenylalanine (DOPA).
      (2) DOPA is converted to melanin.
      (3) Melanosomes are transferred by dendritic processes to keratinocytes.

Melanin: synthesized from tyrosine; packaged in melanosomes

   d. Skin color
      (1) Number of melanocytes is essentially the *same* in all races.
      (2) Melanin is degraded more rapidly in whites than in black Americans.
      (3) In whites, melanosomes are concentrated in the basal layer.
      (4) In black Americans, melanosomes are present throughout all layers.
         - Melanocytes are larger and have more dendritic processes.
   e. Sunlight and adrenocorticotropic hormone stimulate melanin synthesis.
B. Common terms used in dermatology (Table 24-1)

TABLE 24-1:
Common Terms in Dermatology

Term	Definition	Example
Macroscopic		
Macule	Pigmented or erythematous flat lesion on epidermis	Tinea versicolor
Papule	Peaked or dome-shaped surface elevation < 5 mm diameter	Acne vulgaris
Nodule	Elevated, dome-shaped lesion > 5 mm diameter	Basal cell carcinoma
Plaque	Flattened, elevated area on epidermis > 5 mm diameter	Psoriasis
Vesicle	Fluid-filled blister < 5 mm diameter	Varicella (chickenpox)
Bulla	Fluid-filled blister > 5 mm diameter	Bullous pemphigoid
Pustule	Fluid-filled blister with inflammatory cells	Impetigo
Wheal (hive)	Edematous, transient papule or plaque caused by infiltration of dermis by fluid	Urticaria
Scales	Excessive number of dead keratinocytes produced by abnormal keratinization	Seborrheic dermatitis
Microscopic		
Hyperkeratosis	Increased thickness of stratum corneum produces scaly appearance of skin	Psoriasis
Parakeratosis	Persistence of nuclei in stratum corneum layer	Psoriasis
Papillomatosis	Spire-like projections from surface of skin or downward into papillary dermis	Verruca vulgaris
Acantholysis	Loss of cohesion between keratinocytes	Pemphigus vulgaris

II. **Viral Disorders**
  A. **Common warts**
    1. Caused by human papillomavirus (DNA virus)
    2. Common sites are the fingers and soles
    3. Verrucous papular lesions covered by scales (Fig. 24-1)
  B. **Molluscum contagiosum**
    1. Caused by a poxvirus (DNA virus)
    2. Bowl-shaped lesions with central depression filled with keratin (Fig. 24-2)
      • Depression contains viral particles called molluscum bodies.
  C. **Rubeola (measles)**
    1. RNA paramyxovirus
    2. Prodrome
      • Fever, conjunctivitis, runny nose, cough
    3. Koplik spots develop on the buccal mucosa.
      • Koplik spots are red with a white center.
    4. Maculopapular rash develops *after* Koplik spots disappears.
    5. Complications

Measles: rash after
Koplik spots disappear

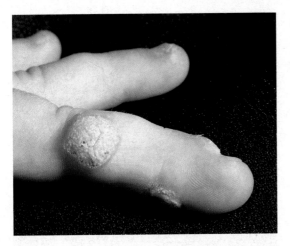

24-1: *Verruca vulgaris (common wart) on the fingers, showing scaling, verrucous papules with interrupted skin lines. (From Lookingbill D, Marks J: Principles of Dermatology, 3rd ed. Philadelphia, WB Saunders, 2000, p 68, Fig. 6-1A.)*

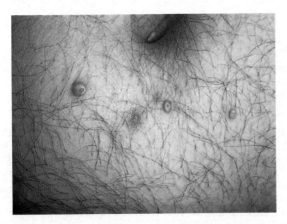

24-2: *Molluscum contagiosum, showing small bowl-shaped lesions with central areas of depression (umbilication). (From Savin J, Hunter JA, Hepburn NC: Diagnosis in Color: Skin Signs in Clinical Medicine. London, Mosby-Wolfe, 1997, p 79, Fig. 2-47.)*

   a. Giant cell pneumonia
   - Warthin-Finkeldey multinucleated giant cells
   b. Acute appendicitis in children
   c. Otitis media
D. Rubella (German measles)
   1. RNA togavirus
   - Produces "3-day measles"
   2. Painful postauricular lymphadenopathy
   3. Maculopapular rash lasts 3 days.
   4. Polyarthritis common in adults.

Rubella: painful postauricular lymphadenopathy

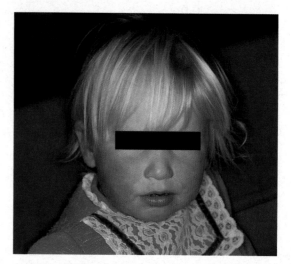

24-3: *Erythema infectiosum in a child showing the "slapped face" appearance. (From Savin J, Hunter JA, Hepburn NC: Diagnosis in Color: Skin Signs in Clinical Medicine. London, Mosby-Wolfe, 1997, p 6, Fig. 1-10.)*

E. **Erythema infectiosum (fifth disease)**
1. Caused by parvovirus B19 (DNA virus)
2. Confluent maculopapular rash
   a. Begins on the cheeks ("slapped face" appearance; Fig. 24-3)
   b. Extends to the trunk

> Other disorders caused by parvovirus B19 include pure red blood cell aplasia and aplastic anemia in chronic hemolytic diseases (e.g., hereditary spherocytosis) and chronic arthritis. Pregnant mothers exposed to a child with the infection may abort the fetus.

F. **Roseola infantum**
1. Caused by human herpesvirus 6 (DNA virus)
2. Maculopapular rash occurs after 3 to 7 days of high fever.
3. High fever may precipitate a febrile convulsion.

G. **Disorders caused by varicella-zoster virus**
1. DNA herpesvirus
   • Remains latent in cranial and thoracic sensory ganglia
2. Varicella (chickenpox)
   a. Rash progresses from macules, to vesicles, to pustules (Fig. 24-4).
      • All stages of development are simultaneously present.
   b. Positive Tzanck test similar to herpes simplex virus (see Chapter 21)
   c. Complications
      (1) Association with Reye syndrome
      (2) Pneumonia, self-limited cerebellitis
3. Herpes zoster (shingles)
   • Painful vesicles follow sensory dermatomes (Fig. 24-5)

Common cause of febrile convulsions: roseola

Herpes zoster: painful vesicles follow sensory dermatomes

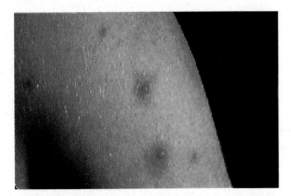

24-4: *Varicella infection of skin showing vesicles surrounded by an erythematous base. (From Goldstein BG: Practical Dermatology, 2nd ed. St. Louis, Mosby, 1997, p 248, Fig. 18-10.)*

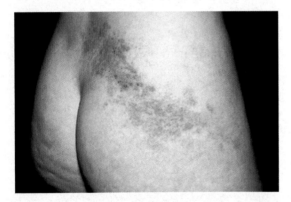

24-5: *Herpes zoster. The erythematous vesicular rash with the characteristic "band" distribution starts from the midline and extends to the lateral trunk. (From Forbes C, Jackson W: Color Atlas and Text of Clinical Medicine, 2nd ed. St. Louis, Mosby, 2003, p 29, Fig. 1-85.)*

III. **Bacterial Disorders**
   A. ***Staphylococcus aureus* skin infections**
      1. Gram-positive coccus
      2. Toxic shock syndrome
         a. Production of toxic shock syndrome toxin (TSST)
            • Superantigen that stimulates release of cytokines
         b. Usually occurs in tampon-using menstruating women
         c. Clinical findings
            (1) Fever, hypotension
            (2) Desquamating, sunburn-like rash
         d. Impetigo
      3. Other infections
         a. Skin abscess
         b. Hidradenitis suppurativa
            • Abscess of apocrine glands in the axilla
         c. Postsurgical wound infection (most common pathogen)

TSST: produces desquamating sunburn-like rash

Scarlet fever: increased risk for developing poststreptococcal glomerulonephritis

B. Scarlet fever
1. Caused by *Streptococcus pyogenes*
   a. Gram-positive coccus
   b. Particular strains produce an erythrogenic toxin.
2. Desquamating, sandpaper-like erythematous rash
   • Develops on the skin and tongue ("strawberry" tongue)
3. Increased risk for developing poststreptococcal glomerulonephritis

C. Impetigo
1. Most often caused by *Staphylococcus aureus*
   • *Streptococcus pyogenes* second most common cause
2. Rash usually begins on the face (Fig. 24-6)
   • Vesicles and pustules rupture to form honey-colored, crusted lesions.
3. Presence of bullae commonly occurs with *Staphylococcus aureus*.

D. Leprosy
1. Caused by *Mycobacterium leprae*
2. Tuberculoid type
   a. Granulomas present
      • Very few acid-fast bacteria are present in the granulomas.
   b. Positive lepromin skin test
      • Indicates intact cellular immunity
   c. Localized skin lesions with nerve involvement
      • Autoamputation of digits
3. Lepromatous type
   a. Absence of granulomas

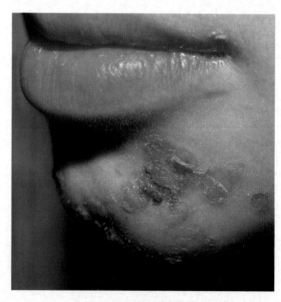

24-6: Impetigo of the face showing "honey-colored" crusts overlying an erythematous base. (From Lookingbill D, Marks J: Principles of Dermatology, 3rd ed. Philadelphia, WB Saunders, 2000, p 217, Fig. 13-9.)

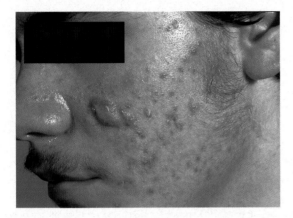

24-7: *Patient with severe facial acne with inflamed papules and cystic lesions. (From Savin J, Hunter JA, Hepburn NC: Diagnosis in Color: Skin Signs in Clinical Medicine. London, Mosby-Wolfe, 1997, p 135, Fig. 5-20.)*

      (1) Numerous bacteria are present in foamy macrophages.
      (2) Macrophages located under a subepidermal zone free of organisms
         • Called the Grenz zone
    b. Negative lepromin skin test
      • Indicates a lack of cellular immunity
    c. Nodular lesions produce the classic leonine facies.
  E. Acne vulgaris
    1. Chronic inflammation of the pilosebaceous unit
    2. Inflammatory type
      a. Abnormal keratinization of the follicular epithelium
      b. Increased sebum production (androgen-dependent)
      c. Bacterial lipase *(Propionibacterium acnes)* produces irritating fatty acids.
         • Produces the inflammatory reaction (Fig. 24-7)
    3. Obstructive type (comedones)
      • Plugging of the outlet of a hair follicle by keratin debris
  F. Acne rosacea
    1. Inflammatory reaction of the pilosebaceous units of facial skin
    2. Pustules and flushing of the cheeks (Fig. 24-8)
    3. Sebaceous gland hyperplasia
      • Produces enlargement of the nose (rhinophyma)

IV. Fungal Disorders
  A. Superficial mycoses (dermatophytoses)
    1. Fungi confined to the stratum corneum or its adnexal structures.

> Acne vulgaris: androgen receptors are located on the sebaceous glands

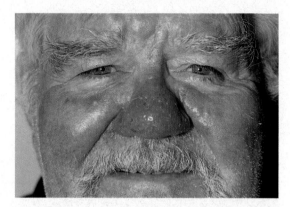

24-8: *Acne rosacea showing pustules and papules superimposed on a background of erythema and telangiectasias (dilated vessels). There is also enlargement of the nose due to sebaceous gland hyperplasia (rhinophyma). (From Lookingbill D, Marks J: Principles of Dermatology, 3rd ed. Philadelphia, WB Saunders, 2000, p 213, Fig. 13-4A.)*

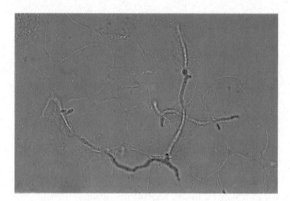

24-9: *Potassium hydroxide preparation of skin scrapings showing hyphae and yeasts. (From Goldstein BG: Practical Dermatology, 2nd ed. St. Louis, Mosby, 1997, p 24, Fig. 3-2.)*

Wood's lamp and potassium hydroxide (KOH)–treated skin scrapings from lesions are commonly used for diagnosis of the dermatophytoses. Wood's lamp (ultraviolet A light) detects fluorescent metabolites produced by organisms (e.g., fungi, some bacteria). KOH preparations identify yeasts and hyphae in the stratum corneum or hair shafts (Fig. 24-9).

2. Tinea capitis
   a. Pathogens
      (1) Most often caused by *Trichophyton tonsurans*
         (a) Infects the inner hair shaft
         (b) Negative Wood's lamp
      (2) *Microsporum canis*
         (a) Infects the outer hair shaft
         (b) Positive Wood's lamp

Trichophyton tonsurans: most common cause of tinea capitis

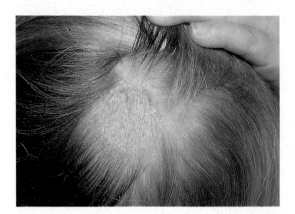

24-10: *Tinea capitis due to Trichophyton tonsurans. Note the area of alopecia (hair loss) with black dots representing broken off hairs and scaling of the skin. (From Goldstein BG: Practical Dermatology, 2nd ed. St. Louis, Mosby, 1997, p 97, Fig. 10-1.)*

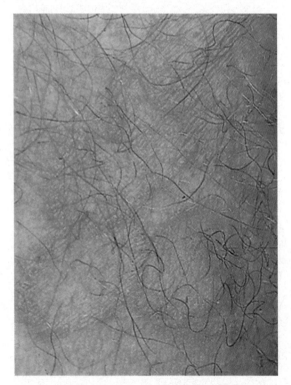

24-11: *Tinea corporis showing annular lesions with erythematous margins and clear centers. (From Forbes C, Jackson W: Color Atlas and Text of Clinical Medicine, 2nd ed. St. Louis, Mosby, 2003, p 97, Fig. 2-57.)*

      b. Circular or ring-shaped patches of hair loss (alopecia)
         • Black dot is present where hair breaks off (Fig. 24-10).
    2. Other infections are most often caused by *Trichophyton rubrum.*
      a. Tinea corporis (body surface) (Fig. 24-11)

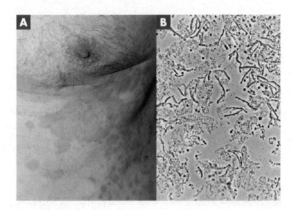

24-12: *Tinea versicolor showing skin with pink-tan patches (**A**) and a potassium hydroxide scraping (**B**) showing short hyphae (resemble "spaghetti") and yeasts (resemble "meatballs"). (From Lookingbill D, Marks J: Principles of Dermatology, 3rd ed. Philadelphia, WB Saunders, 2000, p 227, Figs. 14-2 and 14-3.)*

    b. Tinea pedis ("athlete's foot")
    c. Tinea cruris (groin; "jock itch")
    d. Tinea unguium (nail)
  3. Tinea versicolor
    a. Caused by *Malassezia furfur*
    b. Affected skin does *not* tan ("white spots"); normal skin does.

> *M. furfur:* produces acid that inhibits melanosome transfer to keratinocytes

      (1) Fungus produces acid that inhibits melanosome transfer to keratinocytes.
      (2) Lesions become hyperpigmented and scaly in winter months (Fig. 24-12A).
    c. KOH findings (Fig. 24-12B)
      (1) Short hyphae have the appearance of "spaghetti."
      (2) Yeasts have the appearance of "meatballs."
  4. Infections caused by *Candida albicans*
    a. Intertrigo
      (1) Erythematous rash in body folds
        • KOH shows pseudohyphae and yeast (see Fig. 21-1A)
      (2) Examples—rash under pendulous breasts, diaper rash
    b. Onychomycosis
      • Nail infection
  5. Seborrheic dermatitis
    a. Caused by *M. furfur*
    b. Scaly, greasy dermatitis
    c. Locations
      • Scalp (dandruff), eyebrows, and nasal creases
 B. Sporotrichosis
  1. Caused by *Sporothrix schenckii*
    a. Subcutaneous mycotic infection
    b. Dimorphic fungus
      • Mold in soil, yeast in tissue

> Sporotrichosis: traumatic implantation

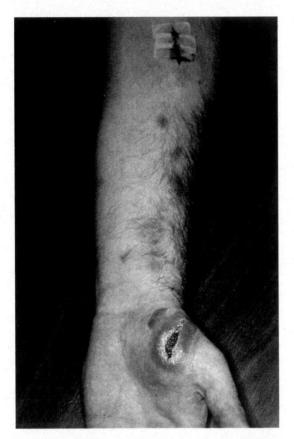

24-13: *Lymphocutaneous sporotrichosis showing a linear array of suppurating subcutaneous nodules. (From Murray PR, Shea YR: Medical Microbiology, 2nd ed. St. Louis, Mosby, 2002, p 163, Fig. 43-14.)*

    2. Traumatic implantation of fungus
- Rose gardening and use of sphagnum moss for packing material

    3. Lymphocutaneous disease
- Chain of suppurating subcutaneous nodules (Fig. 24-13)

V. Benign Noninfectious Disorders
A. Ichthyosis vulgaris
    1. Autosomal dominant
- Most common inherited skin disorder

    2. Defect in keratinization
      a. Causes increased thickness of the stratum corneum
      b. Absent stratum granulosum

    3. Hyperkeratotic, dry skin
- Involves palms, soles, and extensor areas

B. Xerosis
    1. Most common cause of dry skin and pruritus in the elderly
- Due to a decrease in skin lipids

Most common inherited skin disorder: ichthyosis vulgaris

2. Other age-related changes
   a. Decreased number of hair follicles, sweat glands
   b. Decrease in thickness of epidermis
   c. Decreased dermal collagen/elastic tissue
   d. Decreased subcutaneous fat
      • Example—over dorsum of hands
   e. Increased cross-linking of collagen and elastic tissue

C. Polymorphous light eruption
   1. Most common photodermatitis
   2. Positive family history
      • Very common in Native Americans
   3. Rash begins with sun exposure.
      a. Erythematous macules, papules, plaques, or vesicles/bullae
      b. *Not* related to drugs

D. Eczema
   1. Group of inflammatory dermatoses
      • Characterized by pruritus
   2. Acute eczema
      • Weeping, erythematous rash with vesicles
   3. Chronic eczema
      • Dry, thickened skin (hyperkeratosis) caused by continual scratching
   4. Atopic dermatitis
      a. Type I IgE-mediated hypersensitivity reaction
      b. Dermatitis in children
         • Dry skin and eczema on cheeks and extensor and flexural surfaces
      c. Dermatitis in adults
         • Dry skin and eczema on hands, eyelids, elbows, and knees
   5. Contact dermatitis
      a. Allergic contact dermatitis
         (1) Type IV hypersensitivity reaction
         (2) Examples—poison ivy, nickel in jewelry (Fig. 24-14)
      b. Contact photodermatitis
         (1) Ultraviolet light reacts with drugs that have a photosensitizing effect.
         (2) Example—tetracycline

E. Autoimmune skin disorders
   1. Chronic cutaneous lupus erythematosus (see Chapter 3)
      a. Associated with atrophy of the epidermis
      b. DNA–anti-DNA immunocomplex deposition in the basement membrane
         (1) Degeneration of basal cells and hair shafts (alopecia)
         (2) Positive immunofluorescent (IF) band test
            • IF shows complexes deposited along the basement membrane.
      c. Clinical findings
         (1) Erythematous maculopapular eruption
            • Usually over malar eminences and bridge of nose ("butterfly" rash) (see Fig. 3-1)

Atopic dermatitis: type I IgE-mediated hypersensitivity

Contact dermatitis: type IV hypersensitivity; poison ivy, nickel in earrings

Lupus skin involvement: immunocomplexes along basement membrane

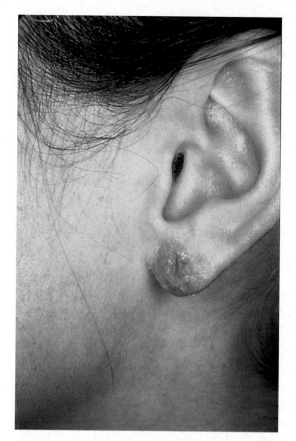

24-14: *Contact dermatitis secondary to nickel in earrings. Note the acute eczematous reaction characterized by a weeping, erythematous rash with vesicle formation. (From Goldstein BG: Practical Dermatology, 2nd ed. St. Louis, Mosby, 1997, p 163, Fig. 14-3.)*

      (2) Skin lesions are exacerbated by ultraviolet light.
  2. Pemphigus vulgaris
    a. IgG antibodies against intercellular attachment sites (desmosomes) between keratinocytes
      • Type II hypersensitivity reaction
    b. Vesicles and bullae develop on skin and oral mucosa.
    c. Intraepithelial vesicles are located *above* the basal layer (suprabasal).
      (1) Basal cells resemble a row of tombstones.
      (2) Acantholysis of keratinocytes in the vesicle fluid
      (3) Positive Nikolsky sign
        • Outer epidermis separates from basal layer with minimal pressure
  3. Bullous pemphigoid
    a. IgG antibodies against the basement membrane
      • Type II hypersensitivity reaction
    b. Vesicles are subepidermal.

Pemphigus vulgaris and bullous pemphigoid: type II hypersensitivity reactions

Dermatitis herpetiformis: associated with celiac disease

(1) Develop on the skin and oral mucosa
(2) *No* acantholytic cells in vesicle fluid
(3) Negative Nikolsky sign

4. Dermatitis herpetiformis (see Fig. 17-14)
   a. IgA–anti-IgA complexes deposit at the tips of the dermal papillae.
      • Produces subepidermal vesicles with neutrophils
   b. Strongly correlated with celiac disease
      • Increase in antireticulin and endomysial antibodies

F. Premalignant skin disorders

1. Actinic (solar) keratosis
   a. Associated with prolonged ultraviolet light exposure
   b. Precursor (squamous dysplasia) of squamous cell carcinoma
      • Squamous cancer occurs in 2% to 5% of cases.
   c. Hyperkeratotic, pearly gray-white appearance

In actinic keratosis, lesions recur after being scraped off.

      (1) Occurs on face, back of neck, dorsum of hands/forearms (Fig. 24-15)
      (2) Commonly recurs when scraped off

2. Lichen planus
   a. Intensely pruritic, scaly, violaceous, flat-topped papules (Fig. 24-16)
      • Usually located on the wrists
   b. Oral mucosa is often involved (50% of cases).
      (1) Produces a fine, white, netlike lesion (Wickham's striae)
      (2) Slight risk of developing squamous cell carcinoma

Lichen planus: associated with hepatitis C

   c. Association with hepatitis C

G. Psoriasis

1. Unregulated proliferation of keratinocytes
   a. Genetic factors involved (30% of cases)
   b. Infection increases risk for disease.
      • Strong association with streptococcal pharyngitis

Psoriasis: erythematous plaques with silver scales

   c. Microcirculatory changes in superficial papillary dermis

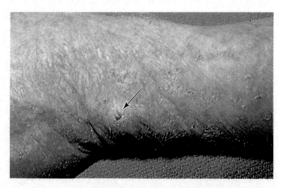

24-15: Actinic (solar) keratosis. Arrow shows a pearly, gray-white hyperkeratotic lesion on dorsum of the wrist. (From Goldstein BG: Practical Dermatology, 2nd ed. St. Louis, Mosby, 1997, p 140, Fig. 13-1.)

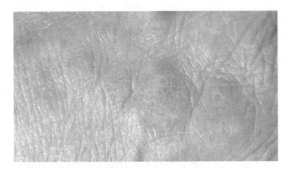

24-16: *Lichen planus showing flat-topped violaceous papules. (From Lookingbill D, Marks J: Principles of Dermatology, 3rd ed. Philadelphia, WB Saunders, 2000, p 201, Fig. 12-7A.)*

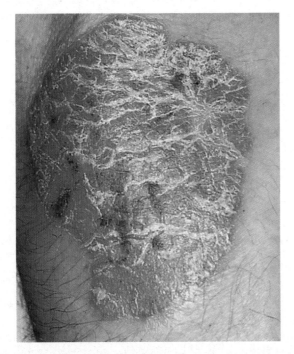

24-17: *Psoriasis involving the elbow showing flat, salmon-colored plaques covered by white to silver-colored scales. (From Forbes C, Jackson W: Color Atlas and Text of Clinical Medicine, 2nd ed. St. Louis, Mosby, 2003, p 87, Fig. 2-15.)*

2. Well-demarcated, flat, elevated salmon-colored plaques (Fig. 24-17)
    a. Covered by adherent white to silver-colored scales
        • Pinpoint areas of bleeding occur when scales are scraped off.
    b. Rash commonly develops in areas of trauma (elbows, lower back).
        • Called Koebner phenomenon
3. Pitting of the nails (Fig. 24-18)
4. Microscopic findings
    a. Hyperkeratosis and parakeratosis

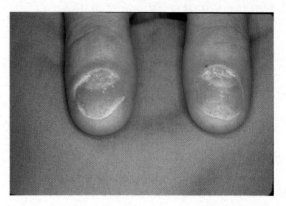

24-18: *Nail changes in psoriasis showing pitting and separation of the distal nail plate (onycholysis). (From Goldstein BG: Practical Dermatology, 2nd ed. St. Louis, Mosby, 1997, p 180, Fig. 14-16.)*

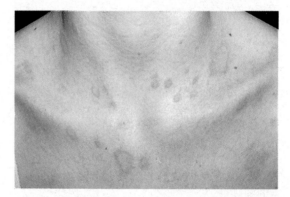

24-19: *Pityriasis rosea showing erythematous, scaly papules and plaques following the lines of cleavage of the skin ("Christmas tree" distribution). The initial herald patch was present in the left supraclavicular region. (From Goldstein BG: Practical Dermatology, 2nd ed. St. Louis, Mosby, 1997, p 177, Fig. 14-13.)*

      b. Elongation of rete pegs
        • Downward extensions of basal layer
      c. Extension of the papillary dermis close to the surface epithelium
        • Blood vessels in dermis rupture when scales are picked off (Auspitz sign).
      d. Neutrophil collections in the stratum corneum
        • Called Munro microabscesses
    5. Treatment modalities
      a. Topical corticosteroids
      b. Ultraviolet light A plus psoralen applied to plaques
      c. Ultraviolet light B plus coal tar applied to plaques
      d. Methotrexate in resistant case

H. Pityriasis rosea
    1. Initially presents as a single, oval-shaped, scaly plaque on the trunk
      • Called the "herald patch"
    2. Days or weeks later, a papular eruption develops on the trunk (Fig. 24-19).

Pityriasis rosea: herald patch followed by rash in "Christmas tree" distribution

    a. Rash follows the lines of cleavage ("Christmas tree" distribution).

    b. Lesions tend to be pruritic.

    c. Rash remits spontaneously in 2 to 10 weeks.

I. Erythema multiforme

    1. Hypersensitivity skin reaction to infection or drugs

        a. Infection associations

         • *Mycoplasma pneumoniae,* herpes simplex virus

        b. Drug associations

         • Sulfonamides, penicillin, barbiturates, phenytoin

    2. Vesicles and bullae have a "targetoid" appearance (Fig. 24-20).

      • Located on the palms, soles, and extensor surfaces

    3. Stevens-Johnson syndrome

      • Erythema multiforme that involves the skin and mucous membranes

J. Erythema nodosum

    1. Inflammatory lesion of subcutaneous fat (panniculitis)

    2. Raised, erythematous, painful nodules

      • Usually located on the anterior portion of the shins (Fig. 24-21)

    3. Common associations

        a. Coccidioidomycosis, histoplasmosis, tuberculosis, leprosy

        b. Streptococcal infection, sarcoidosis

K. Granuloma annulare

    1. Chronic inflammatory dermal disorder

      • Unknown etiology

    2. Occurs in children and adults

      • Female predominance

    3. Begin as erythematous papules

      • Papules evolve into annular plaques (Fig. 24-22).

    4. Occur on the dorsum of the hands and feet

      • Disseminated type may be associated with diabetes mellitus.

    5. Spontaneously resolve within 2 years

      • Recurrence occurs in 40% of cases.

> Erythema nodosum: panniculitis involving anterior portion of shins
>
> Erythema nodosum: most common inflammatory lesion of subcutaneous fat
>
> Granuloma annulare: association with diabetes mellitus

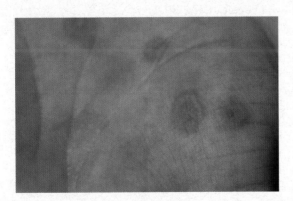

24-20: *Erythema multiforme involving the palms showing target lesions with three zones of color. (From Lookingbill D, Marks J: Principles of Dermatology, 3rd ed. Philadelphia, WB Saunders, 2000, p 267, Fig. 17-3A.)*

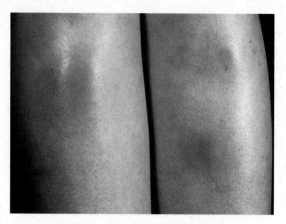

24-21: *Erythema nodosum involving the anterior portion of the shins. Note the raised, erythematous nodular lesions. (From Savin J, Hunter JA, Hepburn NC: Diagnosis in Color: Skin Signs in Clinical Medicine. London, Mosby-Wolfe, 1997, p 8, Fig. 1-14.)*

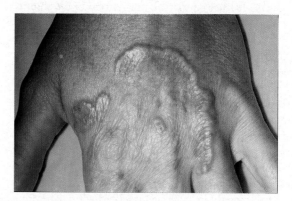

24-22: *Granuloma annulare showing an erythematous, nonscaling, annular plaque on the dorsum of the hands. (From Goldstein BG: Practical Dermatology, 2nd ed. St. Louis, Mosby, 1997, p 312, Fig. 23-4.)*

L. Porphyria cutanea tarda (PCT)
1. Genetic or acquired disease involving porphyrin metabolism
2. Deficiency of uroporphyrinogen decarboxylase
    a. Urine is wine-red color on voiding.
    b. Uroporphyrin I is increased in urine.
3. Associated with hepatitis C and excessive alcohol intake
4. Clinical findings
    a. Photosensitive bullous skin lesions
        (1) Caused by porphyrin metabolites deposited in the skin
        (2) Patients avoid light.
    b. Hyperpigmentation, fragile skin
    c. Increased amounts of lanugo (fine, downy hair)
M. Urticaria
1. Pruritic elevations of the skin
    a. Most often due to mast cell release of histamine

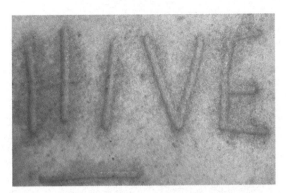

24-23: *Dermatographism showing swelling with the word HIVE. (From Lookingbill D, Marks J: Principles of Dermatology, 3rd ed. Philadelphia, WB Saunders, 2000, p 264, Fig. 17-2.)*

    b. Type I IgE-mediated reactions associated with certain exposure:
      (1) Certain foods (e.g., peanuts)
      (2) Insect bites (e.g., fire ant)
      (3) Drugs (e.g., penicillin, morphine)
  2. Dermatographism (Fig. 24-23)
    • Urticaria develops in areas of mechanical pressure on skin.

Urticaria: exhibits dermatographism

N. Acanthosis nigricans
  1. Verrucoid, pigmented skin lesion
  2. Commonly located in the axilla (Fig. 24-24)
  3. Associated with several factors:
    a. Stomach adenocarcinoma
    b. Multiple endocrine neoplasia syndrome IIb
    c. Insulin receptor deficiency, obesity

VI. Benign Melanocytic Disorders
  A. Solar lentigo
    1. Common finding in elderly individuals
    2. Brown, macules located on sun-exposed areas ("liver spots") (Fig. 24-25)
      • Increased number of melanocytes
    3. *Not* precancerous

Freckles: normal number of melanocytes with increase in melanosomes

  B. Vitiligo
    1. Common in black Americans
    2. Autoimmune destruction of melanocytes
      • Causes localized to extensive areas of skin depigmentation.
    3. Often associated with other autoimmune conditions
      • Examples—Hashimoto's thyroiditis, hypoparathyroidism

Vitiligo: autoimmune destruction of melanocytes

  C. Chloasma
    1. Female predominance
      a. Women taking oral contraceptives
      b. Women who are pregnant ("pregnancy mask")
    2. Macular, hyperpigmented lesions on the forehead and cheeks

Albinism: deficiency of tyrosinase; absent melanin in melanocytes

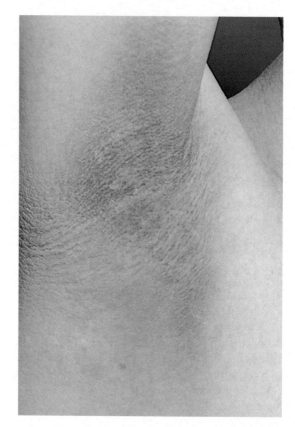

24-24: *Acanthosis nigricans showing a pigmented verrucoid lesion in the axilla. (From Lookingbill D, Marks J: Principles of Dermatology, 3rd ed. Philadelphia, WB Saunders, 2000, p 350, Fig. 25-5.)*

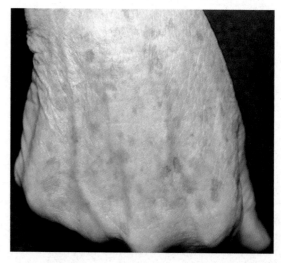

24-25: *Solar lentigo on the dorsum of the hand showing numerous brown macules. (From Lookingbill D, Marks J: Principles of Dermatology, 3rd ed. Philadelphia, WB Saunders, 2000, p 94, Fig. 7-2.)*

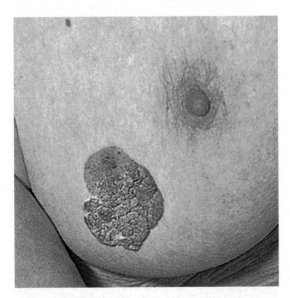

24-26: *Seborrheic keratosis on the breast showing raised, pigmented lesion with a verrucoid surface. (From Forbes C, Jackson W: Color Atlas and Text of Clinical Medicine, 2nd ed. St. Louis, Mosby, 2003, p 110, Fig. 2-107.)*

VII. Neoplastic Skin Disorders

A. Seborrheic keratosis

1. Occurs in individuals older than 50 years of age
2. Benign pigmented epidermal tumor (Fig. 24-26)
   - Coin-like, macular to raised verrucoid lesion with "stuck-on" appearance
3. Leser-Trélat sign
   a. Rapid increase in number of keratoses
   b. Phenotypic marker for stomach adenocarcinoma

B. Keratoacanthoma

1. Male predominance
2. Rapidly growing, benign crateriform tumor with a central keratin plug (Fig. 24-27)
   a. Develops in sun-exposed areas
   b. Mimics a well-differentiated squamous cell carcinoma
3. Regresses spontaneously with scarring

C. Benign epidermal cysts

1. Epidermal inclusion cysts
   a. Derived from the epidermis of the hair follicle
   b. Locations
      - Face, base of ears, and trunk

Leser-Trélat sign: phenotypic marker for stomach adenocarcinoma

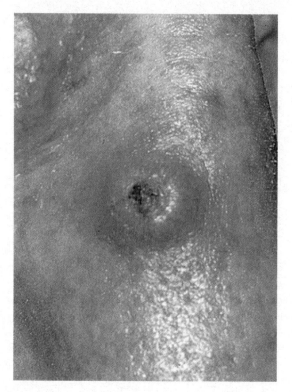

24-27: *Keratoacanthoma showing a crateriform tumor with a central keratin plug. (From Lookingbill D, Marks J: Principles of Dermatology, 3rd ed. Philadelphia, WB Saunders, 2000, p 83, Fig. 6-12.)*

     c. Cyst wall composed of normal epidermis that produces keratin
       • Keratin intermixed with lipid-rich debris
     d. Spontaneous inflammation and rupture may occur.
   2. Pilar cyst (wen)
     a. Derived from hair root sheaths
     b. Located on the scalp and face
     c. Cyst wall lacks stratum granulosum.
       • Keratin has a laminated appearance.
     d. Spontaneous inflammation and rupture may occur.

D. Nevocellular nevus (mole)
   1. Neoplastic melanocytic disorder
   2. Benign tumor of neural crest–derived nevus cells
     • Nevus cells are modified melanocytes.
   3. Begins in early childhood as junctional nevus
     a. Pigmented macular lesion
     b. Nests of nevus cells occur along the basal cell layer.
   4. Junctional nevus develops into a compound nevus.
     a. Usually occurs in children and adolescents
     b. Nevus cells extend into the superficial dermis.
       • Junctional and intradermal components are present.

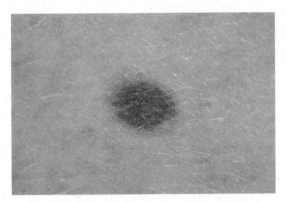

24-28: *Compound nevus showing a pigmented lesion with a papillomatous surface. (From Lookingbill D, Marks J: Principles of Dermatology, 3rd ed. Philadelphia, WB Saunders, 2000, p 94, Fig. 7-4A.)*

    c. Pigmented lesion with a papillomatous surface (Fig. 24-28)

5. Intradermal nevus
   - Develop when a compound nevus loses its junctional component

6. Dysplastic nevus (atypical mole)
   a. May arise sporadically
      - Small risk for developing into a malignant melanoma
   b. May be associated with the dysplastic nevus syndrome
      (1) Autosomal dominant syndrome with more than 100 nevi on the skin
      (2) Dysplastic nevi may develop into malignant melanomas.
      (3) All patients require a yearly dermatologic examination.
   c. Characteristics
      (1) Usually have a diameter greater than 6 mm
      (2) Irregular borders, irregular distribution of melanin

E. **Basal cell carcinoma**
   1. Caused by chronic exposure to ultraviolet light
   2. Raised papule or nodule with a central crater (see Fig. 8-8)
      - Sides of the crater are surfaced by telangiectatic vessels.
   3. Occurs in sun-exposed areas
      - Inner canthus of the eye, upper lip
   4. Locally aggressive, infiltrating cancer that does *not* metastasize
      a. Arises from the basal cell layer of the epidermis
      b. Cords of basophilic-staining basal cells infiltrate the underlying dermis.

F. **Squamous cell carcinoma**
   1. Risk factors
      a. Excessive exposure to ultraviolet light (most common)
      b. Actinic (solar) keratosis
      c. Arsenic exposure
      d. Scar tissue in a third-degree burn

Most common nevus in adults: intradermal nevus

Dysplastic nevus syndrome: marked increase in development of malignant melanoma

Most common malignant skin tumor: basal cell carcinoma

Squamous cell
carcinoma: most common
cancer complicating
immunosuppressive
therapy

    e. Orifice of chronically draining sinus tract

    f. Immunosuppressive therapy

  2. Scaly to nodular lesions

    a. Nodules are often ulcerated.

    b. Majority occur in sun-exposed areas of the body.

      • Examples—ears, lower lip, dorsum of the hands

    c. Usually well-differentiated

      • Minimal risk for metastasis

G. Malignant melanoma

  1. Malignant tumor of melanocytes

  2. Most rapidly increasing cancer worldwide

    • More common in whites than black Americans

  3. Risk factors

    a. Exposure to excessive sunlight at an early age

      • Single most important risk factor

    b. Dysplastic nevus syndrome

    c. History of melanoma in first- or second-degree relative

    d. Xeroderma pigmentosum (see Chapter 8)

  4. Radial growth phase

    a. Initial phase of invasion

    b. Melanocytes proliferate

      (1) Laterally within the epidermis

      (2) Along the dermoepidermal junction

      (3) Within the papillary dermis

    c. *No* metastatic potential in this phase

  5. Vertical growth phase

    a. Final phase of invasion

    b. Malignant cells penetrate the underlying reticular dermis.

    c. Potential for metastasis

ABCD signs of
melanoma: *a*symmetry;
*b*orders irregular; *c*olor
changes; *d*iameter
increased

  6. Types of malignant melanoma

    a. Superficial spreading melanoma (see Fig. 8-9)

      (1) Most common type (70% of cases)

      (2) Develops on lower extremities and back

    b. Lentigo maligna melanoma (4–10% of cases)

      (1) Extension of lentigo maligna (intraepidermal lesion) into the dermis

      (2) Occurs on parts of the face most exposed to the sun (Fig. 24-29)

Most common type of
malignant melanoma:
superficial spreading
melanoma

    c. Nodular melanoma (15–30% of cases)

      (1) *No* radial growth phase

      (2) Directly invades the dermis

      (3) Poor prognosis

    d. Acral lentiginous melanoma (2–8% of cases)

      (1) Located on the palm, sole, or beneath the nail

        • Often confused with a subungual hematoma

      (2) May occur in black Americans

      (3) Poor prognosis

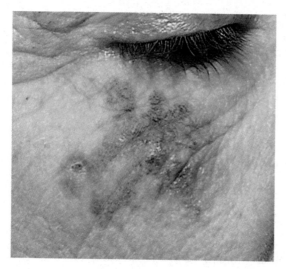

24-29: *Lentigo maligna melanoma on the face showing asymmetry, border irregularity, color variation, and diameter greater than 6 mm. (From Lookingbill D, Marks J: Principles of Dermatology, 3rd ed. Philadelphia, WB Saunders, 2000, p 94, Fig. 7-4B.)*

7. Depth of invasion best determines biologic behavior.
   a. Lesions with less than 0.76 mm invasion do *not* metastasize.
   b. Lesions with greater than 1.7 mm invasion have the potential for lymph node metastasis.
8. Prevention
   • Sunscreen above 15 SPF (controversial)

Management of suspected melanoma: excision of entire tumor

VIII. Hair Disorders
A. Phases of hair growth in succession
1. Anagen phase
   a. Development of new shaft of hair comes from hair bulb.
   b. Hair length is determined in this stage.
2. Catagen phase
   a. Regression of growth site of hair shaft
   b. Resting phase
3. Telogen phase
   a. Regression of hair-producing elements of hair follicle
   b. Followed by anagen phase
4. Hair growth is usually asynchronous.
   • Only a small percentage of hair is lost at any point in time.
5. Estrogen effect on hair growth
   a. Causes synchronous hair growth
   b. All the hairs enter the resting phase at once.

Estrogen: causes synchronous hair growth; risk for massive hair loss

B. Massive hair loss
1. Postpartum
   • Most common cause

2. Oral contraceptive pills
3. Stress
4. Radiation/chemotherapy
   - Inhibition of anagen phase when cells in the hair bulb are dividing

C. Alopecia areata
1. Hairless areas on the scalp
2. Short, underdeveloped hairs in areas of baldness

IX. **Nail Disorders**
   A. Nail anatomy
   1. Lunula
      a. White half-moon–shaped area proximal to the cuticle
      b. Underlying nail bed is partially keratinized, which produces the white color.
   2. Nail plate
      - Attached to the nail bed except distally where it separates from the hyponychium
   3. Nail matrix
      a. Underneath the cuticle (eponychium)
      b. Germinative zone where the nail plate originates
   B. Nail disorders
   1. Psoriasis
      - Greater than 80% have nail pitting.
   2. Iron deficiency
      - Koilonychia (spoon nails)
   3. Infective endocarditis and trichinosis
      - Splinter hemorrhages in nails
   4. Mees' lines
      a. Sign of arsenic poisoning and systemic illness of any kind
      b. Transverse white lines in the nail plate
         - Extend proximally until they are pared off
   5. Subungual hematoma
      - Blood clot under the nail plate due to trauma

25 CHAPTER

Nervous System Disorders

I. **Cerebral Edema, Pseudotumor Cerebri, Herniations, Hydrocephalus**

A. **Cerebral edema**
   1. Subdivided into intracellular and extracellular types
   2. Intracellular edema
      a. Water moves into cells.
      b. Causes
         (1) Dysfunctional Na^+/K^+-ATPase pump (e.g., hypoxia)
         (2) Hyponatremia causing osmotic shift
   3. Extracellular edema
      a. Due to increased vessel permeability
      b. Causes
         (1) Acute inflammation (e.g., meningitis, encephalitis)
         (2) Metastasis, trauma, lead poisoning
         (3) Respiratory acidosis, hypoxemia

> A patient with head trauma is purposely hyperventilated to produce respiratory alkalosis, which causes cerebral vessel constriction. This decreases the risk of increased vessel permeability and cerebral edema. Respiratory acidosis and hypoxemia cause vasodilation of cerebral vessels, which increases cerebral vessel permeability, resulting in cerebral edema.

Respiratory acidosis, hypoxemia: increase cerebral vessel permeability; enhance cerebral edema

   4. Produces signs of increased intracranial pressure (intracranial hypertension)
      a. Papilledema
         • Swelling of the optic disk (Fig. 25-1)
      b. Headache, projectile vomiting *without* nausea
      c. Sinus bradycardia, hypertension
      d. Potential for herniation (see below)

Papilledema: sign of cerebral edema

B. **Pseudotumor cerebri**
   • Benign intracranial hypertension
   1. Increased intracranial pressure
      • Absence of tumor and obstruction to cerebrospinal fluid (CSF) flow
   2. Epidemiology and pathogenesis
      a. Decreased CSF resorption
      b. Commonly occurs in young, obese females
   3. Clinical findings (see above)
   4. Diagnosis
      a. Normal CT and MRI

Pseudotumor cerebri: ↑ intracranial pressure without evidence of tumor or obstruction

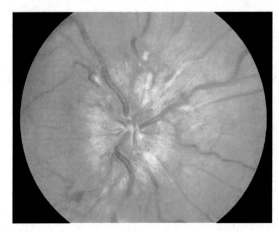

25-1: *Optic disk with papilledema showing loss of the disk margin and hard exudates (white streaks). (From Perkin GD: Mosby's Color Atlas and Text of Neurology. St. Louis, Mosby, 2002, p 160, Fig. 9-4.)*

    b. Increased CSF pressure
       • Usually over 300 mm H$_2$O (normal 70–180)
    c. Decreased CSF protein

C. Cerebral herniation
    1. Pathogenesis
      a. Complication of increased intracranial pressure
      b. Portions of the brain become displaced.
        (1) Openings of dural partitions
        (2) Openings of the skull
    2. Subfalcine herniation
      a. Cingulate gyrus herniates under the falx cerebri.
      b. Causes compression of the anterior cerebral artery (ACA)
    3. Uncal herniation
      a. Medial portion of temporal lobe herniates through tentorium cerebelli.
      b. Complications
        (1) Compression of the midbrain
          • Produces Duret's hemorrhages
        (2) Compression of oculomotor nerve
          (a) Eye is deviated down and out.
          (b) Pupil is mydriatic (dilated).
            • Compression of parasympathetic postganglionic fibers
        (3) Compression of posterior cerebral artery
          • Causes hemorrhagic infarction of occipital lobe
    4. Tonsillar herniation
      a. Cerebellar tonsils herniate into the foramen magnum.
      b. Causes "coning" of the cerebellar tonsils
      c. Produces cardiorespiratory arrest

Uncal herniation: compression of oculomotor nerve

Uncal herniation: midbrain hemorrhage, oculomotor nerve palsy, mydriasis

D. Hydrocephalus
- Increase in the CSF volume causes enlargement of the ventricles.
  1. Production and movement of CSF
     a. Produced by the choroid plexus in the ventricles
     b. Exits fourth ventricle through foramina and enters subarachnoid space
     c. Reabsorbed by the arachnoid granulations into the dural venous sinuses
     d. CSF characteristics
        (1) Lower protein and glucose than serum
        (2) *No* neutrophils, rare mononuclear cells
        (3) Higher chloride level than serum
  2. Communicating (nonobstructive) hydrocephalus
     a. Open communication between ventricles and subarachnoid space
     b. Causes
        (1) Increased CSF production
           - Example—choroid plexus papilloma
        (2) Obstruction in reabsorption of CSF by arachnoid granulations
           - Examples—postmeningitic scarring, tumor
  3. Noncommunicating (obstructive) hydrocephalus
     a. Obstruction of CSF flow out of the ventricles
     b. Causes
        (1) Stricture of the aqueduct of Sylvius
           (a) Most common cause in newborns
           (b) Paralysis of upward gaze (Parinaud's syndrome)
        (2) Tumor in the fourth ventricle
           - Examples—ependymoma, medulloblastoma
        (3) Scarring at the base of the brain
           - Example—tuberculous meningitis
        (4) Colloid cyst in the third ventricle
        (5) Developmental disorders (see section II)
  4. Clinical findings
     a. Newborns
        - Ventricles dilate and enlarge the head circumference.
     b. Adults
        - Progressive dementia, wide-based gait, urinary incontinence
  5. Hydrocephalus ex vacuo
     a. Dilated appearance of the ventricles when the brain mass is decreased
     b. Example—Alzheimer's disease

II. Developmental Disorders
A. Neural tube defects
  1. Pathogenesis
     a. Failure of fusion of the lateral folds of the neural plate
     b. Rupture of a previously closed neural tube
  2. Maternal findings
     - Increased maternal α-fetoprotein in serum or amniotic fluid

> Blockage of aqueduct of Sylvius: most common cause of hydrocephalus in newborns

> Hydrocephalus adults: dementia, gait disturbance, urinary incontinence

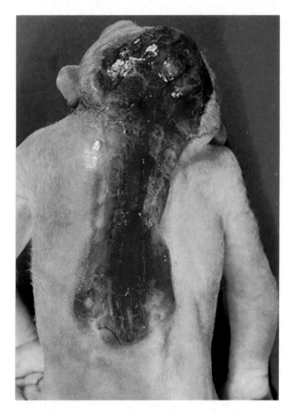

25-2: *Anencephaly showing absence of the brain and opening of the spinal canal. (From Damjanov I: Pathology for the Health-Related Professions, 2nd ed. Philadelphia, WB Saunders, 2000, p 126, Fig. 5-23B.)*

Protection against neural tube defects: folate level must be adequate *before* pregnancy

3. Anencephaly
   a. Complete absence of brain (Fig. 25-2)
   b. Frog-like appearance
   c. Maternal polyhydramnios
4. Spina bifida occulta
   a. Defect in closure of the posterior vertebral arch
   b. Dimple or tuft of hair in the skin overlying L5–S1
5. Meningocele
   a. Spina bifida with cystic mass containing meninges
   b. Most common in lumbosacral region
6. Meningomyelocele
   a. Spinal bifida with cystic mass containing meninges and spinal cord
   b. Most common in lumbosacral region

B. Arnold-Chiari malformation
1. Caudal extension of medulla and cerebellar vermis through foramen magnum
2. Noncommunicating hydrocephalus
3. Platybasia (flattening of base of skull)
4. Meningomyelocele, syringomyelia

C. Dandy-Walker malformation
1. Hypoplasia of the cerebellar vermis
2. Cystic dilation of the fourth ventricle
3. Noncommunicating hydrocephalus

D. Syringomyelia
1. Degenerative disease of spinal cord
    a. Fluid-filled cavity (syrinx) within the cervical spinal cord
    b. Produces cervical cord enlargement
    c. Cavity expands and causes degeneration of spinal tracts.
2. Associated with Arnold-Chiari malformation
3. Clinical findings
    a. Disruption of the crossed lateral spinothalamic tracts
        (1) Loss of pain and temperature sensation in the hands
        (2) Patient can burn hands *without* being aware of the burn.
    b. Destruction of anterior horn cells
        (1) Atrophy of intrinsic muscles of the hands
        (2) Often confused with amyotrophic lateral sclerosis (ALS)
            • *No* sensory changes in ALS

Syringomyelia: ↓ pain and temperature sensation in hands

E. Phakomatoses
1. Neurocutaneous syndromes
    a. Disordered growth of ectodermal tissue
    b. Malformations or tumors of the central nervous system (CNS)
2. Tuberous sclerosis
    a. Autosomal dominant disorder
    b. Mental retardation and seizures beginning in infancy
    c. Angiofibromas on the face
    d. Hypopigmented skin lesions ("ash leaf" lesions)
        • Best identified with Wood's lamp
    e. Hamartomatous lesions
        (1) Astrocyte proliferations in subependyma
            • Look like "candlestick drippings" in the ventricles
        (2) Angiomyolipomas in the kidneys
    f. Rhabdomyoma in the heart

Tuberous sclerosis: mental retardation; hamartomas in brain, kidneys

3. Neurofibromatosis
    a. Autosomal dominant disorder
    b. Café-au-lait macules, pigmented neurofibromas (Fig. 25-3)
    c. Lisch nodules
        • Hamartomas in the iris
    d. Kyphoscoliosis
    e. Optic nerve glioma, meningioma, acoustic neuroma
    f. Pheochromocytoma, Wilms' tumor
        • Both are associated with hypertension.
    g. Neurofibrosarcoma
        • Usually involving large nerve trunks

Neurofibromatosis: associated with pheochromocytoma, acoustic neuromas

4. Sturge-Weber syndrome (see Chapter 9)
    a. Somatic mosaicism or sporadic

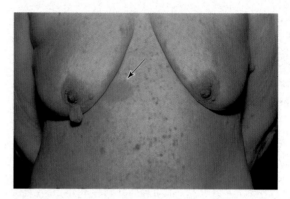

25-3: *Neurofibromatosis showing café-au-lait macule (arrow) and numerous pigmented, pedunculated neurofibromas. (From Forbes C, Jackson W: Color Atlas and Text of Clinical Medicine, 2nd ed. St. Louis, Mosby, 2003, p 104, Fig. 2-86.)*

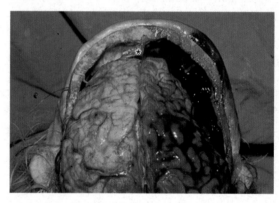

25-4: *Epidural hematoma showing blood between the dura (asterisk) and the bone of the skull. (From Bouloux P-M: Self-Assessment Picture Tests: Medicine, vol. 1. St. Louis, Mosby, 1996, p 14, Fig. 28.)*

      b. Vascular malformation on the face
      c. Ipsilateral arteriovenous malformation in the meninges

III. Head Trauma
  A. Cerebral contusion
    1. Permanent damage to small blood vessels and the surface of the brain

Coup injuries: site of impact

    2. Most often secondary to an acceleration-deceleration injury
    3. Coup injuries occur at the *site* of impact.

Contrecoup injuries: opposite site of impact

    4. Contrecoup injuries occur *opposite* the site of impact.
      • Common sites are at the tips of the frontal and temporal lobes.
  B. Acute epidural hematoma
    1. Arterial bleed creates a blood-filled space between the bone and dura (Fig. 25-4).

Epidural hematoma: temporoparietal skull fracture and tear of middle meningeal artery

    2. Caused by a fracture of the temporoparietal bone
      a. Severance of the middle meningeal artery
      b. Vessel lies between the dura and inner table of bone.
    3. Intracranial pressure increases, leading to herniation and death.

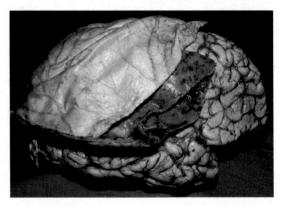

25-5: *Subdural hematoma. The reflected dura shows the outer membrane of an organized venous clot covering the convexity of the brain. (From Damjanov I, Linder J: Pathology: A Color Atlas. St. Louis, Mosby, 2000, p 405, Fig. 19-20.)*

C. Subdural hematoma
1. Venous bleeding between the dura and arachnoid membranes
   a. Most often the result of blunt trauma
      - Examples—car accident, baseball bat
   b. Due to tearing of bridging veins between brain and dural sinuses (Fig. 25-5)
   c. Slowly enlarging blood clot covers the convexity of the brain.
2. Fluctuating levels of consciousness
3. Herniation and death may occur.

Subdural hematoma: tear of bridging veins producing venous blood clot

IV. CNS Vascular Disorders
A. Global hypoxic injury
1. Causes of hypoxic injury (see Chapter 1)
   a. Ischemia secondary to atherosclerosis of the carotid artery
   b. Chronic carbon monoxide poisoning
   c. Chronic hypoxemia (e.g., chronic lung disease)

> Repeated episodes of hypoglycemia have the same effects on the brain as does hypoxic injury. Hypoglycemia most commonly occurs in type 1 diabetes mellitus.

2. Complications
   a. Cerebral atrophy
      (1) Due to apoptosis of neurons in layers 3, 5, and 6 of the cerebral cortex
         - Produces laminar necrosis
      (2) Neurons are the most susceptible cell to hypoxic injury.
   b. Watershed infarcts (see Chapter 1)
      (1) Occur at the junctions of arterial territories
      (2) Example—junction between the anterior and middle cerebral arteries
   c. Cerebrovascular accident (e.g., stroke)

B. Cerebrovascular accidents

1. Atherosclerotic (thrombotic) stroke
    a. Most common type of stroke
    b. Usually pale infarcts (liquefactive necrosis)
        (1) Platelet thrombus develops over a disrupted plaque.
            (a) Middle cerebral artery (MCA)
            (b) Internal carotid artery near the bifurcation
        (2) Reperfusion usually does *not* occur.
            • Hemorrhagic infarction develops if reperfusion occurs.
    c. Most occur in the distribution of the middle cerebral artery (MCA).
    d. Gross and microscopic findings
        (1) Wedge-shaped area of pale infarction
            • Develops at the *periphery* of the cerebral cortex (Fig. 25-6)
        (2) Swelling of the brain occurs.
            (a) Loss of demarcation between gray and white matter
            (b) Myelin begins to break down.
        (3) Gliosis is the reaction to injury.
            (a) Astrocytes proliferate at the margins of the infarct.
            (b) Microglial cells (macrophages) remove lipid debris.
        (4) Cystic area develops after 10 days to 3 weeks.
    e. Clinical findings
        (1) Most strokes are preceded by transient ischemic attacks.
            • Transient neurologic deficits last less than 24 hours.
        (2) Deficits that do *not* resolve within 24 hours are called strokes.
    f. Strokes involving the MCA
        (1) Contralateral hemiparesis and sensory loss in upper extremity
        (2) Expressive aphasia
            • If Broca's area is involved in the dominant (left) hemisphere
        (3) Visual field defects
        (4) Head and eyes deviate *toward* the side of the lesion.
    g. Strokes involving vertebrobasilar arterial system
        (1) Vertigo, ataxia
        (2) Ipsilateral sensory loss in face
        (3) Contralateral hemiparesis and sensory loss in the trunk and limbs

2. Embolic stroke
    a. Source of emboli
        • Most often originate from the left side of the heart (see Chapter 4)
    b. Produces a hemorrhagic infarction
        (1) Most occur in the distribution of the MCA (Fig. 25-7).
        (2) Vessel reperfusion after lysis of embolic material produces hemorrhage.

3. Intracerebral hemorrhage
    a. Most often due to stress imposed on vessels by hypertension
        (1) Branches of lenticulostriate vessels develop Charcot-Bouchard macroaneurysms.
        (2) Rupture of aneurysms produces intracerebral hemorrhage (hematoma).

Atherosclerotic stroke: pale infarction extending to periphery of cerebral cortex

Embolic stroke: hemorrhagic infarction extending to periphery of cerebral cortex

Intracerebral hemorrhage: complication of hypertension

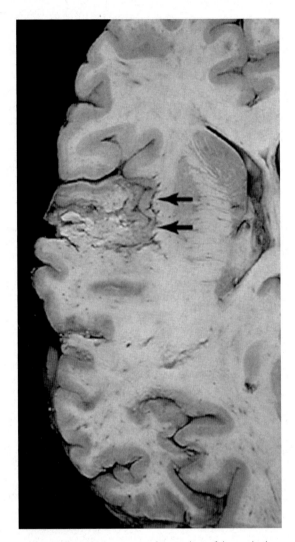

25-6: *Atherosclerotic stroke showing necrotic areas at the periphery of the cerebral cortex. Arrows are located at the line of demarcation between normal and infarcted tissue. (From Damjanov I, Linder J: Pathology: A Color Atlas. St. Louis, Mosby, 2000, p 408, Fig. 19-25A.)*

- Intracerebral hematoma pushes the brain parenchyma aside (Fig. 25-8).
  - b. Common sites of hemorrhage
    - (1) Basal ganglia (35–50% occur in the putamen)
    - (2) Thalamus (10%)
    - (3) Pons and cerebellar hemispheres (10%)
  - 4. Subarachnoid hemorrhage
    - a. Causes
      - (1) Majority are secondary to rupture of a congenital berry aneurysm.

Treatment of hypertension reduces the incidence of stroke by more than 40%.

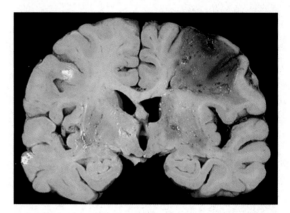

25-7: *Embolic stroke showing a wedge-shaped hemorrhagic infarction along the periphery of the cerebral cortex. (From Damjanov I, Linder J: Anderson's Pathology, 10th ed. St. Louis, Mosby, 1996, p 375, Fig. 17-16.)*

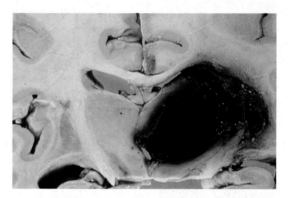

25-8: *Intracerebral hemorrhage, showing a large blood clot within the basal ganglia area of the brain. (From Damjanov I: Pathology for the Health-Related Professions, 2nd ed. Philadelphia, WB Saunders, 2000, p 506, Fig. 21-7.)*

    (2) Bleeding from an arteriovenous malformation is a less common cause.

  b. Congenital berry aneurysm

    (1) May develop from normal hemodynamic stress or hypertension

    (2) Most develop at junctions of communicating branches with main cerebral artery.

      (a) Junction lacks internal elastic lamina and smooth muscle.

      (b) Most common site for berry aneurysm is junction with ACA.

    (3) Rupture releases blood into the subarachnoid space.

      • Blood covers the surface of the brain.

    (4) Blood in the CSF is broken down into bilirubin pigment.

      • Imparts a yellow color to CSF called xanthochromia

  c. Clinical findings

    (1) Sudden onset of severe occipital headache

Subarachnoid hemorrhage: rupture of congenital berry aneurysm

(a) Described as "worst headache ever"
(b) Nuchal rigidity is present.
(2) About 50% of patients die soon after the hemorrhage.
(3) Complications
(a) Further hemorrhage
(b) Hydrocephalus
(c) Permanent neurologic deficits
5. Lacunar infarcts
a. Cystic areas of microinfarction less than 1 cm in diameter
b. Caused by hyaline arteriolosclerosis
- Secondary to either hypertension (most common) or diabetes mellitus
c. Stroke syndromes
(1) Pure motor strokes with or without dysarthria
- Occur if the posterior limb of the internal capsule is involved
(2) Pure sensory strokes
- Occur if the thalamus is involved

Lacunar strokes: caused by hypertension or diabetes mellitus

V. CNS Infections
A. Pathogenesis
1. Hematogenous spread (most common)
2. Traumatic implantation
3. Local extension from nearby infection
4. Ascent of peripheral nerve

CNS infections: most are due to sepsis

B. Meningitis
1. Inflammation of pia matter covering the brain (Fig. 25-9)

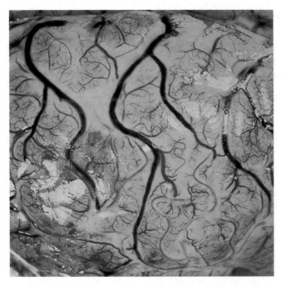

25-9: *Bacterial meningitis showing engorged blood vessels and a creamy exudate covering the surface of the pia mater. (From Perkin GD: Mosby's Color Atlas and Text of Neurology. St. Louis, Mosby, 2002, p 196, Fig. 11-1.)*

TABLE 25-1:
Cerebrospinal Fluid (CSF) Findings in Viral, Bacterial, and Fungal Meningitis

CSF	Bacterial/Fungus	Viral
Total cell count	1000–20,000 cells/mm³	<1000 cells/mm³
Differential count	>90% neutrophils and mononuclear cells	First 24–48 hours, neutrophils, then switches to lymphocytes/monocytes after 48 hours
CSF glucose	Decreased	Normal: exceptions—mumps, herpes
CSF protein	Increased	Increased
Gram stain	Frequently positive (sensitivity 75–80%)	Negative

2. Usually due to hematogenous spread
3. Clinical findings
   - Fever, nuchal rigidity, headache
4. Laboratory findings in viral meningitis (Table 25-1)
   a. Increased CSF protein
      - Due to increased vessel permeability
   b. Increased total CSF leukocyte count
      - Initially neutrophils but converts to lymphocytes in 24 hours
   c. Normal CSF glucose
5. Laboratory findings in bacterial and fungal meningitis (see Table 25-1)
   a. Increased CSF protein
   b. Increased total CSF leukocyte count
   c. Decreased CSF glucose

C. **Encephalitis**
   1. Inflammation of the brain
   2. Clinical findings
      a. Fever, headache
      b. Impaired mental status, drowsiness
D. **Cerebral abscess**
   1. Pathogenesis
      a. Spread from an adjacent focus of infection (e.g., sinuses)
      b. Hematogenous spread (e.g., infective endocarditis)
   2. Single or multiple lesions (Fig. 25-10)
E. **Viral CNS infections (Figs. 25-11 and 25-12; Tables 25-2 and 25-3)**
F. **Bacterial CNS infections (Table 25-4)**
G. **Fungal and parasitic CNS infections (Table 25-5 and Fig. 25-13)**

VI. **Demyelinating Disorders**
   A. **Pathogenesis**
      1. Destruction of normal myelin
         - Example—multiple sclerosis
      2. Production of abnormal myelin
         - Example—leukodystrophy

Meningitis: ↑ CSF protein (viral, bacterial, fungal); ↓ CSF glucose (bacterial, fungal)

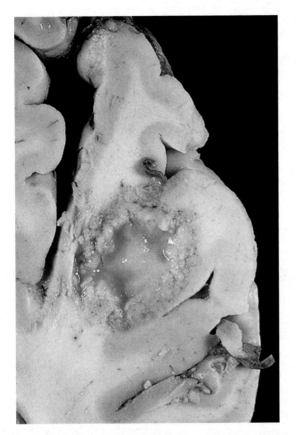

25-10: *Cerebral abscess showing a cystic mass lined by necrotic, purulent material. (From Burger PC, Scheithauer BW, Vogel KS: Surgical Pathology of the Nervous System, 4th ed. London, Churchill Livingstone, 2002, p 121, Fig. 3-17.)*

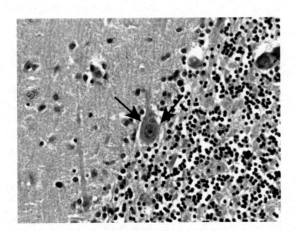

25-11: *Cerebellum in a patient with rabies showing Purkinje cells with intracytoplasmic, eosinophilic inclusions (arrows) called Negri bodies. (From Kumar V, Fausto N, Abbas A: Robbins and Cotran's Pathologic Basis of Disease, 7th ed. Philadelphia, WB Saunders, 2004, p 1375, Fig. 28-25.)*

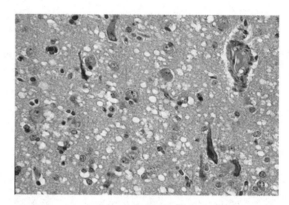

25-12: *Spongiform encephalopathy in Creutzfeldt-Jakob disease showing classic "bubbles and holes" of the neuropil cell bodies. (From Damjanov I, Linder J: Pathology: A Color Atlas. St. Louis, Mosby, 2000, p 412, Fig. 19-41.)*

TABLE 25-2:
Viral Infections of the Central Nervous System

Virus	Disease	Comments
Arboviruses	Encephalitis	Mosquitoes are the vector Wild birds are the reservoir for the virus West Nile virus: crows and other birds are spreading the disease from New York to the West Coast Encephalitis can be fatal
Coxsackievirus	Meningitis	Most common cause of viral meningitis Viral meningitis peaks in late summer and early autumn
Cytomegalovirus	Encephalitis	Most common viral CNS infection in AIDS Primarily intranuclear basophilic inclusions Periventricular calcification in newborns
Herpes simplex virus type 1	Meningitis and encephalitis	Causes hemorrhagic necrosis of temporal lobes
HIV	Encephalitis	Most common cause of AIDS dementia Microglial cells fuse to form multinucleated cells
Lymphocytic choriomeningitis	Meningitis and encephalitis	Endemic in the mouse population Transmission: food or water contaminated with mouse urine/feces Meningoencephalitis: combination of nuchal rigidity and mental status abnormalities (encephalitis) CSF findings: increased protein, lymphocyte infiltrate, normal to decreased glucose
Poliovirus	Encephalitis and myelitis (spinal cord)	Destroys upper and lower motor neurons Causes muscle paralysis
Rabies virus (Fig. 25-11)	Encephalitis	Most often transmitted by raccoon bite (40% of case) Other vectors are dog, skunk, bat, and coyote Virus ascends peripheral nerves Neurons contain intracytoplasmic Negri bodies CNS excitability stage followed by flaccid paralysis

CNS, central nervous system.

TABLE 25-3:
Slow Virus Diseases of the Central Nervous System

Disease	Comments
Creutzfeldt-Jakob disease (Fig. 25-12)	Unconventional slow virus encephalitis due to prions (proteinaceous material devoid of RNA or DNA) Transmitted by corneal transplantation, contact with human brain, use of improperly sterilized cortical electrodes, or ingestion of tissues from cattle with bovine spongiform encephalopathy ("mad cow" disease) Brain has "bubble and holes" spongiform change in cerebral cortex Death usually occurs within 1 year
Progressive multifocal leukoencephalopathy	Conventional slow virus encephalitis due to papovavirus Intranuclear inclusion in oligodendrocytes Occurs in AIDS when CD4 T_H count < 50 cells/μL
Subacute sclerosing panencephalitis	Conventional slow virus encephalitis associated with rubeola (measles) virus Intranuclear inclusions in neurons and oligodendrocytes Death usually occurs within 1–2 years

TABLE 25-4:
Bacterial Infections of the Central Nervous System

Bacterium	Disease	Comments
Group B streptococcus (Streptococcus agalactiae)	Neonatal meningitis	Gram-positive coccus Most common cause of neonatal meningitis Spreads from a focus of infection in maternal vagina
Escherichia coli	Neonatal meningitis	Gram-negative rod Second most common cause of neonatal meningitis
Listeria monocytogenes	Neonatal meningitis	Gram-positive rod with tumbling motility Pathogen found in soft cheese, hot dogs
Neisseria meningitidis	Meningitis	Gram-negative diplococcus Most common cause of meningitis in those between 1 month and 18 years of age
Streptococcus pneumoniae	Meningitis	Gram-positive diplococcus Most common cause of meningitis in patients > 18 years of age
Mycobacterium tuberculosis	Meningitis	Complication of primary tuberculosis Involves base of brain Vasculitis (infarction) and scarring (hydrocephalus)
Treponema pallidum	Meningitis, encephalitis, and myelitis	Spirochete Types of neurosyphilis: Meningovascular: vasculitis causing strokes General paresis: dementia Tabes dorsalis: involves posterior root ganglia and posterior column; causes ataxia, loss of vibration sensation, absent deep tendon reflexes, Argyll-Robertson pupil (pupils accommodate but do not react)

TABLE 25-5:
Fungal and Parasitic Infections of the Central Nervous System

Fungus/Parasite	Disease	Comments
Cryptococcus neoformans	Meningitis and encephalitis	Occurs in immunocompromised host Most common fungal CNS infection in AIDS Budding yeasts visible with India ink
Mucor species	Frontal lobe abscess	Occurs in diabetic ketoacidosis; spreads from frontal sinuses
Naegleria fowleri	Meningoencephalitis	Involves frontal lobes Contracted by swimming in freshwater lakes
Taenia solium (Fig. 25-13)	Cysticercosis	Patient (intermediate host) ingests food or water containing eggs; eggs develop into larval forms (cysticerci) that invade brain, producing calcified cysts causing seizures
Toxoplasma gondii	Encephalitis	Most common CNS space-occupying lesion in AIDS Congenital toxoplasmosis produces basal ganglia calcification

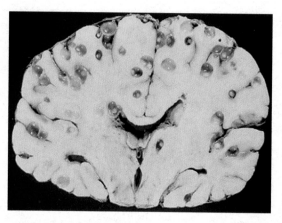

25-13: *Neurocysticercosis showing multiple cysts between the gray and white matter. (From Damjanov I, Linder J: Pathology: A Color Atlas. St. Louis, Mosby, 2000, p 411, Fig. 19-38.)*

    3. Destruction of oligodendrocytes
      • Examples—multiple sclerosis, slow virus infections
  B. Acquired disorders
    1. Multiple sclerosis (MS)
      a. Epidemiology
        (1) Most common demyelinating disease
        (2) Female predominance
          • Occurs most often in women 20 to 40 years of age
        (3) Associated with HLA-DR2
      b. Pathogenesis
        (1) CD8 T-cell destruction of myelin sheaths and oligodendrocytes

        (2) Antibodies directed against myelin basic protein in
            oligodendrocytes

  c. Gross findings
     • Demyelinating plaques occur in white matter of brain/spinal cord
       (Fig. 25-14).

  d. Clinical findings
        (1) Episodic course punctuated by acute relapses and remissions
        (2) Sensory and motor dysfunction
           • Paresthesias, muscle weakness
        (3) Optic neuritis
           (a) Inflammation of the optic nerve
           (b) Blurry vision or sudden loss of vision
        (4) Cerebellar ataxia
        (5) Scanning speech (sound drunk)
        (6) Intention tremor, nystagmus
        (7) Bilateral internuclear ophthalmoplegia
           • Demyelination of medial longitudinal fasciculus

MS: autoimmune destruction of myelin sheath and oligodendrocytes

Bilateral internuclear ophthalmoplegia: pathognomonic for MS

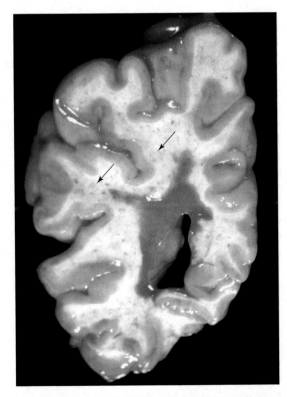

25-14: *Multiple sclerosis showing multiple areas of demyelinated white mater (arrows pointing to brown plaques). (From Kumar V, Fausto N, Abbas A: Robbins and Cotran's Pathologic Basis of Disease, 7th ed. Philadelphia, WB Saunders, 2004, p 1383, Fig. 28-32.)*

e. Laboratory findings
  (1) Increased CSF leukocyte count
    • Primarily T lymphocytes
  (2) Increased CSF protein
    • Primarily an increase in γ-globulins
  (3) Increased CSF myelin basic protein
    • Indicates active disease
  (4) Normal CSF glucose
  (5) High-resolution electrophoresis shows oligoclonal bands.
    (a) Discrete bands of protein in the γ-globulin region
    (b) Sign of demyelination

Oligoclonal bands in CSF electrophoresis: sign of demyelination

2. Central pontine myelinolysis
  a. Most often occurs in alcoholics who have hyponatremia
  b. Rapid intravenous correction causes demyelination in the basis pontis.

Central pontine myelinolysis: due to rapid intravenous correction of hyponatremia

3. Viral infections with direct infection of oligodendrocytes
  • Examples—subacute sclerosing panencephalitis, progressive multifocal leukoencephalopathy

C. **Hereditary disorders**
  • Leukodystrophies are inborn errors of metabolism.
  1. Adrenoleukodystrophy
    a. X-linked recessive disorder
    b. Enzyme deficiency in β-oxidation of fatty acids in peroxisomes
      • Results in accumulation of long-chain fatty acids
    c. Causes generalized loss of myelin in the brain and adrenal insufficiency
  2. Metachromatic leukodystrophy
    a. Autosomal recessive disorder
      • Lysosomal storage disease
    b. Deficiency of arylsulfatase A
      • Results in accumulation of sulfatides
  3. Krabbe's disease
    a. Autosomal recessive disorder
      • Lysosomal storage disease
    b. Galactocerebroside β-galactocerebrosidase deficiency
      • Leads to accumulation of galactocerebroside
    c. Brain shows large, multinucleated, histiocytic cells (globoid cells).

VII. **Degenerative Disorders**
  • Degenerative diseases involve neurons in the brain or spinal cord.
  A. **Alzheimer's disease**
    1. Most common cause of dementia
      a. Presenile (<65 years of age)
      b. Senile (>65 years of age)
      c. Usually sporadic
      d. Approximately 10% of cases have a genetic basis.
    2. Role of β-amyloid (Aβ) protein
      a. Amyloid precursor protein (APP) is normally coded on chromosome 21.

(1) Trisomy 21 (Down syndrome) has a greater increase in APP.

(2) Most Down patients have Alzheimer's disease by 40 years of age.

b. Defects in degradation of APP by secretases cause an increase in Aβ.

(1) α-Secretases cleave APP into fragments that cannot produce Aβ.

(2) β and γ-Secretases cleave APP into fragments that are converted to Aβ.

(3) Aβ deposits in neurons are neurotoxic.
   • They also deposit in the walls of cerebral blood vessels.

c. Apolipoprotein gene E, allele ∈ 4, located on chromosome 19

(1) Codes for a product with a high binding affinity for Aβ

(2) Causes a familial late-onset Alzheimer's disease

3. Role of tau protein

a. Normal function is to maintain microtubules in neurons.

b. Mutations on chromosome 14

(1) Produce a hyperphosphorylated tau protein

(2) Protein causes formation of neurofibrillary (NF) tangles.

4. Gross and microscopic findings

a. Cerebral atrophy with dilation of ventricles (hydrocephalus ex vacuo)

(1) Due to loss of neurons in the temporal, frontal, and parietal lobes

(2) Occipital lobe is usually spared.

b. Presence of NF tangles in the cytoplasm of neurons

(1) NF tangles are pairs of protein-rich neurofilaments.

(2) Best visualized with silver stains

(3) They occur in other disorders.
   • Elderly patients *without* dementia, Huntington's disease

c. Senile plaques

(1) Core of Aβ surrounded by neuronal cell processes containing tau protein (Fig. 25-15)

Alzheimer's disease: ↑ β-amyloid → destruction of neurons

Alzheimer's disease: ↑ density of neurofibrillary tangles and amyloid plaques

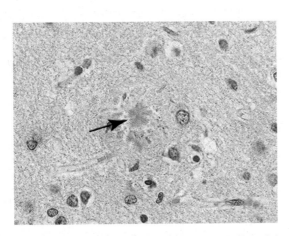

25-15: *Senile plaque (arrow) shows an eosinophilic center with peripherally located distended neuronal processes (neurites). (From Burger PC, Scheithauer BW, Vogel KS: Surgical Pathology of the Nervous System, 4th ed. London, Churchill Livingstone, 2002, p 428, Fig. 8-9.)*

(2) Aβ stains with Congo red (see Chapter 3).

(3) Best visualized with silver stains

    d. Amyloid angiopathy

      (1) Aβ is present in cerebral vessels.

      (2) Causes weakening of vessels

        • Increased risk for hemorrhage

    e. Confirmation of Alzheimer's disease

      (1) Requires postmortem examination of the brain

      (2) Must be widespread presence of NF tangles and senile plaques

  5. Clinical findings

    a. General impairment of higher intellectual function

      • *No* focal neurologic deficits are present.

    b. Patients usually die of an infection.

      • Example—intercurrent bronchopneumonia

B. Parkinsonism

  1. Group of disorders that alter dopaminergic pathways involved in voluntary muscle movement

    a. Striatal system involved in voluntary muscle movement

      • Substantia nigra, caudate, putamen, globus pallidus, subthalamus, thalamus

    b. Dopamine is the principal neurotransmitter in the nigrostriatal tract.

      • Connects the substantia nigra with the caudate and putamen

  2. Idiopathic Parkinson's disease

    a. Occurs between 45 and 65 years of age

      (1) Distribution is equal in men and women.

      (2) Most cases are sporadic.

      (3) Some cases are familial.

    b. Pathophysiology

      (1) Degeneration/depigmentation of neurons in substantia nigra (Fig. 25-16)

      (2) Causes deficiency of dopamine

      (3) Neurons contain intracytoplasmic, eosinophilic bodies called Lewy bodies.

        • Ubiquinated damaged neurofilaments (see Chapter 1)

> Idiopathic Parkinson's disease: depigmentation substantia nigra neurons; ↓ dopamine

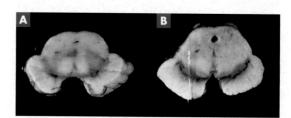

25-16: *Substantia nigra in a patient with Parkinson disease (**A**) and a normal individual (**B**). In Parkinson disease, the specimen is atrophied and the substantia nigra is partially depigmented when compared to the normal. (From Damjanov I, Linder J: Pathology: A Color Atlas. St. Louis, Mosby, 2000, p 419, Fig. 19-67.)*

  c. Clinical findings
     (1) Muscle rigidity
         (a) Slowness of voluntary muscle movement (bradykinesia)
         (b) Cogwheel rigidity on physical examination
     (2) Resting tremor
         (a) "Pill rolling" between thumb and index fingers
         (b) Illegible writing
     (3) Expressionless face, stooped posture
     (4) Shuffling gait
     (5) Dementia in some cases
  3. Other causes of parkinsonism
     a. Encephalitis, ischemia
     b. Chronic carbon monoxide poisoning
        • Causes necrosis of globus pallidus
     c. Wilson's disease
     d. Addiction to MPTP, a derivative of meperidine
        • 1-Methyl-4-phenyl-1,2,3,6-tetrahydropyridine
     e. Antipsychotic drugs (e.g., phenothiazines)
  4. Treatment
     a. Replacement of dopamine
     b. Prevention of reuptake and metabolism of dopamine

C. Huntington's disease
  1. Autosomal dominant disease
     a. Trinucleotide repeat disorder involving chromosome 4 (see Chapter 5)
     b. Delayed appearance of symptoms until 35 to 40 years of age
  2. Atrophy/loss of striatal neurons
     • Caudate, putamen, globus pallidus (Fig. 25-17)
  3. Clinical findings
     • Chorea, muscle rigidity, dementia

Huntington's disease: atrophy of caudate nucleus

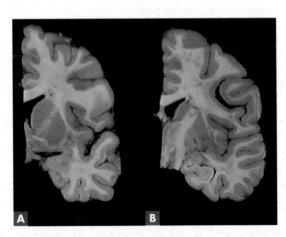

25-17: Huntington disease. Coronal section (**B**) shows atrophy of the caudate, putamen, and globus pallidus when compared with a normal coronal section (**A**). (From Perkin GD: Mosby's Color Atlas and Text of Neurology. St. Louis, Mosby, 2002, p 156, Fig. 8-19A and B.)

D. Friedreich's ataxia
   1. Autosomal recessive disease
      - Trinucleotide repeat disorder
   2. Sites of involvement
      a. Cerebellum
         - Ataxic gait
      b. Posterior and lateral columns of spinal cord
         - Diminished joint sensation, spasticity, respectively
      c. Peripheral neuropathy
      d. Hypertrophic cardiomyopathy

E. Lou Gehrig's disease (ALS)

ALS: degeneration of lower and upper motor neurons

   1. Degenerative disease involving upper and lower motor neurons
   2. Symptoms usually appear between 40 and 60 years of age.
      a. Most cases are sporadic.
      b. Familial cases involve mutations on chromosome 21.
         (1) Defective superoxide dismutase 1
         (2) Produces superoxide free radical injury of neurons
   3. Clinical findings
      a. Upper motor neuron signs
         - Spasticity, Babinski's sign
      b. Lower motor neuron signs
         (1) Muscle weakness
            - Begins with atrophy of intrinsic muscles of the hands
         (2) Eventual paralysis of respiratory muscles
      c. Average survival time is 3 to 5 years.

F. Werdnig-Hoffmann disease
   - Lower motor neuron disease that occurs in children

VIII. Toxic and Metabolic Disorders
   A. Wilson's disease (see Chapter 18)
      1. Autosomal recessive disease
         a. Defect in copper excretion in bile
         b. Defect in synthesis of ceruloplasmin
         c. Leads to liver cirrhosis and excess free copper in blood
      2. CNS findings
         a. Signs of parkinsonism, chorea, and dementia

Wilson's disease: cystic degeneration of putamen

         b. Atrophy and cavitation of basal ganglia, particularly the putamen (Fig. 25-18)
   B. Acute intermittent porphyria (AIP)
      1. Autosomal dominant disorder
      2. Defect in porphyrin metabolism
         a. Deficiency of uroporphyrinogen synthase (porphobilinogen deaminase)
         b. Proximal increase in porphobilinogen (PBG) and δ-aminolevulinic acid (ALA)
         c. Urine is *colorless* when first voided.

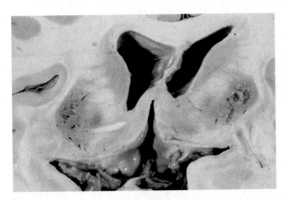

25-18: *Wilson's disease showing cavitary necrosis of the putamen on both sides of the brain. (From Damjanov I, Linder J: Pathology: A Color Atlas. St. Louis, Mosby, 2000, p 413, Fig. 19-43.)*

   (1) Exposure to light causes oxidation of PBG to porphobilin producing port-wine color.
   (2) Classic "window-sill test"
   d. Heme has a negative feedback relationship with ALA synthase.
      • ALA synthase is the rate-limiting enzyme of porphyrin metabolism.
   e. Decreasing heme precipitates porphyric attacks by increasing porphyrin synthesis.
      • Example—drugs enhancing liver cytochrome P-450 system (e.g., alcohol)
 3. Clinical findings
   a. Neurologic dysfunction
      (1) Recurrent bouts of severe abdominal pain simulating acute abdomen
      (2) Often mistaken for a surgical abdomen
         • Patient has "bellyful of scars."
   b. Psychosis, peripheral neuropathy, dementia

Acute intermittent porphyria: "bellyful of scars"

C. Vitamin B$_{12}$ deficiency (see Chapter 11)
 1. Subacute combined degeneration of the spinal cord
   • Posterior column and lateral corticospinal tract demyelination
 2. Dementia, peripheral neuropathy
D. CNS findings associated with alcohol abuse
 1. Cortical and cerebellar atrophy
 2. Central pontine myelinolysis
 3. Wernicke-Korsakoff syndrome
   a. Most often due to thiamine deficiency
   b. Gross and microscopic findings
      (1) Hemorrhages with hemosiderin deposits
         • Mamillary bodies, wall of the third and fourth ventricles (Fig. 25-19)
      (2) Neuronal loss, gliosis, vessel hemorrhage

Wernicke-Korsakoff syndrome: hemorrhage in mamillary bodies

   c. Wernicke's encephalopathy; reversible findings:
      • Confusion, ataxia, nystagmus, ophthalmoplegia (eye muscle weakness)
   d. Korsakoff's psychosis

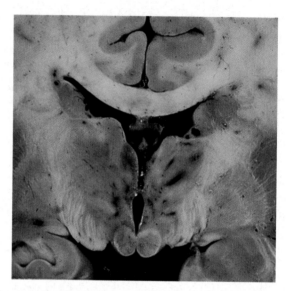

25-19: *Wernicke's encephalopathy showing hemorrhage and discoloration of mamillary bodies and the wall of the third ventricle.*

    (1) Advanced irreversible stage of Wernicke's encephalopathy
       • Targets the limbic system
    (2) Anterograde amnesia (inability to form new memories)
    (3) Retrograde amnesia (inability to recall old memories)

IX. **CNS Tumors**
  A. **Epidemiology**
    1. Primary brain tumors in adults
      a. Approximately 70% occur above the tentorium cerebelli.
      b. In order of decreasing frequency:
        • Glioblastoma multiforme, meningioma, ependymoma
    2. Primary brain tumors in children
      a. Approximately 70% occur below the tentorium cerebelli.
      b. In order of decreasing frequency:
        • Cystic cerebellar astrocytoma, medulloblastoma, brainstem glioma
    3. Risk factors
      • Turcot's syndrome, neurofibromatosis, cigarette smoking
  B. **Astrocytoma**
    1. Accounts for about 70% of all neuroglial tumors
      a. Usually involves frontal lobe in adults
      b. Usually involves the cerebellum in children
      c. Grades I and II are low-grade cancers.
      d. Grades III and IV are high-grade cancers.
    2. Glioblastoma multiforme (GBM)
      a. High-grade astrocytoma
        (1) May arise de novo
        (2) May arise from dedifferentiation of a low-grade astrocytoma

Most common primary CNS tumor in adults: glioblastoma multiforme

Childhood tumors: cystic astrocytoma and medulloblastoma, both in cerebellum

GBM: most common adult primary brain cancer

  b. Hemorrhagic tumor (Fig. 25-20)
    (1) Multifocal areas of necrosis and cystic degeneration
    (2) Commonly cross the corpus callosum
  c. May seed the neuraxis via the CSF
    • Rarely metastasize outside the CNS

C. Meningioma
  1. Most common benign brain tumor in adults
    • Female predominance (tumors have estrogen receptors)
  2. Derived from arachnoidal cells
    • Locations—parasagittal location, olfactory groove, lesser wing of sphenoid
  3. Associated with neurofibromatosis
  4. Gross and microscopic findings (Fig. 25-21)
    a. Firm tumors
      (1) May indent *(not invade)* the surface of brain
      (2) Often infiltrate overlying bone
        • Causes increased bone density
    b. Swirling masses of meningothelial cells encompass psammoma bodies (calcified bodies).

Meningioma: female predominance; psammoma bodies

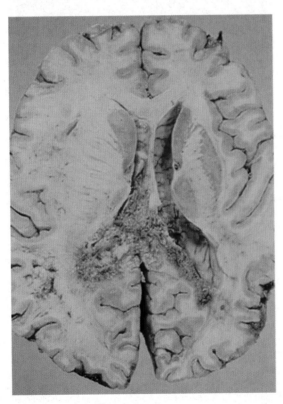

25-20: *Glioblastoma multiforme showing hemorrhage and necrosis in the brain parenchyma and spreading into the adjacent hemisphere via the corpus callosum. (From Damjanov I, Linder J: Anderson's Pathology, 10th ed. St. Louis, Mosby, 1996, p 2750, Fig. 77-120.)*

Ependymoma: fourth
ventricle in children;
cauda equina in adults

Oligodendroglioma:
frontal lobe calcifications
in an adult

5. Common cause of new-onset focal seizures

D. Ependymoma
1. Benign tumor derived from ependymal cells
2. Arises in cauda equina in adults and fourth ventricle in children

E. Medulloblastoma
1. Malignant small cell tumor
   • Primarily occurs in children
2. Arises from the external granular cell layer of the cerebellum (Fig. 25-22)
3. Often seeds the neuraxis and invades the fourth ventricle

F. Oligodendroglioma
1. Benign tumor derived from oligodendrocytes
   • Primarily occurs in adults
2. Frontal lobe tumor that frequently calcifies

G. CNS lymphoma
1. Majority are metastatic high-grade B-cell non-Hodgkin's lymphomas
2. Primary CNS lymphomas

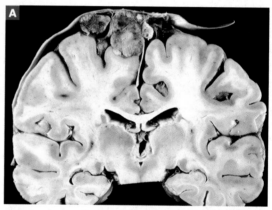

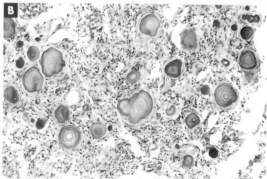

25-21: Gross (**A**) and microscopic (**B**) views of a meningioma. The gross appearance shows a parasagittal multilobular tumor attached to the overlying dura. The tumor compresses the underlying surface of the brain. The microscopic view shows numerous basophilic staining psammoma bodies. (From Kumar V, Fausto N, Abbas A: Robbins and Cotran's Pathologic Basis of Disease, 7th ed. Philadelphia, WB Saunders, 2004, p 1409, Fig. 28-48A and B.)

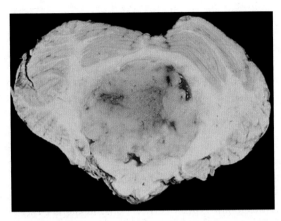

25-22: *Medulloblastoma in the cerebellum showing a centrally located hemorrhagic tumor filling in most of the fourth ventricle. (From Damjanov I, Linder J: Pathology: A Color Atlas. St. Louis, Mosby, 2000, p 424, Fig. 19-82.)*

  a. Most often associated with AIDS
  b. Epstein-Barr virus (EBV)–mediated B-cell lymphomas
  c. Rapidly increasing due to the increase in AIDS
 H. **Metastasis**
  1. Most common brain malignancy
  2. In order of decreasing frequency:
   • Lungs, breast, skin (melanoma), kidney, gastrointestinal tract

X. **Peripheral Nervous System Disorders**
 A. **Peripheral neuropathies**
  1. Associated with demyelination and axonal degeneration.
   a. Demyelination is often segmental.
    • Sensory changes (e.g., paresthesias), often in a "glove and stocking" distribution
   b. Axonal degeneration
    • Muscle fasciculations leading to muscle atrophy
  2. Charcot-Marie-Tooth (CMT) disease
   a. Most common hereditary neuropathy
    • Autosomal dominant disease
   b. Peroneal nerve neuropathy
    (1) Causes atrophy of muscles of lower legs
    (2) Legs have an "inverted bottle" appearance.
  3. Guillain-Barré syndrome (GBS)
   a. Most common acute peripheral neuropathy
   b. Autoimmune demyelination syndrome
    (1) Involves peripheral and spinal nerves
    (2) Common preceding disorders
     • *Mycoplasma pneumoniae* pneumonia, *Campylobacter jejuni* enteritis
   c. Rapidly progressive ascending motor weakness

Primary CNS lymphoma: occurs in AIDS; EBV-mediated cancer

Most common brain malignancy: metastasis

CMT: lower legs have "inverted bottle" appearance

        (1) Less commonly descending motor weakness

        (2) Danger of respiratory muscle paralysis and death

   d. Increased CSF protein

      • Oligoclonal bands present on high-resolution electrophoresis

   e. Majority recover with/without permanent disability.

   f. Treatment is plasmapheresis.

4. Diabetes mellitus

   a. Most common cause of peripheral neuropathy

   b. Due to osmotic damage of Schwann cells (see Chapter 22)

5. Toxin-associated neuropathies

   • Alcohol, heavy metals, diphtheria

6. Idiopathic Bell's palsy

   a. Lower motor neuron palsy causing unilateral facial paralysis

   b. Inflammatory reaction of facial nerve (CN VII)

      • Near the stylomastoid foramen or in the bony facial canal

   c. May be associated with HIV, sarcoidosis, Lyme disease

      • Often bilateral in Lyme disease

   d. Clinical findings (Fig. 25-23)

        (1) Drooping of the corner of the mouth

        (2) Difficulty speaking

        (3) Inability to close the eye

7. Drugs producing peripheral neuropathy

   • Examples—vincristine, hydralazine

8. Vitamin deficiencies producing peripheral neuropathy

   • Examples—deficiency of thiamine, vitamin B_{12}, pyridoxine

B. Schwannoma (neurilemoma)

1. Benign tumor derived from Schwann cells

   a. Cranial nerves (CN) V (trigeminal) and VIII (acoustic) may be involved.

   b. Spinal nerve roots, peripheral nerves may be involved.

2. Acoustic neuroma

   a. Schwannoma of CN VIII

   b. Majority are located in the cerebellopontine angle.

        (1) Encapsulated tumors

        (2) Microscopic view shows alternating dark and light areas (Fig. 25-24).

   c. Clinical findings

        (1) Associated with neurofibromatosis

          • Unilateral or bilateral tumors

        (2) Tinnitus (ringing in the ears)

        (3) Sensorineural deafness

        (4) Sensory changes in CN V distribution

          • Due to tumor impingement on CN V

XI. Selected Eye Disorders (Table 25-6; Figs. 25-25 and 25-26)

XII. Selected Ear Disorders (Table 25-7)

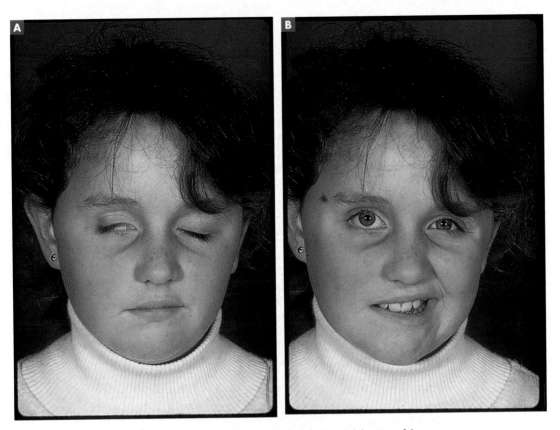

25-23: A and **B,** Right-sided Bell's palsy showing inability to fully close the eye and drooping of the corner of the mouth. (From Perkin GD: Mosby's Color Atlas and Text of Neurology. St. Louis, Mosby, 2002, p 77, Fig. 4-24A and B.)

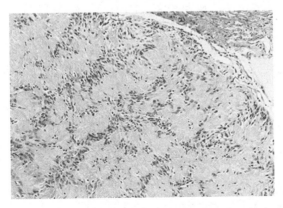

25-24: Acoustic neuroma showing spindle-shaped cells with alternating dark and light areas. (From Damjanov I, Linder J: Pathology: A Color Atlas. St. Louis, Mosby, 2000, p 432, Fig. 19-107.)

TABLE 25-6: Selected Eye Disorders

Eye Disorder	Discussion
Ophthalmia neonatorum	Conjunctivitis in newborn Pathogens: *Neisseria gonorrhoeae* (first week), *Chlamydia trachomatis* (second week)
Bacterial conjunctivitis	Purulent conjunctivitis; pain but *no* blurry vision Pathogens: *Staphylococcus aureus* (most common), *Streptococcus pneumoniae*, *Hemophilus influenzae* (*aegyptius*, pink eye)
Viral conjunctivitis	Watery exudates Adenovirus: viral cause of pink eye, preauricular lymphadenopathy HSV-1: keratoconjunctivitis with dendritic ulcers noted with fluorescein staining
Allergic	Seasonal itching of eyes
Acanthamoeba conjunctivitis	Severe keratoconjunctivitis in patients who do not clean their contact lenses properly
Stye	Infection of eyelid most commonly due to *S. aureus*
Chalazion	Granulomatous inflammation involving the meibomian gland in the eyelid
Orbital cellulitis	Periorbital redness and swelling that is often secondary to sinusitis (e.g., ethmoiditis in children) Pathogens: *S. pneumoniae*, *H. influenzae* Fever, proptosis (eye bulges out), periorbital swelling, ophthalmoplegia (eye movement impaired), normal retinal examination
Pterygium	Raised, triangular encroachment of thickened conjunctiva on the nasal side of the conjunctiva Due to excessive exposure to wind, sun, and sand
Optic neuritis	Inflammation of optic nerve Causes: multiple sclerosis (most common), methanol poisoning Blurry vision or loss of vision, may cause optic atrophy
Central retinal artery occlusion	Causes: embolization of plaque material from ipsilateral carotid or ophthalmic artery; giant cell temporal arteritis involving the ophthalmic artery Sudden, painless, complete loss of vision in one eye, pallor of optic disk, "boxcar" segmentation of blood in retinal veins
Central retinal vein occlusion	Causes: hypercoagulable state (e.g., polycythemia vera) Sudden, painless, unilateral loss of vision, swelling of optic disk, engorged retinal veins with hemorrhage
Glaucoma	Increased intraocular pressure Chronic open angle type: decreased rate of aqueous outflow into the canal of Schlemm; bilateral aching eyes; pathologic cupping of optic disks; night blindness and gradual loss of peripheral vision leading to tunnel vision and blindness Acute angle-closure type: due to narrowing of anterior chamber angle, precipitated by mydriatic agent, uveitis, lens dislocation; severe pain associated with photophobia and blurry vision; red eye with a steamy cornea; pupil fixed and nonreactive to light
Optic nerve atrophy (Fig. 25-25)	Pale optic disk Most commonly due to optic neuritis or glaucoma
Uveitis	Inflammation of uveal tract (iris, ciliary body, choroid) Causes: sarcoidosis, ulcerative colitis, ankylosing spondylitis Pain with blurry vision, miotic pupil, circumcorneal ciliary body vascular congestion, normal intraocular pressure, adhesions between iris and anterior lens capsule

TABLE 25-6:
Selected Eye
Disorders—cont'd

Eye Disorder	Discussion
Macular degeneration	Most common cause of permanent visual loss in the elderly Disruption of Bruch's membrane in the retina Antioxidants decrease risk
CMV retinitis	Most common cause of blindness in AIDS; usually occurs when CD4 T helper cell count < 50 cells/μL Cotton-wool exudates and retinal hemorrhages Rx: ganciclovir or foscarnet
Cataracts	Opacity in the lens Causes: advanced age (most common), diabetes mellitus (osmotic damage), infection (e.g., rubella), corticosteroids Common in congenital infections (e.g., CMV, rubella)
Malignant tumors (Fig. 25-26)	Retinoblastoma in children ("white eye reflex") Malignant melanoma in adults

CMV, cytomegalovirus; HSV, herpes simplex virus; Rx, treatment.

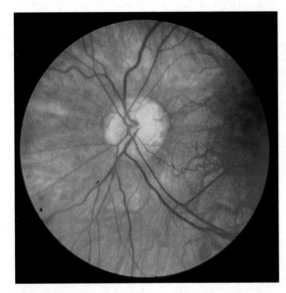

25-25: Optic nerve atrophy showing a pale optic disk. (From Perkin GD: Mosby's Color Atlas and Text of Neurology. St. Louis, Mosby, 2002, p 64, Fig. 4-3.)

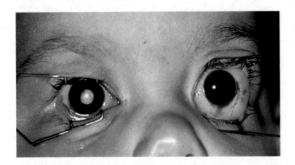

25-26: Retinoblastoma in the right eye of a child showing a white papillary reflex. (From Damjanov I, Linder J: Pathology: A Color Atlas. St. Louis, Mosby, 2000, p 445, Fig. 20-39.)

**TABLE 25-7:
Selected Ear
Disorders**

Ear Disorder	Description and Comments

Meniere's disease	Increased endolymph in inner ear and loss of cochlear hairs
	Dizziness, vertigo, tinnitus, sensorineural hearing loss
	Sensorineural defect
	  Weber test: lateralizes to normal ear (contralateral ear is affected)
	  Rinne test: air conduction > bone conduction in both normal and
	    affected ear

Presbycusis	Most common cause of sensorineural hearing loss in elderly Due to degeneration of cochlear hairs

Otosclerosis	Most common cause of conduction deafness in elderly
	Due to fusion of middle ear ossicles
	Other causes of conduction defects: impacted cerumen in outer ear
	  canal; otitis media
	Conduction defect
	  Weber test: lateralizes to affected ear
	  Rinne test: bone conduction > air conduction

Otitis media	Most common cause of conduction deafness in children Most commonly due to *Streptococcus pneumoniae* Other causes: *H. influenzae, Moraxella catarrhalis*

External otitis	Inflammation of outer ear canal
	"Swimmer's ear: due to *Pseudomonas aeruginosa, Staphylococcus
	  aureus, Aspergillus* species
	Malignant external otitis: severe infection of outer ear canal in
	  patients with diabetes mellitus; *Pseudomonas aeruginosa* most
	  common cause

Common Laboratory Values

Test	Conventional Units	SI Units
Blood, Plasma, Serum		
Alanine aminotransferase (ALT, GPT at 30°C)	8–20 U/L	8–20 U/L
Amylase, serum	25–125 U/L	25–125 U/L
Aspartate aminotransferase (AST, GOT at 30°C)	8–20 U/L	8–20 U/L
Bilirubin, serum (adult): total; direct	0.1–1.0 mg/dL; 0.0–0.3 mg/dL	2–17 μmol/L; 0–5 μmol/L
Calcium, serum (Ca^{2+})	8.4–10.2 mg/dL	2.1–2.8 mmol/L
Cholesterol, serum	Rec: <200 mg/dL	<5.2 mmol/L
Cortisol, serum	8:00 AM: 6–23 μg/dL; 4:00 PM: 3–15 μg/dL	170–630 nmol/L; 80–410 nmol/L
	8:00 PM: ≤50% of 8:00 AM	Fraction of 8:00 AM: ≤0.50
Creatine kinase, serum	Male: 25–90 U/L	25–90 U/L
	Female: 10–70 U/L	10–70 U/L
Creatinine, serum	0.6–1.2 mg/dL	53–106 μmol/L
Electrolytes, serum		
Sodium (Na^+)	136–145 mEq/L	135–145 mmol/L
Chloride (Cl^-)	95–105 mEq/L	95–105 mmol/L
Potassium (K^+)	3.5–5.0 mEq/L	3.5–5.0 mmol/L
Bicarbonate (HCO_3^-)	22–28 mEq/L	22–28 mmol/L
Magnesium (Mg^{2+})	1.5–2.0 mEq/L	1.5–2.0 mmol/L
Estriol, total, serum (in pregnancy)		
24–28 wk; 32–36 wk	30–170 ng/mL; 60–280 ng/mL	104–590 nmol/L; 208–970 nmol/L
28–32 wk; 36–40 wk	40–220 ng/mL; 80–350 ng/mL	140–760 nmol/L; 280–1210 nmol/L
Ferritin, serum	Male: 15–200 ng/mL	15–200 μg/L
	Female: 12–150 ng/mL	12–150 μg/L
Follicle-stimulating hormone, serum/plasma (FSH)	Male: 4–25 mIU/mL	4–25 U/L
	Female:	
	Premenopause, 4–30 mIU/mL	4–30 U/L
	Midcycle peak, 10–90 mIU/mL	10–90 U/L
	Postmenopause, 40–250 mIU/mL	40–250 U/L
Gases, arterial blood (room air)		
pH	7.35–7.45	[H^+] 36–44 nmol/L
PCO_2	33–45 mm Hg	4.4–5.9 kPa
PO_2	75–105 mm Hg	10.0–14.0 kPa
Glucose, serum	Fasting: 70–110 mg/dL	3.8–6.1 mmol/L
	2 hr postprandial: <120 mg/dL	<6.6 mmol/L
Growth hormone–arginine stimulation	Fasting: <5 ng/mL	<5 μg/L
	Provocative stimuli: >7 ng/mL	>7 μg/L

continued

Test	Conventional Units	SI Units
Blood, Plasma, Serum—cont'd		
Immunoglobulins, serum		
IgA	76–390 mg/dL	0.76–3.90 g/L
IgE	0–380 IU/mL	0–380 kIU/L
IgG	650–1500 mg/dL	6.5–15 g/L
IgM	40–345 mg/dL	0.4–3.45 g/L
Iron	50–170 µg/dL	9–30 µmol/L
Lactate dehydrogenase, serum	45–90 U/L	45–90 U/L
Luteinizing hormone, serum/	Male: 6–23 mIU/mL	6–23 U/L
plasma (LH)	Female:	
	Follicular phase, 5–30 mIU/mL	5–30 U/L
	Midcycle, 75–150 mIU/mL	75–150 U/L
	Postmenopause, 30–200 mIU/mL	30–200 U/L
Osmolality, serum	275–295 mOsm/kg	275–295 mOsm/kg
Parathyroid hormone, serum,	230–630 pg/mL	230–630 ng/L
N-terminal		
Phosphatase (alkaline), serum	20–70 U/L	20–70 U/L
(p-NPP at 30°C)		
Phosphorus (inorganic), serum	3.0–4.5 mg/dL	1.0–1.5 mmol/L
Prolactin, serum (hPRL)	<20 ng/mL	<20 µg/L
Proteins, serum		
Total (recumbent)	6.0–8.0 g/dL	60–80 g/L
Albumin	3.5–5.5 g/dL	35–55 g/L
Globulin	2.3–3.5 g/dL	23–35 g/L
Thyroid-stimulating hormone,	0.5–5.0 µU/mL	0.5–5.0 mU/L
serum or plasma (TSH)		
Thyroidal iodine (^{123}I) uptake	8–30% of administered dose/24 hr	0.08–0.30/24 hr
Thyroxine (T$_4$), serum	4.5–12 µg/dL	58–154 nmol/L
Triglycerides, serum	35–160 mg/dL	0.4–1.81 mmol/L
Triiodothyronine (T$_3$), serum (RIA)	115–190 ng/dL	1.8–2.9 nmol/L
Triiodothyronine (T$_3$) resin uptake	25–38%	0.25–0.38
Urea nitrogen, serum (BUN)	7–18 mg/dL	1.2–3.0 mmol urea/L
Uric acid, serum	3.0–8.2 mg/dL	0.18–0.48 mmol/L
Cerebrospinal Fluid		
Cell count	0–5 cells/mm^3	$0–5 \times 10^6$/L
Chloride	118–132 mEq/L	118–132 mmol/L
Gamma globulin	3–12% total proteins	0.03–0.12
Glucose	50–75 mg/dL	2.8–4.2 mmol/L
Pressure	70–180 mm H$_2$O	70–180 mm H$_2$O
Proteins, total	<40 mg/dL	<0.40 g/L
Hematology		
Bleeding time (template)	2–7 min	2–7 min
Erythrocyte count	Male: 4.3–5.9 million/mm^3	$4.3–5.9 \times 10^{12}$/L
	Female: 3.5–5.5 million/mm^3	$3.5–5.5 \times 10^{12}$/L
Erythrocyte sedimentation rate	Male: 0–15 mm/hr	0–15 mm/hr
(Westergren)	Female: 0–20 mm/hr	0–20 mm/hr
Hematocrit (Hct)	Male: 40–54%	0.40–0.54
	Female: 37–47%	0.37–0.47

Test	Conventional Units	SI Units
Hematology—cont'd		
Hemoglobin A$_{\text{IC}}$	≤6%	≤ 0.06%
Hemoglobin, blood (Hb)	Male: 13.5–17.5 g/dL	2.09–2.71 mmol/L
	Female: 12.0–16.0 g/dL	1.86–2.48 mmol/L
Hemoglobin, plasma	1–4 mg/dL	0.16–0.62 mmol/L
Leukocyte count and differential		
Leukocyte count	4500–11,000/mm^3	$4.5\text{–}11.0 \times 10^9$/L
Segmented neutrophils	54–62%	0.54–0.62
Bands	3–5%	0.03–0.05
Eosinophils	1–3%	0.01–0.03
Basophils	0–0.75%	0–0.0075
Lymphocytes	25–33%	0.25–0.33
Monocytes	3–7%	0.03–0.07
Mean corpuscular hemoglobin (MCH)	25.4–34.6 pg/cell	0.39–0.54 fmol/cell
Mean corpuscular hemoglobin concentration (MCHC)	31–37% Hb/cell	4.81–5.74 mmol Hb/L
Mean corpuscular volume (MCV)	80–100 μm^3	80–100 fl
Partial thromboplastin time (activated) (aPTT)	25–40 sec	25–40 sec
Platelet count	150,000–400,000/mm^3	$150\text{–}400 \times 10^9$/L
Prothrombin time (PT)	12–14 sec	12–14 sec
Reticulocyte count	0.5–1.5% of red cells	0.005–0.015
Thrombin time	<2 sec deviation from control	<2 sec deviation from control
Volume		
Plasma	Male: 25–43 mL/kg	0.025–0.043 L/kg
	Female: 28–45 mL/kg	0.028–0.045 L/kg
Red cell	Male: 20–36 mL/kg	0.020–0.036 L/kg
	Female: 19–31 mL/kg	0.019–0.031 L/kg
Sweat		
Chloride	0–35 mmol/L	0–35 mmol/L
Urine		
Calcium	100–300 mg/24 hr	2.5–7.5 mmol/24 hr
Creatinine clearance	Male: 97–137 mL/min	
	Female: 88–128 mL/min	
Estriol, total (in pregnancy)		
30 wk	6–18 mg/24 hr	21–62 μmol/24 hr
35 wk	9–28 mg/24 hr	31–97 μmol/24 hr
40 wk	13–42 mg/24 hr	45–146 μmol/24 hr
17-Hydroxycorticosteroids	Male: 3.0–9.0 mg/24 hr	8.2–25.0 μmol/24 hr
	Female: 2.0–8.0 mg/24 hr	5.5–22.0 μmol/24 hr
17-Ketosteroids, total	Male: 8–22 mg/24 hr	28–76 μmol/24 hr
	Female: 6–15 mg/24 hr	21–52 μmol/24 hr
Osmolality	50–1400 mOsm/kg	
Oxalate	8–40 μg/mL	90–445 μmol/L
Proteins, total	<150 mg/24 hr	<0.15 g/24 hr

questions

DIRECTIONS: Each numbered item or incomplete statement is followed by options arranged in alphabetical or logical order. Select the best answer to each question. Some options may be partially correct, but there is only **ONE BEST** answer.

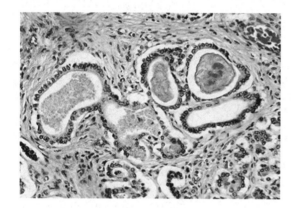

A. Ca^{2+} moving into the cytosol
B. Cytochrome c diffusing out of the mitochondria
C. Intracellular pH increasing
D. Na^+ and H_2O moving into the cytosol
E. Phospholipase damaging the cell membrane

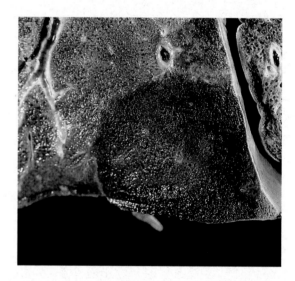

1. A 22-year-old man with cystic fibrosis had type 1 diabetes mellitus and chronic diarrhea characterized by excessive bloating and greasy stools. The figure shows a histologic section of the pancreas obtained at autopsy. Which of the following is responsible for the histologic changes shown in the pancreatic ducts?
A. Atrophy
B. Dysplasia
C. Hyperplasia
D. Hypertrophy
E. Metaplasia

2. A 65-year-old man has a ruptured abdominal aortic aneurysm and is in hypovolemic shock. Which of the following is a reversible cellular event that is most likely to occur in the straight portion of the proximal tubular cells of the kidneys?

3. A 45-year-old woman undergoes cholecystectomy for a gangrenous gallbladder. On postoperative day 4, the patient complains of chest pain on the right side, which increases on inspiration. The first set of arterial blood gases drawn after this complaint shows an increase in arterial pH with a decrease in arterial Po_2. On postoperative day 7, the patient dies. The figure shows a cut section from the right lower lobe of the lung. Which of the following best explains the cause of the decrease in arterial Po_2 on day 4?

A. Diffusion defect
B. Perfusion defect
C. Respiratory acidosis
D. Respiratory alkalosis
E. Ventilation defect

4. A cholecystectomy is performed on a 55-year-old woman, and the incision is not healing properly. When asked about her diet, the woman says that she consumes a diet high in protein but does not eat fruits or vegetables. Which of the following events most likely accounts for the poor wound healing?

A. Decreased synthesis of granulation tissue
B. Decreased synthesis of type III collagen
C. Decreased tensile strength of collagen
D. Defect in fibrillin in elastic tissue
E. Leukocyte adhesion molecule defect

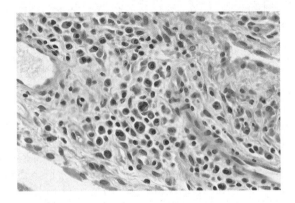

5. A 52-year-old woman has a 10-year history of progressively worsening arthritis in the hands and knees, which has led to ankylosis. The figure shows a histologic section of synovial tissue removed from the knee joint. Which of the following types of inflammation is evident in this tissue?

A. Acute
B. Chronic
C. Granulomatous
D. Pseudomembranous
E. Suppurative

6. A 5-year-old boy with a family history of seasonal allergies develops erythema, itching, and swelling of the skin after a subcutaneous injection of ragweed pollen. Which of the following chemical mediators is most responsible for this skin reaction?

A. Bradykinin
B. Complement
C. Histamine
D. Nitric oxide
E. Prostaglandins

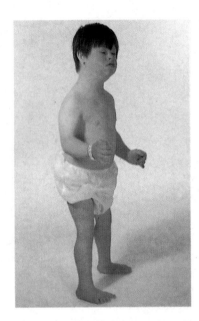

7. The child in the figure has moderately severe mental retardation. Chromosome analysis shows 46 chromosomes. Which of the following types of genetic mutation is responsible for this condition?

A. Balanced translocation
B. Frameshift mutation
C. Microdeletion
D. Nondisjunction
E. Point mutation

8. A 48-year-old man with alcoholic cirrhosis has ascites and dependent pitting edema in the lower legs. Fluid accumulation in the peritoneal cavity and legs occurs by which of the following mechanisms?

A. Decreased plasma oncotic pressure
B. Increased plasma hydrostatic pressure
C. Increased vessel permeability due to histamine
D. Lymphatic obstruction with lymphedema
E. Movement of water into the intracellular compartment

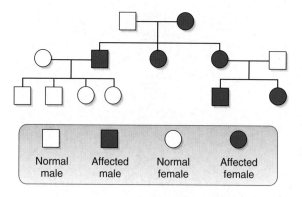

□	■	○	●
Normal male	Affected male	Normal female	Affected female

9. Which of the following clinical disorders is most compatible with the distribution of affected patients shown in the pedigree depicted in the figure?

A. Alport's syndrome
B. Familial hypercholesterolemia
C. Familial polyposis coli
D. Leber's optic neuropathy
E. McArdle's disease

10. A 62-year-old man is involved in a head-on automobile collision and is examined by paramedics at the scene of the accident. His heart rate is 120 beats/minute, and his blood pressure is 80/60 mm Hg. His skin is cold and clammy. Which of the following hemodynamic changes has occurred?

A. Decreased arterial Po_2
B. Decreased hemoglobin concentration
C. Decreased RBC count
D. Increased left ventricular end-diastolic pressure
E. Increased total peripheral arteriolar resistance

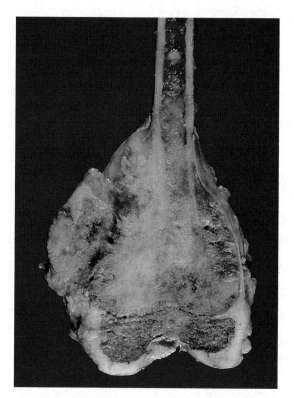

11. The figure shows the distal femur of a 21-year-old woman. When the patient was 2 years old, a cancerous lesion was surgically removed from the right eye. Which of the following regulatory genes is most likely responsible for these eye and bone lesions?

A. *BRCA1* suppressor gene
B. *MYC* proto-oncogene
C. *RAS* proto-oncogene
D. *RB* suppressor gene
E. *TP53* suppressor gene

12. A 24-year-old woman in her first trimester of pregnancy complains of heat intolerance. Physical examination shows an enlarged, nontender thyroid gland. Thyroid function studies show a serum thyroxine (T_4) level of

14 µg/dL and a serum thyroid-stimulating hormone (TSH) level of 3.0 µU/mL. Which of the following best explains the results of these studies?

A. Decreased peripheral conversion of T_4 to triiodothyronine (T_3)
B. Increased release of T_4 from acute thyroiditis
C. Increased synthesis of T_3
D. Increased synthesis of T_4
E. Increased synthesis of thyroid-binding globulin

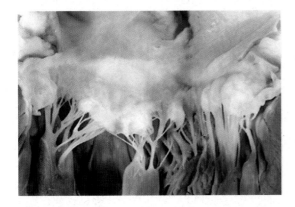

13. The figure shows a valvular lesion on the left side of the heart of a 25-year-old woman, who died in a car accident. Which of the following heart sounds is most likely to be associated with this lesion?

A. Diastolic blowing murmur after S_2
B. Midsystolic click followed by a murmur
C. Opening snap followed by a mid-diastolic rumbling murmur
D. Pansystolic murmur at the apex
E. Systolic ejection murmur

14. An 11-year-old boy has enlarged, nontender testicles, a long face with a prominent jaw, a high arched palate, and protruding ears. The child is in a special educational program at school. Which of the following studies is most useful for evaluation of this patient?

A. Buccal smear
B. DNA analysis of the X chromosome
C. Human chorionic gonadotropin

D. Serum gonadotropins
E. Testicular biopsy

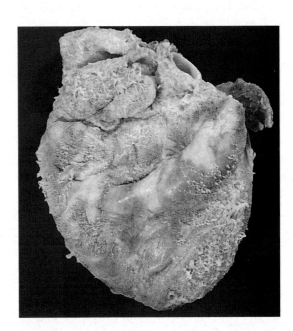

15. A 59-year-old man had an acute anterior myocardial infarction (MI). Six weeks later, he saw his physician because of fever and precordial chest pain that was less severe when he leaned forward. On physical examination, a friction rub was heard over the precordium. The figure shows the heart removed at autopsy. Which of the following mechanisms is most likely involved in the pathogenesis of the abnormality in the heart?

A. Alteration in Starling pressure
B. Immunologic reaction
C. Metastatic disease
D. Rupture of the anterior wall
E. Viral infection

16. A 32-year-old black American medical missionary who recently returned to the United States from a trip overseas is diagnosed with malaria due to *Plasmodium vivax*. After 4 days of therapy with primaquine, he develops fever, chills, low back pain, and dark urine. A complete blood cell count shows a hemoglobin of 6 g/dL, a WBC count of 15,000/mm³, and a platelet count of 450,000/mm³. A corrected reticulocyte count is 10%. A peripheral smear shows polychromasia and numerous RBCs that are missing parts of their membrane. A urine dipstick is positive for blood. Which of the following laboratory findings is most likely to be reported?

A. Abnormal hemoglobin electrophoresis
B. Decreased mean corpuscular hemoglobin concentration
C. Decreased serum ferritin concentration
D. Positive direct Coombs' test
E. Positive Heinz body preparation

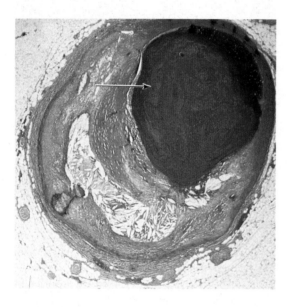

17. The *arrow* in the figure points to an intraluminal mass in a left anterior descending coronary artery of a 56-year-old man who died of an acute myocardial infarction (MI). Which of the following drugs would most likely have been used to prevent the formation of the intraluminal mass?

A. Aspirin
B. Glycoprotein IIb/IIIa inhibitor
C. Heparin
D. Tissue plasminogen activator (tPA)
E. Warfarin

18. A 28-year-old man has a family history of sudden cardiac death at a young age. Physical examination shows a systolic ejection type murmur that decreases in intensity when the patient lies down and increases in intensity when he stands up. An echocardiogram shows abnormal movement of the anterior mitral valve leaflet against an asymmetrically thickened interventricular septum (IVS). Which of the following is the cause of the systolic murmur?

A. Aortic regurgitation
B. Aortic stenosis
C. Hypertrophic cardiomyopathy
D. Mitral stenosis
E. Mitral valve prolapse

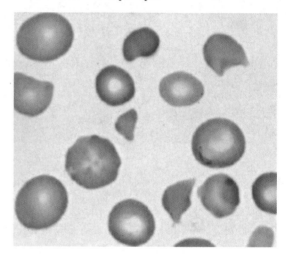

19. A 62-year-old man complains of fatigue. Physical examination shows a harsh systolic ejection murmur, grade 4/6, that radiates into the carotid arteries. Laboratory studies show a mild microcytic anemia. A urine dipstick test is positive for blood. The figure shows a representative section of the peripheral blood smear. Which of the following laboratory studies would most likely identify the cause of the microcytic anemia?

A. Direct Coombs' test
B. Enzyme assay for pyruvate kinase
C. Hemoglobin electrophoresis
D. Osmotic fragility test
E. Serum ferritin test

20. A 42-year-old woman develops fever and dyspnea approximately 24 hours after a cholecystectomy for acute gangrenous cholecystitis. Physical examination shows dullness to percussion, absent vocal tactile fremitus, and absent breath sounds in the right lower lobe of the lung. The diaphragm is elevated, and an inspiratory lag is present on the right side. The trachea is shifted to the right. Which of the following is the most likely diagnosis?
A. Atelectasis
B. Lobar pneumonia
C. Lung abscess
D. Pulmonary infarction
E. Spontaneous pneumothorax

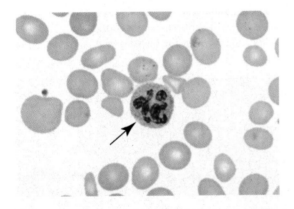

21. A 62-year-old woman complains that her tongue is sore. She reports instability when walking. Physical examination shows atrophy of the tongue papillae, decreased vibratory sensation in both lower extremities, and instability when she stands and closes her eyes. An endoscopic examination indicates chronic atrophic gastritis involving the body and fundus of the stomach. Laboratory studies show a severe macrocytic anemia with pancytopenia. The figure shows a representative section of the peripheral blood smear and a leukocyte abnormality *(arrow).* Which of the following laboratory test findings would most likely be reported?
A. Decreased serum folate
B. Decreased serum gastrin
C. Decreased urine methylmalonic acid

D. Increased antigliadin antibodies
E. Increased vitamin B_{12} absorption after addition of intrinsic factor

22. A 45-year-old man with a 20-year history of alcohol abuse complains of recurrent episodes of forgetfulness and tiredness. Laboratory studies show a serum glucose level of 20 mg/dL and increases in serum insulin and serum C peptide. Which of the following is the most likely cause of this hypoglycemia?
A. Alcohol-induced hypoglycemia
B. Benign tumor of β-islet cells
C. Ectopic secretion of an insulin-like factor
D. Malignant tumor of α-islet cells
E. Patient injection of human insulin

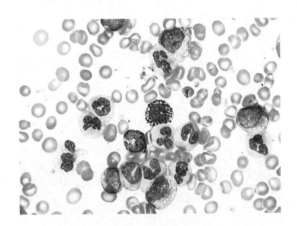

23. A 48-year-old man has fever, weight loss, sweating, and a dragging sensation in the abdomen. Physical examination shows generalized lymphadenopathy and massive hepatosplenomegaly. Laboratory studies reveal a normocytic anemia and thrombocytopenia, and a WBC count of 110,000/mm³. A bone marrow biopsy shows hypercellularity and the presence of neutrophils at all stages of development. Less than 2% of the WBCs in the bone marrow are myeloblasts. The figure shows a representative section of the peripheral blood smear. Which of the following laboratory findings would most likely be positive?

A. Leukocytes for alkaline phosphatase
B. Leukocytes for the CD10 antigen
C. Leukocytes for Philadelphia chromosome
D. Leukocytes for tartrate-resistant acid phosphatase
E. Leukocytes for terminal deoxynucleotidyl transferase

24. Physical examination of a 21-year-old man shows a xanthoma of the Achilles tendon in the right foot and bilateral yellow, raised patches on the eyelids. He has a family history of premature death due to stroke and myocardial infarction by 30 to 40 years of age. Which of the following best explains the pathogenesis of the tendon and skin lesions?
A. Decreased activation of capillary lipoprotein lipase
B. Deficiency of apolipoprotein C-II
C. Deficiency of apolipoprotein E
D. Deficiency of low-density lipoprotein (LDL) receptors
E. Increased synthesis of very low-density (VLDL) lipoprotein

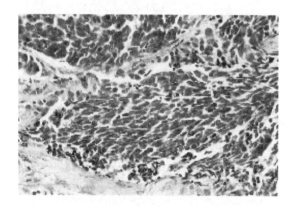

25. A centrally located lung mass is removed from a 58-year-old man who has smoked two packs of cigarettes a day for 30 years. The figure shows an H&E-stained histologic section of the mass. Which of the following endocrinopathies is frequently associated with this type of tumor?
A. Carcinoid syndrome
B. Hypercalcemia
C. Hypocalcemia
D. Inappropriate antidiuretic hormone secretion
E. Polycythemia

26. A 50-year-old man had an acute anterior myocardial infarction (MI) 4 days ago, and he now complains of substernal chest pain with radiation into the left arm and jaw. Physical examination shows no cardiac or pulmonary abnormalities. Laboratory studies show increases in serum creatine kinase MB (CK-MB), serum troponin-I (cTnI), and serum troponin-T (cTnT). Which of the following is the most likely cause of the chest pain?
A. Angina pectoris
B. Pericarditis
C. Reinfarction
D. Right ventricular infarction
E. Rupture of the anterior wall

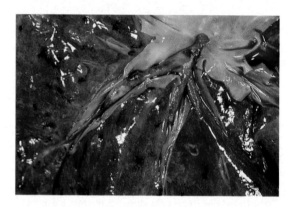

27. The figure shows a lung removed at autopsy from a 72-year-old woman, who died suddenly 5 days after a total hip replacement. Which of the following is the most likely cause of death?
A. Acute pulmonary infarction
B. Acute right-sided ventricular strain
C. Aspiration of gastric contents
D. Disseminated metastasis
E. Nosocomial pneumonia

28. A febrile 5-year-old child complains of chest pain. Physical examination shows painful cervical adenopathy, dry, cracked lips, and erythema and swelling of the hands and feet. A desquamating rash develops on the fingers and toes. Which of the following is a potential complication of the patient's disease?
A. Acute myocardial infarction
B. Aortic arch aneurysm
C. Aortic dissection
D. Infective endocarditis
E. Mitral stenosis

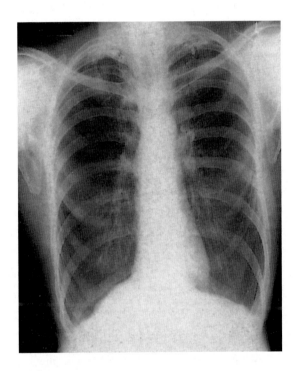

29. A 56-year-old woman who has smoked two packs of cigarettes daily for 35 years has chronic dyspnea. She has an emaciated appearance and pink discoloration of the skin. It is difficult to hear heart and lung sounds. The figure shows the chest radiograph in the patient. Which of the following results of pulmonary function tests would most likely be reported?
A. Decreased functional residual capacity
B. Decreased total lung capacity

C. Increased FEV_{1sec}/FVC ratio
D. Increased residual volume
E. Increased tidal volume

30. A 48-year-old man complains of fever and several fainting spells over the past few months. He states that he faints when he stands up and not when he is lying down. He also complains of pain in the left upper quadrant that is aggravated by inspiration and pain in the right flank. Physical examination shows a normal blood pressure when lying down and sitting up. A late diastolic murmur is heard. The spleen is enlarged and tender, and a splenic friction rub is present. There is right flank pain on percussion. A urine dipstick is positive for blood, and RBCs are present in the urine sediment. Which of the following is the most likely diagnosis?
A. Calcific aortic stenosis
B. Hypertrophic cardiomyopathy
C. Left atrial myxoma
D. Mitral stenosis
E. Pericardial effusion

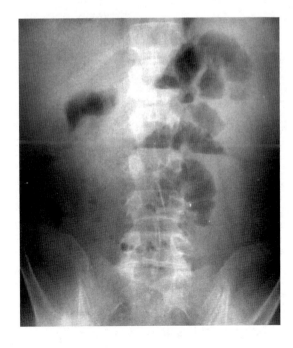

31. A 35-year-old woman complains of colicky abdominal pain and vomiting. She has had previous surgery for endometriosis involving the small bowel. The figure on page 607 shows a plain abdominal radiograph taken of the patient in an erect position. Which of the following is the most likely cause of the abdominal pain?
A. Direct inguinal hernia
B. Intussusception
C. Large bowel infarction
D. Small bowel adhesions
E. Volvulus

32. A newborn child coughs during and after breast-feeding. The stomach is distended and tympanitic. The mother had polyhydramnios during pregnancy. Which of the following is the most likely diagnosis?
A. Choanal atresia
B. Congenital pyloric stenosis
C. Duodenal atresia
D. Esophageal web
E. Tracheoesophageal fistula

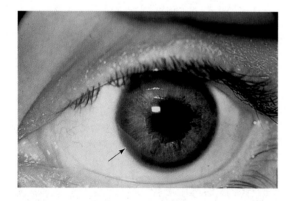

33. A 36-year-old man has a history of chronic liver disease and a movement disorder. The figure shows an abnormality in the cornea of the eye *(arrow)*. Which of the following laboratory findings would most likely be reported?
A. Decreased serum ceruloplasmin
B. Increased percent iron saturation
C. Increased serum iron
D. Increased total serum copper
E. Normal serum prothrombin time

34. A 23-year-old man is scuba diving in 60 ft of water and suddenly develops stabbing chest pain in the left side with dyspnea while coming slowly to the surface. Physical examination of the left lung shows hyperresonance to percussion, deviation of the trachea to the left, elevation of the left diaphragm, absent tactile fremitus, and absent breath sounds. Which of the following is the most likely diagnosis?
A. Decompression sickness
B. Pleural effusion
C. Pulmonary infarction
D. Spontaneous pneumothorax
E. Tension pneumothorax

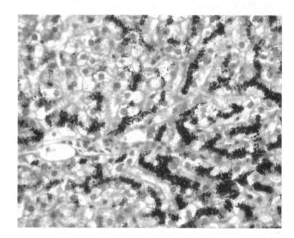

35. A 30-year-old man has type 1 diabetes mellitus, pale gray skin, and chronic diarrhea. His 58-year-old sister has similar problems. His skin is pale gray, and this is most obvious on his hands. A screening test is performed on the patient and is positive. The figure shows a liver biopsy with a Prussian blue stain. Which of the following laboratory findings prompted the liver biopsy?
A. Decreased serum ceruloplasmin
B. Decreased serum iron
C. Decreased small bowel reabsorption of D-xylose
D. Increased serum ferritin
E. Increased total iron-binding capacity

36. A 52-year-old woman has a 20-year history of chronic left-sided and right-sided heart failure. As a child, she had numerous episodes of pharyngitis. At autopsy, the heart showed thickening of the mitral valve leaflets and fusion of the commissures. Which of the following is the most likely cause of the valvular disease?
A. Immune reaction in systemic lupus erythematosus (SLE)
B. Ischemic heart disease
C. Myxomatous degeneration
D. Recurrent bacterial endocarditis
E. Recurrent immune reaction against group A streptococci

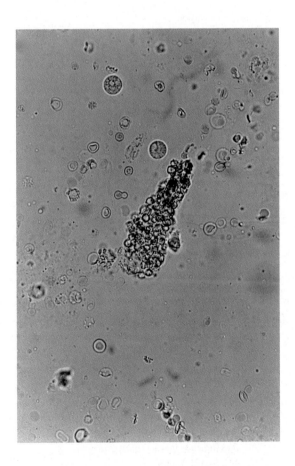

37. A 12-year-old boy has an episodic history of developing pink-staining urine shortly after an upper respiratory infection. The patient is normotensive and afebrile. The urine dipstick test is positive for blood and shows mild to moderate amounts of protein. The antistreptolysin O titer, the anti-DNAase B titer, and the serum antinuclear antibody (ANA) test are all negative. The figure shows the urine sediment. Which of the following is the most likely diagnosis?
A. Diffuse membranous glomerulopathy
B. Glomerulonephritis in systemic lupus erythematosus (SLE)
C. IgA glomerulopathy
D. Minimal change disease
E. Poststreptococcal glomerulonephritis

38. A sexually active 19-year-old woman complains of increased frequency and a burning sensation upon urination. Pelvic examination shows inflammation of the exocervix and an exudate in the cervical os. Urinalysis shows numerous neutrophils but no bacteria. A cervical Pap smear shows numerous lymphocytes and metaplastic squamous cells with vacuoles in the cytoplasm containing an inclusion. Which of the following pathogens is the causal agent?
A. *Candida albicans*
B. *Chlamydia trachomatis*
C. Human papillomavirus (HPV)
D. *Neisseria gonorrhoeae*
E. *Trichomonas vaginalis*

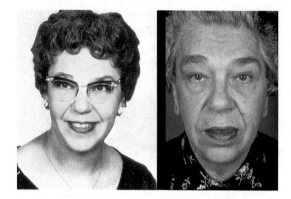

D. Increased plasma ACTH and 11-deoxycortisol after metyrapone stimulation

E. Increased urine 17-hydroxycorticoids with prolonged ACTH stimulation

39. The photograph on the right is a 55-year-old woman and the one on the left is the same woman at age 45. Currently, the patient complains of headaches and dyspnea. Physical examination shows bilateral inspiratory crackles in the lungs and enlarged hands and feet. A chest radiograph shows generalized enlargement of the heart and lung infiltrates consistent with congestive heart failure. Which of the following is the most sensitive screening test for this disorder?

A. Serum cortisol
B. Serum glucose
C. Serum insulin-like growth factor-I
D. Serum prolactin
E. Serum thyroid-stimulating hormone (TSH)

40. A 48-year-old man complains of extreme fatigue, weakness, and light-headedness when he stands up quickly from a seated position. The patient is normotensive when lying down; however, when sitting, his blood pressure drops and his pulse rate increases. There is diffuse brown pigmentation of the buccal mucosa. The physician suspects a disorder involving the adrenal glands. Which of the following laboratory findings would most likely be reported?

A. Decreased plasma ACTH and 11-deoxycortisol after metyrapone stimulation
B. Decreased serum sodium and serum potassium
C. Increased plasma ACTH and decreased serum cortisol

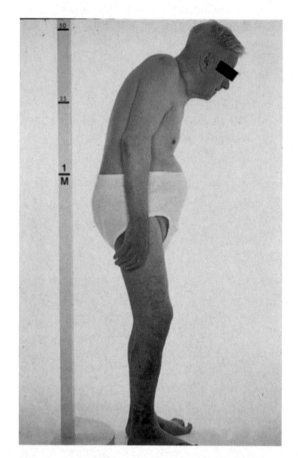

41. The photograph shows a 60-year-old man who has a 45-year history of lower back pain that began in the sacroiliac joints and shifted to the vertebral column. Physical examination reveals a high-pitched early diastolic murmur in the second intercostal space on the right. Which of the following laboratory findings is most likely to be reported?

A. Antibodies against *Borrelia burgdorferi*
B. HLA-B27 genotype
C. Hyperuricemia
D. Positive blood culture
E. Rheumatoid factor

42. For the past 15 years, a 72-year-old woman has experienced a loss in height and has had a chronic backache, resulting in forward curvature of the spine. Radiographs of the vertebral column show decreased bone density and wedge-shaped flattening of the vertebral bodies in the midthoracic region. What is the pathogenesis of this clinical condition?
A. Decreased estrogen
B. Genetic defect in osteoclasts
C. Hypophosphatemia
D. Hypovitaminosis D
E. Metastasis to bone

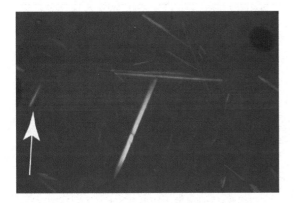

43. A 45-year-old man complains of a sudden onset of pain in his right great toe. Physical examination shows the area to be red and swollen. The total peripheral WBC count is 18,000/mm³, and the differential count shows predominantly neutrophils with greater than 10% band neutrophils. Synovial fluid from the metatarsophalangeal joint is viewed under compensated polarized light (see figure). The *arrow* in the figure is in the direction of the slow ray of the compensator. Which of the following crystals is present in the synovial fluid?
A. Calcium pyrophosphate crystals
B. Cholesterol crystals
C. Hydroxyapatite crystals
D. Negative birefringent crystals
E. Positive birefringent crystals

44. A 25-year-old man develops a pruritic lesion on the trunk. The lesion has an oval shape with an erythematous margin, and the central area has fine white scales. A KOH examination of skin scrapings taken from the leading edge of the lesion is negative for fungal organisms. Shortly thereafter, the patient develops a more widespread truncal eruption that follows the lines of cleavage of the skin. Which of the following is the most likely diagnosis?
A. Eczema
B. Pityriasis rosea
C. Secondary syphilis
D. Tinea corporis
E. Tinea versicolor

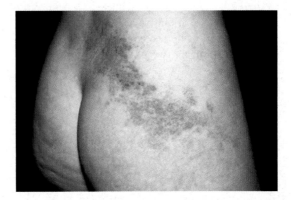

45. The figure shows the L2 dermatome of a 60-year-old woman who is currently being treated for a follicular B-cell malignant lymphoma. Which of the following best characterizes the pathogenesis of this lesion?
A. Photosensitive reaction to a drug
B. Reactivation of a latent virus in the sensory dorsal root ganglia
C. Skin invasion by malignant CD4 helper T cells
D. Toxin-producing strain of *Staphylococcus aureus*
E. Toxin-producing strain of *Streptococcus pyogenes*

46. A 3-year-old boy develops a maculopapular rash on his face 24 hours after the onset of a mild fever and sore throat. The rash causes prominent erythema of the cheeks. The causal agent of this disorder may also cause which of the following complications?
A. Acute lymphocytic leukemia
B. Acute myelogenous leukemia
C. Aplastic anemia
D. B-cell malignant lymphoma
E. Disseminated intravascular coagulation

47. For the past 3 years, a 55-year-old woman has had multiple pigmented, pedunculated tumors and flat, oval, coffee-colored skin patches. She has complained of episodic "attacks" of headache, palpitations, and profuse perspiration. She has recently experienced substernal chest pain during the attacks. Her pulse is 160 beats/minute and the average of three blood pressure readings is 180/120 mm Hg. Which of the following laboratory tests would be most useful in finding the cause of the hypertension?
A. Complete urinalysis
B. Serum electrolytes
C. Urine for free cortisol, 24 hours
D. Urine for 17-ketosteroids, 24 hours
E. Urine for metanephrines, 24 hours

48. A 4-year-old boy has a history of frequent respiratory infections and greasy stools. The child is below the normal percentile for weight and height for age. Physical examination shows nasal polyps and coarse inspiratory crackles in both lung fields that clear with coughing. Which of the following laboratory studies is the next step in determining a diagnosis?
A. Chromosome study
B. Nasal smear for eosinophils

C. Serum IgE level
D. Stool culture
E. Sweat chloride test

49. A 25-year-old intravenous drug abuser develops fever, scleral icterus, and right upper quadrant pain. Laboratory studies show an increase in serum aminotransferases and an increase in the serum bilirubin with approximately equal unconjugated and conjugated bilirubin fractions. The suspected diagnosis is acute hepatitis B. Which of the following hepatitis B profiles is expected?

	HBsAg	HBeAg	IgM– anti-HBc	IgG– anti-HBc	Anti-HBs
A.	Negative	Negative	Negative	Negative	Positive
B.	Negative	Negative	Negative	Positive	Positive
C.	Negative	Negative	Positive	Negative	Negative
D.	Positive	Negative	Negative	Negative	Negative
E.	Positive	Positive	Positive	Negative	Negative

Anti-HBs, anti-HBV surface antibody; HBeAg, hepatitis B e antigen; HBsAg, hepatitis B surface antigen; IgG–anti-HBc, anti-HBV core antibody IgG; IgM–anti-HBc, anti-HBV core antibody IgM.

50. An 85-year-old man has blood group A and is mistakenly given 1 unit of packed RBCs of blood group AB. He does not develop a hemolytic transfusion reaction. In vitro testing of the patient's plasma with test RBCs that are blood group B reveals no agglutination or hemolysis of the RBCs. Which of the following best explains why a hemolytic reaction did not occur?
A. Blood group AB lacks isohemagglutinins
B. Donor unit is packed RBCs
C. Patient does not have anti-B IgM
D. Patient has a B-cell immunodeficiency
E. Patient has a T-cell immunodeficiency

answers

1. **A** (atrophy) is correct. In cystic fibrosis (CF), a three-nucleotide deletion, which codes for phenylalanine, leads to transcription of a defective CF transmembrane conductance regulator (CFTR) for chloride ions. CFTR is *not* processed correctly in the Golgi apparatus and degrades before reaching the cell surface. This causes decreased sodium and chloride reabsorption in sweat glands, which is the basis of the sweat test. However, in other secretions (e.g., pancreatic ducts, bronchioles), there is increased sodium and water reabsorption out of luminal secretions and decreased chloride secretion into luminal secretions leading to thickened, dehydrated secretions lacking sodium chloride and water. In the histologic section, the exocrine ducts of the pancreas contain thick, pink secretions that obstruct and dilate the ducts and compress the ductal epithelium. Duct obstruction, in turn, causes an increase in back pressure on the proximally located exocrine glands, causing a loss of glandular cells by apoptosis and compression atrophy. Atrophy refers to a decrease in tissue mass due to diminished cell size or loss of cells. The patient's chronic diarrhea is due to malabsorption of fats and other nutrients related to a lack of pancreatic enzymes (e.g., lipase). Chronic pancreatitis eventually occurs with destruction of β-islet cells resulting in type 1 diabetes mellitus.

   B (dysplasia) is incorrect. Dysplasia refers to abnormal tissue development. Dysplastic epithelial changes include increased mitoses, lack of cell orientation, and nuclear enlargement with atypical changes in chromatin. These changes are *not* present in the pancreatic ducts.

   C (hyperplasia) is incorrect. Hyperplasia is an increase in cell number. The pancreatic duct epithelium is flattened and atrophic.

   D (hypertrophy) is incorrect. Hypertrophy is an increase in cell size. The pancreatic duct epithelium is flattened and atrophic.

   E (metaplasia) is incorrect. Metaplasia is the replacement of one adult cell type by another in response to injury. The pancreatic duct epithelium is normally cuboidal and has *not* changed to another cell type in the pancreatic biopsy.

2. **D** (Na^+ and H_2O moving into the cytosol) is correct. Blood loss due to a ruptured abdominal aortic aneurysm causes tissue hypoxia (inadequate oxygenation of tissue). The straight portion of the proximal tubule is the part of the nephron that is most sensitive to hypoxia. It responds to loss of O_2 first by decreasing the synthesis of ATP in the mitochondria (decrease in oxidative phosphorylation). This decrease in ATP affects the Na^+, K^+-ATPase pump by allowing Na^+ and H_2O to enter the cytosol, which results in cellular swelling, which is reversible.

   A (Ca^{2+} moving into the cytosol) is incorrect. Lack of ATP causes Ca^{2+} to move out of the mitochondria and the interstitial tissue into the cytosol of the cell. Ca^{2+} activates enzymes in the cell membrane (phospholipase), cytosol (proteases), and nucleus (endonucleases), all of which irreversibly damage the cell.

B (cytochrome c diffusing out of the mitochondria) is incorrect. Movement of cytochrome c out of the mitochondria stimulates apoptosis (death) of the cell.

C (intracellular pH increasing) is incorrect. In tissue hypoxia, anaerobic glycolysis is the key biochemical process used by cells to produce ATP. Lactic acid is the final product of anaerobic glycolysis and reduces the intracellular pH. Intracellular acidosis denatures enzymatic proteins in the cell, leading to coagulation necrosis.

E (phospholipase damaging the cell membrane) is incorrect. Activation of phospholipase by Ca^{2+} irreversibly damages the cell membrane.

3. **B** (perfusion defect) is correct. A perfusion defect occurs when blood flow to the alveoli is obstructed in the presence of normal ventilation of the alveoli. This produces an increase in dead space in the lungs and less exchange of O_2 between the alveoli and pulmonary capillaries resulting in decreased arterial Po_2 (called hypoxemia). In this patient, the perfusion defect is caused by a pulmonary infarction, which produces the wedge-shaped hemorrhagic infarct shown in the gross specimen. The base of the infarct extends to the pleural surface. Pulmonary infarctions are common in nonambulatory hospitalized patients because of blood stasis in the lower extremities, leading to deep venous thrombosis and thromboembolism to the lungs.

A (diffusion defect) is incorrect. A diffusion defect occurs when blood flows to the alveoli, but diffusion of O_2 into the pulmonary capillaries is inhibited by fibrous tissue (as in sarcoidosis), fluid (as in pulmonary edema), or other factors. In this patient, there is a perfusion defect due to a pulmonary infarct.

C (respiratory acidosis) is incorrect. Respiratory acidosis (decreased arterial pH) is caused by retention of CO_2 with a subsequent increase in alveolar Pco_2, decrease in alveolar Po_2, and decrease in arterial Po_2. In a pulmonary

infarction, hypoxemia stimulates peripheral chemoreceptors to increase the rate of ventilation causing respiratory alkalosis (increased arterial pH with a decrease in Pco_2).

D (respiratory alkalosis) is incorrect. Respiratory alkalosis (increased arterial pH with a decrease in Pco_2) is the most common arterial blood gas abnormality in a pulmonary infarction. However, it is the result of hypoxemia and *not* the cause of hypoxemia in the patient.

E (ventilation defect) is incorrect. A ventilation defect occurs when blood flows to the alveoli but O_2 is prevented from entering the alveoli (e.g., atelectasis with collapse of the airways). This produces an intrapulmonary shunt leading to hypoxemia. In this patient, a ventilation defect could *not* have caused the reduced Po_2, because atelectasis of the lung is not hemorrhagic or wedge-shaped and is more likely to be associated with respiratory acidosis rather than respiratory alkalosis.

4. **C** (decreased tensile strength of collagen) is correct. This patient has scurvy (vitamin C deficiency) caused by a diet lacking in fruits and vegetables. Lack of cross-linking in scurvy causes decreased tensile strength in collagen and poor wound healing. Vitamin C (ascorbic acid) is important in the hydroxylation of proline and lysine in the initial phases of collagen synthesis by fibroblasts. The sites of hydroxylation are the anchor sites for the cross-links between the triple helix composed of α-chains.

A (decreased synthesis of granulation tissue) is incorrect. Granulation tissue is produced in patients with scurvy. However, the type III collagen produced lacks tensile strength.

B (decreased synthesis of type III collagen) are incorrect. Type III collagen is produced in scurvy, however, it lacks tensile strength.

D (defect in fibrillin in elastic tissue) is incorrect. A defect in fibrillin is present in Marfan syndrome, causing weakness of elastic tissue, thus weakening the aorta (e.g., aortic dissection) and ligaments. Vitamin C deficiency does *not* produce defects in fibrillin.

E (leukocyte adhesion molecule defect) is incorrect. A defect in neutrophil adhesion molecules (integrins and selectins) prevents neutrophils from adhering to endothelial cells and transmigrating into tissue. Although this interferes with proper wound healing, it usually presents as a congenital defect. Defects in leukocyte adhesion are *not* caused by vitamin C deficiency.

5. **B** (chronic) is correct. A chronic inflammatory infiltrate is shown in the histologic section of synovial tissue. It consists of reactive plasma cells with peripherally located nuclei and perinuclear clearing, as well as lymphocytes with round nuclei and scant cytoplasm. A few of the plasma cells are multinucleated. The patient's clinical history indicates rheumatoid arthritis, a chronic inflammatory disease associated with destruction of articular cartilage caused by an overgrowth of hyperplastic synovial tissue (pannus).

A (acute) is incorrect. Acute inflammation is characterized by the presence of neutrophils, which have multilobed nuclei and granular cytoplasm. Neutrophils are *not* present in the histologic section.

C (granulomatous) is incorrect. Granulomatous inflammation is associated with the formation of well-circumscribed granulomas that contain macrophages, lymphocytes, and multinucleated giant cells. Granulomas are *not* present in the histologic section.

D (pseudomembranous) is incorrect. Pseudomembranous inflammation is mucosal damage induced by bacterial toxins, which produce a shaggy membrane (pseudomembrane) composed of necrotic tissue (e.g., pseudomembranous colitis due to *Clostridium difficile*). Pseudomembrane formation is *not* evident in the histologic section.

E (suppurative) is incorrect. Suppurative inflammation is a type of acute inflammation caused by bacterial pathogens. It is characterized by the excessive production of exudate (pus), containing predominantly neutrophils (*not* lymphocytes).

6. **C** (histamine) is correct. Histamine released from mast cells is the primary chemical mediator of type I hypersensitivity reactions. Histamine contracts the venular endothelial cells and exposes the basement membrane, causing increased vessel permeability and swelling of the tissue. Histamine causes arteriolar vasodilation, which produces redness (rubor) of the skin and increased heat (calor). Histamine also causes pruritus.

A (bradykinin) is incorrect. Activated coagulation factor XII converts high-molecular-weight kininogen to bradykinin. Bradykinin causes vasodilation of arterioles, increased vessel permeability, and pain in acute inflammation. Bradykinin is *not* released from mast cells and is *not* operative in type I hypersensitivity reactions.

B (complement) is incorrect. Complement is synthesized by the liver and has many functions in acute inflammatory reactions. Anaphylatoxins C3a and C5a directly stimulate mast cell release of histamine; however, this is not the mechanism for histamine release from mast cells in type I hypersensitivity reactions.

D (nitric oxide) is incorrect. Nitric oxide (NO), a free radical gas produced mainly by macrophages and endothelial cells, is released during conversion of arginine to citrulline by NO synthase. NO causes arteriolar vasodilation. It is *not* a key chemical mediator in type I hypersensitivity reactions.

E (prostaglandins) is incorrect. Prostaglandins are produced in leukocytes, endothelial cells, and platelets. Arachidonic acid is converted to PGG_2 by cyclooxygenase, and PGG_2 is then converted to PGH_2, the major precursor of prostaglandins that produce vasodilation

(PGE₂, PGI₂), pain (PGE₂), and fever (PGE₂) in acute inflammation. In type I hypersensitivity reactions, prostaglandins further enhance the inflammatory reaction after they are synthesized and released by mast cells. They do *not* produce pruritus.

7.   **A** (balanced translocation) is correct. The child has Down syndrome (epicanthal folds, flat nasal bridge). The presence of 46 chromosomes in the child indicates that a translocated chromosome, inherited from one of the parents, is responsible. Translocation occurs when one part of a chromosome is transferred to a nonhomologous chromosome. In balanced (robertsonian) translocation, the translocated fragment is functional. In this case, the long arm of chromosome 21 was translocated onto chromosome 14 in the mother, creating one long chromosome (14;21). The mother also has one chromosome 14 and one chromosome 21. The father has the normal 46 chromosomes. The affected child has 46 chromosomes with three functional 21 chromosomes including chromosome (14;21) and chromosome 21 from the mother and chromosome 14 and chromosome 21 from the father.

B   (frameshift mutation) is incorrect. The child's facial features are characteristic of Down syndrome, which is *not* caused by a frameshift mutation. In a frameshift mutation, nucleotides are inserted into or deleted from a DNA strand, resulting in synthesis of an abnormal protein product (e.g., Tay-Sachs disease).

C   (microdeletion) is incorrect. The child's facial features are characteristic of Down syndrome, which is *not* caused by microdeletion. Microdeletion involves the loss of a small portion of one chromosome, which can be detected only by high-resolution techniques.

D   (nondisjunction) is incorrect. Nondisjunction refers to unequal separation of chromosomes in the first meiotic phase, resulting in an egg or a sperm with 22 or 24 chromosomes.

Nondisjunction is responsible for most numeric chromosome disorders (e.g., trisomy 21), but because this patient has 46 chromosomes, a balanced translocation is responsible.

E   (point mutation) is incorrect. A point mutation involves the substitution of a single nucleotide base. If the altered DNA codes for the same amino acid, there is no change in the phenotypic effect (silent mutation). If the altered DNA codes for a different amino acid, there is a change in the phenotypic effect (missense mutation). If the altered DNA codes for a stop codon (e.g., UAA), there is premature termination of protein synthesis (nonsense mutation). These are *not* operative in the pathogenesis of Down syndrome.

8.   **A** (decreased plasma oncotic pressure) is correct. Edema is the accumulation of fluid in body cavities (e.g., ascites) and in the interstitial space (e.g., peripheral edema). Edema caused by cirrhosis of the liver involves alterations in vascular hydrostatic pressure and in oncotic pressure. An increase in hydrostatic pressure or a decrease in plasma oncotic pressure (hypoalbuminemia) cause outflow of a protein-poor (<3 g/dL) and cell-poor fluid into body cavities and interstitial spaces. This defines a transudate. In cirrhosis, the portal vein encounters increased resistance to emptying blood into the liver sinusoids (intrasinusoidal hypertension) due to compression of the sinusoids by regenerative nodules and fibrosis. This causes increased hydrostatic pressure (portal hypertension) that contributes to ascites formation. The synthetic function of the liver is compromised in cirrhosis; therefore, hypoalbuminemia occurs, which decreases the plasma oncotic pressure, further contributing to ascites and peripheral edema (dependent pitting edema). Because transudates have decreased protein and cells, they obey the law of gravity and percolate through the interstitial tissue and settle in the most dependent portions of the body (e.g., feet).

B (increased plasma hydrostatic pressure) is incorrect. Increased hydrostatic pressure is involved only in ascites formation. It is *not* involved in dependent pitting edema in the legs.

C (increased vessel permeability due to histamine) is incorrect. Increased vessel permeability due to histamine, which is a marker of acute inflammation, causes a nonpitting type of peripheral edema. The edema fluid is a protein-rich exudate (>3 g/dL) that contains polymorphonuclear leukocytes. Exudates also accumulate in body cavities (e.g., pleural effusion in pneumonia).

D (lymphatic obstruction with lymphedema) is incorrect. Obstruction of lymphatic channels causes leakage of lymphatic fluid into the interstitial space (e.g., filariasis), producing a nonpitting lymphedema. Lymphatic fluid accumulates in body cavities (e.g., chylous effusions in the pleural cavities caused by a tear in the thoracic duct).

E (movement of water into the intracellular compartment) is incorrect. Movement of water between the extracellular fluid (ECF) compartment and the intracellular fluid (ICF) compartment is called osmosis. Alterations in the serum Na^+ concentration in the ECF compartment is the primary cause of water movement between the compartments. In hyponatremia, water moves from the ECF into the ICF compartment, whereas in hypernatremia, water moves from the ICF into the ECF compartment.

9. **D** (Leber's optic neuropathy) is correct. Leber's optic neuropathy is a neurodegenerative disease in which progressive loss of central vision eventually leads to blindness. It has a mitochondrial DNA inheritance pattern, which is shown in the pedigree. Mitochondrial DNA disorders generally involve enzyme deficiencies in oxidative phosphorylation in the mitochondria. Unlike sperm, ova do *not* lose their mitochondria on

fertilization, so affected females transmit the abnormal allele to all their children. However, affected males do *not* transmit it to any of their children, because mitochondria are located in the tail of the sperm, which is lost during fertilization.

A (Alport's syndrome) is incorrect. Alport's syndrome is an X-linked dominant disorder associated with hereditary nephritis and sensorineural hearing loss. X-linked dominant disorders are characterized by a dominant allele that causes both male and female carriers to express the disease. Affected males transmit the abnormal allele to all their daughters. Symptomatic carrier females transmit disease to 50% of their sons and 50% of their daughters. This pattern is *not* shown in the pedigree.

B (familial hypercholesterolemia) is incorrect. Familial hypercholesterolemia is an autosomal dominant disorder involving a deficiency of low-density lipoprotein receptors that leads to severe hypercholesterolemia. Autosomal dominant disorders are characterized by a dominant allele that expresses itself in either the homozygous or the heterozygous state. Only one parent must have the abnormal allele to transmit the disease to the children. A heterozygous parent with disease transmits it to 50% of the children. This pattern is *not* shown in the pedigree.

C (familial polyposis coli) is incorrect. Familial polyposis coli is an autosomal dominant disorder characterized by the development of premalignant polyps in the colon. The disorder eventually progresses to colorectal cancer.

E (McArdle's disease) is incorrect. McArdle's disease is a glycogen storage disease (type V), which all have an autosomal recessive inheritance pattern. In McArdle's disease there is a deficiency of muscle phosphorylase, which renders muscle incapable of metabolizing glycogen to glucose. Therefore, during exercise there is no glucose for anaerobic glycolysis and no accumulation of lactic acid. In autosomal recessive disorders, disease is present only in patients who are homozygous (aa) for the abnormal allele. In most cases, both parents are asymptomatic heterozygous (Aa) carriers. Approximately 25% of their children will express the disease. This pattern of distribution is *not* evident in the pedigree.

10. **E** (increased total peripheral arteriolar resistance) is correct. The patient has hypovolemic shock caused by blood loss (tachycardia with weak pulse; cold, clammy skin; decreased blood pressure). In the initial phase of acute blood loss, the hemoglobin and RBC count are normal, because whole blood that contains both RBCs and plasma is lost. Within a few hours, plasma begins to be replaced and the RBC count and hemoglobin level drop. A decrease in cardiac output causes underfilling of the aortic arch, which activates the sympathetic nervous system, subsequently releasing catecholamines. Catecholamines cause venoconstriction, increased myocardial contraction, increased heart rate, and vasoconstriction of the smooth muscle cells of the peripheral resistance arterioles. Decreased renal blood flow activates the renin-angiotensin-aldosterone system, causing the release of angiotensin II and peripheral arteriolar vasoconstriction. Antidiuretic hormone (ADH) is also released, which produces vasoconstriction of peripheral resistance arterioles. Vasoconstriction of arterioles in the skin shunts blood to more important areas of the body, causing cold, clammy skin.

A (decreased arterial Po_2) is incorrect. In hypovolemic shock, gas exchange in the lung is normal; therefore, the arterial Po_2 is normal (*not* decreased).

B (decreased hemoglobin concentration) is incorrect. Hemoglobin concentration is normal in the early phase of hypovolemic shock resulting from blood loss.

C (decreased RBC count) is incorrect. The RBC count is normal in the early phase of hypovolemic shock resulting from blood loss.

D (increased left ventricular end-diastolic pressure) is incorrect. Left ventricular end-diastolic pressure is decreased (*not* increased) in hypovolemic shock, because there is less blood in the circulation.

11. **D** (*RB* suppressor gene) is correct. The patient has osteosarcoma and a history of retinoblastoma, which together indicate inactivation of the *RB* suppressor gene on chromosome 13. Osteosarcoma is a tumor of the connective tissue that arises from osteocytes. They most commonly occur in the metaphysis of the distal femur or proximal tibia. In the figure, the osteosarcoma appears as a gray-white necrotic tumor in the metaphysis that extends through the cortex into the surrounding connective tissue. Inactivation of the *RB* suppressor gene may be sporadic or inherited as an autosomal dominant trait. In the latter type, one of the alleles on chromosome 13 is inactivated in utero. After birth, only one additional mutation must occur on the remaining allele to produce cancer (one-hit theory). The patient then is at risk for developing a retinoblastoma, the most common malignancy of the eye in children. However, there is also an increased risk for developing an osteosarcoma when the patient is between 10 and 25 years of age.

A (*BRCA1* suppressor gene) is incorrect. The *BRCA1* suppressor gene is involved in DNA repair. Inactivation of the gene is associated with breast cancer in women and prostate cancer in men.

B (*MYC* proto-oncogene) is incorrect. The c-*MYC* and n-*MYC* proto-oncogenes are involved in nuclear transcription. Activation of the c-*MYC* proto-oncogene by a t(8;14) translocation produces Burkitt's lymphoma, whereas activation of the n-*MYC* proto-oncogene produces a neuroblastoma.

C (*RAS* proto-oncogene) is incorrect. The *RAS* proto-oncogene is a signal transducer that generates second messengers. *RAS* is activated by a point mutation and accounts for 30% of human cancers (e.g., cancers of the lung, colon, and pancreas; leukemias). It is *not* associated with retinoblastoma and osteosarcoma.

E (*TP53* suppressor gene) is incorrect. The *TP53* suppressor gene is involved in DNA repair. Inactivation of the gene by a point mutation allows unregulated proliferation of the cell. Although *TP53* accounts for 70% of all cancers (e.g., cancers of the colon, breast, lung, and brain), it is *not* associated with retinoblastoma and osteosarcoma.

12. **E** (increased synthesis of thyroid-binding globulin) is correct. The total serum T_4 level reflects free, unbound, metabolically active T_4 and metabolically inactive T_4 bound to thyroid-binding globulin (TBG). Enlargement of the thyroid gland is normal in pregnancy, and the increase in estrogen that normally occurs during this period stimulates liver synthesis of TBG. T_4 normally occupies one third of the binding sites on TBG, and the additional TBG with its bound fraction increases the total level of T_4 *without* affecting the free T_4. Therefore, the patient is clinically euthyroid, and the serum TSH remains normal.

A (decreased peripheral conversion of T_4 to triiodothyronine) is incorrect. The outer ring deiodinase that normally converts T_4 to T_3 in the periphery is normal in pregnancy.
B (increased release of T_4 from acute thyroiditis) is incorrect. The patient's thyroid gland is nontender, and there is no evidence of thyrotoxicosis. Furthermore, the serum TSH level is normal, indicating that the patient is euthyroid.
C (increased synthesis of T_3) is incorrect. Increased synthesis of T_3 produces signs of thyrotoxicosis and suppression of serum TSH. There is *no* evidence of thyrotoxicosis.

D (increased synthesis of T_4) is incorrect. Increased synthesis of T_4 produces signs of thyrotoxicosis and suppression of serum TSH. There is *no* evidence of thyrotoxicosis.

13. **B** (midsystolic click followed by a murmur) is correct. The figure shows redundancy of the mitral valve, particularly in the posterior leaflet on the right side of the photograph. A systolic click occurs when the valve prolapses into the left atrium during systole and is suddenly restrained by the chordae tendineae. The murmur following the click is caused by mitral regurgitation. Most patients with mitral valve prolapse are asymptomatic. Redundancy of the valve leaflet is due to an increase in dermatan sulfate in the valve causing myxomatous degeneration.

A (diastolic blowing murmur after S_2) is incorrect. A diastolic blowing murmur after S_2 characterizes aortic regurgitation, which causes volume overload of the left ventricle. The aortic valve is *not* shown in the figure.
C (opening snap followed by a mid-diastolic rumbling murmur) is incorrect. An opening snap followed by mid-diastolic rumbling characterizes mitral stenosis, in which the leaflets of the mitral valve appear fibrotic or calcified, unlike those in the specimen. Mitral stenosis is most often caused by chronic rheumatic fever.
D (pansystolic murmur at the apex) is incorrect. A pansystolic murmur at the apex characterizes mitral regurgitation, which causes volume overload of the left ventricle. The mitral regurgitation in mitral valve prolapse follows a systolic click and does occur throughout systole.
E (systolic ejection murmur) is incorrect. A systolic ejection murmur characterizes aortic stenosis, in which the area of the valvular orifice is reduced. The aortic valve is *not* shown in the figure.

14. **B** (DNA analysis of the X chromosome) is correct. The boy most likely has fragile X syndrome. In most cases, inheritance of fragile X syndrome is X-linked recessive, with a fragile site or gap at the end of the long arm of the X chromosome, where there are trinucleotide repeats (CGG). DNA analysis of the X chromosome in lymphocytes identifies the trinucleotide repeats and is considered more sensitive than the fragile X chromosome study. Characteristic findings include mental retardation, enlarged, nontender testicles (present at adolescence, *not* at birth), a long face with a prominent jaw, a high arched palate, and protruding ears.

A (buccal smear) is incorrect. A buccal smear is performed to rule out deficient or extra X chromosomes. Normal females have random inactivation of one of the two X chromosomes. Hence, normal females have one Barr body, and normal males have no Barr bodies. Patients with fragile X syndrome have no Barr bodies.

C (human chorionic gonadotropin) is incorrect. Human chorionic gonadotropin is *not* present in males unless they have choriocarcinoma of the testicle.

D (serum gonadotropins) is incorrect. The patient shows no clinical evidence of hypogonadism (e.g., delayed puberty); therefore, gonadotropins are *not* indicated. Furthermore, they are normal in the fragile X syndrome.

E (testicular biopsy) is incorrect. Testicular biopsy is *not* warranted, because the patient does not have a testicular neoplasm or signs of Klinefelter's syndrome, which is characterized by testicular atrophy.

15. **B** (immunologic reaction) is correct. The figure shows fibrinous pericarditis, in which a layer of fibrin covers the visceral surface of the heart. Because of the MI 6 weeks earlier, an immunologic reaction is the likely cause. In Dressler's syndrome (post-MI syndrome), the patient develops antibodies against the pericardial tissue. The immunologic reaction causes increased vessel permeability, loss of proteins, and production of a fibrinous exudate. Clinical manifestations of Dressler's syndrome include fever, precordial friction rub, and pain that increases on inspiration but lessens when the patient leans forward. Fibrinous pericarditis also may occur in the first week of an acute transmural (Q-wave) infarction. However, the pericarditis is due to increased vessel permeability *not* related to immunologic damage of the pericardium.

A (alteration in Starling pressure) is incorrect. An alteration in Starling pressure refers to increased hydrostatic pressure or decreased oncotic pressure within the vascular compartment. The transudate produced by this change is poor in proteins and cells, unlike the fibrinous exudate (shown in the figure), which is rich in protein and inflammatory cells.

C (metastatic disease) is incorrect. Metastatic disease involving the pericardium produces multiple nodular masses and a fibrinous and hemorrhagic exudate, unlike the lesions shown in the figure.

D (rupture of the anterior wall) is incorrect. A rupture of the anterior wall occurs 3 to 7 days after an acute MI, causing cardiac tamponade and death. These findings are *not* present in the heart.

E (viral infection) is incorrect. Coxsackievirus is the most common cause of pericarditis. This patient's history of MI indicates that an immunologic cause for the pericarditis is more likely.

16. **E** (positive Heinz body preparation) is correct. The patient has an acute hemolytic anemia caused by glucose-6-phosphate dehydrogenase (G6PD) deficiency, an X-linked recessive disorder. G6PD deficiency is most common in black Americans and persons of Mediterranean descent (i.e., Greeks, Italians).

G6PD deficiency leads to decreased synthesis of glutathione (GSH), which is necessary to neutralize H_2O_2, an oxidant product in RBC metabolism. Oxidant stresses that induce hemolysis include infection (most common) and drugs (e.g., primaquine, dapsone, trimethoprim). H_2O_2 accumulation in the RBC damages the RBC membrane (intravascular hemolysis) and denatures hemoglobin, forming discrete inclusions called Heinz bodies. Splenic macrophages often remove damaged RBC membranes, leaving cells with membrane defects, called "bite cells," circulating in the peripheral blood. The screening test of choice in acute hemolysis is a Heinz body preparation, which requires a special supravital stain to identify the Heinz bodies. Enzyme analysis for G6PD is the confirmatory test and must be performed when active hemolysis has subsided.

A (abnormal hemoglobin electrophoresis) is incorrect. The patient does *not* have a hemoglobinopathy, in which a decrease in the synthesis of globin chains (e.g., thalassemia) or the synthesis of an abnormal hemoglobin (e.g., sickle cell anemia) is present. The development of a hemolytic anemia shortly after beginning primaquine therapy rules out a hemoglobinopathy.

B (decreased mean corpuscular hemoglobin concentration) is incorrect. The mean corpuscular hemoglobin concentration, the average hemoglobin concentration in RBCs, is normal in G6PD deficiency, increased in hereditary spherocytosis, and decreased in microcytic anemias.

C (decreased serum ferritin concentration) is incorrect. Serum ferritin, which indicates the status of the iron stores in the macrophages in the bone marrow, is normal in G6PD deficiency, decreased in iron deficiency, and increased in iron overload diseases.

D (positive direct Coombs' test) is incorrect. The direct Coombs' test, which is used to detect IgG and/or complement on RBC membranes, is the screening test of choice for diagnosis of an autoimmune hemolytic anemia. Because G6PD is *not* immune-mediated, the test is normal.

17. **A** (aspirin) is correct. The *arrow* in the figure points to a platelet thrombus (red lesion), which is composed of aggregated platelets bound together by fibrin. Directly underneath the thrombus is a fibrous cap (blue lesion), the pathognomonic lesion of atherosclerosis. Directly beneath the blue fibrous cap is a core of necrotic material containing cholesterol (clear, needle-shaped spaces). There is a small fissure at the edge of the fibrous cap (disrupted plaque) that contains necrotic atheromatous debris. This debris was responsible for initiating the formation of a platelet thrombus in the lumen of the vessel. Aspirin prevents platelet aggregation by inhibiting platelet cyclooxygenase activity. This prevents the production of prostaglandin H_2 and its conversion to thromboxane A_2. Thromboxane A_2 is a potent vasoconstrictor and platelet aggregator.

B (glycoprotein IIb/IIIa inhibitor) is incorrect. Glycoprotein IIb/IIIa inhibitors prevent the attachment of fibrinogen to receptors on the platelet membrane, thus preventing platelet aggregation. Glycoprotein IIb/IIIa inhibitors are very expensive and are most often used to prevent thrombosis after an angioplasty rather than as a routine drug to prevent platelet thrombosis.

C (heparin) is incorrect. Heparin is an anticoagulant that inhibits the formation of fibrin clots, which are most often venous clots that develop in the deep veins of the leg in the lower extremities. However, heparin does *not* prevent platelet aggregation or the formation of platelet thrombi.

D (tissue plasminogen activator) is incorrect. Tissue plasminogen activator (tPA) is used primarily to break up an existing platelet thrombus. It does so by converting plasminogen to plasmin, which breaks up the fibrin strands holding a thrombus together, allowing reperfusion of the heart and preventing further extension of an area of infarction. The drug is *not* used to prevent thrombus formation.

E (warfarin) is incorrect. Warfarin is an anticoagulant that inhibits the formation of venous clots. It does *not* prevent platelet aggregation or the formation of a platelet thrombus.

18. **C** (hypertrophic cardiomyopathy) is correct. Hypertrophic cardiomyopathy is the most common cause of sudden cardiac death in young people. In some cases, inheritance is autosomal dominant. In hypertrophic cardiomyopathy, asymmetric hypertrophy of the IVS causes the anterior leaflet of the mitral valve to be closer to the septum than normal. This narrows the outlet channel for blood flow through the aorta and is the site of obstruction in hypertrophic cardiomyopathy. When systole occurs, the anterior leaflet of the mitral valve is drawn against the IVS and obstructs blood flow, producing a systolic ejection murmur that may easily be confused with aortic stenosis. Aberrant myofibers in the hypertrophied septum and conduction system abnormalities also occur; the latter are responsible for a fatal ventricular arrhythmia and sudden death. Maneuvers that distinguish the systolic ejection murmur in hypertrophic cardiomyopathy versus aortic stenosis involve changing preload. Whenever left ventricular volume (preload) is increased in hypertrophic cardiomyopathy, the intensity of the associated heart murmur decreases, indicating decreased obstruction. Increasing preload expands the left ventricular chamber and opens the outflow channel a little to allow more blood to exit the heart. Preload is increased by lying down (increasing venous return to the right side of the heart) or using drugs that decrease heart rate (e.g., β-blockers, calcium-channel blockers), which increases the length of diastole, causing more

filling of the left ventricle. Standing or holding one's breath (Valsalva maneuver) reduces venous return to the heart, decreases preload, which intensifies the murmur in hypertrophic cardiomyopathy, indicating increased obstruction. In aortic stenosis, increasing preload intensifies the murmur, because the heart has to get more blood out through the stenotic valve. Decreasing preload decreases the intensity of the murmur, because less blood has to exit the stenotic valve.

A (aortic regurgitation) is incorrect. Aortic regurgitation is characterized by an early diastolic murmur directly after the second heart sound. It does *not* cause sudden cardiac death.

B (aortic stenosis) is incorrect. Aortic stenosis is characterized by a systolic ejection murmur. Murmur intensity increases with an increase in preload (decreases in hypertrophic cardiomyopathy) and decreases in intensity with a decrease in preload (increases in hypertrophic cardiomyopathy). Aortic stenosis is *not* associated with sudden cardiac death.

D (mitral stenosis) is incorrect. Mitral stenosis is characterized by the presence of an opening snap followed by a diastolic rumble. It is a complication of recurrent rheumatic fever and does *not* cause sudden cardiac death.

E (mitral valve prolapse) is incorrect. Mitral valve prolapse produces a midsystolic ejection click followed by a murmur. It does *not* cause sudden cardiac death *except* when associated with Marfan syndrome, in which conduction defects are often present.

19. **E** (serum ferritin test) is correct. The systolic ejection murmur indicates aortic stenosis, and the fragmented RBCs (schistocytes) in the peripheral blood indicate the presence of a microangiopathic hemolytic anemia due to intravascular destruction of the RBCs as they hit the stenotic and dystrophically calcified valve. The damaged RBCs are called schistocytes, or fragmented RBCs. The damaged cells release hemoglobin directly into the blood. Haptoglobin, a protein synthesized in the liver, combines with the free hemoglobin to form complexes that are phagocytosed by macrophages in the spleen and completely degraded, causing very low to absent serum haptoglobin levels. The excess hemoglobin in the plasma is now filtered into the urine producing a red color and a positive dipstick for blood. Chronic hemoglobinuria eventually causes iron deficiency and a microcytic anemia. Serum ferritin is the best screening test for iron deficiency. Because ferritin is a soluble iron-binding protein, some ferritin leaks out of bone marrow macrophages and directly reflects the ferritin stores in the bone marrow. In iron deficiency, ferritin stores are decreased; therefore, serum ferritin is also decreased. Aortic stenosis is the most common cause of hemolytic anemia associated with schistocytes.

A (direct Coombs' test) is incorrect. The direct Coombs' test detects the presence of IgG and/or C3b on the surface of RBCs. It is useful when autoimmune hemolytic anemia is suspected. Autoimmune hemolytic anemias are normocytic, and schistocytes are *not* present in the peripheral blood.

B (enzyme assay for pyruvate kinase) is incorrect. When anemia is caused by pyruvate kinase deficiency, the peripheral blood smear shows dehydrated RBCs with thorny projections, unlike the cells shown in the figure. In addition, pyruvate kinase deficiency produces a normocytic (*not* microcytic) anemia.

C (hemoglobin electrophoresis) is incorrect. Hemoglobin electrophoresis detects changes in the concentration of normal and abnormal forms of hemoglobin, such as hemoglobin S in sickle cell disease. There are *no* hemoglobin alterations in microangiopathic hemolytic anemias.

D (osmotic fragility test) is incorrect. The osmotic fragility test is used to confirm a diagnosis of hereditary spherocytosis, in which the osmotic fragility of RBCs is increased. Hereditary spherocytosis is a normocytic anemia, and schistocytes are *not* present in the peripheral blood.

20. **A** (atelectasis) is correct. The most common cause of fever within the first 24 to 36 hours after surgery is atelectasis, which refers to either collapse of a previously inflated lung or incomplete expansion of the lungs on inspiration. Postoperatively, mucous plugs develop in the terminal bronchioles, allowing resorption of air out of the distal respiratory unit through the pores of Kohn. The loss of lung mass causes ipsilateral elevation of the diaphragm and inspiratory lag, because the lung is *not* expanding properly on inspiration, and deviation of the trachea to the ipsilateral side. In addition, vocal tactile fremitus and breath sounds are absent, because no air is entering the lungs.

B (lobar pneumonia) is incorrect. Postoperative pneumonia usually occurs 3 to 10 days after surgery. In lobar pneumonia, productive cough is present and there are signs of lung consolidation due to pus in the alveoli. This causes increased (*not* decreased) vocal tactile fremitus.

C (lung abscess) is incorrect. Aspiration of oropharyngeal contents, the most common cause of a lung abscess, occurs more than 24 hours after surgery. There is usually a cough productive of foul-smelling sputum due to aerobes and anaerobes in the abscess. These findings are *not* present in the patient.

D (pulmonary infarction) is incorrect. Pulmonary thromboembolism usually occurs 5 to 7 days after surgery. Signs of a pulmonary infarction include dyspnea and pleuritic chest pain, the latter *not* present in this patient.

E (spontaneous pneumothorax) is incorrect. Spontaneous pneumothorax involves the collapse of a portion of the lung, which produces hyperresonance (not dullness) to percussion.

21. **E** (increased vitamin B_{12} absorption after addition of intrinsic factor) is correct. The patient has pernicious anemia (PA), an autoimmune disease in which impaired intestinal absorption of vitamin B_{12} is caused by a lack of intrinsic factor. Antibodies directed against parietal cells in the body and fundus cause mucosal damage (chronic atrophic gastritis), achlorhydria (loss of acid production by parietal cells), and a decrease in synthesis of intrinsic factor, which normally forms a complex with vitamin B_{12} in the duodenum that is reabsorbed in the terminal ileum. Neurologic deficits are also present in vitamin B_{12} deficiency, because it is involved in propionic acid metabolism (see answer **C**). The peripheral smear shows a number of large, egg-shaped macro-ovalocytes. The arrow points to a hypersegmented neutrophil (with more than five nuclear lobes), a valuable and early marker of vitamin B_{12} deficiency. Pancytopenia is the rule in PA, because deficiency of the vitamin B_{12} causes decreased production of DNA leading to nuclear enlargement of nucleated hematopoietic cells in the bone marrow. These cells or derivatives from these cells (e.g., mature RBCs, platelets, neutrophils) are often phagocytosed and destroyed by bone marrow macrophages *before* they enter the peripheral blood. In addition, there is increased apoptosis of these enlarged cells. Reabsorption of orally administered vitamin B_{12} after the addition of intrinsic factor confirms the diagnosis of pernicious anemia. This is called the Schilling test.

A (decreased serum folate) is incorrect. Because of the patient's neurologic deficits and the presence of chronic atrophic gastritis of the body and fundus, a folic acid deficiency is excluded.

B (decreased serum gastrin) is incorrect. The patient has achlorhydria (absence of hydrochloric acid), which causes an increase (*not* a decrease) in serum gastrin levels.

C (decreased urine methylmalonic acid) is incorrect. Vitamin B_{12}, unlike folic acid, is involved in propionate fatty acid metabolism (odd-chain fatty acids). Propionyl CoA is converted to methylmalonic CoA, and methylmalonic CoA is converted to succinyl CoA using an enzyme reaction that requires vitamin B_{12} as a cofactor. Deficiency of vitamin B_{12} causes an increase (*not* a decrease) in methylmalonic acid levels (also propionic acid levels) in the urine. These acids are responsible for producing demyelination in the posterior columns and lateral corticospinal tract of the spinal cord (subacute combined degeneration), dementia, and peripheral neuropathy. The patient has decreased vibratory sensation and joint dysequilibrium (cannot stand up with her eyes closed), both of which are signs of posterior column disease.

D (increased antigliadin antibodies) is incorrect. Antigliadin antibodies are diagnostic of celiac disease, which may cause malabsorption of vitamin B_{12}. However, in this patient, pernicious anemia is the cause of the vitamin B_{12} deficiency.

22. **B** (benign tumor of β-islet cells) is correct. Benign tumors of the β-islet cells, or insulinomas, synthesize excess insulin, resulting in fasting hypoglycemia. When preproinsulin in the β-islet cells is delivered to the Golgi apparatus, proteolytic reactions generate insulin and a cleavage peptide called C peptide. Hence, C peptide is a marker for endogenous synthesis of insulin. Both serum insulin and serum C-peptide levels are increased in this patient, thus confirming the presence of an insulinoma.

A (alcohol-induced hypoglycemia) is incorrect. Alcohol is a common cause of hypoglycemia in the fasting state. The increase in NADH in alcohol metabolism causes pyruvate to be converted to lactic acid. This reduces the amount of pyruvate to use as a substrate for gluconeogenesis, which is the primary source of glucose in the fasting state. Alcohol has no direct effect on insulin or C-peptide levels; however, hypoglycemia would decrease serum insulin and C peptide.

C (ectopic secretion of an insulin-like factor) is incorrect. An insulin-like factor that causes hypoglycemia is most often produced by a hepatocellular carcinoma. Hypoglycemia suppresses β-islet cells, resulting in a decrease in serum insulin and C peptide.

D (malignant tumor of α-islet cells) is incorrect. Tumors of α-islet cells secrete glucagon, which produces hyperglycemia (*not* hypoglycemia) by stimulating gluconeogenesis.

E (patient injection of human insulin) is incorrect. Injection of human insulin increases serum insulin and produces hypoglycemia. Hypoglycemia suppresses β-islet cells, causing a decrease in endogenous synthesis of insulin and a corresponding decrease in serum C peptide.

23. **C** (leukocytes for Philadelphia chromosome) is correct. This patient has chronic myelogenous leukemia (CML). CML occurs in patients between 40 and 60 years of age. It is caused by translocation of the *ABL* proto-oncogene on chromosome 9 to chromosome 22 (Philadelphia chromosome), where it forms a fusion gene with the break cluster region. The Philadelphia chromosome is present in over 95% of patients with CML. A small percentage of patients with acute lymphoblastic leukemia also have the Philadelphia chromosome. Detecting the presence of the fusion gene has greater specificity for confirming the diagnosis. The presence of neutrophils in all stages of development and a myeloblast count below 10% in the bone marrow indicate a chronic, *not* an acute, leukemia. The myeloblasts in

CML do *not* contain Auer rods (red splinter to rod-shaped inclusion) even when CML transforms into an acute leukemia. The peripheral blood smear shows a marked increase in the number of leukocytes and basophils (cells with dark granules). Segmented and band neutrophils are prominent, as are myelocytes and metamyelocytes. Leukemias commonly metastasize to the lymph nodes (lymphadenopathy), liver, and spleen (hepatosplenomegaly).

A (leukocytes for alkaline phosphatase) is incorrect. Benign neutrophils contain alkaline phosphatase in the cytoplasmic granules (neoplastic neutrophils do *not*). This patient has CML, in which neoplastic leukocytes are negative for alkaline phosphatase.

B (leukocytes for CD10 antigen) is incorrect. CD10 in leukocytes is the marker for the common acute lymphoblastic leukemia antigen (CALLA), which is present in early pre–B-cell types of acute lymphoblastic leukemia (*not* CML).

D (leukocytes for tartrate-resistant acid phosphatase) is incorrect. Leukemia cells positive for tartrate-resistant acid phosphatase are present in hairy cell leukemia, which is a B-cell leukemia. The leukemia cells have hair-like cytoplasmic projections in the peripheral blood and do *not* contain Auer rods. The stain is negative in CML.

E (leukocytes for terminal deoxynucleotidyl transferase) is incorrect. Terminal deoxy-nucleotidyl transferase is present in early pre–B-cell and T-cell types of acute lymphoblastic leukemia. It is negative in CML.

24. **D** (deficiency of low-density lipoprotein receptors) is correct. The patient has familial hypercholesterolemia, an autosomal dominant disorder associated with a deficiency of LDL receptors. A decrease in LDL receptors causes increased levels of serum cholesterol. Excess

cholesterol deposits in tendons (Achilles tendon in this case) and the eyelids (yellow patches called xanthelasma). It also causes premature atherosclerosis, resulting in strokes and myocardial infarctions between 30 and 40 years of age.

A (decreased activation of capillary lipoprotein lipase) is incorrect. Deficiency of capillary lipoprotein lipase, an enzyme that normally hydrolyses chylomicrons, causes an increase in chylomicrons in children (type I hyperlipo-proteinemia). Hyperchylomicronemia leads to hypertriglyceridemia, causing pancreatitis, hepatosplenomegaly, and papular skin lesions (eruptive xanthomas, *not* tendon xanthomas).

B (deficiency of apolipoprotein C-II) is incorrect. Deficiency of apolipoprotein C-II, the activator of capillary lipoprotein lipase, causes an increase in chylomicrons in children (type I hyperlipoproteinemia). Hyperchylo-micronemia leads to hypertriglyceridemia, causing pancreatitis, hepatosplenomegaly, and papular skin lesions (eruptive xanthomas, *not* tendon xanthomas).

C (deficiency of apolipoprotein E) is incorrect. Chylomicron remnants and intermediate-density lipoproteins normally have apolipoprotein E on their surface. Receptors for apolipoprotein E in hepatocytes remove these remnants from the blood. Deficiency of apolipoprotein E leads to an increase in chylomicron remnants (remnant disease or dysbetalipoproteinemia) and increased levels of both triglyceride and cholesterol (type III hyperlipoproteinemia). There may be yellow deposits of triglycerides and cholesterol in skin creases on the palms (*not* tendons).

E (increased synthesis of very low-density lipoprotein) is incorrect. Increased synthesis of endogenous triglyceride in the liver increases the VLDL fraction in blood (type IV hyperlipoproteinemia. There may be deposits of VLDL fraction and triglycerides in

yellow papular skin lesions (eruptive xanthomas, *not* tendon xanthomas).

25. **D** (inappropriate antidiuretic hormone secretion) is correct. The patient has a small-cell carcinoma of the lung, which presents as a centrally located lung mass. Small-cell carcinomas are neuroendocrine tumors that derive from Kulchitsky cells. The biopsy shows round- to spindle-shaped basophilic cells, increased mitotic activity, and necrotic foci. These tumors may secrete antidiuretic hormone or adrenocorticotropic hormone ectopically, causing hyponatremia or hypercortisolism, respectively. Small-cell carcinomas have a strong association with smoking and have usually metastasized widely by the time they are discovered.

A (carcinoid syndrome) is incorrect. Carcinoid syndrome is caused by secretion of serotonin from a carcinoid tumor that has metastasized to the liver. In most cases, the tumor is located in the terminal ileum. Bronchial carcinoids may secrete serotonin without metastasis, but this is very uncommon. Carcinoid tumors from any site are *not* associated with smoking.

B (hypercalcemia) is incorrect. Primary squamous cell carcinomas of the lung ectopically secrete parathyroid hormone–related protein, causing hypercalcemia. These tumors are centrally located and strongly associated with smoking, but H&E-stained sections show keratin pearls and eosinophilic-staining cells, which are *not* present in the histologic section.

C (hypocalcemia) is incorrect. There are no primary cancers of the lung that produce hypocalcemia, ostensibly by secreting calcitonin, which inhibits osteoclast activity in bone. However, medullary carcinomas of the thyroid secrete calcitonin and hypocalcemia is a potential complication.

E (polycythemia) is incorrect. There are *no* primary cancers of the lung that produce polycythemia, ostensibly by secreting erythropoietin. However, renal cell carcinomas and hepatocellular carcinomas can ectopically secrete erythropoietin producing secondary polycythemia. Renal cell carcinoma is most commonly caused by cigarette smoking, while hepatocellular carcinoma has *no* smoking association.

26. **C** (reinfarction) is correct. After an uncomplicated acute MI, serum CK-MB peaks in 24 hours and returns to normal within 72 hours. Therefore, the presence of CK-MB on day 4, after an MI, indicates reinfarction. Both cTnI and cTnT peak in 24 hours and return to normal within 7 to 10 days following an uncomplicated MI. The presence of cTnI and cTnT on day 4 is expected.

   A (angina pectoris) is incorrect. Angina pectoris causes myocardial ischemia without causing myocardial cell injury. Angina pectoris does *not* lead to an increase in CK-MB, troponin-I, and troponin-T.

   B (pericarditis) is incorrect. Pericarditis is inflammation of the surface lining of the heart, causing precordial chest pain, and it is associated with a pericardial friction rub. Pericarditis does *not* damage the myocardial tissue and therefore does *not* lead to the release of cardiac enzymes.

   D (right ventricular infarction) is incorrect. Isolated right ventricular infarction is extremely rare, because the blood vessels perfusing the right ventricle are usually too small to develop occluding atheromas. Right ventricular infarction produces signs of right-sided heart failure (neck vein distention, dependent pitting edema), which are *not* present in the patient.

   E (rupture of the anterior wall) is incorrect. Rupture caused by necrosis of the myocardial wall usually occurs on days 3 to 7 following an MI. Rupture of the anterior wall produces cardiac tamponade with muffled heart sounds and neck vein distention followed by rapid death. The patient has normal findings on cardiac examination.

27. **B** (acute right-sided ventricular strain) is correct. The figure shows a pulmonary artery thromboembolism (saddle embolus) with extension into all the main pulmonary artery trunks. The site of origin for an embolus of this size is usually one of the femoral veins in the lower extremity. A venous thrombus first developed in the deep veins of the leg and then continued to propagate and eventually extend into the femoral vein, where it dislodged and embolized to the lungs. Thromboembolism is common in the postoperative setting, particularly after a total hip replacement. Sudden occlusion of the mainstem pulmonary arteries produces an acute increase in pulmonary artery pressure and acute right-sided ventricular strain, leading to sudden death (acute cor pulmonale).

   A (acute pulmonary infarction) is incorrect. The figure does *not* show acute changes in the lung parenchyma, such as a hemorrhagic pulmonary infarction. A massive saddle embolus causes death so quickly that there is not enough time for an infarction to occur.

   C (aspiration of gastric contents) is incorrect. Aspiration of gastric contents is common postoperatively. It often precipitates acute respiratory distress syndrome, but it does *not* cause sudden death.

   D (disseminated metastasis) is incorrect. There are no gray-white lesions in the lung parenchyma to suggest either a primary lung cancer or metastatic lung disease as the cause of death.

   E (nosocomial pneumonia) is incorrect. There are no patchy yellow-gray areas in the lung parenchyma to suggest a hospital-acquired pneumonia as the cause of death.

28. **A** (acute myocardial infarction) is correct. The patient has Kawasaki disease (mucocutaneous lymph node syndrome). Characteristic findings include painful cervical lymph nodes, swelling of the hands and feet, a desquamating rash involving the fingers, and vasculitis of the coronary arteries. Vasculitis often leads to coronary artery thrombosis and acute myocardial infarction. The treatment is intravenous gamma globulin. Corticosteroids are contraindicated, because they increase the risk for aneurysms in the coronary arteries.

B (aortic arch aneurysm) is incorrect. Thoracic aneurysms are most often caused by atherosclerosis. Kawasaki disease is *not* associated with inflammation of the aortic arch or the aortic arch vessels.

C (aortic dissection) is incorrect. Kawasaki disease is *not* associated with inflammation of the aortic arch or the aortic arch vessels; therefore, aortic dissections do *not* occur.

D (infective endocarditis) is incorrect. Infective endocarditis is most often caused by an infectious organism such as *Staphylococcus aureus* or *Streptococcus viridans.* Infection of the heart valves does *not* occur in Kawasaki disease.

E (mitral stenosis) is incorrect. Mitral stenosis is most often caused by chronic rheumatic mitral valvulitis. Infection of the heart valves does *not* occur in Kawasaki disease.

29. **D** (increased residual volume) is correct. The patient has a classic history and radiographic findings for emphysema related to smoking cigarettes. The chest radiograph shows hyperinflation in both lung fields, depression of both diaphragms, and a vertically oriented cardiac silhouette. Emphysema is a chronic obstructive pulmonary disease involving permanent enlargement of all or part of the respiratory unit (respiratory bronchioles, alveolar ducts, and alveoli). Elastic tissue destruction in these airways causes trapping of air and distention of the distal air space. This increases the residual volume, which is the volume of air left in the lung after maximal expiration. An increase in residual volume automatically increases total lung capacity, which causes hyperinflation of the lungs, an increase in the anteroposterior diameter, depression of the diaphragms, and vertical orientation of the heart.

A (decreased functional residual capacity) is incorrect. The functional residual capacity is the total amount of air in the lungs at the end of a normal expiration. It is the sum of the expiratory reserve volume (amount of air forcibly expelled at the end of a normal expiration) and the residual volume. An increase in residual volume increases (*not* decreases) the functional residual capacity.

B (decreased total lung capacity) is incorrect. An increase in residual volume automatically increases (*not* decreases) total lung capacity.

C (increased FEV_{1sec}/FVC ratio) is incorrect. In emphysema, lung compliance (ability to fill the lung with air) is increased and elasticity (recoil of the lung) is decreased because of destruction of elastic tissue. The FEV_{1sec}, or the amount of air expelled from the lungs in 1 second after a maximal inspiration, is decreased (e.g., to 1 L from the normal 4 L) because of the trapping of air in the distended distal airways. The FVC, or total amount of air expelled after a maximal inspiration, is also decreased (e.g., to 3 L from the normal 5 L). Therefore, the ratio of FEV_{1sec} to FVC is decreased (*not* increased) in emphysema.

E (increased tidal volume) is incorrect. The patient has emphysema, with increased residual volume. As the residual volume increases, the tidal volume (volume of air that enters or leaves the lungs during normal quiet respiration) is either normal or decreased (*not* increased).

30. **C** (left atrial myxoma) is correct. Cardiac myxomas are the most common primary cardiac tumors in adults. Symptoms include nonspecific complaints such as fever and malaise. The tumor has a ball-valve effect that causes sudden blockage of blood flow through the mitral valve, resulting in episodic fainting spells. A diastolic murmur similar to that of mitral stenosis is also present. Peripheral embolization of tumor also occurs. Infarctions of the spleen cause pain in the left upper quadrant and friction rubs. Infarctions of the kidneys cause flank pain and hematuria.

A (calcific aortic stenosis) is incorrect. Calcific aortic stenosis is associated with a systolic ejection murmur. Angina with exercise occurs because of ischemia of the subendocardium in the concentrically hypertrophied left ventricle. The decreased cardiac output through the stenotic valve causes syncope with exercise. Peripheral embolization does *not* occur.

B (hypertrophic cardiomyopathy) is incorrect. Hypertrophic cardiomyopathy is characterized by asymmetric hypertrophy of the interventricular septum causing findings similar to those described for calcific aortic stenosis. Peripheral embolization does *not* occur.

D (mitral stenosis) is incorrect. Mitral stenosis is a complication of chronic rheumatic fever. Left atrial dilation and thrombus formation with embolization is a common finding. The patient has no history of recurrent rheumatic fever, and physical examination does *not* reveal an opening snap in early diastole.

E (pericardial effusion) is incorrect. A pericardial effusion produces muffled heart sounds and is *not* associated with syncope or with peripheral embolization.

31. **D** (small bowel adhesions) is correct. The patient's history of colicky pain (pain followed by a pain-free interval) is characteristic of a small bowel obstruction. The history of previous abdominal surgery for endometriosis involving small bowel most likely produced adhesion causing small bowel obstruction. Adhesions from previous surgery are the most

common cause of bowel obstruction. The figure shows the classic radiograph of small bowel obstruction, mainly multiple air-fluid levels with a stepladder configuration.

A (direct inguinal hernia) is incorrect. Direct inguinal hernias produce a bulge in the middle of the triangle of Hesselbach, which is located above the inguinal ligament. The bulge appears when the patient is standing and disappears when the patient is lying down. This type of hernia is *not* associated with entrapment of bowel leading to small bowel obstruction.

B (intussusception) is incorrect. An intussusception, or telescoping of a portion of bowel into another portion of bowel, is uncommon in adults. The nidus for intussusception in adults usually is a polyp or cancer. Obstruction and ischemic damage with bloody diarrhea usually are present, neither of which are present in the patient.

C (large bowel infarction) is incorrect. Large bowel infarctions cause bloody diarrhea and localized, noncolicky abdominal pain. The pain is localized to the splenic flexure where there is an overlap between the superior and inferior mesenteric arteries.

E (volvulus) is incorrect. Volvulus occurs when bowel (sigmoid colon or cecum) twists around the mesenteric root, resulting in obstruction and strangulation. The affected bowel is distended and visible on a plain abdominal radiograph.

32. **E** (tracheoesophageal fistula) is correct. In a tracheoesophageal fistula, the proximal esophagus ends blindly. The distal esophagus arises from the trachea, causing the stomach to distend with air. When the infant breast-feeds, milk refluxes into the trachea, causing coughing due to aspiration of milk into the lungs. Polyhydramnios occurs during pregnancy, because the fetus cannot swallow the amniotic fluid and reabsorb it in the duodenum.

A (choanal atresia) is incorrect. Choanal atresia is caused by a bony septum between the nose and the pharynx, which forces the infant to breathe only through the mouth. The cyanosis that develops when the infant is breast-feeding ceases when the infant breaks from the breast and begins crying. Gastric distention or polyhydramnios is *not* associated with choanal atresia.

B (congenital pyloric stenosis) is incorrect. Hypertrophy of the pylorus does *not* present at birth but at approximately 2 to 4 weeks of life. Projectile vomiting of non–bile-stained fluid occurs. *No* polyhydramnios or cough during or after breast-feeding is associated with congenital pyloric stenosis.

C (duodenal atresia) is incorrect. Duodenal atresia (lack of a lumen) occurs just distal to the entry of the common bile duct into the duodenum. Projectile vomiting of bile-stained fluid occurs at birth. Air is present in the stomach and in the duodenum proximal to the opening of the common bile duct. Polyhydramnios occurs during pregnancy, because there is not enough duodenum to reabsorb the amniotic fluid. There is an increased association with Down syndrome.

D (esophageal web) is incorrect. Esophageal webs are uncommon in newborns. They produce dysphagia for solids but not liquids. *No* polyhydramnios or cough during or after breast-feeding is associated with esophageal webs.

33. **A** (decreased serum ceruloplasmin) is correct. The patient has Wilson's disease. A Kayser-Fleischer ring (rusty-colored pigment around the perimeter of the cornea), chronic liver disease, and a movement disorder are features of Wilson's disease, an autosomal recessive disease. Wilson's disease is due to a defect in the hepatocyte transport system for copper secretion into bile. In addition, copper cannot be incorporated into an α_2-globulin to produce ceruloplasmin, which is the binding protein of copper. The total serum copper equals copper that is bound to ceruloplasmin (95% of the total) plus copper that is unbound (free). In Wilson's disease, the total serum copper level is decreased because ceruloplasmin is decreased. However, the free copper level in the serum and urine is increased due to defective excretion in the bile and subsequent accumulation of copper in the serum. Excess copper deposits in Descemet's membrane of the eye and in the basal ganglia, particularly the putamen, result in parkinsonism, or choreiform movements, in some cases.

B (increased percent iron saturation) is incorrect. Movement disorders and deposition of iron in the cornea are *not* associated with disorders of iron metabolism (e.g., hemochromatosis). Hemochromatosis (*not* Wilson's disease) is associated with excess iron reabsorption from the gastrointestinal tract causing an increase in serum iron, decrease in total iron-binding capacity, and increase in percent iron saturation of transferrin, the binding protein for iron.

C (increased serum iron) is incorrect. Hemochromatosis (*not* Wilson's disease) is associated with an increase in the serum iron.

D (increased total serum copper) is incorrect. In Wilson's disease, the total serum copper level is decreased (*not* increased), because ceruloplasmin is decreased.

E (normal serum prothrombin time) is incorrect. The patient has chronic liver disease (chronic hepatitis or cirrhosis). Therefore, the prothrombin time is most likely increased (*not* normal) because of decreased synthesis of coagulation factors in the liver.

34. **D** (spontaneous pneumothorax) is correct. A pulmonary complication of scuba diving is rupture of a preexisting intrapleural bleb or a subpleural bleb, causing a hole in the pleura and a spontaneous pneumothorax. A hole in the pleura causes a loss of negative pressure in the pleural cavity, which collapses all or part of the lung. Physical findings include hyperresonance to percussion, tracheal deviation to the side of the collapse, elevation of the diaphragm, absent breath sounds, and absent vocal tactile fremitus.

A (decompression sickness) is incorrect. Decompression sickness (gas embolism) is a complication of scuba diving. As a diver descends, nitrogen gas under increased pressure moves from the alveoli and dissolves in tissue and blood. Rapid ascent forces nitrogen to come out of the tissue and blood in the form of bubbles, causing ischemic damage. A spontaneous pneumothorax is *not* a complication of gas embolism.

B (pleural effusion) is incorrect. Although a pulmonary thromboembolism leading to a pulmonary infarction and pleural effusion is a complication of scuba diving, it usually occurs when the diver is stationary and in deep water. Physical findings of a pleural effusion include dullness to percussion, deviation of the trachea to the contralateral side, and absent breath sounds.

C (pulmonary infarction) is incorrect. Although a pulmonary thromboembolism leading to a pulmonary infarction and pleural effusion is a complication of scuba diving, it usually occurs when the diver is stationary and in deep water. Clinical findings in a pulmonary infarction are pleuritic chest pain and dyspnea. Physical examination would *not* show hyperresonance to percussion, tracheal deviation to the left, and elevation of the diaphragm.

E (tension pneumothorax) is incorrect. A tension pneumothorax is *not* a common cause of dyspnea in scuba diving. Unlike a spontaneous pneumothorax, a tension pneumothorax is associated with a flap-like pleural tear. Inspiration causes the flap to open and allow air to enter the pleural cavity. However, the flap closes on expiration and prevents the air from leaving the cavity.

Increased intrapleural pressure (greater than the atmosphere) causes compression of the lung (atelectasis) and deviation of the trachea to the contralateral side. The diaphragm is depressed.

35. D (increased serum ferritin) is correct. The patient has early findings of hemochromatosis. Features of hemochromatosis include personal and family history of type 1 diabetes mellitus, cirrhosis (late finding), chronic diarrhea, and a pale gray skin color. Hemochromatosis is an autosomal recessive disease in which increased reabsorption of iron from the small intestine leads to iron overload in the liver (where it causes cirrhosis), pancreas (where it causes diabetes and malabsorption leading to diarrhea), and skin (where it increases the production of melanin). The term *bronze diabetes* is often applied to this condition. Serum ferritin is the usual screening test. Ferritin is a soluble iron-binding protein that binds iron in macrophages in the bone marrow. A small fraction of ferritin circulates in the blood and reflects the bone marrow iron stores. In hemochromatosis, and iron-overload disease, serum ferritin is increased. The biopsy stained with Prussian blue shows numerous blue-colored iron granules in the hepatocytes. The treatment of choice is phlebotomy to reduce the serum ferritin levels. Chelation therapy can also be used.

A (decreased serum ceruloplasmin) is incorrect. Patients with Wilson's disease have decreased serum ceruloplasmin. Wilson's disease, an autosomal recessive disorder, is associated with chronic liver disease and a movement disorder caused by defective secretion of copper into bile and reduced ceruloplasmin synthesis in the liver. Excess copper deposition in tissue does *not* cause skin discoloration or pancreatic insufficiency; however, it does cause cirrhosis.

B (decreased serum iron) is incorrect. Patients with iron overload diseases have an increase in serum iron, ferritin, and percent saturation of transferrin.

C (decreased small bowel reabsorption of D-xylose) is incorrect. D-Xylose absorption is an excellent screening test for small bowel disease as a cause of malabsorption. Small bowel disease (e.g., celiac disease) is characterized by inability to reabsorb orally administered D-xylose into the blood. The mechanism of malabsorption in hemochromatosis is deficiency of pancreatic enzymes (e.g., lipase) due to chronic pancreatitis.

E (increased total iron-binding capacity) is incorrect. Patients with iron overload diseases have an increase in serum iron, ferritin, and percent saturation of transferrin. However, the total iron-binding capacity is decreased because increased iron stores are associated with decreased synthesis of transferrin (binding protein of iron) in the liver. Because transferrin is decreased, total iron-binding capacity is decreased.

36. E (recurrent immune reaction against group A streptococci) is correct. The patient had chronic rheumatic fever and developed mitral stenosis after recurrent infections by group A streptococci. The most common cause of mitral stenosis is rheumatic fever. Antibodies against the M proteins of group A streptococci cross-react with antigens present in valvular tissue as well as other tissues (e.g., skin, joints, basal ganglia). Repeated immune reactions involving the valve led to repair by fibrosis, dystrophic calcification, and eventual stenosis of the valve. Increased resistance to blood emptying into the left ventricle led to atrial dilation and hypertrophy and an increase in pulmonary venous pressure resulting in pulmonary edema and pulmonary venous hypertension. Increased pulmonary vein pressure caused right ventricular hypertrophy and right-sided heart failure. The combination of pulmonary hypertension and right ventricular hypertrophy is called cor pulmonale.

A (immune reaction in systemic lupus erythematosus) is incorrect. SLE produces sterile vegetations on the mitral valve (Libman-Sacks endocarditis); however, this does *not* result in mitral stenosis.

B (ischemic heart disease) is incorrect. Ischemic heart disease produces heart failure, but it does *not* cause mitral stenosis.

C (myxomatous degeneration) is incorrect. Myxomatous degeneration is the characteristic histologic finding in mitral valve prolapse, which is associated with mitral regurgitation rather than mitral stenosis.

D (recurrent bacterial endocarditis) is incorrect. Recurrent bacterial infection of the mitral valve leads to valve destruction, resulting in mitral regurgitation rather than mitral stenosis.

37. C (IgA glomerulopathy) is correct. The urine sediment shows a RBC cast. Dysmorphic RBCs (RBCs with double circle and irregular borders) are also present lying free in the sediment. RBC casts, hematuria with dysmorphic RBCs, and proteinuria are characteristic of a nephritic type of nephropathy. The episodic history of hematuria following upper respiratory infections and the absence of hypertension are characteristic of IgA glomerulonephritis, which is the most common type of nephropathy.

A (diffuse membranous glomerulopathy) is incorrect. Diffuse membranous glomerulopathy is the most common cause of the nephrotic syndrome (proteinuria > 3.5 g/24 hours, fatty casts) in adults. The patient has a nephritic type of glomerulonephritis.

B (glomerulonephritis in systemic lupus erythematosus) is incorrect. A negative serum ANA test excludes glomerulonephritis in SLE.

D (minimal change disease) are incorrect. Minimal change disease is the most common cause of the nephrotic syndrome in children. The patient has a nephritic type of glomerulonephritis.

E (poststreptococcal glomerulonephritis) is incorrect. Negative antistreptolysin O and DNAase B titers and the absence of hypertension exclude acute poststreptococcal glomerulonephritis.

38. **B** *(Chlamydia trachomatis)* is correct. The patient has follicular cervicitis due to *C. trachomatis.* Two distinct forms of the organism that develop in vacuoles within metaplastic squamous cells are the elementary body (metabolically inert but infective) and the reticulate body (metabolically active but *not* infective). Binary fission of the reticulate bodies in the vacuoles of the infected cell results in the production of numerous elementary bodies. Urinalysis findings suggest acute urethral syndrome, which is also due to *C. trachomatis.* The treatment is a 1-g oral dose of azithromycin.

A *(Candida albicans)* is incorrect. *Candida* causes vaginal mucosal inflammation with a white discharge containing yeasts and pseudohyphae. Irritation of the urethra can cause dysuria. Metaplastic squamous cells do *not* contain inclusion bodies.

C (human papillomavirus) is incorrect. HPV produces koilocytotic atypia in squamous cells, which is characterized by a halo surrounding a pyknotic (dense) nucleus. These cells are *not* described in the cervical Pap smear.

D *(Neisseria gonorrhoeae)* is incorrect. *N. gonorrhoeae* causes cervicitis and urethritis. The gram-negative diplococci are *not* visible with Pap stains. Furthermore, the pathogen does *not* produce inclusion bodies in metaplastic squamous cells.

E *(Trichomonas vaginalis)* is incorrect. *Trichomonas* causes cervicitis and urethritis. The pear-shaped organisms have flagella. These organisms are *not* described in the cervical Pap smear.

39. **C** (serum insulin-like growth factor-1) is correct. The photograph on the right shows coarse facial features, enlarged nose, and thick lips. These findings along with the presence of enlarged hands and feet and cardiomyopathy with congestive heart failure is consistent with acromegaly. Pituitary adenomas secreting excess growth hormone are often quite large and extend out of the sella turcica, causing headache, visual field defects, and hydrocephalus. Gigantism occurs if the tumor is present before the epiphyses have fused, whereas acromegaly develops if the epiphyses have closed. Excess growth hormone causes hyperglycemia (growth hormone is gluconeogenic) and increased amino acid uptake in muscle and other tissues. Excess growth hormone also stimulates the liver to synthesize and release excess amounts of insulin-like growth factor-1. This hormone increases linear and lateral bone growth and also causes visceromegaly. Although growth hormone is used as a screening test in cases of suspected acromegaly, insulin-like growth factor-1 is a more sensitive test.

A (serum cortisol) is incorrect. Serum cortisol is a screening test for adrenocortical hypofunction or hyperfunction disorders, neither of which produces the changes noted in this patient.

B (serum glucose) is incorrect. Serum glucose is a screening test for diabetes mellitus, types 1 and 2 (*not* acromegaly). The patient most likely has diabetes mellitus due to excess growth hormone.

D (serum prolactin) is incorrect. Serum prolactin is used to screen patients who have galactorrhea to rule out a prolactinoma (*not* a growth hormone–producing pituitary tumor).

E (serum thyroid-stimulating hormone) is incorrect. TSH is used to screen for thyroid hypofunction and hyperfunction (*not* a growth hormone–producing tumor). TSH is decreased in hyperthyroidism and hypopituitarism and increased in primary hypothyroidism.

40. **C** (increased plasma ACTH and decreased serum cortisol) is correct. Hyperpigmentation of the buccal mucosa, plus a history of fatigue, weakness, and signs of hypovolemia when supine (decreased blood pressure and increased pulse rate), suggests a diagnosis of Addison's disease. Most cases of Addison's disease are due to autoimmune destruction of the adrenal cortex. This produces deficiencies of mineralocorticoids (e.g., aldosterone), glucocorticoids (e.g., cortisol), and sex hormones (e.g., androstenedione, testosterone). Hypocortisolism causes an increase in plasma ACTH due to a negative feedback relationship. ACTH has melanocyte-stimulating properties that increase the synthesis of melanin on the skin and mucosal surfaces. Hypovolemia is related to the loss of sodium in the urine due to aldosterone deficiency.

A (decreased plasma ACTH and 11-deoxycortisol after metyrapone stimulation) is incorrect. Metyrapone is a drug that blocks 11-hydroxylase in the adrenal cortex. This enzyme is normally responsible for conversion of the glucocorticoid 11-deoxycortisol to cortisol. Therefore, a normal response to metyrapone is a decrease in cortisol with a subsequent increase in ACTH and 11-deoxycortisol proximal to the enzyme block. If both plasma ACTH and 11-deoxycortisol are decreased, then hypopituitarism causes hypocortisolism. Hypopituitarism does *not* cause hyperpigmentation. In Addison's disease, the test causes an increased (*not* decreased) plasma ACTH and a decreased 11-deoxycortisol, because the adrenal cortex is destroyed.

B (decreased serum sodium and serum potassium) is incorrect. Aldosterone normally maintains Na^+-K^+ channels in the late distal and collecting tubules that increase sodium reabsorption from urine in exchange for potassium, which is lost in the urine. In Addison's disease, hypoaldosteronism causes Na^+ loss in the urine (which causes hyponatremia) and retention of K^+ (hyperkalemia, *not* hypokalemia).

D (increased plasma ACTH and 11-deoxycortisol after metyrapone stimulation) are incorrect. Metyrapone is a drug that blocks 11-hydroxylase in the adrenal cortex. This enzyme is normally responsible for conversion of the glucocorticoid 11-deoxycortisol to cortisol. Therefore, a normal response to metyrapone is a decrease in cortisol with a subsequent increase in ACTH and 11-deoxycortisol proximal to the enzyme block. In Addison's disease, the test results in an increased plasma ACTH and a decreased (*not* increased) 11-deoxycortisol, because the adrenal cortex is destroyed.

E (increased urine 17-hydroxycorticoids with prolonged ACTH stimulation) is incorrect. The adrenal cortex is destroyed; therefore, urine 17-hydroxycorticoids (cortisol and 11-deoxycortisol) remain decreased after prolonged ACTH stimulation if the patient has Addison's disease. Patients with hypopituitarism have increased 17-hydroxycorticoids in urine after prolonged ACTH stimulation.

41. **B** (HLA-B27 genotype) is correct. The patient has ankylosing spondylitis (AS). The photograph shows the patient in a bent position so that the patient cannot see directly ahead. A radiograph of the spine would show forward curvature of the spine (kyphosis) with ankylosis (fusion) of the lumbar vertebrae ("bamboo spine"). AS begins with pain in the sacroiliac joints and then involves the vertebral column. This disorder, which commonly occurs in males, is part of a related group of disorders called seronegative spondyloarthropathies. These disorders are characterized by a strong association with the HLA-B27 genotype, involvement of the sacroiliac joints, and arthritis that may involve

peripheral joints. The heart murmur in this patient is due to aortitis involving the ascending aorta, which is often associated with aortic regurgitation (high-pitched diastolic murmur). Patient's may also develop uveitis leading to blindness.

A (antibodies against *Borrelia burgdorferi*) is incorrect. Arthritis due to *B. burgdorferi* (causative agent of Lyme disease) does *not* involve the vertebral joints.

C (hyperuricemia) is incorrect. Gouty arthritis, a disorder characterized by underexcretion or overproduction of uric acid, usually involves the peripheral joints (e.g., first metatarso-phalangeal joint), where it causes an erosive type of arthritis. It does *not* involve the sacroiliac joints and vertebral column.

D (positive blood culture) is incorrect. The aortitis in ankylosing spondylitis does *not* have an infectious etiology.

E (rheumatoid factor) is incorrect. Rheumatoid factor is *not* present in ankylosing spondylitis. The term seronegative refers to the fact that rheumatoid factor is *not* present and that AS is *not* a variant of rheumatoid arthritis.

42. A (decreased estrogen) is correct. The patient has severe kyphosis (anterior curvature of the thoracic vertebrae) and a history of chronic backache, suggesting postmenopausal osteoporosis associated with estrogen deficiency. Estrogen normally inhibits the formation and function of osteoclasts and enhances osteoblastic activity (mineralization of bone). Therefore, estrogen deficiency results in increased osteoclastic activity with greater breakdown of bone than formation of bone by osteoblasts. In osteoporosis, there is an overall reduction in osteoid and mineralized bone causing a decrease in bone mass and bone density. Histologically, there is loss of cortical thickness and a reduction in the number and size of trabeculae in bone. Thoracic vertebral bodies become biconcave and develop anterior wedging caused by compression or collapse of bone, resulting in kyphosis (dowager's hump) and nerve root compression (radicular pain). Use of estrogen in preventing osteoporosis is currently under investigation. In lieu of using estrogen, stressing bones with weight lifting and increasing the intake of calcium and vitamin D are helpful in preventing osteoporosis.

B (genetic defect in osteoclasts) is incorrect. Osteopetrosis is a genetic defect in osteoclasts. It is an autosomal dominant or recessive disorder characterized by a defect in osteoclast resorption of bone, resulting in overgrowth and sclerosis of bone. Although it does predispose to fractures, it does *not* produce compression fractures in the vertebra and curvature of the spine.

C (hypophosphatemia) is incorrect. Phosphorus is important in the mineralization of bone. If there is hypophosphatemia, even in the presence of normal, decreased, or increased calcium, bone will *not* be mineralized and osteomalacia (soft bone) will occur. Osteomalacia produces pathologic fractures; however, it does *not* cause vertebral compression fractures.

D (hypovitaminosis D) is incorrect. Hypovitaminosis D, like hypophosphatemia, causes osteomalacia. In osteomalacia, defective mineralization of bone is accompanied by an increase in nonmineralized osteoid. Total bone mass eventually decreases. In osteoporosis, bone mass is also decreased; however, the mineral content of the *remaining* bone is normal.

E (metastasis to bone) is incorrect. The vertebral column is the most common site for bone metastasis. Most metastases occur in the lumbar vertebrae and result in osteolytic lesions (radiolucent) or osteoblastic lesions (radiodense). In osteoporosis, bone density is decreased (osteopenia), and compression fractures of the vertebrae are the key finding.

43. **D** (negative birefringent crystals) is correct. Inflammation of the metatarsophalangeal joint of the great toe is the classic presentation of acute gouty arthritis, which is characterized by the deposition of monosodium urate (MSU) crystals in the joint. MSU crystals have negative birefringence, which is defined by certain color changes that occur in the crystals when they are examined under compensated polarized light. In the figure, the background is red, and the crystals are yellow and blue. MSU crystals are yellow when aligned parallel to the slow ray of the compensator in the microscope, which is the case in this patient.

A (calcium pyrophosphate crystals) is incorrect. Calcium pyrophosphate crystals are either needle- or rhomboid-shaped in synovial fluid and show positive birefringence when viewed under compensated polarized light. They are blue (*not* yellow) when aligned parallel to the slow ray of the compensator. Calcium pyrophosphate deposit disease most commonly involves the knee joint.

B (cholesterol crystals) is incorrect. Cholesterol crystals are associated with chronic inflammatory joint effusions (e.g., rheumatoid arthritis). The crystals are *not* needle-shaped and do *not* exhibit birefringence.

C (hydroxyapatite crystals) is incorrect. Hydroxyapatite crystals are associated with degenerative osteoarthritis. They are not needle-shaped and do not exhibit birefringence.

E (positive birefringent crystals) are incorrect. Positive birefringence is defined when crystals are viewed under compensated polarized light. If the crystals are blue when aligned parallel to the slow ray of the compensator, they exhibit positive birefringence.

44. **B** (pityriasis rosea) is correct. The patient has pityriasis rosea, a dermatitis of unknown etiology. This eruptive dermatitis begins with an oval lesion ("herald patch") with an erythematous margin. The central area has fine white scales. Within 1 to 2 weeks, a more widespread eruption follows the lines of cleavage of the skin ("Christmas tree" distribution).

A (eczema) is incorrect. Eczema does *not* have a herald patch or a rash with a "Christmas tree" distribution.

C (secondary syphilis) is incorrect. The palms, soles, and mucous membranes (condyloma latum) are affected in secondary syphilis. There is *no* herald patch or a rash with a "Christmas tree" distribution.

D (tinea corporis) is incorrect. Tinea corporis is caused by *Trichophyton rubrum*, which is a superficial dermatophyte. The KOH examination is negative; therefore, the diagnosis of tinea corporis is excluded.

E (tinea versicolor) are incorrect. Tinea versicolor is caused by *Malassezia furfur*, which is a superficial dermatophyte. The KOH examination is negative; therefore, the diagnosis of tinea veriscolor is excluded.

45. **B** (reactivation of a latent virus in the sensory dorsal root ganglia) is correct. The patient has shingles, caused by the varicella-zoster virus. The figure shows the "band" distribution that is characteristic of this vesiculobullous skin disorder. The virus remains latent in the sensory dorsal root ganglia after the primary infection.

A (photosensitive reaction to a drug) is incorrect. Photosensitive drug eruptions develop in areas of exposure to sunlight (e.g., face, neck, hands). They do *not* involve a specific dermatome.

C (skin invasion by malignant CD4 helper T cells) is incorrect. The plaques and nodular lesions of cutaneous T-cell lymphoma (mycosis fungoides) do *not* follow a dermatome.

D (toxin-producing strain of *Staphylococcus aureus*) is incorrect. *S. aureus* is a toxin-producing agent that causes toxic shock syndrome. The rash does *not* involve a dermatome. The toxin produces an erythematous rash that desquamates.

E (toxin-producing strain of *Streptococcus pyogenes*) is incorrect. *S. pyogenes* produces an erythrogenic toxin that causes scarlet fever. The erythematous rash desquamates and does *not* follow dermatomes.

46. **C** (aplastic anemia) is correct. The child has erythema infectiosum, or fifth disease, which is caused by parvovirus B19. The rash causes erythema of the cheeks, giving the child a "slapped face" appearance. If a patient has chronic hemolytic anemia (e.g., hereditary spherocytosis), the virus can infect either a trilineage stem cell, resulting in a self-limited aplastic anemia, or an erythroid stem cell, resulting in a pure red blood cell aplasia.

A (acute lymphocytic leukemia) is incorrect. Parvovirus B19 has *not* been associated with the development of any leukemia.

B (acute myelogenous leukemia) is incorrect. Parvovirus B19 has *not* been associated with the development of any leukemia.

D (B-cell malignant lymphoma) is incorrect. Parvovirus B19 has *not* been associated with the development of any type of malignant lymphoma.

E (disseminated intravascular coagulation) is incorrect. Activation of the intrinsic or extrinsic coagulation system must occur to produce intravascular clotting. Parvovirus B19 does *not* cause tissue damage (release of tissue thromboplastin) or endothelial cell damage (activation of factor XII) to initiate disseminated intravascular coagulation.

47. **E** (urine for metanephrines, 24 hours) is correct. This patient has neurofibromatosis complicated by hypertension due to a pheochromocytoma. The skin lesions in neurofibromatosis include pigmented, pedunculated tumors (neurofibromas) and flat, shaped, coffee-colored patches (café-au-lait patches). Neurofibromatosis is an autosomal dominant neurocutaneous disorder with increased incidence of pheochromocytoma (unilateral or bilateral) and central and peripheral nervous system tumors (e.g., meningioma, acoustic neuroma). The classic triad of headache, palpitations, and excessive perspiration is highly predictive of a pheochromocytoma. Catecholamine excess may cause subendocardial ischemia resulting in angina (as occurred in this patient). Hypertension is characterized as sustained, sustained with paroxysms (most common), or paroxysmal only. A 24-hour urine test for metanephrines (most sensitive test) and a 24-hour test for vanillylmandelic acid are most often used as screening tests.

A (complete urinalysis) is incorrect. Although a urinalysis is useful in the workup of hypertension related to renal disease, it does *not* provide adequate information in screening for a pheochromocytoma.

B (serum electrolytes) is incorrect. Serum electrolytes are most useful in diagnosing primary aldosteronism (*not* a pheochromocytoma). The benign adrenocortical adenomas arise in the zona glomerulosa of the adrenal cortex. Excess aldosterone causes hypernatremia, hypokalemia, and metabolic alkalosis. A pheochromocytoma is *not* associated with any electrolyte abnormalities.

C (urine for free cortisol, 24 hours) is incorrect. Increase in urine free cortisol is a characteristic finding in Cushing syndrome, which is associated with hypertension. The patient does *not* have any of the classic findings for Cushing syndrome—moon facies, truncal obesity, and purple abdominal striae. The urine free cortisol is normal in a pheochromocytoma.

D (urine for 17-ketosteroids, 24 hours) is incorrect. Increased urine 17-ketosteroids (dehydroepiandrosterone and androstenedione) is a characteristic finding in Cushing syndrome. It is *not* increased in a pheochromocytoma.

48. **E** (sweat chloride test) is correct. The patient has cystic fibrosis, which is an autosomal recessive disease characterized by a deficiency of cystic fibrosis transport regulator that normally regulates sodium and chloride ions in secretions. The sweat chloride test detects the presence of defective chloride transport by measuring increased amounts of chloride in the sweat. Clinical findings of cystic fibrosis include recurrent respiratory infection caused by thickened secretions and malabsorption caused by thickened secretions blocking exocrine ducts in the pancreas. Nasal polyps are frequently present in children.

A (chromosome study) is incorrect. Chromosome studies are generally reserved for prenatal diagnosis of cystic fibrosis. The defect occurs on chromosome 7 (three-nucleotide deletion), and specialized techniques are required to identify the abnormal gene locus.
B (nasal smear for eosinophils) is incorrect. Allergic polyps occur in patients with allergic rhinitis associated with IgE antibody–mediated disease (type I hypersensitivity). Allergic polyps mainly develop in adults and are *not* seen in children. The patient has no signs of allergic rhinitis (e.g., nasal stuffiness, seasonal variation).
C (serum IgE level) is incorrect. Allergic polyps occur in patients with allergic rhinitis associated with IgE antibody–mediated disease (type I hypersensitivity). Allergic polyps mainly develop in adults and are *not* seen in children. Serum IgE levels are normal in cystic fibrosis.
D (stool culture) is incorrect. The history of greasy stools in the patient is a sign of

malabsorption and *not* an invasive enterocolitis due to a microbial pathogen. Therefore, this test would *not* be useful in diagnosing cystic fibrosis.

49. **E** is correct. The presence of a mixed hyperbilirubinemia (increase in unconjugated and conjugated bilirubin) and an increase in the serum transaminases in an intravenous drug abuser are markers of the icteric phase of acute hepatitis B. HBsAg, HBeAg, and IgM–anti-HBc are positive. HBsAg first appears in the serum 2 to 8 weeks before symptoms develop and is the last antigen marker to disappear if recovery occurs. HBeAg is an infective particle that appears shortly after HBsAg and disappears before it. IgM–anti-HBc is a nonprotective antibody that appears shortly after HBsAg and is a marker of acute hepatitis.

A is incorrect. The presence of anti-HBs and the absence of HBsAg, HBeAg, IgM–anti-HBc and IgG–anti-HBc indicate immunization with hepatitis B vaccine. Anti-HBs is a protective antibody.
B is incorrect. The presence of anti-HBs and IgG–anti-HBc and the absence of HBsAg, HBeAg, and IgM–anti-HBc indicate recovery from hepatitis B. Anti-HBs is a protective antibody, and anti-HBc-IgG develops after 6 months.
C is incorrect. The presence of IgM–anti-HBc and the absence of HBsAg, HBeAg, IgG–anti-HBc, and anti-HBs indicate that the patient is in the "window phase" of recovery from hepatitis B when all the antigens have disappeared and their corresponding antibodies have not yet had time to develop.
D is incorrect. The presence of HBsAg and the absence of HBeAg, IgM–anti-HBc, IgG–anti-HBc, and anti-HBs are characteristic of the earliest phase of acute hepatitis B.

50. **C** (patient does not have anti-B IgM) is correct. Elderly individuals frequently lose their isohemagglutinins (e.g., anti-A IgM, anti-B IgM). The patient is blood group A and should have anti-B IgM isohemagglutinins in the plasma. However, in vitro testing showed that reacting his plasma with test blood group B RBCs did *not* produce agglutination or hemolysis. Therefore, the infusion of donor group AB RBCs did *not* produce a hemolytic transfusion reaction because the patient has no anti-B IgM antibodies to attach to the B antigen on the donor's RBCs.

A (blood group AB lacks isohemagglutinins) is incorrect. Although patients with blood group AB lack isohemagglutinins (anti-A IgM, anti-B IgM), if the patient receiving the AB blood is blood group A (have anti-B IgM antibodies), blood group B (have anti-A IgM antibodies) or blood group O (have anti-A and anti-B IgM antibodies) a hemolytic transfusion reaction will occur. Blood group AB people are universal recipients, *not* universal donors. A universal recipient means that AB people lack isohemagglutinins in their plasma and can be transfused blood group AB, A, B, or O blood. People who are blood group O are universal donors, because they lack A and B antigens on the surface of their RBCs. Therefore, transfusion of O packed RBCs into A, B, or AB individuals does *not* produce a hemolytic transfusion reaction. However, blood group O people can only receive blood group O blood, because blood group O people have anti-A and anti-B IgM antibodies to attack A, B, or AB blood.

B (the donor unit is packed RBCs) is incorrect. Whether the donor unit is packed RBCs or whole blood, plasma is present in both types of transfusion. If antibodies are present in the plasma in either preparation that could cause a hemolytic anemia, a hemolytic transfusion reaction will occur. However, this patient has no anti-B-IgM to hemolyze the donor blood group AB RBCs.

D (patient has a B-cell immunodeficiency) is incorrect. Elderly patients do *not* lack B cells; however, there is a decrease in the synthesis of isohemagglutinins, which are natural (*not* atypical) IgM antibodies.

E (patient has a T-cell immunodeficiency) is incorrect. Hemolytic transfusion reactions are antibody-mediated type II hypersensitivity reactions and do *not* involve T cells.

questions

DIRECTIONS: Each numbered item or incomplete statement is followed by options arranged in alphabetical or logical order. Select the best answer to each question. Some options may be partially correct, but there is only **ONE BEST** answer.

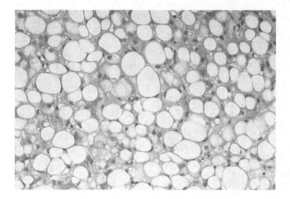

1. A 58-year-old man with a 10-year history of alcohol abuse complains of tenderness in the right upper quadrant. Physical examination shows tender hepatomegaly. Serum bilirubin is normal; however, serum aspartate aminotransferase is preferentially increased. The figure shows a histologic section of the liver obtained on biopsy. Which of the following best explains the pathogenesis of the liver disease?
A. Decreased hydrolysis of fat in adipose cells
B. Decreased synthesis of fatty acids
C. Decreased synthesis of very low density lipoprotein
D. Increased synthesis of glycerol 3-phosphate
E. Increased β-oxidation of fatty acids

2. The retina of a 35-year-old man who has a 15-year history of type 1 diabetes mellitus shows microaneurysms and retinal hemorrhages. Which of the following is the pathogenesis of the lesions in the retina?
A. Increased intraocular pressure
B. Inflammation of the optic nerve
C. Microangiopathy
D. Nonenzymatic glycosylation
E. Osmotic damage

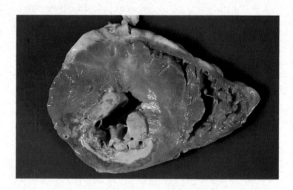

3. A 75-year-old man is admitted to the hospital with severe substernal chest pain that radiates into the left arm and jaw. On day 5 of hospitalization, he develops a ventricular arrhythmia and dies. The figure shows a transverse section of the heart at autopsy. The left ventricle shows which of the following types of necrosis?
A. Caseous necrosis
B. Coagulation necrosis
C. Enzymatic fat necrosis
D. Fibrinoid necrosis
E. Liquefactive necrosis

4. A 22-year-old woman who is anxious about her upcoming wedding has numbness and tingling at the tips of her fingers. Her right hand shows adduction of the thumb into the palm when provoked by inflating the sphygmomanometer cuff. Which of the following is most likely responsible for these findings?
A. Diabetic ketoacidosis
B. Nephrotic syndrome
C. Primary hyperparathyroidism
D. Respiratory alkalosis
E. Sarcoidosis

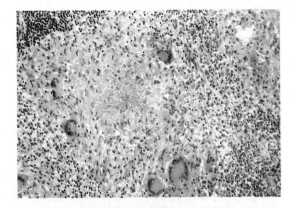

5. A 45-year-old woman has fever, night sweats, and weight loss. The figure shows a histologic section of tissue removed from the right apex of the lung. Which of the following best describes the type of necrosis that is present?
A. Caseous necrosis
B. Coagulation necrosis
C. Enzymatic fat necrosis
D. Fibrinoid necrosis
E. Liquefactive necrosis

6. A 10-year-old boy has muscle weakness that became symptomatic 5 years ago. When placed in a prone position, he must "walk" his hands to his feet and up the front of his legs to stand. Serum creatine kinase was initially increased at birth but is progressively decreasing with age. Which of the following is the pathogenesis of this clinical disorder?

A. Antibodies against acetylcholine receptors
B. Deficiency of dystrophin
C. Demyelinating disorder
D. Inflammatory myopathy
E. Motor neuron disorder

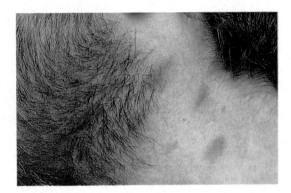

7. The figure shows painless and nonpruritic lesions on the left side of the neck of a 25-year-old man with AIDS. Similar lesions are also present on the hard palate. Which of the following is the most likely causal organism?
A. *Bartonella henselae*
B. Cytomegalovirus
C. Epstein-Barr virus
D. Human herpesvirus 8
E. Human immunodeficiency virus

8. A 4-year-old boy has a history of pathologic fractures since birth. Physical examination shows blue discoloration of the sclerae in both eyes. Which of the following is the most likely diagnosis?
A. Ehlers Danlos syndrome
B. Marfan syndrome
C. Osteogenesis imperfecta
D. Osteopetrosis
E. Vitamin D–dependent rickets

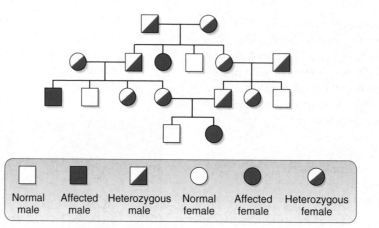

Normal male | Affected male | Heterozygous male | Normal female | Affected female | Heterozygous female

9. Which of the following clinical disorders is most compatible with the distribution of affected patients shown in the pedigree above?
   A. Glucose-6-phosphate dehydrogenase (G6PD) deficiency
   B. Hereditary spherocytosis
   C. Hemochromatosis
   D. Neurofibromatosis
   E. Type 2 diabetes mellitus

10. A 9-month-old girl has an infection on her face that began as erythematous macules. She later develops pustules that rupture and cause honey-colored crusted lesions. The girl's 5-year-old brother develops similar lesions. Which of the following is the causal agent?
    A. *Staphylococcus aureus*
    B. Herpes simplex virus type 1
    C. *Malassezia furfur*
    D. *Propionibacterium acnes*
    E. *Trichophyton rubrum*

11. The figure to the right shows two children, each with a different nutritional disorder. Which of the following findings would most likely be reported only in the crying child on the left?
    A. Decrease in serum albumin
    B. Decrease in somatic protein stores
    C. Decrease in subcutaneous fat
    D. Decrease in total calorie intake
    E. Defects in cell mediated immunity

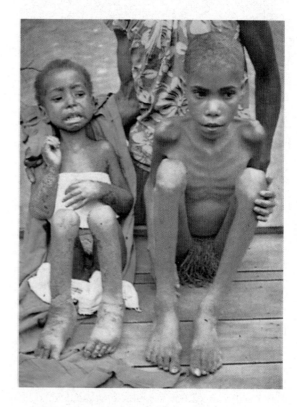

12. A 26-year-old woman has retro-orbital pain and blurry vision in the right eye. Physical examination shows flame hemorrhages around the disk vessels and a swollen optic disk. After treatment with systemic corticosteroids, the patient's vision is restored to normal. A few

months later, the patient has slurry speech, an ataxic gait, and weakness and paresthesias in the arms and legs that eventually remit without sequelae. Which of the following findings is most likely present in the cerebrospinal fluid (CSF)?

A. Decreased glucose
B. Increased neutrophils
C. Normal protein
D. Oligoclonal bands
E. Positive Gram stain

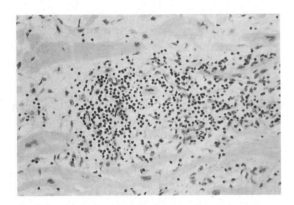

13. A 28-year-old man has fever, fatigue, difficulty breathing, and substernal chest pain while walking or at rest. The patient has a history of alcohol abuse. Physical examination shows bibasilar inspiratory crackles, distention of the jugular neck veins, hepatomegaly, and dependent pitting edema. A chest radiograph shows generalized cardiac enlargement. Laboratory studies reveal an increase in cardiac-specific troponins. The figure shows a histologic section of myocardial tissue. Which of the following is the most likely cause of the heart disease?

A. Acute rheumatic fever
B. Coronary artery thrombosis
C. Ischemic heart disease
D. Toxin-induced myocarditis
E. Viral myocarditis

14. For the past few months, a 26-year-old man with AIDS has experienced progressive loss of visual acuity in both eyes. Intraocular pressure is normal. The CD4 helper T-cell count is

48 cells/mm^3. Examination of the retinas of both eyes shows white areas with indistinct borders. Which of the following pathogens is the most likely causal agent?

A. *Candida albicans*
B. Cytomegalovirus
C. Herpes simplex virus type 1
D. Human immunodeficiency virus
E. *Toxoplasma gondii*

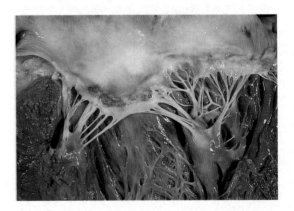

15. A 22-year-old woman saw her physician because of a severe sore throat. Three weeks later, she complained of fever, pains in the knees, and a rash on the arms that consisted of a circular ring of erythema around normal skin. Other findings on physical examination included bibasilar inspiratory crackles, an S$_3$ heart sound, and a pansystolic murmur at the apex that radiated into the axilla. Both murmur and S$_3$ heart sound increased in intensity on expiration. The figure shows the opened left side of the heart. Which of the following is the most likely diagnosis?

A. Acute bacterial endocarditis
B. Acute rheumatic fever
C. Libman-Sacks endocarditis
D. Nonbacterial thrombotic endocarditis
E. Subacute bacterial endocarditis

16. The umbilical cord of a 6-week-old male infant has not sloughed off. The cord is removed surgically and histologic sections show an absence of neutrophil margination along the umbilical vessels and absence of neutrophil transmigration into interstitial tissue. Which of the following defects of neutrophil function is most likely responsible?

A. Absent respiratory burst
B. Leukocyte adhesion molecule defect
C. Myeloperoxidase deficiency
D. Opsonization defect
E. Phagocytosis defect

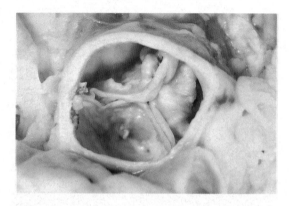

17. The figure shows the aortic side of an unopened aortic valve of a 62-year-old man, who died in a car accident. Which of the following complications commonly occurs with the aortic valvular lesion?

A. Acute myocardial infarction (MI)
B. Aortic dissection
C. Hemolytic anemia
D. Hypertension
E. Stroke syndrome

18. A 2-year-old boy with Bruton's agamma-globulinemia has recurrent pneumonia caused by *Streptococcus pneumoniae*. Which of the following defects is the most likely cause of increased susceptibility to bacterial infections?

A. Leukocyte adhesion molecule defect
B. Neutrophil chemotactic defect
C. Neutrophil membrane-associated protein defect
D. Neutrophil microbicidal defect
E. Neutrophil opsonization defect

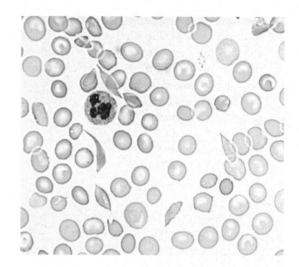

19. A 25-year-old black American man has fever and pain in the lower right thigh. A radiograph of the thigh shows irregular lucency in the metaphysis and thickening of the periosteum of the distal right femur. The figure shows his peripheral blood smear. Which of the following pathogens is most likely responsible for lesion in the femur?

A. *Pseudomonas aeruginosa*
B. *Salmonella paratyphi*
C. *Staphylococcus aureus*
D. *Streptococcus pneumoniae*
E. *Streptococcus pyogenes*

20. A 25-year-old woman with AIDS has recurrent candidiasis and a *Pneumocystis jiroveci* pneumonia. Which of the following laboratory test results is expected?

A. Hypergammaglobulinemia
B. Increase in CD4 helper T-cell/CD8 suppressor T-cell ratio
C. Intact cellular immunity
D. Normal phytohemagglutinin assay
E. Normal skin reaction to intradermal injection of *Candida*

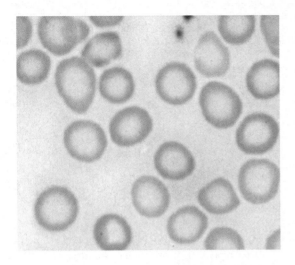

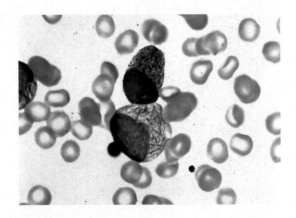

21. A 23-year-old black American woman with a history of dysfunctional uterine bleeding complains of fatigue when exercising. Laboratory studies show a mild microcytic anemia and increased RBC distribution width (RDW). The figure shows a representative section of the peripheral blood smear. Which of the following investigative studies would be most useful in defining the type of anemia that is present?
A. Bone marrow aspiration biopsy
B. Hemoglobin electrophoresis
C. Osmotic fragility test
D. Serum ferritin test
E. Sickle cell screening

22. A 26-year-old man is scuba diving off the coast of Bermuda in water 30 to 60 ft deep when he develops problems with his air tank and must ascend quickly to the surface. One hour later, he has pain in the muscles and joints in the legs. Which of the following is most likely responsible for these symptoms?
A. Deep venous thrombosis
B. Disseminated intravascular coagulation
C. Fat embolization
D. Hemorrhage into muscles and joints
E. Nitrogen gas embolism

23. A 22-year-old man has blood oozing from his nose and mouth. Physical examination shows petechiae and ecchymoses over most of his body. There is generalized lymphadenopathy and hepatosplenomegaly. Laboratory studies show a normocytic anemia and thrombocytopenia and a WBC count of 32,000/mm³. There are increases in D-dimers and in prothrombin and partial thromboplastin times. The figure shows a peripheral blood smear. This patient is most likely to have which chromosome translocation?
A. t(8;14)
B. t(9;22)
C. t(12;21)
D. t(14;18)
E. t(15;17)

24. Five days ago, a 68-year-old woman with a history of chronic ischemic heart disease and severe osteoarthritis had a total hip replacement. During the surgery, she received three units of packed RBCs. Which of the following is the chief risk factor for pulmonary thromboembolic disease?
A. Age of the patient
B. Decreased cardiac output
C. Decreased hemoglobin concentration
D. Immobilization
E. Turbulent blood flow

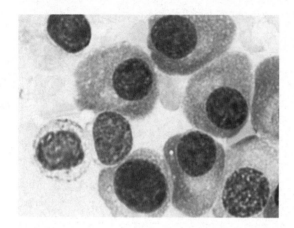

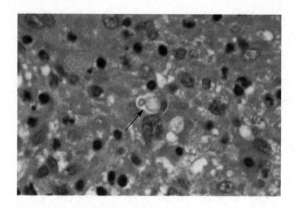

25. A 62-year-old woman has pain in the lower lumbar spine, pelvis, and sternum. Initial laboratory studies show a normocytic anemia with rouleaux. Serum blood urea nitrogen (BUN) is 80 mg/dL, and serum creatinine is 8 mg/dL. The figure shows a representative section of a bone marrow aspirate. Which of the following additional laboratory findings is most likely to be reported?
A. Decreased erythrocyte sedimentation rate
B. Decreased serum calcium level
C. Increased prothrombin time
D. Monoclonal protein spike on serum protein electrophoresis
E. Normal bleeding time

26. A 58-year-old man with small cell carcinoma of the lung complains of a headache and blurry vision. Examination shows swelling of the optic nerve. MRI of the head shows cerebral edema, but no there is evidence of metastatic disease. The serum Na^+ level is 115 mEq/L. Which of the following is the most appropriate nonpharmacologic treatment for this patient?
A. Decrease intake of Na^+ and H_2O
B. Decrease intake of Na^+, maintain intake of H_2O
C. Decrease intake of H_2O, maintain intake of Na^+
D. Increase intake of Na^+ and H_2O
E. Maintain intake of Na^+ and H_2O

27. A 46-year-old man develops pneumonia shortly after repainting a bridge. The figure shows an H&E-stained biopsy from the lung. The *arrow* depicts the pathogen responsible for the pneumonia. Which of the following pathogens is depicted in the histologic section?
A. *Aspergillus fumigatus*
B. *Coccidioides immitis*
C. *Cryptococcus neoformans*
D. *Histoplasma capsulatum*
E. *Pneumocystis jiroveci*

28. A 58-year-old man complains of frequent headaches and generalized itching after bathing. Physical examination shows congestion of the retinal vessels, a ruddy complexion, and splenomegaly. Initial laboratory studies show an RBC count of 8.0 million/mm^3, a WBC count of 15,000/mm^3, and a platelet count of 500,000/mm^3. The WBC differential count shows an increase in normal-appearing segmented neutrophils. Which of the following sets of laboratory results is most likely to be reported?

	RBC Mass	Plasma Volume	O_2 Saturation	EPO Concentration
A.	Increased	Increased	Normal	Decreased
B.	Increased	Normal	Decreased	Increased
C.	Increased	Normal	Normal	Increased
D.	Normal	Decreased	Normal	Normal

EPO, erythropoietin.

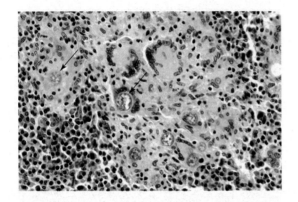

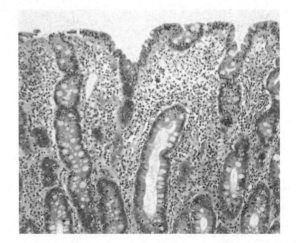

29. Shortly after a trip to the desert in the southwestern United States, a 58-year-old archaeologist develops a dry cough, fatigue, and painful nodules in the lower extremities. The figure shows a biopsy of the lung. The *arrows* point to the pathogen causing the respiratory disorder. What is the most likely diagnosis?
A. Aspergillosis
B. Coccidioidomycosis
C. Cryptococcosis
D. Histoplasmosis
E. Tuberculosis

30. A routine physical examination of an asymptomatic 21-year-old black American woman is normal. However, urinalysis shows RBCs with no casts present in the urine sediment. The patient states that she occasionally has had blood in her urine. A urine culture is negative, a peripheral smear is normal, and renal ultrasonography is normal. Laboratory studies show a serum blood urea nitrogen of 10 mg/dL, serum creatinine of 1.0 mg/dL, hemoglobin of 14.0 g/dL, and mean corpuscular volume of $82 \mu m^3$. Which of the following is the next best step in the workup?
A. Bone marrow examination
B. Cystoscopy
C. Renal biopsy
D. Serum ferritin
E. Sickle cell screen

31. A 22-year-old woman with a history of chronic diarrhea describes her stools as greasy. She recently developed a pruritic vesicular lesion on her elbow. The figure shows an endoscopic biopsy of the jejunum. Which of the following would be most useful in confirming the diagnosis?
A. Antigliadin antibodies
B. Antinuclear antibodies
C. Fecal smear for leukocytes
D. Stool for ova and parasites
E. Stool osmotic gap

32. A 2-day-old newborn male infant with respiratory distress syndrome (RDS) has a continuous harsh murmur that is heard over the entire precordium. Which of the following sets of oxygen saturation (SaO_2) values in the cardiac chambers and vessels is most likely present in this patient?

	RA	RV	PA	PV	LV	Ao
Normal SaO_2	75	75	75	95	95	95
A.	75	75	75	95	95	95
B.	75	80	80	95	95	95
C.	80	80	80	95	95	95
D.	75	75	80	95	95	95
E.	75	75	75	95	80	80

RA, right atrium; RV, right ventricle; PA, pulmonary artery; PV, pulmonary vein; LV, left ventricle; Ao, aorta.

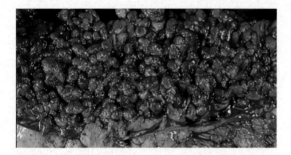

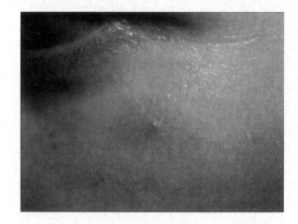

33. A 38-year-old man has a family history of colectomies between 35 and 40 years of age. The figure shows a portion of a total colectomy specimen from this patient. Which of the following best characterizes this disorder?
A. Complication of Crohn's disease
B. Complication of ulcerative colitis
C. Inactivation of a suppressor gene
D. Oral mucosal pigmentation
E. X-linked recessive inheritance pattern

34. An afebrile 50-year-old man complains of watery diarrhea and weight loss over the past 6 months. He states that his face often becomes flushed. Physical examination shows an enlarged, nodular liver. A pansystolic murmur along the parasternal border that increases in intensity with inspiration is heard. A fecal smear of stool is negative. Which of the following laboratory studies is most useful for confirming the diagnosis?
A. Blood cultures
B. Liver function tests
C. Serum electrolytes
D. Stool cultures
E. Urine test for 5-hydroxyindoleacetic acid (HIAA)

35. A 42-year-old man with a history of alcohol abuse has a distended abdomen and dependent pitting edema. The figure shows a lesion on the face. Which additional physical finding in this patient has the same pathogenesis as the skin lesion?
A. Ascites
B. Asterixis
C. Caput medusae
D. Esophageal varices
E. Gynecomastia

36. A 30-year-old woman states that she feels no pain in her hands and frequently burns them. Physical examination shows decreased pain and temperature sensation in the upper extremities, no deep tendon reflexes in the upper extremities, and atrophy of the intrinsic muscles of the hands. Which of the following is the most likely diagnosis?
A. Amyotrophic lateral sclerosis
B. Guillain-Barré syndrome
C. Multiple sclerosis
D. Syringomyelia
E. Vitamin B_{12} deficiency

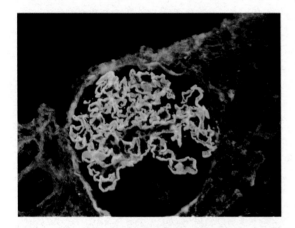

37. A 25-year-old man develops hemoptysis. A few weeks later, he experienced sudden onset of acute renal failure and died. Prior to his death, urinalysis showed mild proteinuria, hematuria, and RBC casts. The figure shows an immunofluorescence study of a representative glomerulus in a section of kidney removed at autopsy. Which of the following is the most likely diagnosis?
   A. Diffuse membranous glomerulopathy
   B. Focal segmental glomerulosclerosis
   C. Goodpasture syndrome
   D. IgA glomerulopathy
   E. Minimal change disease

38. Physical examination of a 72-year-old man shows severe hypertension, an epigastric bruit, and diminished amplitude of pedal pulses. Plasma renin activity is increased. An angiogram of the renal arteries shows decreased uptake of dye and a small kidney on the left side and normal uptake of the dye and a normal-sized kidney on the right side. Which of the following best describes the pathogenesis of the hypertension?
   A. Adrenal tumor that produces excess aldosterone
   B. Adrenal tumor that produces excess catecholamines

   C. Essential hypertension with bilateral nephrosclerosis
   D. Unilateral renal artery stenosis caused by atherosclerosis
   E. Unilateral renal artery stenosis caused by fibromuscular hyperplasia

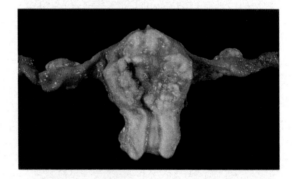

39. An obese 55-year-old woman has post-menopausal bleeding. Menopause occurred at age 51. A hysterectomy and bilateral salpingo-oophorectomy is performed (see figure). Which of the following is the most likely pathogenesis of the lesion in the endometrial cavity?
   A. Adenomyosis
   B. Herpes simplex virus type 2 (HSV-2) infection
   C. Human papillomavirus (HPV) infection
   D. Multiparity
   E. Unopposed estrogen exposure

40. A 50-year-old man with ischemic heart disease has signs of both left- and right-sided heart failure. Which of the following is characteristic of both types of heart failure?
   A. Bibasilar inspiratory crackles
   B. Decreased cardiac output
   C. Dependent pitting edema
   D. Paroxysmal nocturnal dyspnea
   E. Passive congestion in the liver

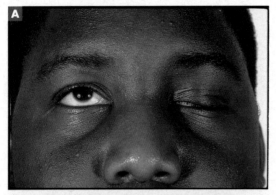

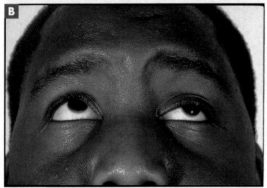

A. Cortisol
B. Epinephrine
C. Glucagon
D. Growth hormone
E. Insulin

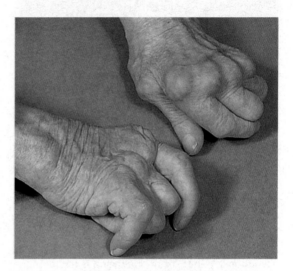

41. A 25-year-old black American man states that he is extremely tired and has drooping of his left eye and double vision toward the end of the workday. He also has difficulty swallowing solids and liquids and states that food seems to "stick near my Adam's apple." The figure shows the patient before (**A**) and after (**B**) a special test. Which of the following terms best describes his clinical disorder?
A. Demyelinating
B. Electrolyte
C. Motor neuron
D. Neuromuscular
E. Primary muscular

42. A 25-year-old woman with poorly controlled gestational diabetes mellitus gives birth to a male infant who develops jitteriness and seizures 3 hours after birth. Which of the following hormones is the most likely cause of these symptoms?

43. A 54-year-old woman states that for the past 12 years the pain in her hands has progressively worsened to the point where she cannot effectively use both hands (see figure). Which of the following laboratory findings is most likely to be reported?
A. Antibodies against *Borrelia burgdorferi*
B. Antibodies against double-stranded DNA
C. HLA-B27 genotype
D. Hyperuricemia
E. Rheumatoid factor

44. Colonoscopic studies show a 3-cm annular mass in the sigmoid colon of a 62-year-old man. Multiple biopsies show a poorly differentiated adenocarcinoma. A colectomy is performed, and a few nodular lesions on the surface of the liver are apparent. A frozen section shows a poorly differentiated adenocarcinoma. Gross and microscopic findings of the colectomy specimen show a mucosally derived cancer that has invaded through the muscle wall and out into the serosal fat. There is metastasis in 3 of 15 mesenteric lymph nodes directly beneath the tumor. Which of the following most influences the patient's prognosis?

A. Age of the patient
B. Differentiation of the tumor
C. Extent of invasion
D. Liver involvement
E. Lymph node involvement

A. Iron deficiency
B. Sickle cell trait
C. Sideroblastic anemia
D. α-Thalassemia
E. β-Thalassemia

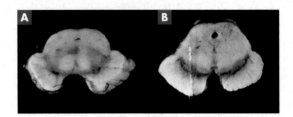

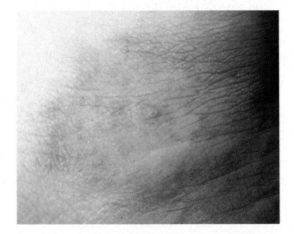

45. A febrile 30-year-old woman sees her physician because of a rash on the thigh (see figure) that developed at the site where she was bitten by an insect when on a camping trip about 4 weeks ago. The woman lives in the northeastern United States. Which of the following is the most likely causal pathogen?

A. *Babesia microti*
B. *Borrelia burgdorferi*
C. *Borrelia recurrentis*
D. *Ehrlichia chaffeensis*
E. *Rickettsia rickettsii*

46. A 22-year-old asymptomatic black American woman has had a mild microcytic anemia since early childhood. Her menstrual history is normal. Physical examination is normal. Laboratory studies show a slightly decreased hemoglobin concentration and an increased RBC count. Hemoglobin electrophoresis is normal. Serum ferritin is normal. Which of the following is the most likely diagnosis?

47. A 65-year-old man with an expressionless face and stooped posture shuffles when walking. He has constant tremor of the thumbs and index fingers of both hands at rest. Physical examination shows increased rigidity of the arm muscles when resisting extension of the arm. All deep tendon reflexes are normal. Part A of the figure shows a midbrain from a patient with similar signs and symptoms. Part B of the figure shows a normal midbrain for comparison. Which of the following best explains the pathogenesis of this disorder?

A. Degeneration of dopaminergic substantia nigra neurons
B. Increased γ-secretase activity
C. Loss of striatal neurons in the caudate nucleus
D. Presence of apolipoprotein gene E, allele ε4
E. Presence of hyperphosphorylated tau protein

48. A 75-year-old man with prostate hyperplasia and urinary retention has been hospitalized for spiking fever, tachypnea, and dyspnea. Physical examination shows bilateral inspiratory crackles. A chest radiograph shows bilateral interstitial and alveolar infiltrates. An arterial blood gas shows severe hypoxemia and respiratory acidosis. Which of the following is the most likely diagnosis of the respiratory disorder?

A. Acute respiratory distress syndrome
B. Congestive heart failure

C. Lobar pneumonia caused by gram-negative bacteria

D. Multiple pulmonary infarcts

E. Pneumonia caused by *Streptococcus pneumoniae*

49. A 2-year-old boy accidentally ingests rat poison. Physical examination shows bleeding from the mouth and gastrointestinal tract. Which of the following sets of laboratory test results is most likely to be reported?

	Platelet Count	Bleeding Time	PT	PTT
A.	Decreased	Prolonged	Normal	Normal
B.	Normal	Normal	Normal	Prolonged
C.	Normal	Normal	Prolonged	Prolonged
D.	Normal	Prolonged	Normal	Normal
E.	Normal	Prolonged	Normal	Prolonged

PT, prothrombin time; PTT, partial thromboplastin time.

50. A febrile 65-year-old man with prostate hyperplasia and urinary retention develops endotoxic shock. Within 24 hours, he has oozing of blood from all needle puncture sites, extensive ecchymoses and petechiae, and gastrointestinal bleeding. Laboratory studies show hemoglobin 9 g/dL, platelet count 75,000/mm³, prothrombin time (PT) 20 seconds, partial thromboplastin time (PTT) 50 seconds, D-dimer positive. Which of the following is the most likely diagnosis?

A. Autoimmune thrombocytopenia

B. Circulating anticoagulant

C. Disseminated intravascular coagulation (DIC)

D. Primary fibrinolysis

E. Thrombotic thrombocytopenic purpura

answers

1. **D** (increased synthesis of glycerol 3-phosphate) is correct. Glycerol 3-phosphate (G3-P) synthesis increases in alcoholics, because of increased production of NADH in alcohol metabolism. An increase in NADH causes dihydroxyacetone phosphate to convert to G3-P, which is then used as the substrate for the synthesis of triglyceride. The figure shows excess triglyceride as clear spaces in the cytosol of hepatocytes. The fatty change shown in the figure is typical of alcoholic liver disease. The hepatomegaly and the preferential increase in serum aspartate aminotransferase (AST) found in this patient are also characteristic of alcohol injury to the liver.

A (decreased hydrolysis of fat in adipose cells) is incorrect. Hydrolysis of fat (triglyceride) in adipose to fatty acids and glycerol is enhanced (*not* decreased) by alcohol. An increase in fatty acids and glycerol increases (*not* decreases) the synthesis of triglyceride in the liver.

B (decreased synthesis of fatty acids) is incorrect. Because the primary substrate for fatty acid synthesis (acetyl CoA) is a by-product of alcohol metabolism, the synthesis of fatty acids increases (*not* decreases) in alcoholics. An increase in fatty acids provides more substrate for the synthesis of triglyceride in the liver.

C (decreased synthesis of very low-density lipoprotein, VLDL) is incorrect. When triglyceride is synthesized in the liver, it is packaged into VLDL with the aid of apolipoprotein B-100. In alcoholics, increased synthesis of triglyceride automatically increases VLDL in the hepatocyte and in the peripheral blood.

E (increased β-oxidation of fatty acids) is incorrect. β-Oxidation of fatty acids occurs in the mitochondrial matrix. Alcohol damages the mitochondria in hepatocytes, which decreases (*not* increases) β-oxidation and increases the concentration of fatty acids, which enhances the synthesis of triglyceride in the liver.

2. **E** (osmotic damage) is correct. Microaneurysms are due to osmotic damage of the pericytes that surround the retinal vessel. Pericytes contain aldose reductase, which converts glucose to sorbitol. Sorbitol is osmotically active and draws water into the pericyte, leading to its destruction. This weakens the vessel wall, causing formation of a microaneurysm. Rupture of aneurysms can cause retinal detachment and neovascularization of the retina, resulting in blindness. Diabetes is the most common cause of blindness in the United States.

A (increased intraocular pressure) is incorrect. An increase in intraocular pressure occurs in glaucoma. It may be due to a narrow anterior chamber angle or to abnormal drainage of the aqueous fluid through the trabecular meshwork. Pathologic cupping of the optic nerve usually is seen in longstanding glaucoma. This change is *not* present in the patient.

B (inflammation of the optic nerve) is incorrect. Optic neuritis (inflammation of the optic nerve) is most commonly due to multiple sclerosis. The optic disk is swollen, and flame hemorrhages are seen surrounding the disk. These changes are *not* present in the patient.

C (microangiopathy) is incorrect. Microangiopathy is a finding in patients with diabetes mellitus and signals the deposition of increased type IV collagen in the basement membrane of small vessels. These changes usually occur in the kidneys rather than in the retina.

D (nonenzymatic glycosylation) is incorrect. Nonenzymatic glycosylation occurs in patients with diabetes mellitus. It refers to the binding of glucose to amino acids in protein within the basement membrane of vessels and in proteins such as hemoglobin. In blood vessels, it causes increased vessel permeability in arterioles, leading to hyaline arteriolosclerosis. These changes are most prominent in the kidneys and are *not* responsible for producing microaneurysms in the retina in diabetics.

3. **B** (coagulation necrosis) is correct. Coagulation necrosis occurs when arterial blood flow suddenly ceases, which in this patient followed thrombosis of the right coronary artery. An infarct is the gross manifestation of coagulation necrosis that is present in underlying tissue. The gross specimen shows an extensive pale yellow infarct in the left ventricle, which involves the posterior wall and papillary muscle (the round structure projecting into the ventricular lumen). This area of the left ventricle is in the distribution of the right coronary artery. The infarct is pale because of the density of dead myocardial tissue, which prevents the infiltration of blood from necrotic blood vessels.

A (caseous necrosis) is incorrect. Caseous necrosis refers to the gross appearance of soft, cheese-like material within a granuloma. It occurs primarily in mycobacterial infections (e.g., tuberculosis) and systemic fungal infections (e.g., histoplasmosis).

C (enzymatic fat necrosis) is incorrect. Enzymatic fat necrosis appears as chalky white areas of saponified fat in an area of pancreatic inflammation (e.g., acute pancreatitis). It does *not* occur in cardiac muscle.

D (fibrinoid necrosis) is incorrect. Fibrinoid necrosis occurs in small muscular arteries, arterioles, venules, and glomerular capillaries. Immunologic damage to these vessels causes leakage of plasma proteins into the wall of the vessels. It is commonly associated with small vessel vasculitis in hypertension and with deposits of antigen-antibody complexes in vessel walls in immunocomplex disease.

E (liquefactive necrosis) is incorrect. Liquefactive necrosis typically appears as an area of soft tissue with a liquid center. Unlike the coagulation necrosis shown in the gross specimen, liquefactive necrosis is associated with softening of tissue caused by the release of hydrolytic enzymes from neutrophils (as in acute inflammation) or from the cells in tissue (as in cerebral infarction).

4. **D** (respiratory alkalosis) is correct. The patient has developed tetany due to anxiety-induced respiratory alkalosis. Adduction of the thumb into the palm plus numbness and tingling at the tips of the fingers are classic signs of tetany. Tetany is due to a decreased concentration of ionized calcium in the blood. This increases neuromuscular excitability by bringing the threshold potential of neuromuscular tissue closer to the resting membrane potential. Therefore, less of a stimulus is required to initiate the action potential, which results in sustained muscle contractions. Total serum calcium represents calcium bound to albumin (40%), calcium bound to phosphorus and citrate (13%), and free, ionized calcium (47%). In respiratory alkalosis, there are more negative charges on albumin, due to less hydrogen ions on the COOH groups of acidic amino acids. These groups become COO^- and bind to some of the ionized calcium, which lowers the ionized level *without* affecting the total serum calcium.

A (diabetic ketoacidosis) is incorrect. In states of acidosis (e.g., diabetic ketoacidosis), less calcium is bound to albumin (more COOH groups are present), causing an increase in ionized calcium and a corresponding decrease in neuromuscular excitability.

B (nephrotic syndrome) is incorrect. In the nephrotic syndrome, serum albumin is markedly decreased due to loss of albumin in the urine. Although this decreases the total calcium level (calcium bound to albumin plus ionized calcium), the ionized calcium level remains unchanged and tetany does *not* occur.

C (primary hyperparathyroidism) is incorrect. Conditions associated with hypercalcemia (e.g., primary hyperparathyroidism) have an increase in the ionized calcium level, causing a corresponding decrease in neuromuscular excitability.

E (sarcoidosis) is incorrect. Conditions associated with hypercalcemia (e.g., sarcoidosis) also increase the ionized calcium level, causing a corresponding decrease in neuromuscular excitability.

5. **A** (caseous necrosis) is correct. Caseous necrosis typically appears as a well-circumscribed granuloma with amorphous, granular material in the center, as shown in the histologic section. The granuloma is surrounded by an inflammatory infiltrate consisting of CD4 T lymphocytes, activated macrophages (epithelioid cells), and a few multinucleated giant cells. Caseous necrosis occurs primarily in patients with mycobacterial infection (tuberculosis in this patient) or systemic fungal infection (e.g., histoplasmosis).

B (coagulation necrosis) is incorrect. Coagulation necrosis is usually associated with cessation of arterial blood flow to tissue, often evidenced by the presence of an infarct and the persistence of cellular outlines in the dead tissue. These features are *not* present in the histologic section.

C (enzymatic fat necrosis) is incorrect. Enzymatic fat necrosis occurs in the pancreas, in adipose tissue in and around an area of inflammation (as in acute pancreatitis). It does *not* occur in the lung.

D (fibrinoid necrosis) is incorrect. Fibrinoid necrosis occurs only in small muscular arteries, arterioles, venules, and glomerular capillaries. It is often associated with small vessel vasculitis in hypertension or with deposits of antigen-antibody complexes in vessel walls in immunocomplex disease.

E (liquefactive necrosis) is incorrect. Liquefactive necrosis appears as an area of soft tissue with a liquid center. The inflammatory infiltrate is usually composed of neutrophils that release hydrolytic enzymes, causing softening of the tissue. The inflammatory infiltrate in the histologic section is composed of cells with round nuclei rather than multilobed nuclei.

6. **B** (deficiency of dystrophin) is correct. The patient has Duchenne's muscular dystrophy, an X-linked recessive disorder with a deficiency of dystrophin. Dystrophin normally anchors actin to membrane glycoprotein. To move into a standing position from a prone position, he must "walk" his hands to his feet and up the front of his legs and then move to a standing position (Gower's maneuver). There is generalized muscle atrophy and pseudohypertrophy of the calf muscles and an increase in serum creatine kinase. Weakening and wasting of proximal pelvic muscles produce a classic waddling gait.

A (antibodies against acetylcholine receptors) is incorrect. IgG antibodies against acetylcholine receptors occur in myasthenia gravis, an autoimmune disease (type II hypersensitivity reaction) that causes progressive muscle weakness. Serum creatine kinase is normal in myasthenia.

C (demyelinating disorder) is incorrect. Demyelinating disorders are uncommon in children. They cause muscle weakness and sensory changes (paresthesias). They do *not* cause an increase in serum creatine kinase.

D (inflammatory myopathy) is incorrect. Polymyositis and dermatomyositis are examples of inflammatory myopathies that cause pain and muscle atrophy. These diseases are uncommon muscle diseases in children; however, they are associated with an increase in serum creatine kinase. The muscle groups involved in these disorders are different from those in Duchenne's muscular dystrophy.

E (motor neuron disorder) is incorrect. Degeneration of upper or lower motor neurons (e.g., Werdnig-Hoffmann disease) is uncommon in children and would *not* be expected to increase serum creatine kinase.

7. **D** (human herpesvirus 8) is correct. The lesions shown on the neck are typical of Kaposi sarcoma, a vascular malignancy closely associated with human herpesvirus 8. Kaposi sarcoma is the most common malignancy in patients with AIDS. Lesions appear most often on the skin but may also occur in the intestinal tract, particularly on the hard palate.

A *(Bartonella henselae)* is incorrect. *B. henselae* is a gram-negative bacterium that causes bacillary angiomatosis, a disease that occurs almost exclusively in patient's with AIDS. It produces highly vascular skin lesions that can mimic the lesions of Kaposi sarcoma. Systemic signs of the infection include fever, lymphadenopathy, and hepatomegaly. These findings are *not* present in this patient.

B (cytomegalovirus) is incorrect. Cytomegalovirus (CMV) is *not* an oncogenic virus and does *not* produce vascular lesions on the skin or in the gastrointestinal tract. In patients with AIDS, CMV is the most common cause of blindness, biliary tract disease, and pancreatitis.

C (Epstein-Barr virus) is incorrect. In patients with AIDS, Epstein-Barr virus does *not* cause vascular skin lesions, although it may cause hairy leukoplakia (glossitis), primary central nervous system lymphoma, and Burkitt's lymphoma.

E (HIV) is incorrect. HIV is *not* oncogenic and does *not* produce vascular skin lesions. In patients with AIDS, it is associated with generalized lymphadenopathy, destruction of CD4 helper T cells, and many central nervous system findings (e.g., AIDS dementia).

8. **C** (osteogenesis imperfecta) is correct. This child has osteogenesis imperfecta, which is characterized by a history of pathologic fractures throughout life. This autosomal dominant disease is associated with a defect in the synthesis of type I collagen. Blue discoloration of the sclerae is due to visualization of the choroidal veins beneath the collagen-deficient sclerae. Bone is a type I collagen-based matrix that is mineralized with calcium, phosphorus, and magnesium. Decreased synthesis of type I collagen results in structurally weak bone with a decrease in bone mass and density (secondary osteoporosis), resulting in pathologic fractures.

A (Ehlers Danlos syndrome) is incorrect. EDS is a mendelian connective tissue disorder with defects in collagen synthesis and structure. Clinical findings include hyperelastic skin, hypermobility of joints, aortic dissection, mitral valve prolapse, and rupture of the colon. Pathologic fractures and blue sclerae do *not* occur in EDS.

B (Marfan syndrome) is incorrect. Marfan syndrome is an autosomal dominant disorder due to a defect in fibrillin, a component of elastic tissue. The key ocular manifestation is dislocation of the lens. Pathologic fractures and blue sclerae do *not* occur in Marfan syndrome.

D (osteopetrosis) is incorrect. Osteopetrosis is an autosomal dominant or recessive disorder that is characterized by a defect in osteoclast resorption of bone, resulting in the overgrowth and sclerosis of bone (marble bone disease). Primary clinical findings include pathologic fractures, anemia, and visual and auditory defects. Blue sclerae are *not* present in osteopetrosis.

E (vitamin D–dependent rickets) is incorrect. Vitamin D–dependent rickets is an autosomal recessive disorder. It is associated with a deficiency of 1α-hydroxylase, resulting in a deficiency of $1,25\text{-}(OH)_2D_3$, which is the active form of vitamin D. Hypovitaminosis D, or rickets, is characterized by defective mineralization of bone accompanied by an increase in nonmineralized osteoid. Pathologic fractures may occur; however, blue sclera is *not* a feature of the disease.

9. **C** (hemochromatosis) is correct. Hemochromatosis, a disorder involving excessive reabsorption of iron from the gastrointestinal tract, has an autosomal recessive inheritance pattern, as shown in the pedigree. In autosomal recessive disorders, disease is present only in patients who are homozygous for the abnormal allele (e.g., aa), and both parents must have the abnormal allele to transmit the disease to their children. In most cases, the parents are asymptomatic heterozygous carriers (e.g., Aa). They have a 25% chance of having a normal child (AA), a 50% chance of having children who are asymptomatic carriers (Aa), and a 25% chance of having a child with the disease (aa).

A (glucose-6-phosphate dehydrogenase deficiency) is incorrect. Deficiency of G6PD is an X-linked recessive disorder associated with hemolytic anemia induced by infection or oxidant drugs (e.g., primaquine). X-linked recessive disorders are expressed in males, whereas females with the abnormal allele are usually asymptomatic carriers. The pedigree does *not* show this pattern of inheritance.

B (hereditary spherocytosis) is incorrect. Hereditary spherocytosis is an autosomal dominant disorder associated with splenomegaly and hemolytic anemia. Autosomal dominant disorders are characterized by a dominant allele that expresses itself in either the homozygous or the heterozygous state. Only one parent must have the abnormal allele for the disease to be transmitted to the children. A heterozygous parent with disease will transmit it to 50% of the children. The pedigree does *not* show this pattern of inheritance.

D (neurofibromatosis) is incorrect. Neurofibromatosis is an autosomal dominant disorder characterized by café-au-lait spots and pedunculated neurofibromas on the skin.

E (type 2 diabetes mellitus) is incorrect. Type 2 diabetes is an example of multifactorial (polygenic) inheritance, which does *not* have the pattern shown in the pedigree. Multifactorial inheritance involves the additive effect of two or more gene mutations of small effect conditioned by environmental and other nongenetic factors.

10. **A** (*Staphylococcus aureus*) is correct. The child has impetigo, which causes honey-colored crusted lesions that cover shallow ulcerations of the skin. *Staphylococcus aureus* is the most common cause of this superficial skin lesion followed by *Streptococcus pyogenes* Impetigo is highly contagious, which explains why the child's brother develops similar lesions.

B (herpes simplex virus type 1) is incorrect. Herpes simplex virus type 1 produces vesicles and pustules on the vermilion border of the lip. It does *not* produce honey-colored crusted lesions on the face.

C (*Malassezia furfur)* is incorrect. *M. furfur,* a superficial dermatophyte, causes tinea versicolor and seborrheic dermatitis (dandruff). It does *not* produce honey-colored crusted lesions on the face.

D *(Propionibacterium acnes)* is incorrect. *P. acnes* is an anaerobe involved in producing the inflammatory reaction associated with acne vulgaris. It does *not* produce honey-colored crusted lesions on the face.

E *(Trichophyton rubrum,)* is incorrect. *T. rubrum,* a superficial dermatophyte, causes tinea corporis (body), tinea cruris (groin), and tinea pedis (foot). It does *not* produce honey-colored crusted lesions on the face.

11. **A** (decrease in serum albumin) is correct. The crying child on the left has kwashiorkor, and the child on the right has marasmus. Both conditions are examples of protein-energy malnutrition. Kwashiorkor is caused by decreased protein intake, which decreases the serum albumin level. The total calorie intake is normal because of increased intake of carbohydrates. A decrease in albumin decreases the plasma oncotic pressure, resulting in dependent edema (see figure). In marasmus, serum albumin levels are usually normal in spite of diminished intake of calories.

B (decrease in somatic protein stores) is incorrect. Somatic protein stores represent the protein in muscle. In marasmus, somatic protein stores are decreased, resulting in muscle wasting in the extremities (child on the right). In kwashiorkor, somatic proteins are relatively intact; however, the visceral protein stores (e.g., in the liver) are decreased.

C (decrease in subcutaneous fat) is incorrect. In marasmus, subcutaneous fat is absent; in kwashiorkor, it is normal.

D (decrease in total calorie intake) is incorrect. In marasmus, the total calorie intake is decreased; in kwashiorkor, the total calorie intake is normal but deficient in protein.

E (defects in cell mediated immunity) is incorrect. Defects in cell-mediated immunity (type IV hypersensitivity) are present in both kwashiorkor and marasmus.

12. **D** (oligoclonal bands) is correct. The patient has multiple sclerosis, an autoimmune disease characterized by destruction of the myelin sheaths due to antibodies directed against myelin basic protein. The episodic course of acute relapses with optic neuritis (blurry vision), scanning speech, cerebellar ataxia, and sensory and motor dysfunction, followed by remissions, are characteristic of this disease. The demyelinating plaques in multiple sclerosis occur in the white matter of the cerebral cortex. The plaques usually have a perivenular distribution and are accompanied by a perivascular lymphoid and plasma cell infiltrate with microglial cells containing phagocytosed myelin. CSF shows an increase in CSF protein. High-resolution electrophoresis of CSF shows discrete bands of immunoglobulins in the γ-globulin region called oligoclonal bands. They are indicative of a demyelinating process.

A (decreased glucose) is incorrect. The CSF glucose is normal in multiple sclerosis.

B (increased neutrophils) is incorrect. CD8 T lymphocytes (*not* neutrophils) are increased in the CSF in multiple sclerosis.

C (normal protein) is incorrect. The CSF protein is increased (*not* normal) in multiple sclerosis.

E (positive Gram stain) is incorrect. The Gram stain is negative (*not* positive) for microbial pathogens in multiple sclerosis.

13. **E** (viral myocarditis) is correct. The histologic section shows an extensive lymphocytic infiltrate (round nuclei) and dissolution of myocardial fibers, which are characteristic of a viral-induced acute myocarditis. Clinical findings include left-sided heart failure (dyspnea, bibasilar inspiratory crackles); right-sided heart failure (neck vein distention, hepatomegaly, dependent pitting edema); and, myocardial damage (increased cardiac-specific troponin levels). Coxsackievirus is the most common viral cause of myocarditis. In this patient, the myocarditis has produced congestive (dilated) cardiomyopathy.

A (acute rheumatic fever) is incorrect. A patient with rheumatic fever would have a history of group A streptococcal infection, which this patient does *not* have. Other features of acute rheumatic fever, such as polyarthritis and erythema marginatum, are also absent in this patient.

B (coronary artery thrombosis) is incorrect. Histologic features of thrombosis leading to a myocardial infarction include coagulation necrosis (loss of nuclei and cross-striations) and a neutrophilic infiltrate (*not* present in the histologic section).

C (ischemic heart disease) is incorrect. Chronic ischemic heart disease is associated with replacement of myocardial tissue by collagen, which is *not* shown in the histologic section.

D (toxin-induced myocarditis) is incorrect. Diphtheria produces a toxin-induced myocarditis. The inflammatory infiltrate in the histologic section is more compatible with infection than toxin-induced damage to the heart.

14. **B** (cytomegalovirus) is correct. The patient has retinitis due to cytomegalovirus (CMV). Examination of the retina shows white areas with indistinct borders (cotton wool exudates) that represent retinal infarctions due to a CMV vasculitis. CMV retinitis is the most common cause of blindness in patients with AIDS and occurs when the CD4 helper T-cell count is less than 50 cells/mm^3.

A *(Candida albicans)* is incorrect. *C. albicans* can cause retinitis in AIDS; however, CMV is the overall most common cause of retinitis.

C (herpes simplex virus type 1) is incorrect. Herpes simplex virus type I can cause retinitis in AIDS; however, CMV is the overall most common cause of retinitis.

D (HIV) is incorrect. HIV has *not* been implicated as a cause of retinitis leading to blindness.

E *(Toxoplasma gondii)* is incorrect. *T. gondii* can cause retinitis in AIDS; however, CMV is the overall most common cause of retinitis.

15. **B** (acute rheumatic fever) is correct. This patient developed acute rheumatic fever several weeks after group A streptococcal pharyngitis. The figure shows small, sterile vegetations along the line of closure of the mitral valve. The lesions are associated with valvular inflammation (i.e., fibrinoid necrosis) caused by acute rheumatic fever. Clinical findings include sore throat, followed within several weeks by fever, joint pain, subcutaneous nodules, and skin changes (erythema marginatum, as in this case). The pansystolic murmur at the apex is caused by mitral regurgitation due to endocarditis, and the bibasilar inspiratory crackles and S$_3$ heart sounds are caused by left-sided heart failure due to myocarditis, which decreases the force of contraction. Cardiac damage is caused by antibodies against the streptococcal M proteins, which cross-react with antigens in the heart and other tissues (i.e., type II hypersensitivity reaction). Blood cultures are negative because rheumatic fever causes immunologic damage to the heart. The serum antistreptolysin O titers are increased and are useful in confirming the diagnosis.

A (acute bacterial endocarditis) is incorrect. In acute bacterial endocarditis (ABE), vegetations are usually bulky and are associated with gross evidence of valvular destruction or disruption of the chordae tendineae cordis. In this case, the lesions are uniformly small and line the entire closing margin of the valve. In addition, ABE is not associated with pharyngitis, polyarthritis, and erythema marginatum.

C (Libman-Sacks endocarditis) is incorrect. Libman-Sacks endocarditis occurs in a minority of patients who have systemic lupus erythematosus (SLE). This patient has none of the classic findings of SLE (e.g., malar rash).

D (nonbacterial thrombotic endocarditis) is incorrect. Nonbacterial thrombotic endocarditis produces sterile lesions on the mitral valve similar in appearance to those shown in the figure. However, it is usually associated with mucin-secreting adeno-carcinomas and *not* with any of the other signs and symptoms that are present in this patient.

E (subacute bacterial endocarditis) is incorrect. Subacute bacterial endocarditis is most often caused by *Streptococcus viridans* because of its low virulence. *S. viridans* seeds previously damaged valves. The autopsy specimen shows *no* evidence of previous damage to the mitral valve.

16. **B** (leukocyte adhesion molecule defect) is correct. A congenital leukocyte adhesion molecule defect prevents separation of the umbilical cord. Adhesion molecules activated on neutrophils include selectins and β-integrins (CD11 and CD18 positive). Selectins are responsible for rolling of the neutrophils in the venules, and β-integrins cause neutrophils to adhere to venules (margination). Neutrophils then release collagenase, dissolve basement membranes between contracted endothelial cells in venules, and transmigrate into the interstitial tissue. Deficiency of either type of adhesion molecule causes an absence of neutrophil adhesion (margination) and an absence of neutrophils in the interstitial tissue, because neutrophils must adhere to endothelium before they can transmigrate. Other findings in leukocyte adhesion defects include an increase in the absolute neutrophil count, problems with wound healing, and severe gingivitis.

A (absent respiratory burst) is incorrect. The respiratory (oxidative) burst in neutrophils and monocytes is part of the O_2-dependent myeloperoxidase (MPO) system for killing bacteria. Activated NADPH oxidase in the cell membrane oxidizes reduced NADPH, converting molecular O_2 to superoxide free radicals ($O_2^{\cdot}$). The respiratory burst is the energy released in this reaction. In chronic granulomatous disease, an X-linked recessive disease caused by absence of NADPH oxidase, the respiratory burst is absent, resulting in a defect in microbicidal activity. A functioning O_2-dependent MPO system is *not* required for cord separation because it does *not* affect neutrophil adhesion or transmigration.

C (myeloperoxidase deficiency) is incorrect. In the O_2-dependent MPO system, $O_2^{\cdot}$ is converted to peroxide (H_2O_2) by superoxide dismutase in the phagolysosomes of neutrophils and monocytes. MPO catalyzes a reaction that combines H_2O_2 with Cl^- to form hypochlorous free radicals that kill the phagocytosed bacteria. Deficiency of MPO results in a defect in microbicidal activity; however, it does *not* affect neutrophil adhesion and transmigration.

D (opsonization defect) is incorrect. IgG and C3b are opsonizing agents that bind to the surface of bacteria. Receptors for IgG and C3b are located on the plasma membranes of phagocytic leukocytes. Binding of the opsonized bacteria to leukocytes facilitates phagocytosis of the bacteria. A deficiency of IgG or C3 produces a defect in phagocytosis; however, it has *no* effect on neutrophil adhesion or transmigration.

E (phagocytosis defect) is incorrect. Leukocyte phagocytic defects include defects in opsonization and defects in the formation of phagolysosomes. Phagolysosomes are produced by fusion of lysosomes containing hydrolytic enzymes with phagosomes. In Chédiak-Higashi syndrome, a defect in lysosomal degranulation into phagosomes is present. Leukocytes contain large azurophilic granules (lysosomes) in the cytosol, because the lysosomes have never been emptied. Defects in opsonization or in formation of phagolysosomes have *no* adverse effect on neutrophil adhesion or transmigration.

17. **C** (hemolytic anemia) is correct. The figure shows a tricuspid aortic valve with severe aortic stenosis. The commissures have fused, and multiple fibrotic calcium deposits protrude into the sinuses of Valsalva. A common complication of aortic stenosis is an intravascular hemolytic anemia with schistocytes (fragmented RBCs), which may lead to chronic iron-deficiency anemia from loss of hemoglobin in the urine. Serum haptoglobin levels are often zero, because haptoglobin combines with free hemoglobin in the plasma and is removed from the circulation by splenic macrophages.

A (acute myocardial infarction) is incorrect. The figure shows severe aortic stenosis. Acute MI is *not* a common complication of aortic stenosis. However, aortic stenosis is the most common valvular lesion associated with angina with exercise. Concentric hypertrophy of the left ventricle occurs in aortic stenosis and the thickened muscle does *not* receive sufficient blood flow during exercise resulting in angina.

B (aortic dissection) is incorrect. The figure shows severe aortic stenosis. Aortic dissection is associated with hypertension and connective tissue disorders leading to cystic medial degeneration. It is *not* a complication of aortic stenosis, in which neither hypertension nor connective tissue disorders are present.

D (hypertension) is incorrect. The figure shows severe aortic stenosis, which does *not* produce hypertension. In aortic stenosis, the diminished area of the stenotic valve orifice eventually leads to a decrease in stroke volume and cardiac output, which reduces systolic pressure but has *no* effect on diastolic pressure.

E (stroke syndrome) is incorrect. The figure shows severe aortic stenosis. There is *no* increased incidence of stroke in patients with aortic stenosis. However, aortic stenosis is the most common valvular lesion associated with syncope with exercise. This is because the stroke volume is not sufficient to perfuse the brain when the patient is exercising.

18. **E** (neutrophil opsonization defect) is correct. Bruton's agammaglobulinemia is an X-linked disorder characterized by failure of pre-B cells to develop into B cells. This produces hypogammaglobulinemia, because there are insufficient numbers of B cells to be antigenically stimulated to become plasma cells. Deficiency of IgG produces an opsonizing defect. The antigen recognition site of IgG attaches to the bacteria, and the Fc portion of the immunoglobulin attaches to receptors in the plasma membrane of phagocytic leukocytes. This facilitates the phagocytosis of bacteria by triggering engulfment of bacteria by pseudopods and eventual formation of a phagocytic vacuole.

A (leukocyte adhesion molecule defect) is incorrect. A defect in neutrophil adhesion molecules (i.e., selectins and integrins) prevents neutrophils from adhering to endothelial cells and transmigrating into tissue. Immunoglobulins are *not* involved in the activation of leukocyte adhesion molecules or in their function.

B (neutrophil chemotactic defect) is incorrect. Movement of neutrophils toward the site of acute inflammation is called *chemotaxis*. Chemical mediators (e.g., C5a, leukotriene B_4) bind to neutrophil receptors causing release of calcium, which increases neutrophil motility. Immunoglobulins are *not* involved in neutrophil chemotaxis.

C (neutrophil membrane-associated protein defect) is incorrect. Neutrophil membrane-associated protein defects occur in Chédiak-Higashi syndrome. This defect interferes with the fusion of lysosomes that contain hydrolytic enzymes with phagosomes in the cytosol of phagocytic leukocytes, producing phagolysosomes. Immunoglobulins are *not* involved in membrane fusion and the formation of phagolysosomes.

D (neutrophil microbicidal defect) is incorrect. A leukocyte defect in killing bacteria usually involves a defect in the O_2-dependent myeloperoxidase (MPO) system (e.g., deficiency of NADPH oxidase or MPO deficiency). Activation of this system eventually results in the formation of hypochlorous free radicals in phagolysosomes that kill bacteria. Immunoglobulins are *not* involved in the proper function of the O_2-dependent MPO system.

19. **B** *(Salmonella paratyphi)* is correct. This patient has *Salmonella* osteomyelitis. The peripheral blood smear shows sickle cells (dense, boat-shaped RBCs) and numerous target cells (RBCs with a bull's-eye appearance). Sickle cell disease is the most common hemolytic disease in black Americans and is due to a missense mutation resulting in replacement of glutamic acid by valine in the sixth position of the β-globin chain. The radiographic findings in the lower right femur (a periosteal reaction and lytic lesion in the metaphysis) are indicative of osteomyelitis, which in sickle cell disease is most often caused by *S. paratyphi*. *Staphylococcus aureus* is the usual pathogen in patients *without* sickle cell disease.

A *(Pseudomonas aeruginosa)* is incorrect. *P. aeruginosa* is a common cause of localized osteomyelitis associated with puncture of the foot in patients wearing rubber footwear. It is *not* a common cause of osteomyelitis in sickle cell disease.

C *(Staphylococcus aureus)* is incorrect. *S. aureus* is the most common cause of osteomyelitis in patients *without* sickle cell disease.

D *(Streptococcus pneumoniae)* is incorrect. In sickle cell disease, *S. pneumoniae* is a common cause of septicemia when the spleen becomes dysfunctional from repeated infarctions; however, it is *not* a common cause of osteomyelitis.

E *(Streptococcus pyogenes)* is incorrect. *S. pyogenes* is *not* the most common cause of osteomyelitis in sickle cell disease.

20. **A** (hypergammaglobulinemia) is correct. AIDS is the most common acquired immunodeficiency in the United States. It is caused by human immunodeficiency virus-1 (HIV-1), which is an RNA retrovirus containing reverse transcriptase. The virus infects CD4 T_H cells. Epstein-Barr virus (EBV) and cytomegalovirus infections are common in AIDS. They are potent polyclonal stimulators of B cells, which produce a polyclonal gammopathy (benign increase in γ-globulins); however, because patients are unable to mount an antibody response to a new antigen, they are still susceptible to bacterial infections.

B (increase in CD4 helper T-cell/CD8 suppressor T-cell ratio) is incorrect. The virus attacks and destroys CD4 helper T cells; therefore, the decreasing the CD4 helper T-cell count (less than 200 cells/μL) and reversing the CD4 helper T-cell/CD8 suppressor T-cell ratio from a normal of 2:1 to less than 1:2.

C (intact cellular immunity) is incorrect. The virus attacks and destroys CD4 helper T cells, thus impairing cell-mediated immunity (type IV hypersensitivity).

D (normal phytohemagglutinin assay) is incorrect. The virus attacks and destroys CD4 helper T cells, thus impairing cell-mediated immunity (type IV hypersensitivity). Therefore, in vitro stimulation of T-cell response to phytohemagglutinin, a potent T-cell mitogen, is impaired (*not* normal).

E (normal skin reaction to intradermal injections of *Candida*) is incorrect. Cellular immunity is impaired in AIDS. Therefore, intradermal injections of *Candida* does *not* elicit the expected T-cell immune response. This lack of immune response is called anergy. Defective cellular immunity is responsible for *Pneumocystis jiroveci* lung infection, which is the most common initial presentation in AIDS, and other opportunistic infections.

21. **D** (serum ferritin test) is correct. The patient's clinical and laboratory findings are consistent with the diagnosis of an iron-deficiency anemia, which can be confirmed by the serum ferritin test. The peripheral blood smear shows RBCs with notable central areas of pallor, which indicate decreased hemoglobin concentration. Strong evidence of iron deficiency is given by the increased RBC distribution width (RDW, increased size variation in RBCs) and the patient's history of dysfunctional uterine bleeding (menorrhagia), which is the most common cause of iron deficiency in women younger than 50 years of age. The RDW is increased in iron deficiency because there is a mixed population of normocytic and microcytic RBCs. The other causes of microcytic anemia (e.g., anemia of chronic disease, thalassemia) are *not* as likely to have this size variation in RBCs and have a normal RDW. The serum ferritin test is the best screening test for iron-related disorders, because serum ferritin levels correlate with the amount of iron stored in the bone marrow.

A (bone marrow aspiration biopsy) is incorrect. The patient has a microcytic anemia. A bone marrow aspiration biopsy is *rarely* indicated in workups for microcytic anemias, because serum tests (e.g., ferritin, hemoglobin electrophoresis) are available to identify the various causes of microcytic anemia.
B (hemoglobin electrophoresis) is incorrect. Hemoglobin electrophoresis identifies changes in the concentration of normal and abnormal forms of hemoglobin. Of the microcytic anemias, the only one that is likely to show an abnormal hemoglobin electrophoresis is β-thalassemia, in which there is a decrease in hemoglobin A (2α,2β) and a corresponding increase in hemoglobins A2 (2α,2δ) and hemoglobin F (2α,2γ). The patient does *not* have β-thalassemia, because the clinical

history is more compatible with iron deficiency from menorrhagia and the RDW is increased (normal RDW in thalassemia).
C (osmotic fragility test) is incorrect. The osmotic fragility test is used to confirm a diagnosis of hereditary spherocytosis, in which the osmotic fragility of RBCs is increased. Hereditary spherocytosis is a normocytic (*not* microcytic) anemia, and spherocytes are *not* present in the peripheral blood of this patient.
E (sickle cell screening) is incorrect. Although the patient is of black American descent, sickle cell anemia is unlikely, because it is usually normocytic (*not* microcytic) and because sickle cells are *not* present in the peripheral blood.

22. **E** (nitrogen gas embolism) is correct. The patient has decompression sickness (gas embolism), which is a complication of scuba diving. As a diver descends, the atmospheric pressure increases by 1 atmosphere (760 mm Hg) for every 33 feet of water. Under increased pressure, nitrogen gas moves from the alveoli through the blood and dissolves in tissue and blood. Rapid ascent forces nitrogen to move out of tissue and blood as bubbles. It forms gas emboli in the blood that obstruct blood vessels, causing ischemic damage to bone (e.g., aseptic necrosis of the femoral head), spinal cord (hemiparesis), and other tissues. Gas bubbles within skeletal muscle and supporting tissues around joints cause a painful condition called the bends. Treatment involves recompression in a compression chamber to force the gas bubbles back into solution followed by slow decompression to prevent them from re-forming.

A (deep venous thrombosis) is incorrect. Increased atmospheric pressure under water may cause stasis and thrombus formation in the deep veins of the leg, potentially causing pulmonary thromboembolism. Leg pain in deep venous thrombosis develops while under water.

B (disseminated intravascular coagulation) is incorrect. Disseminated intravascular coagulation (DIC) is caused by in vivo activation of the coagulation system, resulting in the formation of fibrin clots throughout the microvasculature. DIC is *not* a complication of scuba diving.

C (fat embolization) is incorrect. Fat embolization is most often caused by traumatic fractures of the long bones (e.g., femur) and pelvis. Microglobules of fat from the bone marrow and adipose tissue lodge in the microvasculature throughout the body, producing ischemic damage to tissue. Fat embolization is *not* a complication of scuba diving.

D (hemorrhage into muscles and joints) is incorrect. Hemorrhage into muscles and joints is a complication of a severe coagulation factor deficiency (e.g., hemophilia A). Such hemorrhage is *not* associated with nitrogen gas embolism.

23. **E** (t(15;17)) is correct. This patient has acute promyelocytic leukemia (APL) complicated by disseminated intravascular coagulation (DIC). The peripheral blood smear shows a hypergranular promyelocyte filled with multiple intertwining Auer rods. Auer rods are present *only* in variants of acute myelogenous leukemia. Patients with APL have a characteristic t(15;17) translocation, which causes an abnormality in retinoic acid metabolism. DIC is invariably present in APL, because the release of procoagulant from the granules of the promyelocytes activates the coagulation system cascade. DIC causes multiple coagulation factor deficiencies (prolonged prothrombin time and partial thromboplastin time), thrombocytopenia (which causes petechiae and ecchymoses), and activation of the fibrinolytic system (increased D-dimers). Leukemias commonly metastasize to the lymph nodes (generalized lymphadenopathy), liver, and spleen (hepatosplenomegaly). Treatment of APL with retinoic acid causes maturation of the promyelocytes; however, relapses invariable occur, leading to death.

A (t8;14) is incorrect. A t(8;14) translocation is associated with Burkitt's lymphoma, which is a malignancy involving B cells. The Epstein-Barr virus increases the risk for this translocation by stimulating increased mitotic activity of the B cell when the virus attaches to the CD21 receptor on the membrane. Increased cell divisions increase the risk for a translocation.

B (t9;22) is incorrect. A t(9;22) translocation is associated with chronic myelogenous leukemia, in which myeloblasts with Auer rods are *not* present. The *ABL* proto-oncogene on chromosome 9 is translocated to chromosome 22 where it fuses with the break cluster region to form a fusion gene. Chromosome 22 is called the Philadelphia chromosome.

C (t12;21) is incorrect. A t(12;21) translocation has prognostic significance in acute lymphoblastic leukemia. When present, the prognosis is favorable.

D (t14;18) is incorrect. A t(14;18) translocation is associated with a follicular B-cell lymphoma. The translocation causes overexpression (increased activity) of the *BCL2* family of genes. The protein product of the gene prevents apoptosis of the cell by preventing cytochrome *c* from leaving the mitochondria. Therefore, the translocation ensures immortality of the B cells in the germinal follicles of lymph nodes.

24. **D** (immobilization) is correct. The three main causes of intravascular thrombus formation are endothelial cell injury (e.g., cigarette smoking), stasis of blood flow (e.g., post-surgery), and hypercoagulability (e.g., use of oral contraceptives, hereditary factor deficiencies). Stasis of blood flow is the most common cause of venous thrombus formation, which most often occurs in the deep veins below the knee. Stasis of blood causes endothelial cell injury and local activation of the coagulation system, resulting in the formation of an adherent, occlusive, firm, dark red fibrin clot that entraps RBCs, WBCs, and platelets. The clot propagates toward the heart and may break off once it reaches the femoral vein, which is the most common site of pulmonary thromboembolic disease.

A (age of the patient) is incorrect. The incidence of venous clots does *not* increase with age.

B (decreased cardiac output) is incorrect. Decreased cardiac output may occur in ischemic heart disease complicated by congestive heart failure, which causes stasis of venous blood, predisposing the patient to deep venous thrombosis. However, immobilization is a greater risk factor for developing thromboembolism.

C (decreased hemoglobin concentration) is incorrect. Decreased hemoglobin concentration decreases the viscosity of blood and reduces (*not* increases) the risk of thrombosis.

E (turbulent blood flow) is incorrect. Turbulent blood flow contributes to endothelial damage causing arterial thrombosis. Arterial thrombi usually develop on top of atherosclerotic plaques that rupture. Thrombi are composed of platelets fused by fibrin. Turbulence does *not* predispose to venous clots.

25. **D** (monoclonal protein spike on serum protein electrophoresis) is correct. The patient has multiple myeloma complicated by renal failure. The bone marrow aspirate shows immature plasma cells with eccentric nuclei and perinuclear clearing. The cytoplasm stains blue with a Wright-Giemsa stain, indicating increased synthesis of protein. A monoclonal spike in the γ-globulin region can be expected on serum protein electrophoresis. The spike is caused by a single immunoglobulin (usually IgG) and its corresponding light chain (usually κ), which are secreted by clones derived from a single neoplastic plasma cell. The other plasma cell clones are suppressed. Renal failure, a common complication of multiple myeloma, is diagnosed when serum BUN and serum creatinine levels are raised and the ratio of these values is less than 15:1. Excess light chains, called Bence Jones protein, are usually present in the urine. In this case, renal failure is due to the formation of casts composed of Bence Jones protein blocking the tubular lumens and inciting a foreign body giant cell reaction.

A (decreased erythrocyte sedimentation rate) is incorrect. The increased weight of RBCs in rouleaux (RBCs stacked together like coins) causes them to settle faster in plasma and increases (*not* decreases) the erythrocyte sedimentation rate (ESR). The ESR is *not* a very specific test and is *not* a key test used to diagnose plasma cell malignancies.

B (decreased serum calcium level) is incorrect. The patient has multiple myeloma, which causes osteolytic lesions. This is due to the release of interleukin 1 from malignant plasma cells. This cytokine activates osteoclasts causing lytic lesions wherever malignant plasma cells are located. These lesions tend to increase (*not* decrease) serum calcium levels.

C (increased prothrombin time) is incorrect. In multiple myeloma, coagulation studies, including prothrombin time, are normal. Rouleaux does *not* affect the percentage or function of the coagulation factors.

E (normal bleeding time) is incorrect. In multiple myeloma, the bleeding time is usually prolonged, because rouleaux interferes with platelet aggregation.

26. **C** (decrease intake of H_2O, maintain intake of Na^+) is correct. The patient has the syndrome of inappropriate antidiuretic hormone (SIADH) caused by ectopic secretion of antidiuretic hormone (SIADH) by a primary small cell carcinoma of the lung. ADH normally concentrates urine by reabsorbing H_2O that is free of electrolytes in the collecting tubules of the kidneys back into the blood. Therefore, an excess of ADH causes increased reabsorption of H_2O, which enters the extracellular fluid (ECF) and produces a dilutional hyponatremia. In hyponatremia, an osmotic gradient between the ECF and intracellular fluid (ICF) causes H_2O to move into the ICF, producing cerebral edema. Because there is no excess of Na^+ in the ECF and the primary problem is reabsorbing too much water, the most effective nonpharmacologic treatment is to restrict H_2O intake.

A (decrease intake of Na^+ and H_2O) is incorrect. In SIADH, hyponatremia is caused by the addition of pure H_2O to the ECF, *not* by a gain of Na^+ (may increase serum Na^+). Therefore, only water is restricted.
B (decrease intake of Na^+, maintain intake of H_2O) is incorrect. Decreasing intake of Na^+ and maintaining intake of H_2O is used to treat hypernatremia due to a hypertonic gain of Na^+.
D (increase intake of Na^+ and H_2O) is incorrect. Increasing Na^+ intake may increase the serum Na^+; however, it would be short-lived because plasma volume and glomerular filtration rate are increased in SIADH, causing increased loss of Na^+ in the urine. Increasing water intake only increases the dilutional hyponatremia.
E (maintain intake of Na^+ and H_2O) are incorrect. Water intake must be restricted in SIADH.

27. **C** *(Cryptococcus neoformans)* is correct. This patient has cryptococcosis caused by *C. neoformans*. The biopsy shows a single cryptococcus yeast with a narrow-based bud. Cryptococcosis is commonly contracted by exposure to pigeon excreta, which is often found under bridges where pigeons roost. *C. neoformans* produces granulomatous inflammation with caseous necrosis in the lungs.

A *(Aspergillus fumigatus)* is incorrect. *A. fumigatus* produces narrow-angled septate hyphae and fruiting bodies with chains of parallel aligned conidia, unlike the yeast form of *C. neoformans* shown in the histologic section.
B *(Coccidioides immitis)* is incorrect. In the lungs, *C. immitis* produces spherules containing endospores, unlike the yeast form of *C. neoformans* shown in the histologic section. *C. immitis* pneumonia is contracted primarily in the desert regions of the southwestern United States, particularly in Arizona, New Mexico, and southern California.
D *(Histoplasma capsulatum)* is incorrect. The yeast forms of *H. capsulatum* are phagocytosed by macrophages, unlike the yeast form of *C. neoformans* shown in the histologic section. Histoplasmosis is common in immunocompromised patients (e.g., in those with AIDS), spelunkers (cave explorers) living in the Ohio-Tennessee Valley area of the United States, and chicken farmers.
E *(Pneumocystis jiroveci)* is incorrect. On silver staining, *P. jiroveci* appears as cysts with centrally located dots, unlike the yeast form of *C. neoformans* shown in the histologic section. *P. jiroveci* usually produces pneumonia in patients with HIV when the CD4 T-cell count is about $200/mm^3$.

28. **A** (RBC mass increased, plasma volume increased, O_2 saturation normal, EPO decreased) is correct. The patient has polycythemia vera, a myeloproliferative disease involving a neoplastic proliferation of trilineage myeloid stem cells in the bone marrow. This produces an increase in production of RBCs, neutrophils, and platelets, as in this patient. In polycythemia vera (PV), which is an absolute polycythemia, the total number of RBCs in the body in mL/kg (RBC mass) is increased. This is inappropriate, because there is *no* hypoxic stimulus for an increase in RBC production in PV. The RBC count (RBCs/mm^3 blood) is also always increased if the RBC mass is increased. An increase in plasma volume accompanies the increase in RBC mass, unlike in other types of polycythemia. The O_2 saturation is normal, because the percentage of binding sites on heme occupied by O_2 remains the same. EPO is decreased because the O_2 content of blood is increased: O_2 content $= 1.34 \times$ hemoglobin $\times O_2$ saturation $+$ arterial Po_2. The O_2 content of blood has a negative feedback relationship with EPO. Absolute leukocytosis and thrombocytosis commonly accompany the increase in RBCs. This patient's pruritus after bathing is caused by the increase in histamine released from excess numbers of mast cells in the skin.

B (RBC mass increased, plasma volume normal, O_2 saturation decreased, EPO increased) is incorrect. These laboratory findings are signs of an appropriate type of absolute poly-cythemia related to a hypoxic stimulus for EPO release (decreased O_2 saturation). Examples include obstructive and restrictive lung disease, cyanotic congenital heart disease, and living at high altitudes. Note that the plasma volume is normal in other types of absolute polycythemia, unlike PV in which it is increased.

C (RBC mass increased, plasma volume normal, O_2 saturation normal, EPO increased) is incorrect. These laboratory findings are signs of an inappropriate type of absolute polycythemia (normal O_2 saturation) related to ectopic or inappropriate secretion of EPO. Examples include renal disease (e.g., cancer,

cystic disease, hydronephrosis) and ectopic secretion of EPO from a hepatocellular carcinoma.

D (RBC mass normal, plasma volume decreased, O_2 saturation normal, EPO normal) is incorrect. These laboratory findings are signs of a relative, as opposed to absolute, type of polycythemia in which a decrease in plasma volume hemoconcentrates RBCs in the peripheral blood. This increases the RBC count *without* affecting RBC mass. Any cause of volume depletion (e.g., excessive sweating, severe diarrhea) leads to a relative polycythemia.

29. **B** (coccidioidomycosis) is correct. This patient has coccidioidomycosis caused by *Coccidioides immitis*. This infection occurs in desert regions of the southwestern United States, particularly in Arizona, New Mexico, and southern California. It is contracted by inhalation of arthrospores in the dust. The biopsy shows granulomatous inflammation, with multinucleated giant cells and an intact spherule *(arrows)* containing endospores. Erythema nodosum commonly occurs in coccidioidomycosis. It produces painful nodules in the lower extremities due to inflammation of subcutaneous fat.

A (aspergillosis) is incorrect. *Aspergillus fumigatus* produces narrow-angled septate hyphae with fruiting bodies, unlike the spherules containing endospores of *C. immitis*.

C (cryptococcosis) is incorrect. *Cryptococcus neoformans* has yeast forms with narrow-based buds, unlike the spherules containing endospores of *C. immitis*.

D (histoplasmosis) is incorrect. *Histoplasma capsulatum* has yeast forms phagocytosed by macrophages, unlike the spherules containing endospores of *C. immitis*. Histoplasmosis is endemic in the Ohio River and central Mississippi River valleys.

E (tuberculosis) is incorrect. *Mycobacterium tuberculosis* is an acid-fast bacterium that is usually phagocytosed by alveolar macrophages. Acid-fast stains are necessary to visualize *M. tuberculosis*.

30. **E** (sickle cell screen) is correct. The patient most likely has sickle cell trait, which causes recurrent microscopic hematuria. In sickle cell trait, the percentage of sickle hemoglobin is 40% to 45%, and the remainder of hemoglobin is mostly hemoglobin A. There are no sickle cells in the peripheral smear in sickle cell trait; therefore, a sickle cell screen is required to induce sickling of RBCs containing sickle hemoglobin. The O_2 tension in the renal medulla is low enough to induce sickling of RBCs in the peritubular capillaries. This causes microinfarctions in the renal medulla leading to hematuria. There is also the potential for renal papillary necrosis and subsequent loss of both concentration and dilution.

A (bone marrow examination) is incorrect. A bone marrow examination is *not* warranted, because the patient does *not* have bone marrow–related anemia or evidence of intrinsic bone marrow disease.
B (cystoscopy) is incorrect. If the sickle cell screen is negative, a cystoscopy may be necessary to determine the cause of the hematuria.
C (renal biopsy) is incorrect. If the sickle cell screen is negative, a renal biopsy may be necessary to rule out primary renal disease, particularly IgA glomerulonephritis, which is commonly associated with episodic hematuria.
D (serum ferritin) is incorrect. Although serum ferritin is decreased in the early stages of iron deficiency when anemia is *not* present, hematuria usually is *not* associated with any of the microcytic anemias.

31. **A** (antigliadin antibodies) is correct. This patient has celiac disease. The figure shows villous atrophy (flat mucosa) and hyperplastic glands with an increased number of chronic inflammatory cells in the lamina propria. These findings, plus the history of chronic diarrhea with greasy stools, are features of celiac disease, an autoimmune disease that has antibodies against the gliadin fraction in gluten, which is present in wheat products. The vesicular lesion on the patient's elbow is dermatitis herpetiformis, an autoimmune skin disease that has an almost 100% correlation with underlying celiac disease. Other antibodies present in celiac disease include antiendomysial and antireticulin antibodies. Treatment of celiac disease is to restrict gluten containing products.

B (antinuclear antibodies) is incorrect. The antibodies in celiac disease are *not* directed against nuclear proteins.
C (fecal smear for leukocytes) is incorrect. A fecal smear for leukocytes is used for evaluating diarrhea that may be caused by invasive microbial pathogens (e.g., *Campylobacter jejuni, Shigella sonnei*). The presence of leukocytes presumes an invasive enterocolitis (*not* celiac disease).
D (stool for ova and parasites) is incorrect. Testing the stool for ova and parasites is recommended in the workup of a patient with chronic diarrhea. Giardiasis is the most common cause of chronic diarrhea associated with malabsorption; however, the characteristic pear-shaped organisms are *not* present in the biopsy.
E (stool osmotic gap) is incorrect. A stool sample to calculate the osmotic gap is used for high-volume diarrheal states when a secretory or osmotic type of diarrhea is suspected. Secretory diarrheas are characterized by isotonic diarrheal fluid (e.g., due to certain types of laxatives, enterotoxigenic bacteria), whereas osmotic diarrheas are characterized by hypotonic stool because of the presence of osmotically active solutes (e.g., lactase deficiency with an excess of lactose). The stool osmotic gap is calculated with the following formula: 300

mOsm/kg (value used to represent normal POsm) − 2 × (random stool Na$^+$ + random stool K$^+$). A gap <50 mOsm/kg from the POsm is a secretory diarrhea. A gap >100 mOsm/kg from the POsm is an osmotic diarrhea.

32. **D** (step up of Sao$_2$ in pulmonary artery) is correct. The patient has the classic machinery murmur (continuous murmur) of a patent ductus arteriosus (PDA). This neonate has hypoxemia (decreased arterial Po$_2$) secondary to RDS; therefore, closure of the ductus is *not* stimulated. When oxygenated blood (Sao$_2$ 95%) is shunted into a chamber or vessel with venous blood (Sao$_2$ 75%), there is a step-up of Sao$_2$ (~80%) in the venous blood; this is called a left-to-right shunt. Similarly, when venous blood is shunted into a chamber or vessel with oxygenated blood, there is a step-down of the Sao$_2$ (~80%) leading to clinical cyanosis; this is called a right-to-left shunt. In PDA, there is a left-to-right shunt causing blood to flow from the aorta (where pressure is high) through the PDA to the pulmonary artery (where pressure is low), which causes a step-up of Sao$_2$ in the pulmonary artery.

A (normal Sao$_2$ values) is incorrect. The patient has a heart murmur consistent with a PDA; therefore, there will be a step-up of Sao$_2$ in the pulmonary artery.

B is incorrect. A step-up of Sao$_2$ in the right ventricle and pulmonary artery characterizes a ventricular septal defect (VSD), or left-to-right shunt. VSD is the most common type of congenital heart disease. If a VSD is *not* corrected, cyanosis, or Eisenmenger's syndrome, may eventually occur. This is due to volume overload in the right side of the heart from the left-to-right shunt causing pulmonary hypertension and right ventricular hypertrophy. When pressure in the right heart is greater than the pressure in the left heart, the shunt reverses and becomes right-to-left causing a step-down in Sao$_2$

in the left ventricle and aorta and cyanosis.

C is incorrect. A step-up of Sao$_2$ in the right atrium, right ventricle, and pulmonary artery characterizes an atrial septal defect (ASD, or left-to-right shunt), which is most often the result of a patent foramen ovale. If an ASD is *not* corrected, cyanosis and Eisenmenger's syndrome may eventually occur.

E is incorrect. A step-down of Sao$_2$ in the left ventricle and aorta characterizes tetralogy of Fallot (right-to-left shunt), which is the most common type of cyanotic congenital heart disease. It consists of an overriding aorta (least common defect), VSD, pulmonary stenosis, and right ventricular hypertrophy. The degree of pulmonary stenosis determines the severity of the right-to-left shunt. If the stenosis is *not* severe, then most of the venous blood enters the pulmonary artery and is oxygenated; hence, the patient is often acyanotic. However, when the stenosis is severe, most of the venous blood is shunted through the VSD into the left ventricle (right-to-left shunt), leading to cyanosis.

33. **C** (inactivation of a suppressor gene) is correct. The figure shows the mucosal surface of the colon covered by numerous, sessile adenomas. These findings, plus the family history of colectomies between 35 and 40 years of age, suggest familial polyposis. Familial polyposis is an autosomal dominant disorder characterized by inactivation of the adenomatous polyposis coli suppressor gene on chromosome 5.

A (complication of Crohn's disease) is incorrect. Crohn's disease is a chronic granulomatous ulceroconstrictive disease that involves only the colon in 20% of cases. There is an increased incidence of the disease in first-degree relatives. The inflammation is transmural and produces skip lesions throughout the gastrointestinal tract. Therefore, a total colectomy at an early age is *not* a treatment option in Crohn's disease, although there is minimal risk for developing colorectal cancer. Furthermore, the nodules on the mucosal surface in the figure are true polyps and do not represent cobblestoning (mucosa surrounded by areas of ulceration).

B (complication of ulcerative colitis) is incorrect. Ulcerative colitis is a chronic ulceroinflammatory disease that begins in the rectum and may spread continuously to involve the entire colon up to the ileocecal valve. There is an increased incidence of the disease in first-degree relatives. Ulcerative colitis is characterized by extensive areas of mucosal and submucosal ulceration. Islands of inflamed and hemorrhagic mucosa representing pseudopolyps are interspersed between the areas of ulceration. These findings are *not* present in the colectomy specimen.

D (oral mucosal pigmentation) is incorrect. Peutz-Jeghers syndrome is an autosomal dominant polyposis with hamartomatous polyps located primarily in the small bowel (not colon) and stomach. It is characterized by increased melanin pigmentation of the lips and buccal mucosa. There is *no* increased risk of colorectal cancer.

E (X-linked recessive inheritance pattern) is incorrect. Familial polyposis is an autosomal dominant disorder. There are *no* X-linked polyposis syndromes.

34. **E** (urine test for 5-HIAA) is correct. The patient has the signs and symptoms of carcinoid syndrome (facial flushing, diarrhea, tricuspid regurgitation). In carcinoid syndrome, a carcinoid tumor that secretes serotonin metastasizes to the liver. Although the appendix is the most common site for carcinoid tumors, they do *not* metastasize to the liver and produce the carcinoid syndrome. Most tumors causing the carcinoid syndrome arise in the terminal ileum. When carcinoid tumors metastasize to the liver, tumor nodules release serotonin directly into tributaries of the hepatic vein, which allows serotonin to enter the systemic circulation. Serotonin causes vasodilation of arterioles (causes facial flushing) and increases bowel motility (causes diarrhea). Serotonin is also fibrogenic causing the tricuspid valve leaflets to fibrose producing tricuspid regurgitation (pansystolic murmur that increases with inspiration). The metabolic end product of serotonin is 5-HIAA.

A (blood cultures) is incorrect. Blood cultures would show that the patient's tricuspid regurgitation is *not* caused by infectious endocarditis, which usually occurs in intravenous drug abuse.

B (liver function tests) is incorrect. Liver function tests are usually normal in the presence of liver metastasis caused by focal, rather than diffuse, involvement of the liver parenchyma. Furthermore, liver function tests are *not* useful in diagnosing the carcinoid syndrome.

C (serum electrolytes) is incorrect. The diarrhea in carcinoid syndrome is a secretory type (isotonic loss of fluid). Serum electrolytes in secretory diarrheas show hypokalemia and metabolic acidosis, due to loss of potassium and bicarbonate in diarrheal fluid. Serum electrolytes are *not* useful in confirming the diagnosis of carcinoid syndrome.

D (stool cultures) is incorrect. Stool cultures to rule out an invasive type of diarrhea are *not* warranted, because a fecal smear for leukocytes is negative.

35. **E** (gynecomastia) is correct. This patient has cirrhosis of the liver (history of alcohol abuse, protuberant abdomen, and dependent pitting edema). The skin lesion on the face is a spider telangiectasia. It contains a central spiral arteriole with a group of small vessels radiating from the arteriole. Spider angiomas are associated with hyperestrinism, which is most often caused by cirrhosis. In cirrhosis, the dysfunctional liver is unable to metabolize estrogen or 17-ketosteroids (e.g., androstene-dione), which are aromatized in the adipose cells to weak estrogen compounds. Hyperestrinism in men causes gynecomastia (development of breast tissue in males) and female secondary sex characteristics (palmar erythema, soft skin, female hair distribution).

A (ascites) is incorrect. Development of ascites in cirrhosis is multifactorial. Factors that contribute to the development of ascites include portal hypertension (increase in hydrostatic pressure), hypoalbuminemia (decrease in oncotic pressure), secondary aldosteronism (salt retention), and increased lymphatic drainage into the peritoneal cavity.
B (asterixis) is incorrect. Asterixis, or flapping tremor, refers to the inability to sustain posture. It is a sign of hepatic encephalopathy, which is caused by an increase in ammonia and false neurotransmitters (e.g., γ-aminobenzoic acid).
C (caput medusae) is incorrect. Caput medusae, or dilated periumbilical veins, are associated with increased venous pressure caused by portal hypertension, which is a complication of cirrhosis.
D (esophageal varices) is incorrect. Esophageal varices are dilated left gastric coronary veins. These veins normally drain the distal esophagus and proximal stomach and empty into the portal vein. An increase in portal vein pressure leads to dilation of the left gastric coronary vein and an increased risk for rupture.

36. **D** (syringomyelia) is correct. The patient has syringomyelia, which is a degenerative disease that produces a fluid-filled cavity in the cervical spinal cord, causing cervical cord enlargement. As the cavity expands, it destroys the crossed lateral spinothalamic tracts (loss of pain and temperature sensation) and anterior horn cells (atrophy of intrinsic muscles of the hand).

A (amyotrophic lateral sclerosis) is incorrect. Amyotrophic lateral sclerosis (ALS) is a degenerative disease that causes the destruction of upper and lower motor neurons. Sensory abnormalities do *not* occur.
B (Guillain-Barré syndrome) is incorrect. Guillain-Barré syndrome is the most common acute peripheral neuropathy. It is an autoimmune demyelination syndrome that involves peripheral and spinal nerves. It produces rapidly progressive ascending motor weakness, which is *not* present in this patient.
C (multiple sclerosis) is incorrect. Multiple sclerosis is an autoimmune disease that causes destruction of myelin and myelin-producing cells (e.g., oligodendrocytes, Schwann cells). Features include blurry vision (optic neuritis), paresthesias, spastic paraparesis, intention tremors, nystagmus, ataxia, and scanning speech. Loss of pain and temperature sensation and signs of lower motor neuron disease do *not* occur.
E (vitamin B_{12} deficiency) is incorrect. Vitamin B_{12} deficiency produces a macrocytic anemia and subacute combined degeneration of the spinal cord. Myelopathy involving the posterior columns causes a loss of proprioception (joint sensation) and vibratory sensation. Myelopathy involving the lateral corticospinal tract causes upper motor neuron disease with signs of spasticity. Loss of pain and temperature sensation and atrophy of the intrinsic muscles of the hand do *not* occur.

37. **C** (Goodpasture syndrome) is correct. Goodpasture syndrome is more common in men and is associated with IgG anti–basement membrane antibodies that are directed against pulmonary capillary and glomerular capillary basement membranes. The figure shows uninterrupted (linear) smooth immunofluorescence along the glomerular basement membrane. Pulmonary involvement with hemoptysis usually occurs before renal failure. Renal failure is most often due to crescentic glomerulonephritis, which is associated with a nephritic presentation (hematuria, RBC casts, mild proteinuria), as in this case.

A (diffuse membranous glomerulopathy) is incorrect. Diffuse membranous glomerulopathy is the most common cause of the nephrotic syndrome in adults (pitting edema, fatty casts). It is an immunocomplex disorder with deposition of immunocomplexes in a subepithelial location, which produce granular immunofluorescence.

B (focal segmental glomerulosclerosis) is incorrect. Focal segmental glomerulosclerosis is most often associated with AIDS and with intravenous heroin addiction. It causes the nephrotic syndrome. Glomerular injury is due to cytokine damage of the visceral epithelial cells. It is *not* an immunocomplex disease; therefore, the immunofluorescent study is negative.

D (IgA glomerulopathy) is incorrect. IgA glomerulonephritis is an immunocomplex type of glomerulonephritis associated with episodic bouts of microscopic or macroscopic hematuria. The immunocomplexes produce granular immunofluorescence primarily located in the mesangium.

E (minimal change disease) is incorrect. Minimal change disease is the most common cause of the nephrotic syndrome in children. Cytokine damage to the basement membrane causes a loss of the negative charge, resulting in a selective loss of albumin in the urine. Patients usually are normotensive. It is *not* an immunocomplex disease; therefore, the immunofluorescent study is negative.

38. D (unilateral renal artery stenosis caused by atherosclerosis) is correct. The patient has renovascular hypertension. In men older than 50 years of age, it is most often caused by an atherosclerotic plaque narrowing the orifice of the renal artery. A decrease in renal blood flow activates the renin-angiotensin-

aldosterone (RAA) system, resulting in hypertension caused by renal retention of sodium by aldosterone and vasoconstriction of the peripheral resistance arterioles by angiotensin II. Plasma renin activity (PRA) is increased in the affected kidney and decreased in the contralateral kidney. This is due to an increase in plasma volume related to increased retention of sodium by aldosterone. An increase in plasma volume increases renal blood flow to the uninvolved kidney, leading to suppression of the RAA system. Narrowing of the orifice of the renal artery produces an epigastric bruit, causing atrophy of the affected kidney.

A (adrenal tumor that produces excess aldosterone) is incorrect. An adrenal adenoma that produces aldosterone (primary aldosteronism) causes hypertension due to retention of sodium. Plasma renin activity is decreased (*not* increased), and an epigastric bruit is *not* present.

B (adrenal tumor that produces excess catecholamines) is incorrect. An adrenal tumor that produces catecholamines causing hypertension of adults is a pheochromocytoma, which is a benign tumor arising from the adrenal medulla. Classic findings associated with pheochromocytomas, such as sweating, anxiety, and paroxysms of hypertension, are *not* present in this patient.

C (essential hypertension with bilateral nephrosclerosis) is incorrect. Nephrosclerosis is the renal disease associated with essential hypertension. It is caused by hyaline arteriolosclerosis of arterioles in the kidneys that leads to loss of tubules and glomeruli, causing atrophy of both kidneys. It is *not* associated with an epigastric bruit.

E (unilateral renal artery stenosis caused by fibromuscular hyperplasia) is incorrect. Fibromuscular hyperplasia of the renal arteries is the primary cause of renovascular hypertension in women (*not* men) between the ages of 30 and 50 years.

39. **E** (unopposed estrogen exposure) is correct. The figure shows a hemorrhagic and necrotic tumor filling the endometrial cavity and extending through the wall of the uterus. This patient has endometrial carcinoma, which is most often due to unopposed estrogen exposure. Excessive estrogen stimulation of the endometrial mucosa initially causes endometrial hyperplasia, which becomes atypical and progresses to cancer. Early menarche and late menopause, obesity (patient is obese), taking estrogen without progesterone, and nulliparity are potential risk factors for endometrial adenocarcinoma. They are the most common overall gynecologic tumor (excluding breast carcinoma). The majority present as postmenopausal bleeding. Obesity is a risk factor in the menopausal period, because of increased aromatization of adrenal cortex–derived androstenedione to estrone in the adipose cells.

A (adenomyosis) is incorrect. Adenomyosis is the presence of normal endometrial glands and stroma within the myometrium. It is due to invagination of the stratum basalis into the myometrial tissue. It causes thickening of the myometrial tissue, leading to menstrual irregularities. However, it is *not* a risk factor for endometrial carcinoma.

B (herpes simplex virus type 2 infection) is incorrect. HSV-2 is *not* an oncogenic virus.

C (human papillomavirus infection) is incorrect. High-risk types of HPV (e.g., types 16 and 18) predispose females to squamous cell carcinoma (*not* adenocarcinoma) of the vulva, vagina, and cervix.

D (multiparity) is incorrect. Multiparity reduces the risk of cancer because progesterone opposes hyperestrinism.

40. **B** (decreased cardiac output) is correct. The heart fails when it cannot pump blood delivered to it by the venous system. Therefore, cardiac output is decreased whether the heart failure is left-sided or right-sided.

A (bibasilar inspiratory crackles) is incorrect. Bibasilar inspiratory crackles are a sign of left-sided heart failure, a "forward" heart failure causing a decreased cardiac output and backup of blood in the left ventricle, left atrium, and pulmonary capillaries. Increased pulmonary capillary hydrostatic pressure causes fluid (transudate) to enter the interstitium of the lung and eventually the alveoli (pulmonary edema). Air entering alveoli containing fluid produces inspiratory crackles that are best heard at the bases of both lungs.

C (dependent pitting edema) is incorrect. Dependent pitting edema is a sign of right-sided heart failure, a "backward" heart failure causing systemic venous congestion. The increase in hydrostatic pressure in the venous system causes fluid (transudate) to leak into the interstitial space through the venules, leading to dependent pitting edema.

D (paroxysmal nocturnal dyspnea) is incorrect. Paroxysmal nocturnal dyspnea is a sign of left-sided heart failure, which occurs primarily at night when the patient is supine in bed. At this time, gravity does not impede blood flow to the right side of the heart, and fluid from the interstitial space enters the venous system. Excess blood enters the failed left ventricle and backs up into the lungs, causing pulmonary edema and dyspnea, which awakens the patient. Symptoms resolve when the patient stands up and gravity decreases venous return to the right side of the heart.

E (passive congestion in the liver) is incorrect. Passive congestion in the liver is a sign of right-sided heart failure, a "backward" heart failure causing systemic venous congestion. The increase in hydrostatic pressure in the venous system causes blood to enter the hepatic vein and back up into the central veins, leading to passive congestion in the liver.

41. **D** (neuromuscular) is correct. The patient has myasthenia gravis, which is characterized by drooping eyelids, history of tiredness, diplopia (double vision), and dysphagia for solids and liquids in the upper esophagus. This autoimmune disorder is characterized by the production of IgG antibodies that react against acetylcholine receptors in the neuromuscular junction of striated muscle (type II hypersensitivity reaction). The most common initial presentation is muscle weakness involving the ocular muscles, resulting in ptosis and diplopia toward the end of the day. Note drooping of the left eye in part A of the figure. Other muscle groups eventually become involved. The IgG antibodies are produced in the thymus, where there are prominent germinal follicles (B-cell hyperplasia). Dysphagia for solids and liquids occurs in the upper esophagus, because the primary muscle for motility is striated muscle. The confirmatory test is the Tensilon test. Tensilon inhibits acetylcholine esterase, causing an increase in acetylcholine in the synapse, enough to bind to receptors causing a reversal of the muscle weakness (see part B of the figure).

A (demyelinating) is incorrect. Multiple sclerosis is the most common demyelinating disorder. It is *not* associated with drooping eyelids or motor problems in the esophagus.
B (electrolyte) is incorrect. Hypokalemic periodic paralysis is a genetic disease that causes muscle weakness and paralysis. Attacks produce a sudden onset of generalized muscle weakness and often are provoked by strenuous exercise or a high-carbohydrate meal. This kind of history is *not* present in this patient.
C (motor neuron) is incorrect. Amyotrophic lateral sclerosis is an example of an upper and lower motor neuron disorder. Muscle weakness begins in the hands and progresses throughout the body. The muscle weakness is *not* reversed with Tensilon.
E (primary muscular) is incorrect. A primary muscular disorder mainly involves defects in skeletal muscle rather than defects in the transmission of the nerve impulse to muscle

(e.g., muscular dystrophy with a deficiency of dystrophin). Weakness is *not* reversed with Tensilon in primary muscle disorders.

42. **E** (insulin) is correct. Neonatal hypoglycemia (jitteriness and seizures) is caused by hyperinsulinism related to the poor glycemic control in the mother with gestational diabetes mellitus. After delivery, the source of the fetal hyperglycemia is removed, and the increased insulin levels cause a drastic reduction in the blood glucose levels. This emphasizes the need to infuse these patients with glucose after birth.

A (cortisol) is incorrect. Cortisol is increased in newborns because of the stress of the delivery. It is a gluconeogenic hormone and causes hyperglycemia, which does *not* produce jitteriness or seizures.
B (epinephrine) is incorrect. Epinephrine is increased in newborns because of the stress of the delivery. It causes hyperglycemia by increasing glycogenolysis in the liver. Hyperglycemia does *not* produce jitteriness or seizures.
C (glucagon) is incorrect. Glucagon is a gluconeogenic hormone and causes hyperglycemia, which does *not* produce jitteriness or seizures.
D (growth hormone) is incorrect. Growth hormone is increased in newborns because of the stress of the delivery. It is a gluconeogenic hormone and causes hyperglycemia, which does *not* produce jitteriness or seizures.

43. **E** (rheumatoid factor) is correct. The patient has rheumatoid arthritis. The figure shows swelling of the metacarpophalangeal joints and ulnar deviation in both hands. Joint destruction is initiated by the secretion of cytokines from CD4 helper T cells that cause B-cell proliferation and the release of chemical mediators from macrophages and synovial cells in the joint. The B cells synthesize IgM autoantibodies that react against the Fc portion of IgG, producing rheumatoid factor immunocomplexes. The immunocomplexes activate the complement system, causing the release of chemotactic factors that attract neutrophils into the joint, leading to acute synovitis. Over the ensuing months and years, chronic synovitis develops, characterized by synovial tissue hyperplasia, chronic inflammation, and vascular proliferation. The synovial tissue forms a pannus that extends over the articular cartilage, resulting in destruction of the cartilage, fibrosis, and eventual ankylosis (fusion) of the joint.

A (antibodies against *Borrelia burgdorferi*) is incorrect. *B. burgdorferi* is the causal agent of Lyme disease and is transmitted by a tick. A destructive arthritis in large joints (e.g., knee) occurs in late stages of the disease. The joint disease does *not* involve the hands and produce ulnar deviation.
B (antibodies against double-stranded DNA) is incorrect. Anti–double-stranded DNA bodies are antinuclear antibodies that are specific for systemic lupus erythematosus (SLE). The arthritis in SLE does involve the joints in the hands; however, it is seldom deforming.
C (HLA-B27 genotype) is incorrect. The HLA-B27 genotype is associated with a group of rheumatoid factor–negative (seronegative) spondyloarthropathies that target the sacroiliac joint and the vertebral column (e.g., ankylosing spondylitis). Rheumatoid arthritis is associated with the HLA-DR4 genotype.
D (hyperuricemia) is incorrect. Gout is associated with the deposition of monosodium urate crystals in joints, usually the metatarsophalangeal joint of the great toe. It does *not* produce ulnar deviation of the hands.

44. **D** (liver involvement) is correct. The tumor-node-metastasis (TNM) system is used to stage cancers arising from epithelial tissues. T refers to the size and nuclear features of the tumor; N refers to the presence or absence of

lymph node metastasis; and M refers to the presence or absence of metastasis to sites other than lymph nodes, such as the liver. M is the most important prognostic factor. The presence of distant metastases implies that the cancer has already infiltrated through regional lymph nodes draining the cancer and has entered the bloodstream.

A (age of the patient) is incorrect. Age of the patient is the least important risk prognostic factor of the choices listed.
B (differentiation of the tumor) is incorrect. Differentiation or grade of the tumor describes the histologic appearance of the tumor. If the tumor has recognizable features, such as keratin in squamous cells or glands, then the tumor is well differentiated or low grade. If the tumor has no histologic features with characteristics identifying the tissue of origin, then the tumor is poorly differentiated, anaplastic, or high grade. The extent of differentiation is a less important prognostic factor than the M of the TNM system.
C (extent of invasion) is incorrect. The extent of invasion of the tumor is a less important prognostic factor than the M of the TNM system.
E (lymph node involvement) is incorrect. Lymph node involvement (N) is the second most important prognostic factor; however, M is more important because it implies that the tumor has metastasized to lymph nodes and entered efferent lymphatics to gain access to the blood stream for hematogenous dissemination to other sites.

45. **B** *(Borrelia burgdorferi)* is correct. The figure shows an erythematous expanding rash with concentric circles separated by clear spaces. This is erythema chronicum migrans, which is the pathognomonic skin lesion of early Lyme disease. The disease is transmitted to humans by the bite of an *Ixodes* tick that carries the gram-negative spirochete *B. burgdorferi*.

A *(Babesia microti)* is incorrect. *B. microti* is a protozoan carried by the *Ixodes* tick. It parasitizes RBCs and causes a mild hemolytic anemia that may occur concurrently with Lyme disease. There is *no* skin rash in babesiosis.

C *(Borrelia recurrentis)* is incorrect. *B. recurrentis* is a spirochete that is transmitted to humans by the bite of a tick called *Dermacentor andersoni.* This tick also carries the rickettsial organisms *Ehrlichia chaffeensis* and *Rickettsia rickettsii.* *B. recurrentis* is the causative agent of relapsing fever, which is associated with a high fever and a petechial rash (*not* a rash with concentric circles) that covers the trunk and extremities.

D *(Ehrlichia chaffeensis)* is incorrect. *E. chaffeensis* is a tick-transmitted rickettsial pathogen that is the causal agent of ehrlichiosis. The organism parasitizes leukocytes and causes fever and multisystem disease. *No* rash is associated with the infection.

E *(Rickettsia rickettsii)* is incorrect. *R. rickettsii* is a tick-transmitted pathogen that is the causative agent of Rocky Mountain spotted fever, which is characterized by fever, multisystem disease, and a petechial rash (*not* a rash with concentric circles) that begins on the palms and spreads to the trunk.

46. **D** (α-thalassemia) is correct. α-Thalassemia is an autosomal recessive disorder that involves decreased production of α-globin chains, causing a microcytic anemia with decreased synthesis of hemoglobin A ($2\alpha2\beta$), hemoglobin A_2 ($2\alpha2\delta$), and hemoglobin F ($2\alpha2\gamma$). For unexplained reasons, the RBC count is increased in all the thalassemias, and it is decreased in all other microcytic anemias (e.g., iron deficiency anemia). Hemoglobin electrophoresis is normal, because the proportion of each of the hemoglobins remains the same. α-Thalassemia involves the synthesis of globin chains, and serum ferritin, which correlates with bone marrow iron stores, is normal.

A (iron deficiency) is incorrect. Iron deficiency is the most common cause of a microcytic anemia. RBC count is decreased, and serum ferritin is decreased.

B (sickle cell trait) is incorrect. Sickle cell trait does *not* cause anemia.

C (sideroblastic anemia) is incorrect. Sideroblastic anemias are a group of microcytic anemias that are caused by a defect in the synthesis of heme (iron plus protoporphyrin) in the mitochondria of developing RBC normoblasts. Iron accumulates in the mitochondria of nucleated RBCs and produces ringed sideroblasts, which are easily identified in a bone marrow aspirate. RBC count is decreased, and serum ferritin is increased in these anemias.

E (β-thalassemia) is incorrect. In β-thalassemia, hemoglobin A ($2\alpha2\beta$) is decreased, because β-globin chain synthesis is decreased. There is a corresponding increase in hemoglobin A_2 ($2\alpha2\delta$) and hemoglobin F ($2\alpha2\gamma$), because α-, δ-, and γ-chain synthesis is normal. The hemoglobin electrophoresis is normal in this patient, thus excluding β-thalassemia.

47. **A** (degeneration of dopaminergic substantia nigra neurons) is correct. The patient has Parkinson's disease. Figure A shows atrophy and depigmentation of the substantia nigra when compared with the normal midbrain (figure B). Degeneration of neurons of the substantia nigra causes a loss of dopamine, the principal neurotransmitter of afferents in the nigrostriatal tract that connects the substantia nigra with the caudate and putamen. This interrupts voluntary muscle movement, resulting in muscle rigidity (cogwheel rigidity) and other extrapyramidal signs (resting tremor with "pill rolling" of the thumbs and index fingers).

B (increased γ-secretase activity) is incorrect. An increase in γ-secretases causes increased cleavage of amyloid precursor protein into fragments that are converted into β-amyloid protein, which is toxic to neurons in the brain causing Alzheimer's disease (*not* parkinsonism).

C (loss of striatal neurons in the caudate nucleus) is incorrect. Loss of striatal neurons in the caudate nucleus occurs in Huntington's disease. This autosomal dominant trinucleotide repeat disorder is characterized by chorea, extrapyramidal signs, and dementia.

D (presence of apolipoprotein gene E, allele ε4) is incorrect. Apolipoprotein gene E, allele ε4, makes a product that has a high affinity for β-amyloid protein. This concentrates the protein and causes late-onset Alzheimer's disease (*not* parkinsonism).

E (presence of hyperphosphorylated tau protein) is incorrect. Hyperphosphorylated tau protein increases the formation of neurofibrillary tangles (protein-rich neurofilaments), which are prominent findings in the brain of patients with Alzheimer's disease (*not* parkinsonism).

48. **A** (acute respiratory distress syndrome) is correct. Urinary retention due to prostate hyperplasia has led to sepsis (most often due to *Escherichia coli*) and endotoxic shock, which is the most common cause of acute respiratory distress syndrome. Alveolar macrophages and damaged endothelial cells release cytokines that cause neutrophil adhesion to the pulmonary capillaries. Neutrophils transmigrate into the alveoli and destroy type I and type II pneumocytes. Destruction of type II pneumocytes causes loss of surfactant and collapse of the alveoli. An exudate leaks into the interstitium and alveoli, where hyaline membranes are formed. Clinical findings include dyspnea, tachypnea, and inspiratory crackles. Chest radiography shows interstitial and alveolar infiltrates. Arterial blood gases show hypoxemia and respiratory acidosis.

B (congestive heart failure) is incorrect. Congestive heart failure is most often caused by ischemic heart disease. It is *not* associated with fever and septicemia.

C (lobar pneumonia caused by gram-negative bacteria) is incorrect. A chest radiograph in a lobar pneumonia shows consolidation of a lobe in the lung rather than interstitial and alveolar infiltrates in both lungs.

D (multiple pulmonary infarcts) is incorrect. Pulmonary infarctions produce hypovascular areas at the periphery of the lung, hypoxemia, and respiratory alkalosis, *not* respiratory acidosis.

E (pneumonia caused by *Streptococcus pneumoniae*) is incorrect. *S. pneumoniae* is the most common cause of typical community-acquired, *not* nosocomial pneumonia. Pneumonia caused by *S. pneumoniae* is *not* an outcome of urinary retention.

49. **C** (platelet count normal, bleeding time normal, PT prolonged, PTT prolonged) is correct. Rat poison contains warfarin, an anticoagulant that inhibits epoxide reductase, which normally converts inactive vitamin K to active vitamin K. Lack of active vitamin K renders vitamin K–dependent coagulation factors, such as prothrombin, factor VII, factor IX, and factor X, nonfunctional. Bleeding from the mouth and gastrointestinal tract is a sign of overanticoagulation. Warfarin does *not* affect platelet production or function; therefore, the platelet count and bleeding time (test of platelet function) are normal. The PT evaluates the activity of coagulation factors in the extrinsic system (factor VII) to the formation of a fibrin clot in the final common pathway (factor X, factor V, prothrombin, fibrinogen). The PTT evaluates the activity of the coagulation factors in the intrinsic system (factor XII, factor XI, factor IX, factor VIII) to the formation of a fibrin clot. Both the PT and PTT are prolonged, because factor X and prothrombin are present in the final common pathway. The best treatment for this patient is infusion of fresh frozen plasma, which contains functional vitamin K–dependent factors (i.e., factors that have been γ-carboxylated by vitamin K).

A (platelet count decreased, bleeding time prolonged, PT normal, PTT normal) is incorrect. A decreased platelet count (thrombocytopenia) prolongs the bleeding time, because the end of the bleeding time is marked by the formation of a temporary platelet plug. Signs of thrombocytopenia include petechiae and ecchymoses. Both PT and PTT are normal in thrombocytopenia, because coagulation factors are normal. Warfarin does *not* affect the platelet count or platelet function.

B (platelet count normal, bleeding time normal, PT normal, PTT prolonged) is incorrect. A normal platelet count, normal bleeding time, normal PT, and a prolonged PTT indicate a factor deficiency in the intrinsic coagulation system (e.g., factor VIII deficiency). A normal PT indicates that there are *no* coagulation factor deficiencies in the final common pathway. Warfarin prolongs both the PT and PTT.

D (platelet count normal, bleeding time prolonged, PT normal, PTT normal) is incorrect. A prolonged bleeding time associated with a normal platelet count, normal PT, and normal PTT indicates a defect in platelet function. The most common cause of a prolonged bleeding time is aspirin or other nonsteroidal anti-inflammatory drugs. Warfarin does *not* affect platelet production or function.

E (platelet count normal, bleeding time prolonged, PT normal, PTT prolonged) is incorrect. The most common cause of a prolonged bleeding time and prolonged PTT is von Willebrand disease. Warfarin does *not* affect the bleeding time, which evaluates platelet function.

50. **C** (disseminated intravascular coagulation) is correct. The endotoxins in endotoxic shock (most often due to *Escherichia coli* sepsis) damage tissue, causing the release of tissue thromboplastin. This activates the extrinsic coagulation system, causing DIC. Fibrin clots are produced in the microcirculation that obstruct blood flow and consume coagulation factors, causing bleeding from needle puncture sites and the gastrointestinal tract. Factors that are consumed in a fibrin clot are fibrinogen (factor I), prothrombin (factor II), and factors V and VIII. Because coagulating factors present in the final common pathway are consumed (fibrinogen, prothrombin, factor V), there is prolongation of the PT and PTT. Platelets are trapped in the fibrin clots leading to thrombocytopenia, which produces petechiae and ecchymoses. The fibrinolytic system is activated, and plasmin cleaves the fibrin strands holding the fibrin clots together. Fibrin strands are held together by cross-links, and cleaved fragments with cross-links are detected in the D-dimer assay, which is the most sensitive test for diagnosing DIC.

A (autoimmune thrombocytopenia) is incorrect. DIC is associated with fibrin clots, multiple coagulation factor deficiencies, activation of the fibrinolytic system, and thrombocytopenia. Therefore, conditions that produce thrombocytopenia, such as autoimmune thrombocytopenia, do *not* explain all the clinical and laboratory findings that are present in this patient.

B (circulating anticoagulant) is incorrect. Circulating anticoagulants are antibodies that destroy coagulation factors (e.g., factor VIII), causing prolongation of the PTT and/or PT. However, these antibodies do *not* destroy platelets or produce fibrin clots that obstruct the microcirculation, causing the bleeding from the needle puncture sites and the gastrointestinal tract.

D (primary fibrinolysis) is incorrect. Primary fibrinolysis is very rare. Only the fibrinolytic system is activated. Therefore, clinical findings are primarily those related to coagulation factor deficiencies (e.g., fibrinogen, factor V, factor VIII). The platelet count is normal, and D-dimers are *not* present because there are no fibrin clots.

E (thrombotic thrombocytopenic purpura) is incorrect. DIC is associated with fibrin clots, multiple coagulation factor deficiencies, activation of the fibrinolytic system, and thrombocytopenia. Therefore, conditions that produce thrombocytopenia, such as thrombotic thrombocytopenic purpura, do *not* explain all the clinical and laboratory findings that are present in this patient.

Figure Credits

Corin B: Pathology of the Lungs. London, Churchill Livingstone, 1999.
Figure accompanying Test 1, Question 25
Figure accompanying Test 2, Question 27

Damjanov I, Linder J: Anderson's Pathology, 10th ed. St. Louis, Mosby, 1996.
Figures accompanying Test 1, Questions 5 and 17
Figure accompanying Test 2, Question 3

Damjanov I, Linder J: Pathology: A Color Atlas. St. Louis, Mosby, 2000.
Figures accompanying Test 1, Questions 1, 11, 13, 15, 23, and 27
Figures accompanying Test 2, Questions 13, 15, 17, 23, 31, 33, 39, and 47

Damjanov I: Pathology for the Health-Related Professions, 2nd ed. Philadelphia, WB Saunders, 2000.
Figure accompanying Test 1, Question 39

Forbes C, Jackson W: Color Atlas and Text of Clinical Medicine, 2nd ed. St. Louis, Mosby, 2003.
Figures accompanying Test 1, Questions 7, 29, 37, 41, and 45
Figures accompanying Test 2, Questions 7, 11, and 43

Henry JB: Clinical Diagnosis and Management by Laboratory Methods, 20th ed. Philadelphia, WB Saunders, 2001.
Figure accompanying Test 1, Question 43

Hoffbrand AV: Color Atlas: Clinical Hematology, 3rd ed. St. Louis, Mosby, 2000.
Figures accompanying Test 2, Questions 19 and 25

Katz DS: Radiology Secrets. Philadelphia, Hanley & Belfus, 1998.
Figure accompanying Test 1, Question 31

Kumar V, Fausto N, Abbas A: Robbins and Cotran's Pathologic Basis of Disease, 7th ed. Philadelphia, WB Saunders, 2004.
Figures accompanying Test 1, Questions 3, 21, and 35
Figures accompanying Test 2, Questions 5, 29, and 37

Lookingbill D, Marks J: Principles of Dermatology, 3rd ed. Philadelphia, WB Saunders, 2000.
Figure accompanying Test 2, Question 45

MacSween RNM, Burt AD, Portmann BC: Pathology of the Liver, 4th ed. London, Churchill Livingstone, 2002.
Figure accompanying Test 2, Question 1

Naeim F: Atlas of Bone Marrow and Blood Pathology. Philadelphia, WB Saunders, 2001.
Figure accompanying Test 1, Question 19
Figure accompanying Test 2, Question 21

Perkin GD: Mosby's Color Atlas and Text of Neurology. St. Louis, Mosby, 2002.
Figure accompanying Test 1, Question 33
Figure accompanying Test 2, Question 41

Savin J, Hunter JA, Hepburn NC: Diagnosis in Color: Skin Signs in Clinical Medicine. London, Mosby-Wolfe, 1997.
Figure accompanying Test 2, Question 35

Index

Note: Page numbers followed by f indicate figures; those followed by t indicate tables; and those followed by b indicate boxed material.